Doppler Ultrasound in
Obstetrics and Gynecology

Doppler Ultrasound in Obstetrics and Gynecology

Editors

Joshua A. Copel, M.D.

Department of Obstetrics and Gynecology
Yale University School of Medicine
New Haven, Connecticut

Kathryn L. Reed, M.D.

Department of Obstetrics and Gynecology
University of Arizona School of Medicine
Tucson, Arizona

Raven Press ✿ New York

Raven Press, Ltd., 1185 Avenue of the Americas, New York, New York 10036

Printed and bound in Singapore

Library of Congress Cataloging-in-Publication Data

Doppler ultrasound in obstetrics and gynecology/editors, Joshua A. Copel and
    Kathryn L. Reed.
       p.   cm.
    Includes bibliographical references and index.
    ISBN 0-7817-0206-2:
     1. Doppler ultrasonography.   2. Ultrasonics in obstetrics.
   3. Fetus—Ultrasonic imaging.   I. Copel, Joshua A.   II. Reed,
   Kathryn L.
    [DNLM: 1. Genital Diseases, Female—diagnosis.   2. Obstetrics.
   3. Ultrasonography—methods.   WP 141 D692 1994]
   RG527.5.U48D66   1994
   618′.047543—dc20
   DNLM/DLC
   for Library of Congress   93-48969

9 8 7 6 5 4 3 2 1

For Alix, Rachel, and David,
with thanks to my father, Joseph W. Copel, M.D.,
for starting me along the academic road.
J.C.

To Goldman for his benevolence,
and to the ones whose connections
made this work possible.
K.R.

Contents

IV. Fetal Echocardiography

Contributors

Alfred Z. Abuhamad, M.D.
Department of Obstetrics and Gynecology
Division of Maternal-Fetal Medicine
Eastern Virginia Medical School
825 Fairfax Avenue
Norfolk, Virginia 23507-1912

S. L. Adamson, Ph.D.
Mount Sinai Hospital
600 University Avenue
Toronto, Ontario M5G 1X5
Canada

Michael Applebaum, M.D.
Director of Ultrasound
Associate Director of Reproductive Medicine
The University of Health Sciences
3333 Greenbay Road
North Chicago, Illinois 60064

Ph. Arbeille, M.D., Ph.D.
Unité INSERM
316-CHU Trousseau
37044-Tours-
France

Domenico Arduini, M.D.
Via dei Malvezzi, 6
00191 Roma
Italy

Kirk W. Beach, M.D.
Department of Surgery
University of Washington
Seattle, Washington 98195

Mark S. Cartier, RDMS
Department of Radiology
University of Tennessee, Memphis
465 Jefferson Avenue
Memphis, Tennessee 38163

Joshua A. Copel, M.D.
Department of Obstetrics and Gynecology
Yale University School of Medicine
333 Cedar Street
New Haven, Connecticut 06510

Gordon Crvenkovic, M.D.
Department of Obstetrics and Gynecology
Cedars-Sinai Medical Center
UCLA School of Medicine
8700 Beverly Boulevard
Los Angeles, California 90048

Jeanne Anne Cullinan, M.D.
Departments of Radiology and Radiological
*   Sciences and Obstetrics and Gynecology*
Vanderbilt University Medical Center
Nashville, Tennessee 37232

Michael Y. Divon, M.D.
Department of Obstetrics and Gynecology
Jack D. Weiler Hospital
The Albert Einstein College of Medicine
Bronx, New York 10467

Susan Pamela Drblik, M.A.
The Fetal Cardiology Unit
Service of Cardiology and Pulmonary
*   Medicine*
Department of Pediatrics
Sainte-Justine Hospital
University of Montreal
Montreal, Quebec
Canada

Sturla H. Eik-Nes
National Center for Fetal Medicine
Department of Obstetrics and Gynecology
Trondheim University Center
N-7006 Trondheim
Norway

Donald S. Emerson, M.D.
Department of Radiology
University of Tennessee, Memphis
465 Jefferson Avenue
Memphis, Tennessee 38163

Dan Farine, M.D.
Department of Obstetrics and Gynecology
University of Toronto
Mount Sinai Hospital
600 University Avenue
Toronto, Ontario M5G 1X5
Canada

A. Fignon, M.D.
Station INRA-PRM.D.
Nouzilly 37380 Monnaie
France

Arthur C. Fleischer, M.D.
Departments of Radiology and Radiological
  Sciences and Obstetrics and Gynecology
Vanderbilt University Medical Center
Nashville, Tennessee 37232-2675

Jean-Claude Fouron, M.D.
The Fetal Cardiology Unit
Service of Cardiology and Pulmonary
  Medicine
Department of Pediatrics
Sainte-Justine Hospital
University of Montreal
Canada

Steven G. Gabbe, M.D.
Department of Obstetrics and Gynecology
The Ohio State University
Means Hall
1654 Upham Drive
Columbus, Ohio 43210-1228

Andree Gruslin-Giroux, M.D.
Department of Obstetrics and Gynecology
Ottawa General Hospital
501 Smyth Road
Ottawa, Ontario K1L 8L6
Canada

A. A. Hill, M.A.Sc.
Mount Sinai Hospital
600 University Avenue
Toronto, Ontario M5G 1X5
Canada

James C. Huhta, M.D.
Department of Obstetrics and Gynecology
University of Pennsylvania School of
  Medicine
Pennsylvania Hospital
Philadelphia, Pennsylvania 19107

T. W. A. Huisman, M.D.
Department of Obstetrics and Gynecology
Academic Hospital Rotterdam-Dijkzigt
Erasmus University Rotterdam
Dr. Molewaterplein 40
3015 GD Rotterdam
The Netherlands

Beth Y. Karlan, M.D.
Department of Obstetrics and Gynecology
Cedars-Sinai Medical Center
UCLA School of Medicine
700 Beverly Boulevard
Los Angeles, California 90048

Edmond N. Kelly, M.B.
Department of Pediatrics
University of Toronto
Mount Sinai Hospital
600 University Avenue
Toronto, Ontario M5G 1X5
Canada

Charles S. Kleinman, M.D.
Department of Pediatrics
Yale University School of Medicine
333 Cedar Street
New Haven, Connecticut 06510

Torvid Kiserud, M.D.
National Center for Fetal Medicine
Department of Obstetrics and Gynecology
Trondheim University Center
N-76006 Trondheim
Norway

Mark B. Landon, M.D.
Department of Obstetrics and Gynecology
The Ohio State University
Means Hall
1654 Upham Drive
Columbus, Ohio 43210-1228

P. Leguyader, M.D.
Département Obstetrique et Gynecologie
Hôpital de Lamentin 97232
Lamentin
France

Marco Liberati, M.D.
Department of Obstetrics and Gynecology
Yale University School of Medicine
333 Cedar Street
New Haven, Connecticut 06510

A. Locatelli, M.D.
Station INRA-PMRD
Nouzilly 37380 Monnaie
France

Abraham Ludomirski, M.D.
Director of Research
Department of Obstetrics and Gynecology
Division of Maternal-Fetal Medicine
Pennsylvania Hospital
800 Spruce Street
Philadelphia, Pennsylvania 19107

Giancarlo Mari, M.D.
Department of Obstetrics and Gynecology
Yale University School of Medicine
333 Cedar Street
New Haven, Connecticut 06510

Dev Maulik, M.D., Ph.D.
Department of Obstetrics and Gynecology
Winthrop University Hospital
Mineola, New York 11501

Charles M. McCurdy, Jr., M.D.
Department of Obstetrics and Gynecology
University of Arizona Health Sciences
  Center
Tucson, Arizona 85724

Robert W. McDonald
Oregon Health Sciences University
3181 SW Sam Jackson Park Road
Portland, Oregon 97201

Kenneth J. Moise, Jr., M.D.
Department of Obstetrics and Gynecology
Division of Maternal-Fetal Medicine
Baylor College of Medicine
One Baylor Plaza
Houston, Texas 77030

Robert J. Morrow, M.D.
Mount Sinai Hospital
600 University Avenue
Toronto, Ontario, M5G 1X5
Canada

Carl Nimrod, M.B.
Department of Obstetrics and Gynecology
Ottawa General Hospital
501 Smyth Road
Ottawa, Ontario K1L 8L6
Canada

John S. Pellerito, M.D.
(current address)
Department of Diagnostic Radiology
North Shore University Hospital
300 Community Drive
Manhasset, New York 11030

Lawrence D. Platt, M.D.
Department of Obstetrics and Gynecology
Cedars-Sinai Medical Center
UCLA School of Medicine
8700 Beverly Boulevard
Los Angeles, California 90048

Raphael N. Pollack, M.D.
Department of Obstetrics and Gynecology
The Sir Mortimer B. Davis Jewish General
  Hospital
McGill University
Montreal, Quebec
Canada

Kathryn L. Reed, M.D.
Department of Obstetrics and Gynecology
University of Arizona School of Medicine
1501 North Campbell Avenue
Tucson, Arizona 86724

Rosemary E. Reiss, M.D.
Department of Obstetrics and Gynecology
The Ohio State University
1654 Upham Drive
Columbus, Ohio 43210-1228

Mary Jo Rice, M.D.
Department of Pediatrics
Oregon Health Sciences University
3181 SW Sam Jackson Park Road
Portland, Oregon 97201

J. W. Knox Ritchie, M.D.
Department of Obstetrics and Gynecology
University of Toronto
92 College Street
Toronto, Ontario M5G 1L4
Canada

Giuseppe Rizzo, M.D.
Clinica Ostetrica e Ginecologica
Universita di Roma "Tor Vergata"
Policlinco Nuovo S. Eugenio
P. le Umanesimo, 10
00144 Roma
Italy

Carlo Romanini, M.D.
Department of Obstetrics and Gynecology
Università di Roma "Tor Vergata"
Policlinco Nuovo S. Eugenio
P. le Umanesimo, 10
00144 Roma
Italy

Siegfried Rotmensch, M.D.
Department of Obstetrics and Gynecology
Golda Meir Medical Center
Petach Tikvah
Israel

Greg Ryan, M.B.
Department of Obstetrics and Gynecology
University of Toronto
Mount Sinai Hospital
600 University Avenue
Toronto, Ontario M5G 1X5
Canada

David J. Sahn, M.D.
Oregon Health Sciences University
3181 SW Sam Jackson Park Road
Portland, Oregon 97201

Joaquin Santolaya-Forgas, M.D., Ph.D.
Department of Obstetrics and Gynecology
University of Illinois College of Medicine
840 S. Wood Street
Chicago, Illinois 60612

Elizabeth P. Schneider, M.D.
Department of Obstetrics and Gynecology
Cornell University Medical College
North Shore University Hospital
300 Community Drive
Manhasset, New York 11030

Harold Schulman, M.D.
4605 North A1A
Vero Beach, Florida 32963

Norman H. Silverman, M.D.
Department of Pediatrics
University of California, San Francisco
San Francisco, California 94143

Cindy Smrt, RT, RDMS
Department of Obstetrics and Gynecology
Cedars-Sinai Medical Center
UCLA School of Medicine
8700 Beverly Boulevard
Los Angeles, California 90048

Kenneth J. W. Taylor, M.D., Ph.D.
Department of Diagnostic Imaging
Division of Ultrasound
Yale University School of Medicine
333 Cedar Street
New Haven, Connecticut 06510

Jorge E. Tolosa, M.D. M.Sc.
Department of Obstetrics and Gynecology
University of Pennsylvania School of
* Medicine*
Pennsylvania Hospital
Philadelphia, Pennsylvania 19107

Brian J. Trudinger, M.D.
Department of Obstetrics and Gynecology
The University of Sydney at Westmead
* Hospital*
Westmead, New South Wales 2145
Australia

J. van Eyck, M.D., Ph.D.
Department of Obstetrics and Gynecology
Academic Hospital Rotterdam-Dijkzigt
Erasmus University Rotterdam
Dr. Molewaterplein 40
3015 GD Rotterdam
The Netherlands

J. W. Wladimiroff, M.D., Ph.D.
Department of Obstetrics and Gynecology
Academic Hospital Rotterdam-Dijkzigt
Erasmus University Rotterdam
Dr. Molewaterplein 40
3015 GD Rotterdam
The Netherlands

Foreword

Many years ago, researchers realized that continuous-wave Doppler could be used to monitor the fetal heart rate without applying a scalp electrode directly to the fetus. Only recently, however, was the Doppler concept applied to the evaluation of the uterine and fetal circulation. The advent of color Doppler has taken us to a new level in the investigation of the fetal heart and small-vessel and "slow-flow" circulation. Now all that remains is to determine the best ways to apply the techniques clinically.

It has taken some time to convince the medical community that it was worthwhile to pursue fetal Doppler investigation. Yes, it was possible to obtain waveforms from various maternal and fetal vessels, but did it really add anything to what we already knew? When the initial results emerged the investigators were branded as zealots, and the findings were subject to skepticism. An interesting era evolved in Doppler history in which a diagnostician had to pick sides between the Doppler skeptics and the Doppler enthusiasts. There seemed to be no middle ground.

The Food and Drug Administration (FDA) also needed convincing. Although peak pulse intensities were no higher than generated through standard two-dimensional ultrasound examinations, the longer pulses required to assess changes in frequency resulted in more time in which a transducer was energized and less time for a transducer to "listen" for returning echoes. This appreciable change in duty cycle produced average ultrasound intensities that were far above anything previously used in diagnostic ultrasound.

Two developments resulted in the ability to move forward clinically with Doppler. Manufacturers were able to decrease the average intensities of their machines to reasonable levels, and the FDA set more liberal and rational, limits for Doppler intensities for clinical examinations. However, the FDA had to be convinced of the clinical efficacy of Doppler in fetal investigation. Fortunately, after a series of educational forums involving different disciplines, various medical societies, and industry, the FDA formally condoned the use of Doppler in the clinical evaluation of two conditions: intrauterine growth retardation and fetal cardiac abnormalities.

The pathway of Doppler investigation has taken a few wrong turns. For example, spurred on by a search for a better diagnostic tool in the evaluation of intrauterine growth retardation, some investigators attempted to diagnose small-for-date fetuses with Doppler. Not surprisingly, the sensitivity of such an approach was not optimal. The point was that the best way to tell if a fetus was too small was to assess its size through conventional two-dimensional ultrasound. However, if one wanted to know if a small baby was small because of inadequate placental and fetal perfusion, then Doppler could be very helpful.

Another unfortunate trend was to tout Doppler as the only tool to evaluate fetal condition. Yet, although many are still trying to replace one test or another with Doppler, it seems to this middle grounder (now strongly leaning to the side of the enthusiasts) that its benefit is greatest when used in conjunction with other tests.

This book explores fetal Doppler ultrasound to the fullest. The contributors are leaders in the field and have been well chosen by Drs. Copel and Reed for their expertise in the areas covered. Since investigators from many countries have contributed to the Doppler evolution, it is not surprising that this text has an international flavor. It seems that no important fetal, maternal, or placental area has been overlooked in this comprehensive reference book.

John C. Hobbins
Denver, 1994

Preface

Over the past 10 years, Doppler ultrasound has gone from being an exotic research tool to a common component of prenatal sonography. Many papers have been published on its applications, sessions are devoted to it at scientific meetings, and an international society for perinatal applications has emerged.

Despite all of the attention, we frequently hear the question, "What is the real value of Doppler in Ob-Gyn?"

In first outlining this book, our goal was to tap the knowledge of those with the most experience with different Ob-Gyn Doppler applications to develop a comprehensive text. For many of the chapters, we contacted a senior author but asked that a junior colleague be the primary author, so that the views of both the experienced "professor" and the researcher in the trenches could be included.

We decided not to review the basics of the Doppler equation, believing that those attracted to this book would already know the fundamentals. On the other hand, we thought that more advanced physics would be useful as a reference. The familiar obstetric indices are discussed as they relate to flow hemodynamics rather than just by their clinical correlation to pathologic states. The remainder of the organization of the book is self-explanatory, covering various gynecologic applications, followed by the familiar and the esoteric obstetric uses.

As time went on it became apparent that the book was evolving beyond our expectations. While redundancies were present, it was in these exact areas that the opinions of the authors were most prominent, and any editorial excision of these overlaps would remove much of the flavor and controversy. In the end, we decided to be permissive and inclusive, and we believe that the result is a stronger text that allows the experience of the diverse authors to show.

We are grateful to Craig Percy from Raven Press for shepherding this book along, and to Joanne Porto and Kim Falyer for helping to keep everything straight. We also thank our associates and fellows for tolerating our distractions as this project went on. Finally, we are most appreciative of the efforts that went into the text and illustration preparation by the authors, without whom this book could not have succeeded. Finally, we will always fondly recall the encouragement and friendship of the late Drs. Lewis Shenker and Peter Grannum who we wish had been here to be part of this project.

Joshua A. Copel
Kathryn L. Reed

Doppler Ultrasound in
Obstetrics and Gynecology

Doppler Ultrasound in Obstetrics and Gynecology,
edited by Joshua A. Copel and Kathryn L. Reed.
Raven Press, Ltd., New York © 1995.

CHAPTER 1

Principles of Doppler Signal Processing and Hemodynamic Analysis

Dev Maulik

Doppler ultrasound offers a unique noninvasive technology for investigating the circulatory system. Doppler velocimetry has been extensively used to investigate fetal, fetoplacental, and uteroplacental circulations. There is ample evidence associating abnormal Doppler findings with complications of pregnancy and an adverse perinatal outcome. The application of Doppler ultrasound is not new in obstetric practice; it has been in use for many years for detecting fetal heart activity and for external electronic surveillance of the fetal heart rate. However, this level of Doppler technology generates only Doppler shift audio output. Doppler ultrasound velocimetry, on the other hand, requires a comprehensive analysis of the Doppler signal involving application of advanced technology with varying degrees of complexity and sophistication. In addition, clinical utilization of the Doppler information depends on appropriate analysis and hemodynamic interpretation of the Doppler waveform. It is apparent that a basic understanding of the various aspects of Doppler signal processing and Doppler frequency shift waveform analysis is essential for any critical evaluation of the utility and the limitations of the clinical applications of the technology. This chapter presents a general perspective on this subject.

THE DOPPLER SIGNAL

When a beam of energy waves encounters a reflector smaller than its wavelength, the incident energy waves are reflected in all directions (Fig. 1). This is known as *scattering.* A portion of the scattered energy will be reflected back to the source. This is called *backscattering.*

This phenomenon is also observed when an ultrasound beam intersects blood flow in a vessel; it is scattered in all directions (1–3) and is also backscattered to the transmitting transducer. The phenomenon of ultrasound scattering is analogous to scattering of light by gas molecules in the upper atmosphere and is called *Rayleigh scattering* (4,5). In blood, the primary sources of ultrasonic scattering are the circulating red blood cells. Theoretical and experimental evidence suggests that the scattering is caused by fluctuations in red cell concentration and not by the red cells acting as individual scatterers (3). The greater the fluctuations in red cell concentration, the more intense the scattering. The moving red cells also cause Doppler shift of the scattered ultrasound. The shift is proportional to the speed of red cell movement. The

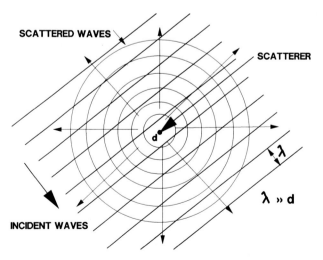

FIG. 1. Ultrasound scattering. Schematic presentation of the principles of ultrasound scattering. λ, wavelength of the incident beam; *d*, scatterer. Note that scattering occurs when the reflector is significantly smaller than the wavelength.

D. Maulik: Dept. of Ob/Gyn, UMKC School of Medicine, Kansas City, MO 64108, USA.

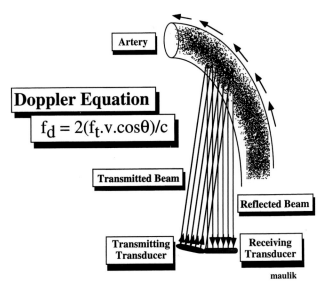

Doppler Equation

$$f_d = 2(f_t \cdot v \cdot \cos\theta)/c$$

Artery

Transmitted Beam

Reflected Beam

Transmitting Transducer

Receiving Transducer

maulik

FIG. 2. The Doppler equation: f_d, Doppler shift; f_t, transducer frequency; v, velocity of blood flow; θ, angle of insonation; and c, velocity of sound in tissue.

relationship between the Doppler frequency shift and blood flow velocity is expressed by the equation (Fig. 2):

$$f_d = \frac{2(f_c \cdot \cos\theta \cdot v)}{c}$$

where f_d is the Doppler frequency shift, f_c is the carrier or transducer frequency, θ is the angle between the incident ultrasonic beam and the axis of the blood flow, v is blood flow velocity, and c is the velocity of sound in tissue. It is clear that the velocity of blood flow can be determined from this equation if the values of the angle and of the Doppler shift are known, and if it is assumed that the transducer frequency and the velocity of sound remain constant. The total Doppler frequency shift signal represents the summation of multiple Doppler frequency

shifts backscattered by millions of red cells. The red cells travel at different speeds, and the number of red cells traveling at these speeds also varies. The Doppler signal, therefore, is composed of a range of frequencies with varying amplitude. In the returning echoes, the Doppler signals from blood flow are mixed with the carrier frequency. Moreover, these also contain high-amplitude, low-frequency signals generated by the movement of tissue structures and high-frequency noise generated by instrumentation. Further processing is obviously necessary before they can be of any practical utility.

DOPPLER SIGNAL PROCESSING

The processing of the Doppler signal involves sequential steps (Fig. 3) consisting of amplification, demodulation, spectral processing, and display. These are described below.

The returning signal is first amplified by the receiver. The Doppler-shifted frequencies are then extracted from the total received echoes which, as mentioned above, also contain the carrier frequency. This process is known as *demodulation*. There are various methods of demodulation (6). Of these, the phase quadrature procedure is most commonly employed. In this technique, the incoming signals are mixed with both the direct and the quarter of a cycle (90°) phase-shifted master oscillator frequencies, and are then filtered. Both low- and high-pass filters are used; the former removes high-frequency signals due to noise, whereas the latter eliminates the low-frequency signals from slower moving structures such as the pulsating vessel wall. The demodulated and filtered outputs are in phase quadrature form and require further separation according to the flow direction. This is achieved by frequency domain processing in which they are mixed with outputs of a quadrature oscillator. The resultant outputs are completely separated accord-

RECEIVER　　**DEMODULATOR**　　**SPECTRAL ANALYZER**　　**CRT**

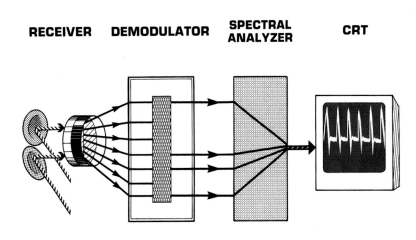

COLLECTS DATA　　**ISOLATES DATA**　　**QUANTIFIES DATA**　　**DISPLAYS DATA**

FIG. 3. Schematic presentation of the steps of Doppler signal processing.

ing to whether the flow is toward the transducer or away from the transducer. With the pilot frequency of the quadrature oscillator providing the baseline, the flow toward the transducer is presented as the positive Doppler shift and the flow away as the negative Doppler shift. The demodulated Doppler signal is displayed as variations of amplitude over time (Fig. 4). It does not, however, provide any orderly quantification of the frequency components of the signal.

The next step is Doppler spectral analysis, which involves processing and quantification of the frequency and power content of the signal. The Doppler spectrum is the orderly array of the constituent frequencies of the signal. This process is known as spectral analysis because it separates and displays the range of frequencies that constitutes the Doppler signal. In addition, the average amplitude of the signal at each frequency level is also quantified. The amplitude approximately represents the number of scatterers traveling at a given speed and is also known as the power of the spectrum. A full spectral processing that provides comprehensive information on both the frequency and its average power content is called the power spectrum analysis. As circulation is a pulsatile phenomenon, the speed of flow varies with time and so does the Doppler frequency shift generated by the flow. Spectral processing must therefore estimate temporal changes in the Doppler power spectrum.

Of the various approaches for spectral processing, Fourier analysis and autoregression techniques are commonly used at present. Of these, Fourier-based approaches are commonly used for Doppler spectral analysis, whereas autoregression techniques are usually employed for two-dimensional Doppler flow mapping. These are briefly discussed below.

Fourier Transform Spectral Analysis

Fourier transform is a mathematical analytic algorithm that converts a complex waveform into a summa-tion of its constituent sine and cosine waves of appropriate frequency, amplitude, and phase. Baron Jean Baptiste Fourier, a French mathematician and physicist of the Napoleonic era, first described this approach in 1807. Fourier analysis has been a powerful tool for spectral analysis of periodic or temporally varying signals by transforming these signals into continuous integral functions of time and frequency domains. This process is known as the continuous Fourier transform. For practical implementation, a modified version of the continuous Fourier transform is used in which samples are drawn so that a finite or discrete series of frequency points are chosen for analysis. This is called the discrete Fourier transform. The fast Fourier transform (FFT) is an algorithm for rapid digital implementation of the discrete Fourier transform (7). FFT processing significantly reduces computational need and is a highly effective tool for power spectral analysis of the Doppler signal (8,9). FFT-based Doppler analysis has been used extensively for assessing various circulatory systems including carotid (10) and umbilical arterial (11) hemodynamics, and is the current industry standard for Doppler ultrasound devices used in medical diagnostic applications.

The number of discrete frequency components that are usually analyzed varies from 64 to 512. Maulik et al. described a 256-point FFT analysis for umbilical arterial velocimetry giving a frequency resolution of 31.25 Hz (1.23 cm/sec) (11). For most perinatal applications, a 64-point FFT analysis is adequate. The initial step involves sampling the demodulated signal at given intervals and digitizing the sampled signals to convert them to numeric values. This is achieved by an analog-to-digital converter. In the next step, the digitized data are processed by the FFT processor, which determines the power spectrum of the sample. Each spectrum is computed over a time window and a number of consecutive overlapping time windows are averaged in order to prevent spectral loss. This procedure, however, also inevitably compromises the spectral resolution. It should be appreciated that the FFT-derived power spectrum is an

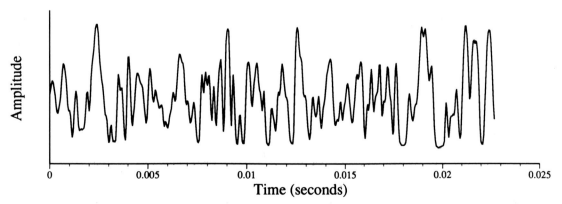

FIG. 4. Actual recording of the demodulated acoustic Doppler signal prior to spectral processing. The vertical axis represents the amplitude; the horizontal axis is the time.

approximation of the true spectrum, is rather noisy, and demonstrates a considerable amount of variance. The latter can be reduced to some extent by various windowing and averaging techniques (12). Figure 5 shows a three-dimensional display of the Doppler power spectrum from the umbilical artery generated by FFT processing.

There are basic limitations of the Fourier approach that cannot simply be eliminated by further processing. The Doppler frequency spectrum from an arterial circulation varies with the changing hemodynamics of the cardiac cycle. The duration of the Doppler signal sample for FFT analysis during which the frequency spectrum can be considered constant is very limited. A shorter length of the sample will improve the temporal resolution of the spectrum. However, the shorter the duration of the Doppler data segment, the worse the frequency resolution. For example, a signal segment of 5 msec will give a resolution of only 200 Hz, whereas increasing the duration to 20 msec will improve the resolution down to 50 Hz. Prolonging the duration, on the other hand, will introduce temporal uncertainty regarding the frequency spectrum, especially in perinatal applications where shorter cardiac cycles produce faster temporal changes in the flow velocity. Another major source of ambiguity for the FFT-based spectrum is related to the phenomenon of transit time broadening, also known as intrinsic spectral broadening. When an ultrasound beam of limited width interrogates a single scatterer moving at a constant speed, the Doppler spectrum will have a range of frequencies rather than a single frequency representing a single ve-

locity. This is caused by amplitude fluctuation of the returning echo producing a range of frequencies distributed around the centroid Doppler shift frequency. The shorter the beam width, the shorter the transit time of the scatter and the broader the frequency distribution. With multiple scatterers, as is the situation with blood flow, random fluctuations in red cell density will contribute to transit time broadening. The situation is worse with short gate-pulsed Doppler ultrasound applications, whereby a scatterer can traverse only a part of the beam of the transmitted short pulse. The consequent transit time broadening effect will generate a significant degree of ambiguity regarding the true distribution of velocity in the sample volume.

Chirp Z Analysis

Like FFT analysis, Chirp Z analysis is also a discrete Fourier transform–based Doppler signal processing technique. This technique allows fast spectral processing of the Doppler signals utilizing analog techniques as opposed to the digital approach of FFT. Doppler devices utilizing Chirp Z processing require less energy and offer a wide dynamic signal processing range.

Autoregression Analysis

Although Fourier-based methods dominate, alternative approaches for Doppler spectral processing are available. These methods are theoretically capable of elimi-

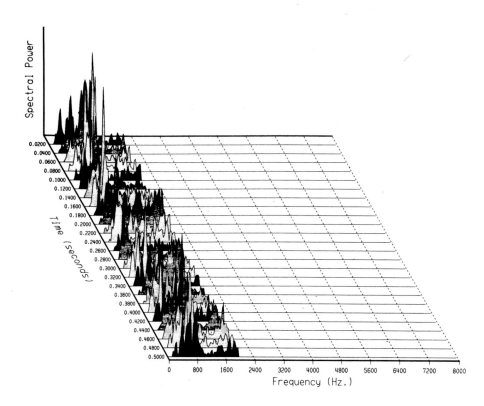

FIG. 5. Three-dimensional display of Doppler frequency shift power spectra as a function of time. From Maulik et al. (11).

nating many of the inherent disadvantages of the FFT method. Kay and Marple comprehensively described the autoregression approach for spectral analysis (13). Such procedures have been widely used in spectral analysis of speech and frequency-dependent phenomena. The autoregression method acts as a digital filter and assumes the signal at a given time to be the sum of the previous samples. In contrast to power quantification of the discrete frequencies in the FFT analysis, autoregression allows power quantification of all the frequencies of the spectrum. Moreover, it produces cleaner spectra and better frequency resolution than those generated by FFT processing. Variations of the autoregressive method have been used for two-dimensional Doppler flow mapping. These include the autocorrelation algorithm that was implemented in the original color flow mapping technology and the more recently introduced maximum entropy spectral analysis. Kierney and Zimmerman (14) described an autoregression-based Doppler spectral analysis for neonatal hemodynamic assessment (Fig. 6).

High- and Low-pass Filter

As discussed above, the Doppler signal consists not only of blood flow–generated frequency shifts but also contains signals from other sources. These include high-amplitude low-frequency signals, known as "clutter,"

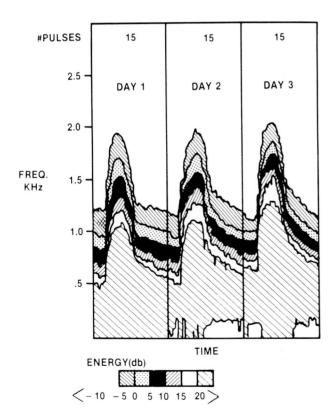

FIG. 6. Autoregression-based averaged spectra of 15 pulses in the same newborn on days 1, 2, and 3 of life. From Kierney et al. (14).

produced by the movement of tissue structures, and high-frequency noise generated by instrumentation. These additional signals are removed by digital filtering. For high-frequency noise, low-pass filtering is used, whereas for clutter signals, high-pass filtering is used. The latter should be used with caution, as a high setting may eliminate end-diastolic frequency shifts from the umbilical or uteroplacental circulations.

The Doppler Waveform

The Doppler power spectrum contains an immense amount of hemodynamic information from the target circulation and is usually displayed as a sonogram (Fig. 7). In this sonographic display, the vertical axis shows the magnitude of frequency shift, the horizontal axis represents the temporal change, and the brightness of the spectrum is indicative of the amplitude or the power of the spectrum. During real-time Doppler interrogation, the spectral display scrolls from the left of the screen to the right with time as progressively newer spectral information is added to the display.

Although the full-power spectral display of the Doppler signal as described above provides a comprehensive account of the dynamics of flow velocity, often more limited and focused spectral information based on the various envelope definitions of the Doppler frequency shift waveform is used (Fig. 8). Such envelope definitions are derived utilizing either an analog or a digital approach. The latter is used almost universally at the present time. Of the various envelopes, the maximum and mean frequency shift waveforms are most commonly used in clinical applications. Many devices allow superimposition of the maximum or mean frequency envelopes over the spectral display waveform. It should be noted that most Doppler descriptor indices are based on the maximum frequency shift values (see below). Under the perfect circumstances of complete and uniform insonation of the target vessel, mean frequency provides an indirect estimate of mean flow velocity; corrected for angle of insonation it will yield actual velocity values. The accuracy of mean frequency measurement is dependent on the velocity profile and is compromised when a vessel is incompletely insonated. The maximum frequency has the advantage of being relatively less affected by noise and is not dependent on the velocity profile of the target circulation. Of the additional definitions of Doppler envelope, the first moment of the Doppler spectral distribution is of particular interest. Theoretically, the first moment represents the integrated cell count–velocity product within the sample volume and is therefore indicative of instantaneous volumetric flow. This, however, assumes that the target vessel is uniformly insonated. It has been demonstrated (15) that under experimental conditions the first moment provides a more linear measure of the

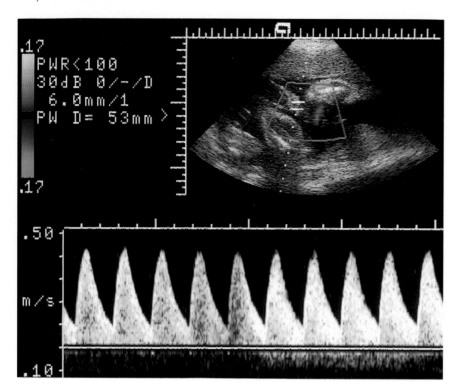

FIG. 7. Doppler sonogram from the umbilical artery. Pulsed wave Doppler was used. Upper panel shows the placement of the Doppler sample volume (*horizontal lines*) in the umbilical artery as depicted by color flow mapping. Lower panel shows the Doppler sonogram. The vertical axis represents the magnitude of the Doppler frequency shift. The brightness is indicative of the intensity or the amplitude of the Doppler power spectrum; the horizontal axis indicates the time.

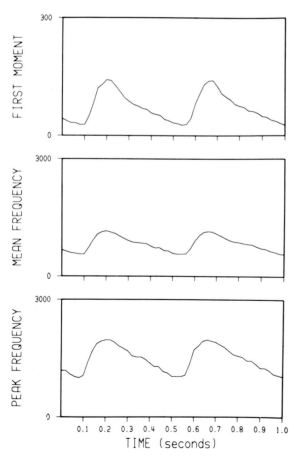

FIG. 8. Typical variation of peak (envelope), mean frequency (Hz), and the first moment (arbitrary units) through the fetal cardiac cycle. The Doppler signal was obtained from the umbilical arteries. From Maulik et al. (11).

actual flow than the maximum or mean flow velocity. This approach has been used to investigate umbilical arterial circulation by Maulik et al. (11). Because of practical limitations, the clinical utility of this technique remains undetermined.

Hemodynamic Information from Doppler

The Doppler frequency shift reflects but does not directly measure blood velocity. Doppler ultrasound can generate a wide range of hemodynamic information from the simple recognition of the presence of flow to the velocity profile of flow, quantification of flow, and assessment of downstream vascular impedance. These are briefly discussed below.

Determination of Velocity Profile

A full spectral display is capable of providing information on the velocity profile of the target circulation. In a flat velocity profile, most red cells travel at the same speed. This generates a slender band of Doppler frequency shift as demonstrated in Fig. 9, which shows Doppler spectra from the fetal pulmonary artery. Note the spectral narrowing at early systole and relative broadening in end diastole. This phenomenon illustrates the cardiac cycle–related changes in the velocity profile. In a parabolic velocity profile, the red cells travel at varying speeds with the cells at the center of the vessel traveling at the greatest velocity and those near the vascular wall

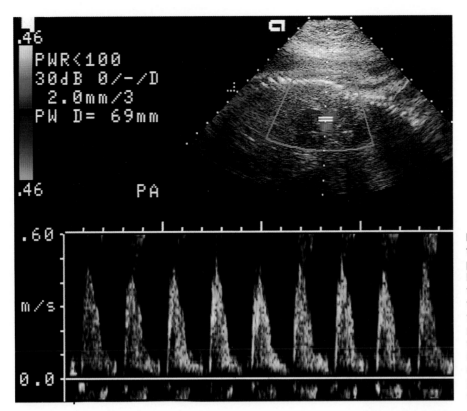

FIG. 9. Doppler waveform from the fetal pulmonary artery just beyond the pulmonic valve. Upper panel shows the Doppler color flow mapping placed in the pulmonic artery. Lower panel shows the spectral Doppler waveforms from the target location. Note the spectral narrowing in the ascending limb of the waveform caused by the uniform velocity distribution because of ventricular ejection. Also note the relative spectral broadening during late systole and diastole.

at the least velocity. Such a wide distribution of red cell velocities causes broadening of the Doppler spectral display. This is seen in the umbilical arterial Doppler waveform shown in Fig. 7.

Flow Quantification

Doppler ultrasound velocimetry is one of the two non-invasive techniques for flow quantification in humans (the other being the recently introduced time domain processing approach). Instantaneous flow can be measured by integrating the mean velocity across the vascular lumen with the vascular cross-sectional area according to the following equation:

$$Q_t = A_t \cdot V_t$$

where Q_t is the instantaneous flow, A_t the vascular cross-sectional area at the instant of the velocity measurement, and V_t the spatial mean velocity across the vascular cross-sectional area at the instant of the measurement. The spatial mean velocity can be determined from the Doppler mean frequency shift if the angle between the sonic beam and the flow axis is known. There are several approaches to Doppler-based flow measurement. These include the uniform insonation method, the multigated velocity profile method, the assumed velocity profile method, and the attenuation compensation method. A detailed discussion of these is beyond the scope of this chapter. Doppler flowmetric technique has been used to measure umbilical venous flow (16), descending aortic

flow (17), and fetal right and left ventricular outputs (18). An example of its application is presented in Fig. 10. The clinical usefulness of Doppler velocimetry for quantifying flow is limited as it suffers from several sources of error (19). One of the critical concerns is the accuracy of measuring the vascular cross-sectional area, especially of the smaller fetal vessels. As estimation of the area involves squaring the radius ($A = \pi r^2$, where A is the cross-sectional area and r is the radius), any error in measuring the vessel diameter is significantly amplified in the calculation of volume flow. Another important source of inaccuracy is the error in determining the angle of insonation. In addition, there are transcendent limitations in accurately determining the instantaneous mean velocity. For example, the mean frequency shift as measured by the uniform insonation method merely approximates the true mean velocity because of numerous sources of error. The main problem is related to the technical difficulties in achieving uniform insonation because of beam inhomogeneity or a beam width that is narrower than the vessel diameter. Similarly, other techniques suffer from a variety of deficiencies. These limitations have restricted the usefulness of Doppler-based flow estimation in clinical practice.

Doppler Waveform Analysis and the Doppler Indices

Because of the problems related to volume flow assessment, there has been a need to seek alternative ways of investigating vascular flow dynamics using the Doppler

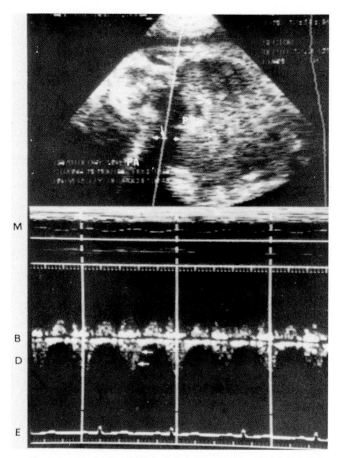

FIG. 10. Doppler characterization of pulmonary artery (PA) flow and measurement of right ventricular stroke volume in a normal fetus. (**top**) The Doppler sample volume, indicated by a short transverse bar (*oblique arrow*) was placed along an M-line cursor in the midlumen of the PA imaged by two-dimensional echocardiography. Maximal inner PA diameter (*d*) (*horizontal arrows*) at the level of the Doppler sample volume measured 0.9 cm. The cross-sectional area at this level was calculated as 0.636 cm^2 ($3.14d^2/4$). PV, pulmonary valve. (**bottom**) The Doppler frequency shifts (*D*) obtained from the PA. Deflection above the baseline (*B*) represents flow toward the transducer and that below the baseline denotes flow away from the transducer. As would be expected, the predominant flow is directed away from the transducer toward the distal PA and is characterized by sharp peaks with rapidly accelerating and decelerating slopes. The maximal area under the flow curve for one cardiac cycle was measured in kHz/sec (vertical distance between the two horizontal arrows = 0.5 kHz) and converted into maximal velocity curve area (s-cm/sec) (*A*) using the instrument calibration factor $K = 25.667 \text{ cm/sec-kHz}$. Multiplying *A* by the PA cross-sectional area gave the stroke volume of 3.76 ml. Cardiac output was then calculated by multiplying the stroke volume by the fetal heart rate. The *vertical lines* represent 1-sec time markers. M = M-mode tracing. E = maternal electrocardiogram. From Maulik et al. (18).

method. The maximum Doppler frequency shift waveform represents the temporal changes in the peak velocity of the red cell movement during the cardiac cycle. It is therefore under the influence of both upstream and downstream circulatory factors (20). The objective has

been to obtain information specifically related to distal circulatory hemodynamics. Techniques have been developed for analyzing this waveform in an angle-independent manner. Most of these analytic techniques involve deriving Doppler indices (DIs) or ratios from the various combinations of the peak systolic, end-diastolic, and temporal mean values of the maximum frequency shift envelope. Because these parameters are taken from the same cardiac cycle, these ratios are virtually independent of the angle of isonation. A unique characteristic of the uteroplacental, fetoplacental, and cerebral circulations in the fetus is the continuing forward flow during diastole so that the perfusion of vital organs is uninterrupted throughout the cardiac cycle. This feature develops progressively in the fetoplacental circulation. The essential effects of this phenomenon include not only a progressive increase in the end-diastolic component of the flow velocity but also a concomitant decrease in the pulsatility, which is the difference between the maximum systolic and the end-diastolic components. The pulsatility of the flow velocity was originally investigated using Doppler ultrasound in the peripheral vascular system. Gosling and King were the first to develop the pulsatility index (PI) as a measure of the systolic–diastolic differential of the velocity pulse (21). The PI was first derived from the Fourier transform data and is known as the Fourier PI. Subsequently, a simpler version, the peak-to-peak PI (Fig. 11), was introduced based on the peak systolic frequency shift (*S*), the end-diastolic frequency shift (*D*), and the temporal mean frequency shift over one cardiac cycle (*A*):

$$\text{PI} = \frac{S - D}{A}$$

Almost at the same time, Pourcelot reported a similar index called the resistance index (RI) (22). This also gave an angle-independent measure of the pulsatility:

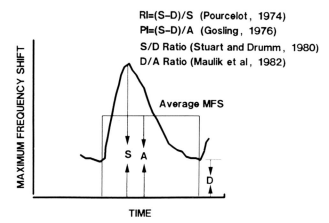

RI=(S–D)/S (Pourcelot, 1974)
PI=(S–D)/A (Gosling, 1976)
S/D Ratio (Stuart and Drumm, 1980)
D/A Ratio (Maulik et al, 1982)

FIG. 11. Doppler indices estimated from the maximum frequency shift envelope. S, peak systolic frequency shift; D, end-diastolic frequency shift; and A, temporal averaged frequency shifts over one cardiac cycle. From Yarlagadda et al. (41).

$$RI = \frac{S - D}{S}$$

where S represents the peak systolic and D the end-diastolic frequency shift. Stuart et al. (23) described a more simple index of pulsatility called the A/B ratio, which is also known as the S/D ratio:

$$\frac{S}{D}$$

where S represents the peak systolic and D represents the end-diastolic maximum frequency shift. Because the variations in the end-diastolic frequency shift appear to be the most relevant component of the waveform, Maulik et al. (18) suggested the direct use of this parameter normalized by the mean value of the maximum frequency shift envelope over the cardiac cycle:

$$\frac{D}{A}$$

where D represents the end-diastolic frequency shift and A represents the mean value of the maximum frequency shift during one cardiac cycle.

Attempts have also been made to analyze the Doppler waveform in a more comprehensive manner. Maulik et al. (11) described a comprehensive feature characterization of a coherently averaged Doppler waveform from the umbilical artery (Fig. 12). The parameters measured included the PI and the normalized systolic slope and end-diastolic velocity. In 1983 Campbell et al. (24) reported a technique for normalization of the whole waveform, called the *frequency index profile* (19). Thompson et al. (25) described yet another technique of comprehensive waveform analysis, which involved a four-parameter curve fitting analysis of an averaged waveform. More recently, Marsal and coworkers reported the use of a classification system based on the PI value and the end-diastolic flow characteristics (26). This classification system was superior to other measures of the waveform in predicting fetal distress and operative delivery due to fetal distress. However, most of these techniques have not been thoroughly evaluated, and currently there is no evidence that they offer any advantages over the simpler Doppler indices. Of the various indices, the PI, RI, and S/D ratio have been used most extensively in obstetric practice.

Hemodynamic Basis of Doppler Waveform Analysis

Studies in this area have, in general, looked for any correlation between the commonly used Doppler indices and independently measured parameters of central and peripheral hemodynamics. The latter included the heart rate, the peripheral resistance, and the components of arterial input impedance. In addition, the relationship between placental angiomorphologic changes and the Doppler indices has been investigated by several workers. This section summarizes these findings and also presents a brief description of basic hemodynamic concepts relevant to Doppler validation studies.

Experimental Approaches for the Hemodynamic Validation of the Doppler Indices

Experimental procedures in this area often require not only the direct measurement of relevant hemodynamic parameters such as pressure and flow but also controlled alterations of the circulatory state. Such interventions are too invasive to be performed in human pregnancy because of risks to the mother and the fetus. This has led to the utilization of physical and animal models. *In vitro* circulatory simulation exemplifies the physical model and has been used widely to investigate complex hemodynamic phenomena. Nonbiological materials are used for prototyping circulatory systems for this type of simulation. In an intact organism, it may be difficult to perform comprehensive hemodynamic measurements without profoundly altering the physiologic state of the preparation. Indeed, it may be impossible to conduct certain hemodynamic experiments *in vivo* because of the inherent complexities of modelling. It is also well recognized that the fundamental hydrodynamic principles are equally applicable to the explanation of circulatory phenomena in a physical simulation and in a biological system. The principles of *in vitro* simulation for hemodynamic studies have been comprehensively reviewed by Hwang (27). More specifically, hemodynamic parameters for designing an *in vitro* circulatory system for validating the Doppler indices have been reviewed by Maulik and Yarlagadda (28). Regarding animal models, lamb fetuses and newborns have been used in both acute and

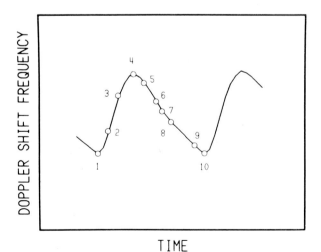

FIG. 12. Reference points in a typical velocity envelope waveform obtained from the umbilical arteries. (1) Trough. (2–3) Ascending slope. (4) Peak. (5–6) Initial descending slope. (7) Inflexion point. (8–9) Final descending slope. (10) Trough. From Maulik et al. (11).

chronic preparations. These models have been utilized traditionally to elucidate the circulatory phenomenon in human fetuses.

Arterial Input Impedance: Basic Concepts and Relevance to Doppler Waveform Analysis

In this section, the relevant aspects of peripheral circulatory dynamics are briefly reviewed. Specifically, the basic principle of arterial input impedance and its relevance to Doppler waveform analysis are discussed. Traditionally, opposition to flow has been expressed in terms of peripheral resistance (Z_{pr}), which is the ratio of the mean pressure to mean flow:

$$Z_{pr} = \frac{P_m}{Q_m}$$

where P_m and Q_m represent mean pressure and mean flow, respectively. Although peripheral resistance has been the prevalent concept for describing the opposition to flow, it is applicable only to steady nonpulsatile flow conditions. Flow of blood in the arterial system, however, is a pulsatile phenomenon driven by myocardiac contractions with a periodic rise and fall of pressure and flow associated with systole and diastole of the ventricles. The pressure and flow pulses thus generated are profoundly affected by the downstream circulatory conditions, specifically the opposition to flow offered by the rest of the arterial tree distal to the measurement point in the peripheral vascular bed. The idea of vascular impedance provides the foundation for understanding this complex phenomenon in a pulsatile circulation. Vascular impedance is analogous to electrical impedance in an alternating current system. It has been shown by Womersley (29) that the equations dealing with electrical impedance are applicable for solving the problems of vascular impedance. It should be noted in this context that the idea of vascular resistance is analogous to the principle of electrical resistance in direct current electrical transmissions.

Closely related to impedance is the phenomenon of wave reflection in a vascular tree. The shape of pressure and flow waves at a specific vascular location results from the interaction of the forward propagating (orthograde) waves with the reflected backward propagating (retrograde) waves (30,31):

$$P_m = P_o + P_r$$
$$Q_m = Q_o + Q_r$$

where P is pressure, Q is flow, m is the measured wave, o is the orthograde wave, and r is the retrograde wave. The presence of reflected pressure and flow waves in arterial circulation has been long recognized by hemodynamicists. However, comprehensive analysis and under-

standing of the phenomenon was facilitated by use of the analogy of the theory of electrical current transmission. The existence of wave reflections in the circulatory system is evident from the observation that as one samples along the arterial tree from the heart to the periphery, the pulsatility of pressure waves progressively increases and that of the flow or flow velocity waves declines. Consequently, pressure and flow waves acquire distinctly differing configurations as they propagate down the arterial tree. The phenomenon has been analyzed mathematically by separating the observed pressure and flow waves into their constituent ortho- and retrograde components (28). It should be noted that the forward propagating waves of pressure and flow demonstrate the same configuration. However, when wave reflection occurs, the retrograde flow waves are inverted, but not the retrograde pressure waves. Consequently, the observed pressure waves, which are produced by the summation of orthograde and retrograde waves, show an additive effect; in contrast, the observed flow (or flow velocity) waves demonstrate a subtractive effect (Fig. 13). In the absence of wave reflection, both the waves would have the same shape. Wave reflections arise whenever there is a significant alteration or mismatch in vascular impedance in a circulation. Current evidence suggests that the arterial–arteriolar junctions serve as the main source of wave re-

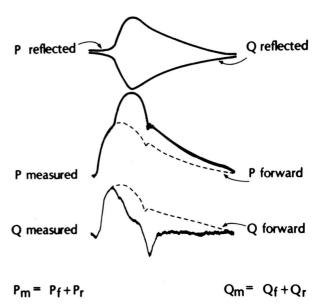

Pm = Pf + Pr   **Qm = Qf + Qr**

FIG. 13. The influence of pulse wave reflections on ascending aortic pressure (*P*) and flow (*Q*) waveforms. Incident or forward (f) and backward or reflected (r) pressure and flow waves are summed to yield measured (m) pressure and flow waveforms. The forward pressure and flow waves are identical, and so are the reflected waves except that the reflected flow wave is inverted with impact to the reflected pressure wave. From Nichols et al. Age related changes in left ventricular/arterial coupling. In: *Ventricular/Vascular Coupling*, Yin FCP, ed., New York, Springer-Verlag, 79–114.

flections in an arterial system. Vasodilation increases impedance and wave reflection, and vasoconstriction decreases impedance and wave reflection. As the Doppler wave represents the flow velocity wave, it is apparent that downstream impedance and wave reflection play a central part in modulating the configuration of this waveform and therefore the descriptor indices. An in-depth discussion of arterial impedance and wave reflection is beyond the scope of this chapter. However, relevant impedance parameters are described briefly below.

The input impedance of an arterial system (20) at a specific vascular site is the ratio between pulsatile pressure and pulsatile flow at that location. As the pressure and flow waves are complex in shape, they are first converted by Fourier analysis to their constituent sinusoidal harmonic components (Fig. 14). Two parameters are generated: the modulus and the phase (Fig. 15). The former is the magnitude of the pressure–flow harmonic ratios as a function of frequency; the units of measurement for the modulus are $dynes \cdot sec \cdot cm^{-3}$ for velocity and $dynes \cdot sec \cdot cm^{-5}$ for volume flow. The impedance phase expresses the phase relation between the pressure and the flow waves as a function of frequency. The phase is measured in negative or positive radians.

Other useful descriptors of vascular impedance include the following:

1. Impedance at zero frequency, which is the peripheral resistance and represents the steady nonpulsatile component of vascular impedance
2. Characteristic impedance, which reflects the properties or characteristics of the arterial system such as the cross-sectional area, wall thickness, and vasculoelasticity (any discontinuity or change in these properties gives rise to reflections of pressure and flow waves), and
3. The reflection coefficient, which expresses the magnitude of the phenomenon of wave reflection in an arterial tree

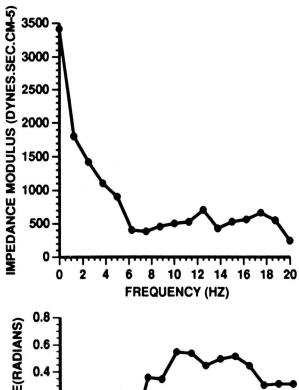

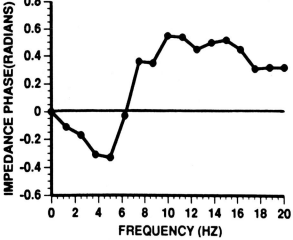

FIG. 15. Arterial input impedance. Upper panel shows the values of the impedance modulus (*vertical axis*) as the function of frequency (*horizontal axis*). Lower panel shows the phase (*vertical axis*) of the impedance as the function of frequency (*horizontal axis*).

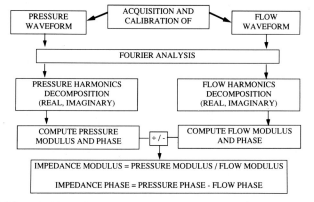

FIG. 14. Flow diagram depicting the steps of impedance analysis based on the Fourier series approach.

The above well-established hemodynamic concepts provide the bases for hemodynamic interpretation of fetal Doppler waveforms in various physiologic and pathologic states. As the arterial Doppler wave represents the arterial flow velocity wave, it is apparent that downstream impedance and wave reflection are among the principal modulators of the waveform and therefore of the descriptor indices. As gestation progresses, umbilical arterial Doppler waveforms demonstrate a continuing increase in the end-diastolic frequency shifts (Fig. 16). This is attributable to a progressive decline in the fetoplacental vascular impedance. The latter is necessarily associated with diminished wave reflections, although it has not been feasible to study the phenomenon directly.

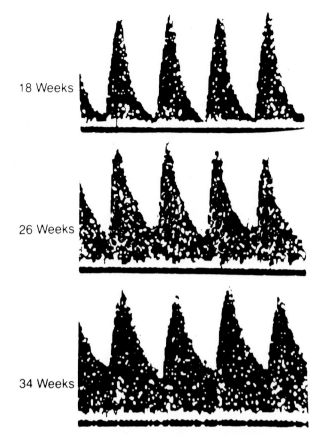

18 Weeks

26 Weeks

34 Weeks

FIG. 16. Changes in the umbilical arterial Doppler frequency shift waveforms with the progression of gestation. Note the continuing increase in the end-diastolic frequency shift that results in progressive decline in the pulsatility. From Maulik D, Yarlagadda P, Willoughby L. Doppler assessment of fetoplacental circulation. *Trophoblast Res* 1988;3:293.

Doppler Indices and Peripheral Resistance

The investigations in this field aimed at establishing a hemodynamic foundation for the Doppler indices in terms of peripheral vascular resistance. Both *in vitro* and *in vivo* models were used. The experimental approach essentially consisted of increasing the circulatory resistance and analyzing the changes in the indices.

Spencer et al. (32) used an *in vitro* flow model to validate the Doppler indices in terms of peripheral resistance (mean pressure/mean flow). The flow was reduced in a stepwise fashion using a clamp. The decline in flow led to increases in RI, PI, and the *S/D* ratio. The pressure and the pressure waveform remained unchanged. The authors noted that the rises in the Doppler indices reflected the increasing peripheral resistance; the RI and PI had a mostly linear increase, whereas the *S/D* ratio demonstrated an exponential increase. Maulik et al. (33) investigated the relationship between the various umbilical arterial Doppler indices and the umbilical arterial resistance in fetal lambs. The hemodynamic perturbation was induced by mechanical constriction of the um-

bilical artery. The mechanical constrictions resulted in declines in flow by 74–89% and increases in pressure by 8–23%. The correlation between the Doppler indices and the hemodynamic parameters are shown in Table 1, which indicates that in well-defined obstruction to downstream flow the indices highly correlate with the downstream hemodynamic parameters including the peripheral resistance ($p < 0.005$).

Trudinger et al. (34) studied the consequences of chronic embolization of the umbilical circulation on umbilical arterial *S/D* ratio and umbilical circulatory resistance in fetal lambs. Chronic embolization resulted in (a) increased fetoplacental vascular resistance (0.25–0.35 mm Hg · ml · min), (b) increased umbilical arterial *S/D* ratios, and (c) significant declines ($p < 0.05$) in the umbilical total flow and in the umbilical-to-splanchnic flow ratio (3.36–1.53). The authors concluded that the umbilical artery flow velocity waveform *S/D* ratio measures the reflection coefficient at the peripheral vascular bed of the placenta. It should be noted, however, that the reflection coefficient, which has a precise hemodynamic definition (see above), was not measured in these experiments and no correlations were performed between the hemodynamic parameters and the indices. Nevertheless, the study established a relationship between chronic circulatory alteration and the umbilical arterial Doppler waveform. The above findings were corroborated by Morrow et al. (35) who observed progressive increases in the umbilical arterial pulsatility consequent to fetoplacental arterial embolization. In this study involving chronically catheterized sheep fetuses, the umbilical arterial *S/D* ratio correlated significantly ($r = 0.76$, $p = 0.001$) with placental resistance derived from aortic–inferior vena caval pressure gradient and mean peak velocity.

One of the limitations of these studies was that resistance rather than impedance was used to assess peripheral circulatory state in a pulsatile flow system. Vascular input impedance, however, is the hemodynamic parameter of choice in assessing the opposition to flow in a pulsatile circulation. In contrast, peripheral resistance is applicable only to the nonpulsatile component of a circulation and as such constitutes one of the parameters of arterial impedance.

TABLE 1. *Correlation coefficients and Doppler indices vs. hemodynamic parameters: Constriction experiments*

Parameter	S/D	PI	RI
Z_{pr}	0.95	0.89	0.88
Q	−0.91	−0.96	−0.97
P	0.81	0.84	0.82

S/D, systolic–diastolic ratio; PI, pulsatility index; RI, resistance index; Z_{pr}, peripheral resistance; Q, volumetric flow; P, pressure.

All significant at $p < 0.005$.

TABLE 2. *Alterations of circulatory parameters in response to vasodilation and vasoconstriction*[a]

Parameter	Baseline	Hydralazine	Norepinephrine
Heart rate (beats/min)	132 ± 15	164 ± 14*	82 ± 10*
Mean arterial blood pressure (mm Hg)	78 ± 5	55 ± 5*	122 ± 8*
Mean volumetric flow, descending aorta (ml/min)	319 ± 21	405 ± 28*	138 ± 22*

[a] Data are means ± SEM.
* Significant difference from baseline parameter < 0.005.

Doppler Indices and Input Impedance

There has been a relative dearth of studies investigating the relation between the Doppler indices and vascular impedance. However, a few recent studies (36–38) have addressed this in an *in vitro* model and a neonatal lamb model.

Maulik et al. (36) used an *in vitro* circulatory simulation system for hydrodynamic validation of the Doppler indices. The *in vitro* system consisted of a ventricular pump, an "arterial" line, a proximal "arterial" compliance unit, a "fetal placental vascular" branching model, a systemic bypass circuit, and a "venous" line for the return of the perfusate into an "atrial" reservoir that was connected to the pump. The impedance to flow was progressively increased by sequentially occluding the vessels of the branching model. All the indices correlated significantly ($p < 0.01$) with the peripheral resistance and reflection coefficient; this indicates that the changes in the peripheral resistance and in the wave reflections from the downstream circulation are expressed by the changes in the Doppler waveform as described by the indices. This study indicated that, within the general confines of a hydrodynamic model characterized by an increasing downstream opposition to a pulsatile flow and by a constant pump function, the descriptor indices of the Doppler waveform are capable of reflecting the state of the downstream flow impedance.

The correlation between vascular impedance and Doppler indices was also investigated in *in vivo* models. Downing et al. (38) developed a pharmacologic model of hemodynamic alteration using chronic term neonatal lamb preparations. General anesthesia was used for the initial surgical preparation, which allowed *in situ* placement of a 4-MHz continuous wave Doppler transducer and a transit time flow transducer on the infrarenal descending aorta. A pressure transducer was introduced up to the level of the flow probe via the left femoral artery. Each animal was allowed to recover for 4 days following which experimental intervention was initiated. Following baseline recording of the blood pressure, heart rate, aortic flow rate, and Doppler waveforms, either vasodilation or vasoconstriction was produced with the administration of hydralazine or norepinephrine, respectively. The following parameters were measured: peripheral vascular resistance, characteristic impedance, reflection

coefficient, and PI. Basic hemodynamic changes are shown in Table 2. As evident, vasodilation led to tachycardia, hyperperfusion, and hypotension. Opposite changes were noted with vasoconstriction. Significant increases in PI, peripheral vascular resistance, characteristic impedance, and reflection coefficient were seen in response to the administration of norepinephrine, and decreases in PI were noted with the administration of hydralazine. Figure 17 depicts the changes in the PI and reflection coefficient and Fig. 18 the changes in the input impedance moduli and phase. As evident, the impedance modulus curve showed distinct changes with vasoconstriction and vasodilation. Further analysis of the data showed a statistically significant correlation between PI and peripheral resistance (Fig. 19). However, changes in PI did not significantly correlate with the changes in characteristic impedance and reflection coefficient.

The next study investigated this issue. The experimental model was the same as in the previous study. The experimental protocol, however, ensured that the heart rate changes due to vasoactive interventions were pharmacologically suppressed by trimethophan during vasodilation or atropine methyl bromide during vasoconstriction. The results are presented in Table 3. In response to both vasodilation and vasoconstriction without controlling the reflex heart rate responses, aortic PI was highly and positively correlated with peripheral re-

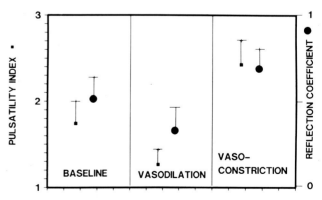

FIG. 17. Responses of PI and R_c to vasodilation with hydralazine and vasoconstriction with norepinephrine. PI and R_c increased significantly from baseline in response to hydralazine; however, R_c was not significantly affected. From Downing et al. (37).

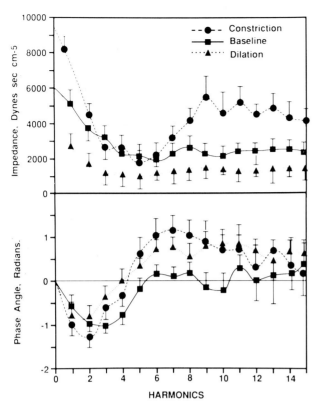

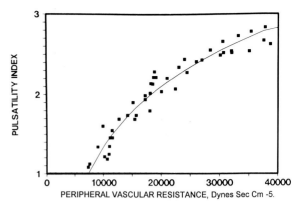

FIG. 19. Correlations between peripheral vascular resistance and PI during baseline, vasodilation, and vasoconstriction conditions ($r = 0.97$; $p < 0.001$). Points represent pooled data from each experiment. From Downing et al. (37).

FIG. 18. Impedance moduli and phase angle during baseline, vasodilation, and vasoconstriction with hydralazine and norepinephrine, respectively. Each curve represents the mean ± SEM impedance moduli for all study animals. From Downing et al. (37).

sistance ($r = 0.78$, $p < 0.001$), but not with characteristic impedance. However, when the reflex heart rate responses were inhibited, the changes in PI correlated well with peripheral resistance and characteristic impedance ($r = 0.92$, 0.95; $p < 0.001$). It is reasonable to conclude from these findings that PI reflects the state of downstream circulation independent of the changes in the heart rate. However, the heart rate does influence PI in the pharmacologically altered hemodynamic state and should therefore be taken into consideration.

Doppler Indices and the Central Circulation

As stated at the outset, central circulation potentially influences the Doppler waveform and should be an im-

portant consideration in interpreting the changes in Doppler indices. The clinical significance of fetal heart rate effect on the indices has been somewhat controversial. Although earlier studies did not find any significant effect of the heart rate on the Doppler indices (25), several subsequent reports refuted this (39,40). However, there is no evidence at present that correcting the indices for fetal heart rate improves their diagnostic efficacy when the baseline heart rate remains within the normal range. The mechanism of the heart rate effect on the Doppler indices has been well studied in animal and *in vitro* models. It is well recognized in clinical practice that when the heart rate drops, the diastolic phase of the cardiac cycle is prolonged, resulting in a decrease in the end-diastolic frequency shift. This obviously increases the pulsatility of the waveform, which is reflected in the descriptor indices such as the PI or the *S/D* ratio.

This phenomenon was clearly demonstrated in ovine fetal models in which fetal bradycardia was experimentally induced by either acute uteroplacental flow occlusion (41,42) or maternal hypoxia. The Doppler indices measured were the RI, *S/D* ratio, and PI. The duration of the cardiac cycle and its systolic and diastolic times were approximated from the Doppler waveform. In the uteroplacental flow insufficiency model, the transient occlusion of the maternal common uterine artery produced statistically significant ($p < 0.005$) increases in the Doppler indices and cardiac cycle time. However, these increases in the Doppler indices disappeared ($p > 0.05$)

TABLE 3. *Hemodynamic parameters and Doppler indices in drug-induced vasodilation and vasoconstriction with and without heart rate changes*

	Control	Hydralazine	Hydralazine trimethophan	Phenylephrine	Phenylephrine atropine MB
HR	128 ± 10	186 ± 12	130 ± 8	65 ± 7	126 ± 8
PI	1.91 ± 13	1.50 ± 21	1.71 ± 13	2.54 ± 19	2.28 ± 0.21
Z_{pr}	39,960 ± 8728	12,350 ± 1210	10,460 ± 961	65,380 ± 8130	60,840 ± 7590
Z_o	4010 ± 340	1683 ± 350	1333 ± 410	8960 ± 760	7683 ± 630

when the latter were corrected for the changes in the cardiac cycle time (Fig. 20). Furthermore, it was noted that the diastolic time was the main component of the changes in the cardiac cycle time (Fig. 21), and the Doppler indices demonstrated a higher correlation with diastolic time than with systolic time. The effect of heart rate was also investigated in a chronic ovine model in which changes in the umbilical arterial Doppler waveform in response to acute maternal hypoxemia were assessed. During the periods of maternal hypoxemia, the fetal heart rate decreased (<80 beats/min) and umbilical arterial Doppler indices increased ($p < 0.001$). Furthermore, the Doppler indices were highly but negatively correlated with alterations in the fetal heart rate ($p < 0.001$). Analysis of the Doppler waveform phase intervals revealed nearly constant systolic intervals while diastolic intervals varied inversely with the heart rate alterations. Moreover, the umbilical arterial Doppler indices, when corrected for the fetal heart rate changes, were relatively unchanged from baseline measurements. Both the studies confirmed that the fetal cardiac cycle and, therefore, the fetal heart rate, plays an important role in shaping the umbilical arterial Doppler waveform. Furthermore, this effect is mediated predominantly via the changes in the diastolic phase of the cardiac cycle. There is also evidence that the fetal heart rate may affect the ability of the Doppler waveform analysis to reflect completely the changes in the downstream impedance (38). It should be noted that there is a paucity of information on the central circulatory factors other than heart rate influencing the Doppler waveform.

Legarth and Thorup (43,44) utilized an *in vitro* model of circulation in which they studied the influence of central and peripheral circulation on the Doppler waveform. The *in vitro* model allowed independent control

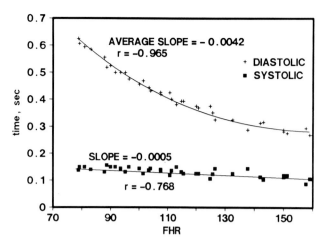

FIG. 21. Correlation between systolic and diastolic components of the Doppler waveform and cardiac cycle time (T). Note that the slope of the cardiac cycle time vs. diastolic time is approximately nine times greater than the slope of the cardiac cycle time vs. systolic time. From Maulik et al. (42).

over pulse rate, volumetric flow, stroke volume, pressure, and peripheral resistance. The authors observed that the velocity indices changed with the pulse rate, although flow and peripheral resistance were constant. They also noted that the rising slope of the Doppler waveform did not correlate with cardiac contractality as measured by the changes in pressure (the first maximum derivative of the intraventricular pressure $-dP/dt$). This finding is intriguing and deserves further investigation. Regarding the effect of resistance on the rising slope, the two parameters did not correlate when the flow was kept constant. However, when the pressure was kept constant, the rising slope increased significantly with resistance.

These studies emphasize the importance of the contribution of the central circulatory changes to alterations in the Doppler waveform.

Angiomorphologic Validation of Doppler Waveform Analysis

A number of investigators reported fetoplacental morphologic changes in relation to umbilical arterial velocimetry and pregnancy complications, including fetal growth compromise. Giles et al. (45) correlated fetoplacental histopathologic changes with an umbilical arterial *S/D* ratio in women with normal and complicated pregnancies. A statistically significant decrease ($p < 0.01$) in the modal small arterial count (arteries in the tertiary stem villi measuring less than 90 m in diameter) was observed in abnormal pregnancies with an abnormal Doppler index. The authors suggested fetoplacental vasoobliterative pathologic processes as the underlying cause of an abnormal Doppler waveform. A similar ob-

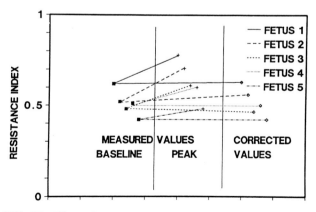

FIG. 20. Effect of variations in the cardiac cycle time (T) correction on the resistance index. The three divisions in these figures correspond to baseline, measured peak, and corrected values, respectively. Note that the differences between the baseline and the measured peak values (all significant at $p < 0.005$) disappeared when corrected for fetal heart rate (none significant at $p = 0.05$). From Maulik et al. (41).

servation was reported in relation to angiomorphologic pathology of the uteroplacental vascular bed and the uteroplacental Doppler waveform. Voigt and Baker (46) performed placental bed biopsies in pregnancies complicated by preeclampsia or otherwise presumed fetal growth retardation delivered by cesarean section. Similar biopsies were also performed in a control group of healthy pregnancies delivered by cesarean section for labor dysfunction or malpresentation. Figure 22 summarizes the results. The uteroplacental PI predicted abnormal uteroplacental angiomorphology with an accuracy of 90%, a sensitivity of 90%, and a specificity of 95%.

Based on these observations, the following vascular and hemodynamic mechanism may be suggested for abnormal Doppler waveform. Fetoplacental or uteroplacental vasoobliterative pathology results in an increase in the arterial impedance that is necessarily associated with enhanced pressure and flow velocity wave reflections. The reflected flow velocity waves propagating backward will change the shape of arterial flow velocity waves. One may identify this by Doppler insonation of the appropriate vascular bed and by demonstrating abnormal Doppler waveforms and indices.

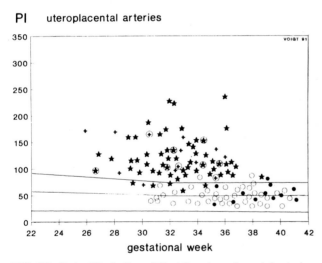

FIG. 22. Pulsatility indices (PI) of the uteroplacental arteries, measured prior to delivery, plotted on our reference curve. The curve is shown in the format of percentiles (3rd, 50th, 97th percentile). The cases with normal placental bed biopsies are marked by open circles, those with pathologic classification by stars. The PI values in the 25 excluded cases are also plotted to show their distribution among the selected suitable cases, which fulfilled the histologic criteria of a true placental bed biopsy. Healthy cases are marked by filled circles, the pathologic cases by crosses. PI values in the group with uteroplacental insufficiency but no hypertension are marked by encircled stars and crosses, showing that they are similar to the group with hypertension. Exclusion of the unsuitable cases did not bias the results. From Voigt and Becker (46).

Sources of Variance of the Doppler Indices

The configuration of an arterial Doppler waveform is modulated by hemodynamic and nonhemodynamic factors (47). The hemodynamic modulators may be short term or long term in nature. Examples of the former include any acute changes in the impedance or in the heart rate; examples of long-term changes in the impedance include those encountered in the umbilical circulation with the progression of pregnancy. The nonhemodynamic modulators are those related to the examiners and to the devices, and constitute the error component of the variance in the Doppler indices. Interobserver and intraobserver variations are the main illustrations of such errors. As an example of the hemodynamic modulation of Doppler waveforms from a circulation, we briefly discuss the hemodynamic sources of variance of the umbilical arterial Doppler indices. Of the various vascular systems of the fetus, the umbilical circulation has been most widely investigated in this regard. The most remarkable influence on the umbilical arterial Doppler indices is that of the duration of pregnancy. As gestation advances, the fetoplacental circulation undergoes a consistent increase in the end-diastolic velocity and a concomitant decrease in the pulsatility. This is reflected in the Doppler indices (48). The S/D ratio, PI, and RI decrease, and the D/A ratio increases throughout pregnancy (Fig. 23). The most likely explanation is that this circulation experiences a progressive fall in the impedance with advancing gestation, especially after the 20th week. During the last trimester of pregnancy, the gestational age effect contributes to 33–46% of the variance of the Doppler indices. The indices are also affected by fetal breathing, fetal heart rate, and the location of measurement. Breathing changes the maximum frequency shift waveform (49). Thus, indices measured during fetal breathing are unreliable. Therefore it is important to assess umbilical arterial Doppler waveforms only during fetal apnea. The influence of fetal heart rate on the indices was discussed earlier. Regarding the effect of the site of Doppler interrogation in the cord on the indices, it has been shown using pulsed Doppler that a variance of 29–46% exists between the velocity samples from the fetal end of the umbilical cord and those from the placental end (45). This may be attributed to the greater proximity of the placental end of the cord to the low-impedance fetoplacental circulation. Obviously, with the continuous wave Doppler, such discrimination of the measurement site is not possible.

SUMMARY

Doppler frequency shifts from an arterial circulation not only represent but also are proportional to the speed

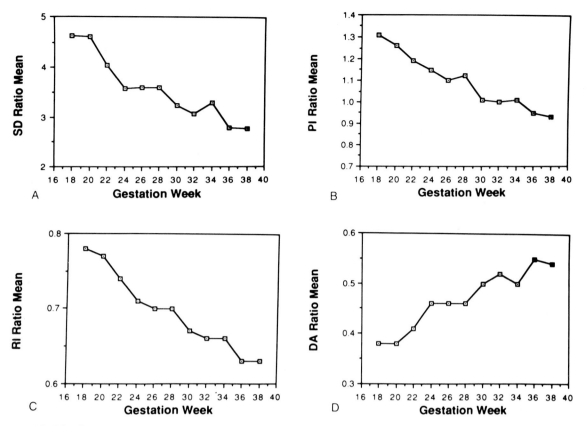

FIG. 23. Changes in the Doppler indices with the progression of gestation. Changes in the *S/D* ratio, PI, and RI, and *D/A* ratio are depicted in panels **A, B, C,** and **D,** respectively. From Maulik D. Basic principles of Doppler ultrasound as applied in obstetrics. *Clin Obstet Gynecol* 1989;32(4):628–644.

of arterial blood flow. The signals generated by Doppler insonation, however, require systematic processing before they can be clinically utilized. The steps of this processing include demodulation, which separates the Doppler frequency shift signals from the returning echoes, and spectral processing, which generates a Doppler power spectrum by quantifying and sorting the frequency shifts according to their magnitude and amplitude content. Of the various methods of spectral processing, fast Fourier transform remains the most widely used technique. Doppler velocimetry offers a wide range of hemodynamic information. For perinatal applications, assessment of the downstream hemodynamic state is of primary importance. This is primarily achieved by Doppler waveform analysis, which generates indices describing the pulsatility of the wave. Although the analytic techniques are based on accepted hemodynamic principles, the data on hemodynamic validation of the Doppler indices became available only recently. As summarized above, the Doppler indices can reflect impedance to flow downstream from the measurement point. However, the effect of fetal heart rate changes on the diastolic phase of the cardiac cycle may confound this capability of the indices.

REFERENCES

1. Sigelman RA, Reid JM. Analysis and measurement of ultrasound backscattering from ensemble of scatterers excited by sinewave bursts. *J Acoust Soc Am* 1973;53:1351.
2. Rschvekin SN. *A course of lectures on the theory of sound.* Oxford: Pergamon; 1963.
3. Shung KK, Sigelman RA, Reid JM. Scattering of ultrasound by blood. *JEEE Trans Biomed Eng* 1976;23:460.
4. Lord Rayleigh. Scientific papers 8 and 9. *Philadelphia Magazine* 1981;107:274.
5. van de Hulst HC. *Light scattering by small particles.* New York: Dover; 1982.
6. Evans DH, McDicken WN, Skidmore R, Woodcock JP. *Doppler ultrasound: Physics, instrumentation and clinical applications.* Chichester, UK: Wiley; 1989.
7. Cooley JW, Tukey JW. An algorithm for the machine calculation of complex Fourier series. *Math Comp.* 1985;19:297.
8. Brigham EO. *The fast Fourier transform.* Englewood Cliffs, NJ: Prentice Hall; 1974.
9. Macpherson PC, Meldrum SJ, Tunstall-Pedoe DS. Angioscan: A spectrum analyzer for use with ultrasonic Doppler velocimeters. *J Med Eng Technol* 1981;5:84.
10. Johnstone KW, Brown PM, Kassam M. Problems of carotid Doppler scanning which can be overcome by using frequency analysis. *Stroke* 1982;13:660.
11. Maulik D, Saini VD, Nanda NC, Rosenzweig MS. Doppler evaluation of fetal hemodynamics. *Ultrasound Med Biol* 1982;8:705.
12. Welch PD. The use of fast Fourier transform for the estimation of power spectra: A method based on time averaging over

short, modified periodograms. *IEEE Trans Audio Electoacoust* 1967;AU-15:7073.

13. Kay SM, Marple SL. Spectrum analysis: A modern perspective. *Proc IEEE* 1981;69:1380.

14. Kierney CMP, Zimmerman GH III. Approaches to Doppler velocity analysis. In: Maulik D, McNellis D., eds. *Doppler measurement of maternal and fetal hemodynamics.* Perinatology Press; Ithaca, NY: 1987:79.

15. Saini VD, Maulik D, Nanda NC, Rosenzweig MS. Computerized evaluation of blood flow measurement indices using Doppler ultrasound. *Ultrasound Med Biol* 1983;9:657–660.

16. Gill RW. Pulsed Doppler with B-mode imaging for quantitative blood flow measurements. *Ultrasound Med Biol* 1979;5:223.

17. Eik Nes SH, Brubakk AO, Ulstein MK. Measurement of human fetal blood flow. *Br Med J* 1980;28:283.

18. Maulik D, Nanda NC, Saini VD. Fetal Doppler echocardiography: Methods and characterization of normal and abnormal hemodynamics. *Am J Cardiol* 1984;53:572.

19. Gill RW. Measurement of blood flow by ultrasound: Accuracy and sources of error. *Ultrasound Med Biol* 1985;11:625–641.

20. McDonald D. *Blood flow in arteries.* Baltimore: William & Wilkins; 1974.

21. Gosling RG, King DH. Ultrasound angiology. In: Harcus AW, Adamson J, eds. *Arteries and veins.* Edinburgh: Churchill-Livingstone.

22. Pourcelot L. Applications clinique de l'examen Doppler transcutane. In: Pourcelot L, ed. *Velocimetric Ultrasonore Doppler.* Paris: INSERM; 1974:213.

23. Stuart B, Drumm J, FitzGerald DE, Diugnan NM. Fetal blood velocity waveforms in normal pregnancy. *Br J Obstet Gynaecol* 1980;87:780.

24. Campbell S, Diaz-Recasens J, Griffin DR, et al. New Doppler technique for assessing uteroplacental blood flow. *Lancet* 1983;1:675.

25. Thompson RS, Trudinger BJ, Cook CM. Doppler ultrasound waveforms in the fetal umbilical artery: Quantitative analysis technique. *Ultrasound Med Biol* 1985;11:707.

26. Marsal K. Ultrasound assessment of fetal circulation as a diagnostic test: A review. In: Lipshitz J, Maloney J, Nimrod C, Carson G, eds. *Perinatal development of the heart and lung.* Ithaca, NY: Perinatology Press; 1987.

27. Hwang NHC. *Cardiovascular flow dynamics and measurements.* Baltimore: University Park Press; 1977.

28. Maulik D, Yarlagadda P. In vitro validation of Doppler waveform indices. In: Maulik D, McNellis D, eds. *Doppler Ultrasound Measurement of Maternal-Fetal Hemodynamics.* Ithaca, NY: Perinatology Press; 1987:257–282.

29. Womersley JR. The mathematical analysis of the arterial circulation in a state of oscillatory motion. Wright Air Development Centre, Technical Report WADC-TR56-614; 1957.

30. Westerhof N, Sipkema P, Van den Bos GC, Elzinga G. Forward and backward waves in the arterial system. *Cardiovasc Res* 1972;6:648–656.

31. Murgo JP, Westerhof N, Giolma JP, Altobelli SA. Manipulation of ascending aortic pressure and flow wave reflections with Valsalva maneuver: Relationship to input impedance. *Circulation* 1981;63:122–132.

32. Spencer JAD, Giussani DA, Moore PJ, Hanson MA. In vitro validation of Doppler indices using blood and water. *J Ultrasound Med* 1991;10:305.

33. Maulik D, Yarlagadda P, Nathanielsz PW, Figueroa JP. Hemodynamic validation of Doppler assessment of fetoplacental circulation in a sheep model system. *J Ultrasound Med* 1989;8:177.

34. Trudinger BJ, Stevens D, Connelly A, et al. Umbilical artery velocity waveform and placental resistance: the effects of embolization of the umbilical circulation. *Am J Obstet Gynecol* 1987;157:1443.

35. Morrow RJ, Adamson SL, Bull SB, Knox Ritchie JW. Effect of placental embolization on the umbilical arterial velocity waveform in fetal sheep. *Am J Obstet Gynecol* 1989;161:1055.

36. Maulik D, Yarlagadda P. Hemodynamic validation of the Doppler indices: An in vitro study. Abstract; Int Perinat Dop Soc, 3rd Congress, Malibu, CA.

37. Downing GJ, Yarlagadda AP, Maulik D. Comparison of the pulsatility index and input impedance parameters in a model of altered hemodynamics. *J Ultrasound Med* 1991;10:317.

38. Downing GJ, Maulik D. Correlation of the pulsatility index (PI) with input impedance parameters during altered hemodynamics (abstract). *J Mat-Fet Invest* 1991;1:114.

39. Mires G, Dempster J, Patel NB, et al. The effect of fetal heart rate on umbilical artery flow velocity waveform. *Br J Obstet Gynaecol* 1987;94:665.

40. Yarlagadda P, Willoughby L, Maulik D. Effect of fetal heart rate on umbilical arterial Doppler indices. *J Ultrasound Med* 1989;8:215.

41. Maulik D, Downing GJ, Yarlagadda P. Umbilical arterial Doppler indices in acute uteroplacental flow occlusion. *Echocardiography* 1990;7:619.

42. Downing GJ, Yarlagadda P, Maulik D. Effects of acute hypoxemia on umbilical arterial Doppler indices in a fetal ovine model. *Early Human Dev* 1991;25:1.

43. Legarth J, Thorup E. Characteristics of Doppler blood velocity waveforms in a cardiovascular in vitro model. I. The model and the influence of pulse rate. *Scand. J Clin Lab Invest* 1989;49:451–457.

44. Legarth J, Thorup E. Characteristics of Doppler blood velocity waveforms in a cardiovascular in vitro model. II. The influence of peripheral resistance, perfusion pressures and blood flow. *Scand J Clin Lab Invest* 1989;49:459–464.

45. Giles WB, Trudinger JB, Baird PJ. Fetal umbilical artery flow velocity waveforms and placental resistance: Pathologic correlation. *Br J Obstet Gynaecol* 1985;92:31.

46. Voigt HJ, Becker V. Uteroplacental insufficiency: Comparison of uteroplacental blood flow velocimetry and histomorphology of placental bed. *J Matern Fetal Invest* 1992;2:251–255.

47. Maulik D, Yarlagadda P, Youngblood JP, Willoughby L. Components of variability of umbilical arterial Doppler velocimetry: a prospective analysis. *Am J Obstet Gynecol* 1989;160:1406.

48. Reuwer PJHM, Nuyen WC, Beijer HJM, et al. Characteristics of flow velocities in the umbilical arteries assessed by Doppler ultrasound. *J Obstet Gynecol Reprod Biol* 1984;17:397.

49. Eik Nes SH, Marsal K, Bruback AU, Ulstein M. Ultrasonic measurements of human fetal blood flow in aorta and umbilical vein: Influence of fetal breathing movements. *Adv Ultrasound* 1982;2:233.

Doppler Ultrasound in Obstetrics and Gynecology,
edited by Joshua A. Copel and Kathryn L. Reed.
Raven Press, Ltd., New York © 1995.

CHAPTER **2**

Fetal Hemodynamics and Flow Velocity Indices

Ph. Arbeille, P. Leguyader, A. Fignon, A. Locatelli, and Dev Maulik

PERIPHERAL FETAL FLOW ASSESSMENT

Accessibility to the main fetal hemodynamics by Doppler has led to the development of various hemodynamic indices. The amplitude of the end-diastolic flow in the fetal vessels is directly related to vascular resistance in the area supplied by these vessels (1). In order to quantify the vascular resistances, various indices [which measure the proportion of systolic flow within the total forward flow (M) during one cardiac cycle, or the relative amplitude of systolic (S) to diastolic (D) flow], have been proposed: $PI = (S - D)/M$ (2), $R = D/S$ (3), $RI = (S - D)/S$ (4), $R = S/D$ (5). Most of these parameters change as the resistance to flow into the vascular territory investigated [$(S - D)/M$, $(S - D)/S$, S/D]. Therefore, for these indices, any abnormally increased values are displayed above the upper limit of the normal range (Figs. 1 and 2a). On the contrary, the D/S index decreases as the resistance to flow increases. Such an increase in vascular resistance may be due to vascular disease (placental infarction or fibrosis) or to distal arteriolar vasoconstriction (brain response to increased pO$_2$ or to drugs). Conversely, abnormally decreased resistance to flow values are displayed below the lower limit of the normal range of the index for $(S - D)/M$, $(S - D)/S$, S/D (Figs. 1 and 2b) and above the upper limit for the D/S index. The decrease in flow resistance may be due to the existence of arteriovenous shunts or to an arteriolar vasodilation (brain adaptation to hypoxia or to drugs).

Ph. Arbeille and A. Fignon: Unité INSERM 316, CHU Trousseau, 37044 Tours, France.

P. Leguyader: Dept. Obstetrique and Gynecologie, Hopital de Lamentin, 97232 Lamentin, France.

A. Locatelli: Station INRA-PRMD, Nouzilly, 37380 Monnaie, France.

D. Maulik: Dept. of Ob/Gn, UMKC School of Medicine, Kansas City, MO 64108, USA.

In order to assess the vascular resistance when there is no diastolic flow in the artery (umbilical, renal artery), we also use an extended resistance index (ERI) that takes into account either the amplitude of the end-diastolic flow or the duration of the forward flow. This index is expressed as follow: $R = (S - D)/S \times (T \times t)$, where T is the cardiac cycle duration and t the duration of the forward flow (Fig. 3). When the forward flow extends to the next systolic peak, the ratio (T/t) is 1 and the index is usually expressed as $R = (S - D)/S$. As the vascular resistance increases, the amplitude of the diastolic component decreases to zero and the index R increases to 1. If the resistance increases more, we observe a reduction in the duration of the diastolic perfusion. The ratio T/t becomes greater than 1, and consequently the resistance index rises. Conversely, when the vascular resistance decreases (placental development), the duration of the diastolic flow (within the umbilical artery) increases progressively until the end-diastolic flow amplitude becomes greater than zero. This ERI has been validated *in vitro* on a hydrodynamic system. The results of this test demonstrate that the extended index changes in proportion to the vascular resistance even if there is no diastolic flow. The extended index as one of the classical indices is virtually angle independent. On the classical resistance index the systolic as well as the diastolic amplitude are affected to the same extent by the angle variations. On the ERI, we take into consideration the time duration of the forward flow and the time duration of the cardiac cycle, which are not angle-dependent.

About the same time an index of peripheral fetal flow distribution was proposed. This parameter, based on the comparison of the brain (R_c) and the placental (R_p) resistances, is expressed as either R_c/R_p (6,7) or R_p/R_c (8). By measuring the flow redistribution between the placenta and brain, these cerebroplacental ratios (in case of pathologic pregnancies) take into account the placental

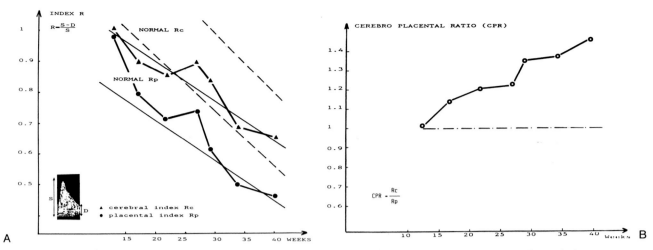

FIG. 1. A: Evolution of the cerebral (R_c) and placental vascular resistances (R_p) on the same fetus during a normal gestation. The fluctuations in parallel of the two indices are related to the variations of the fetal heart rate. Note that the cerebral resistances are superior to the placental resistances at any gestational age. **B:** Evolution of the cerebroplacental ratio during a normal gestation ($R_c > R_p \rightarrow R_c/R_p$ always superior to 1).

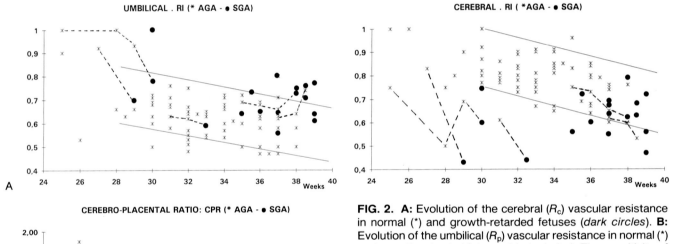

FIG. 2. A: Evolution of the cerebral (R_c) vascular resistance in normal (*) and growth-retarded fetuses (*dark circles*). **B:** Evolution of the umbilical (R_p) vascular resistance in normal (*) and growth-retarded fetuses (*dark circles*). The sensitivity of these indices for the detection of IUGR is about 60%. **C:** Cerebroplacental ratio on normal (*) and growth-retarded fetuses (*dark circles*). The sensitivity of this index for the detection of IUGR is about 85%. The population consists of 90 hypertensive pregnancies, with 17 (19%) moderate IUGR. S, systolic peak; D, end-diastolic velocity; R, resistance index. Arrows show the evolution of the Doppler index when measured several times during the gestation. One can note that strong variation of the index from the "normal to a pathologic stage" may occur within a short time.

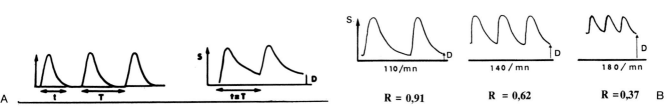

FIG. 3. A: Modified Pourcelot resistance index for the evaluation of the vascular resistances, even in the case of absent end-diastolic flow. $R = [(S - D)/S] \times (T/t)$. T, cardiac cycle duration; t, time of forward flow; S and D, maximum systolic and end-diastolic amplitude. **B:** Effect of the heart rate on the end-diastolic flow and on the resistance index.

disturbances due to the vascular disease at this level, and the cerebral response (vasodilation) to the hypoxia induced by placental dysfunction. In normal pregnancies the diastolic component in the cerebral arteries is lower than in the umbilical arteries at any gestational age. Therefore, the cerebrovascular resistance remains higher than the placental one and the cerebroplacental ratio ($CPR = R_c/R_p$) is greater than 1 (Figs. 1 and 2c). The CPR (R_c/R_p) becomes less than 1 if any flow redistribution in favor of the brain occurs. The R_p/R_c ratio changes in the opposite direction. The CPR is not heart rate–dependent, like the resistance indices. It is well known that an elevation of the fetal heart rate increases the end-diastolic velocity and therefore decreases the resistance index (Fig. 3b). On the other hand, the diminution of the heart rate increases the value of the index. This effect of the heart rate is eliminated by the use of the CPR because both indices R_c and R_p, are measured on the same fetus with the same heart rate. Figure 1 shows, in a normal pregnancy, the fluctuations of both the placental and the umbilical indices (due to the heart rate variations) and the stability of the CPR. Finally, it was demonstrated that the normal range of the CPR is limited by a single lower cutoff value of 1:1.1, at least for the second half of pregnancy (Fig. 1).

During the past 10 years the objective was to check if whether a simple relationship exists between these indices, measuring the variations of the diastolic flow in one artery, or the fetal flows distribution, and the development of intrauterine growth retardation (IUGR) or hypoxia, and if one or a combination of these indices could be used as a predictor of the fetal outcome.

CLINICAL APPLICATION OF THE FETAL DOPPLER INDICES

Umbilical Circulation

Umbilical flow and IUGR

Until now, most of the clinical applications of the fetal Doppler method have been concerned with the investi-

gation of placental arterial hemodynamics. Several studies have already demonstrated the possibilities and the limits of using umbilical Doppler for the assessment of fetal growth (9–20). Most of these studies used the S/D ratio, the $RI = (S - D)/S$, or the $PI = (S - D)/M$, measured on the umbilical arterial Doppler velocity waveform. All these umbilical vascular resistance indices, when greater than the upper limit of the normal range (>2 SD), are frequently associated with IUGR. The sensitivity of this method in this application is generally about 65–70%.

Umbilical Flow and Fetal Outcome

When used as a predictor of fetal well-being several authors showed that only strong disturbances of the umbilical arterial flow, such as absent end-diastolic flow, are frequently associated with acute fetal patency, but in this case it is still difficult to evaluate the degree of hypoxia and fetal distress, according to the reduction in placental perfusion (21–24).

There are several reasons for these results, but we have to keep in mind that umbilical Doppler detects only local hemodynamic abnormalities, which are not in all cases associated with a deterioration of the placental function. These indices measure the resistance to flow, due to the presence of vascular disease at the placental level, and are not influenced by other central hemodynamic parameters like fetal volemia or fetal hypoxia. Therefore, one can easily imagine that placental vascular disease exists (reduction of arteriolar density, limited infarctions, fibrosis) without inducing any fetal hypoxia. Conversely, the alteration of the mother-to-fetus oxygen exchange may be disturbed without any placental hemodynamic lesion. The fetal cerebral circulation was then investigated, the objective being to study the brain response to placental dysfunction and to test the sensitivity of cerebral Doppler as a predictor of fetal outcome.

Cerebral Circulation

The main intracerebral arteries, such as the anterior cerebral artery (6,7,25) and the internal carotid artery

(26), are easy to identify from the well-known intracranial anatomic structures. The reduced diastolic flow in these vessels at the beginning of the second half of the pregnancy (20–25 weeks) develops progressively later on. The increase in the diastolic component as the pregnancy progresses is interpreted as a decrease in the cerebral resistance due to brain development, and the same Doppler indices for the placenta are used for the evaluation of the cerebrovascular resistance changes (Figs. 1 and 2b).

Cerebral Flow and Hypoxia

The Doppler indices measured on the spectrum of the main fetal cerebral arteries are sensitive to any vasoconstriction or vasodilation of the brain vessels. The increase in the diastolic cerebral flow is interpreted as a vasomotor response (vasodilation) to hypoxia. Even if hypoxia is confirmed in most of the cases, it remains difficult to quantify and to follow up this hypoxia (27,28). Comparisons between the cerebral Doppler index and the measurement of pO_2, pCO_2, pH, and O_2 content by cordocentesis have demonstrated a good correlation between pO_2 and the cerebral Doppler index during the early development of hypoxia (the cerebral index decreases with the pO_2). Nevertheless when acidosis appears we observe an increase in the cerebrovascular resistance index due to a decrease in the diastolic flow (29,30).

In a first approach it appears difficult using the cerebral index to quantify hypoxia, but if in fetuses with abnormally decreased cerebral resistance index we measure the cerebral index every 2 days, one can expect to follow up evolution of the hypoxia through the cerebrovascular changes:

First case. The cerebrovascular index decreases progressively, as in normal fetuses, so the hypoxia seems to be compensated by brain hyperperfusion.

Second case. The cerebral index decreases significantly and becomes more and more pathologic; hypoxia develops but the fetus is probably not acidemic.

Third case. The cerebral index, which was much lower than the normal limit, increases and enters the normal range again. In this case the capability of the brain vessels to vasodilate has been overloaded, hypoxia is decompensated, and the fetus becomes acidemic.

These hypotheses are still under clinical evaluation, but so far it is clear that it is hazardous to use only the absolute value of the cerebral Doppler index for the assessment of hypoxia and to make the decision of delivery. Only the evolution of the cerebral index or the CPR over several days may provide information on the development of fetal hypoxia. Nevertheless, a good correlation has been found between the existence of signifi-

cantly decreased (<0.2 SD) cerebral resistance and the development of postasphyxial encephalopathy in the neonate (31). In this study, the specificity and sensitivity of cerebral Doppler as a predictor of neonatal outcome were about 75% and 87%, respectively.

Regional Cerebral Flow

With the color Doppler technology it is now possible to investigate the main cerebral arteries and to evaluate vascular resistance in various brain vascular areas supplied by these arteries (32). In normal fetuses the resistance index was significantly higher in the middle cerebral artery than in the anterior and posterior cerebral arteries. In pathologic pregnancies with cerebral vasodilation (decreased cerebral index), the sensibility of cerebral Doppler was not dependent on the choice of the cerebral artery explored.

Cerebral Flow Reactivity

When the cerebral Doppler index is lower than the normal range or when the CPR points to a fetal flow redistribution, the fetus is considered hypoxic, but it is difficult to evaluate the consequences of this exposure to hypoxia on the brain structures and on cerebral functions (27,31).

The **oxygen test** (maternal oxygenation administration) was used to test fetal brain reactivity (33–35). During oxygen treatment the cerebral index was measured at the level of the internal carotid. In fetuses with brain sparing (cerebral resistance below normal), but that did not develop fetal distress, the oxygen treatment induced an increase in cerebral resistance. On the contrary, those fetuses with cerebral vasodilation that did not respond to

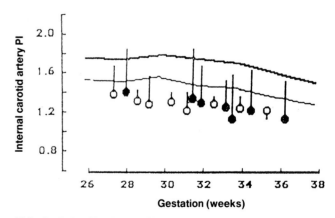

FIG. 4. Pulsatility index (PI) from the internal carotid artery before (*circles*) and 20 min after (*top of vertical lines*) maternal administration of 60% humidified oxygen. Open circles indicate those fetuses that developed acute fetal distress. Normal range for gestation is shown as the mean − 1 SD. From Arduini et al. (33).

the oxygen test (no cerebral resistance increase) developed fetal distress (Fig. 4). The sensitivity of the oxygen test when used as a predictor of imminent fetal distress is about 70% (33). The positive cerebral response proves a maintained placental transfer; this condition could justify the intrauterine treatment of fetuses with long-term maternal oxygen therapy. Conversely, the absence of vascular response to the oxygen test means that either the placental transfer and/or the cerebral reactivity is impaired.

The cerebrovascular resistance of the fetus is also sensitive to the *variation of CO2* content in the air inspired by the mother. A recent study (36) demonstrated that a mixture with 2% CO_2 induces a decrease in fetal cerebral resistance but does not affect the fetal heart rate or the umbilical flow.

The *effect of nicotine* on fetal cerebral flows and reactivity has been studied in pregnant ewes receiving a daily dose of nicotine equivalent to 20 cigarettes (37). The results showed the absence of a decrease in the vascular resistance at the end of the gestation, as normally observed (Fig. 5). This phenomenon, more evident on the cerebral than in the placental vessels, could be interpreted as a cerebral vasoconstriction or as delayed brain development. In addition to these hemodynamic findings, it was observed that there was a higher percentage of stillborns in the nicotine group (63%) than in the control group (13%). The newborns in the nicotine group showed an abnormal cerebrovascular response when submitted to a CO_2 inhalation test (no cerebral vasodilation). The conclusion of the study was that repeated administration of nicotine is responsible for abnormal brain vascular development, with loss of cerebral reactivity, and poor fetal outcome. These results lead to the hypothesis that if fetal hypoxia develops in "nicotine fetuses," the capability of the brain vessels to adapt by vasodilation will be reduced because of nicotine's vasoconstrictive effect and because of the deleterious effects of the drug on the growth and maturation of the brain structures.

Cerebral and Umbilical Circulations

Cerebroplacental Ratio (CPR) and IUGR

The comparison of the cerebral and the placental vascular resistance for the assessment of IUGR was proposed in 1986 (6) and the results confirmed in 1987 (7,8). In pathologic pregnancies (hypertensive pregnancies, for example) with IUGR we frequently observe a reduction in placental perfusion and an increase in flow toward the brain. This phenomenon, called the *brain sparing effect,* is supposed to compensate fetal hypoxia and is associated most of the time with fetal growth retardation. The main advantage of comparing placental and cerebrovascular resistance is that we take into account first the existence of placental disease, which can be responsible for an alteration of the maternal to fetal exchanges, and second the cerebral hemodynamic consequences of these abnormalities.

Nevertheless, the CPR may become pathologic by various situations: (a) there is an increase in the placental resistances but no hypoxia and a normal cerebral perfusion; (b) the placental resistances are normal but hypoxia exists and so the cerebral resistance is abnormally decreased; (c) both placental and cerebral resistances are abnormal; and (d) both indices are within their normal range but the cerebral index is lower than the placental one (Fig. 6). All of these combinations describe a fetal flow redistribution and are associated in most cases with IUGR. Several studies based on the same philosophy, using either the ratio between the anterior cerebral artery index and the umbilical index (CPR = R_c/R_p), which is pathologic when less than 1 (Figs. 1 and 2c) (6,7,38,39), or the ratio between the umbilical index and the internal carotid index ($I = R_p/R_c$), which is pathological when greater than 1 (8,25), demonstrated a sensitivity of approximately 86% and a specificity of about 98%.

The CPR has been tested on hypertensive pregnancies with severe IUGR, idiopathic IUGR, or twin gestations (40), and showed the same accuracy in all these cases. Presently, this parameter is the most widely used in clinical practice.

Recently, the CPR was also tested on a population of pregnancy-induced hypertensives with only moderate

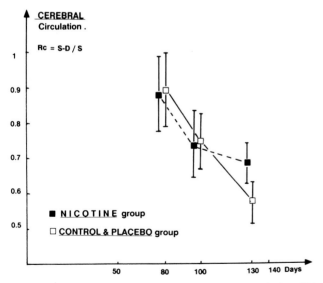

FIG. 5. Variations of the fetal cerebral resistance index (R_c) on lamb fetuses all during the gestation (140 days). On the control-placebo group the cerebral index decreases progressively until the end of the gestation, but not on the nicotine group submitted to repeated maternal injections of nicotine since gestation day 30.

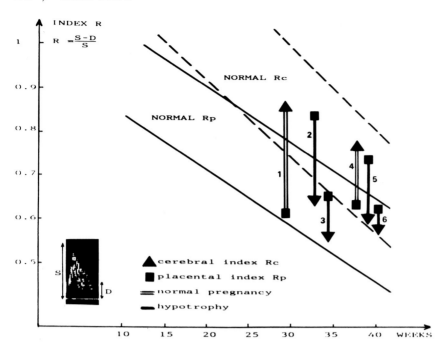

FIG. 6. Different R_c and R_p values associated either with a normal fetus (CPR = $R_c/R_p > 1$) or with an IUGR (CPR < 1). (1–4), Normal R_p and R_c (CPR > 1), *normal fetus*. (2) Abnormal R_c and R_p (CPR < 1), IUGR. (3) Abnormal R_c; normal R_p (CPR < 1), IUGR. (5) Normal R_c; abnormal R_p (CPR < 1), IUGR. (6) Normal R_c; normal R_p (CPR < 1), IUGR.

IUGR (41). The objective was to check the sensitivity of this parameter in the detection of fetal flow redistribution at an early stage of development of IUGR, on a population with only moderate IUGR (Figs. 2a–c). The population consisted of 90 hypertensive pregnant mothers, aged 26.33 ± 5.3 years. The patients were included in the study when blood pressure measured higher than 140/90. All patients were treated by labetalol and dihydralazine. Of the 90 neonates, 73 (81%) were normal growth and 17 (19%) were growth-retarded. The duration of gestation (mean ± SEM) was 38.2 ± 1.35 weeks for the normal growth group and 36.4 ± 3.1 for the growth-retarded group. Eighty-two pregnancies (91.2%) were delivered normally, and 8 (8.8%) required a cesarean section (4, or 4.4%, because of fetal distress and 4, or 4.4%, for other reasons such as placenta praevia). Five of the 17 IUGR fetuses showed abnormal fetal heart rate (dip I or II), and 8 had an abnormal Apgar score.

Doppler investigation of the fetal cerebral, renal, and umbilical arteries was performed three to four times during the pregnancy, the last examination being performed approximately a week before delivery (1.7 weeks ± 1.3). The vascular resistance in the brain (R_c), the kidney (R_r), and the placenta (R_p) were evaluated using the resistance index and the CPR. Eighty-eight percent of the growth-retarded fetuses had an abnormal CPR, but only 41% an abnormal umbilical index and 53% an abnormal cerebral index (Fig. 2a–c). In the normal growth fetuses, 97% had a normal CPR as well as normal umbilical and cerebral indices.

This high sensitivity and specificity of CPR as a predictor of IUGR confirms that, even at the early stage of development of IUGR, the fetal flows redistribution in favor of the brain always exists and is detectable by Doppler. Nevertheless, this adaptation of the fetus may have several origins, such as hypoxia, malnutrition, and hypovolemia, and the role of these factors has to be investigated in animal or computerized models.

Cerebroplacental Ratio (CPR) and Perinatal Outcome

Kjellmer et al. (42) demonstrated in animals that IUGR is generally associated with cerebral metabolism disturbances (monoamines) and delayed development of the brain. Moreover, Fouron et al. (43) showed that in the case of fetal flow redistribution there is a reverse diastolic flow into the aortic arch that confirms the presence, in the flow moving to the brain, of hypoxic blood coming from the right ventricle. This phenomenon probably limits the beneficial effect of the brain-sparing reflex. Therefore, the CPR was tested as an indicator of adverse perinatal outcome. Gramellini et al. (39) found, in a population of 45 growth-retarded fetuses, a sensitivity of 90% for the CPR when used as a predictor of poor perinatal outcome, compared with 78% for the middle cerebral artery and 83% for the umbilical artery indices. In this study, the parameters taken into account to evaluate fetal well-being were fetal heart rate, gestational age, birth weight, cesarean rate, umbilical vein pH, 5-min Apgar score, incidence of admission to the neonatal intensive care unit, and neonatal complications.

Cerebroplacental Ratio (CPR) and Hypoxia

Induced hypoxia on lamb fetuses has demonstrated a very sensitive and rapid brain vasodilation. The fetal ce-

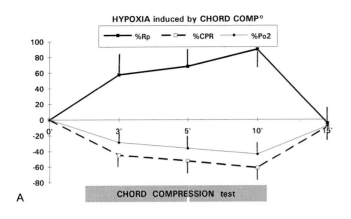

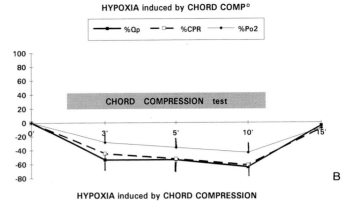

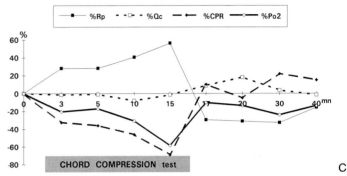

FIG. 7. Variations in % from the pretest value of the (**A**) umbilical vascular resistances (R_p), the cerebroplacental ratio (CPR), and the fetal pO_2, (**B**) the umbilical flow volume (Q_p), the CPR, and the fetal pO_2, on lamb fetuses, during a period of cord compression. The CPR decreases in proportion to the fetal pO_2 and the umbilical flow volume. (**C**) Variations of the umbilical vascular resistances (R_p), the cerebral resistances (R_c), the cerebral flow (Q_c), the CPR, and the fetal pO_2. Note that the CPR follows the pO_2 changes very closely.

rebral and umbilical flows were assessed by Doppler sensors implanted on the fetus (44) during fetal hypoxia induced by cord compression, aorta compression, and drug injection.

Cord compression ($n = 8$) decreases the venous return and the umbilical arterial flow, which induces hypoxia instantaneously and simulates fetal central hypovolemia. During such a compression of 10 min duration, the cerebrovascular resistances decrease and the cerebral flow Q_c is maintained, or only slightly decreased. Simul-

taneous recordings of the cerebral and umbilical Doppler waveforms together with the pO_2 show that the CPR decreases proportionally with the pO_2. The umbilical flow Q_p decreases in the same direction but to a greater extent (Fig. 7a,b). The pH and heart rate stay normal. In the case of progressive cord compression (progressive changes of the umbilical resistances), the CPR follows very closely the changes in fetal pO_2 (Fig. 7c).

Aorta compression ($n = 6$) reduces the uterine flow and induces fetal hypoxia after about 30 sec. After 1 min of

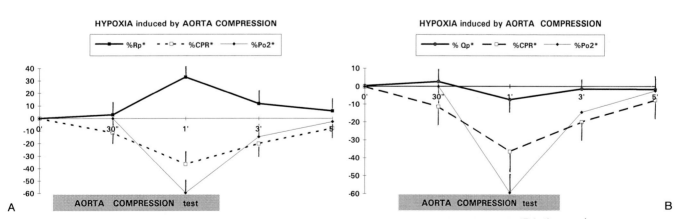

FIG. 8. Variations in % from the pretest value of the (**A**) umbilical vascular resistances (R_p), the cerebroplacental ratio (CPR), and the fetal pO_2, (**B**) the umbilical flow volume (Q_p), the CPR, and the fetal pO_2, on lamb fetuses, during a period of maternal aorta compression. The CPR decreases in proportion with the fetal pO_2 as in the cord compression, but the variations of this parameter are of lower amplitude. In this case the umbilical flow volumes do not change.

compression, the heart rate drops, so the compression is interrupted. The heart rate recovers 30 sec after the end of the compression, and the pH does not change during the test. The umbilical flow remains stable; however, the umbilical resistances increase and the cerebral resistances decrease. As in the previous case, the CPR follows the variations of the fetal pO_2, but the amplitude of its variations is weaker than during the cord compression (Fig. 8).

Propranolol (4 μg/kg) was injected to pregnant ewes intravenously ($n = 3$). From the first minute postinjection, the umbilical resistances increase and the cerebral resistances decrease (44). In this study, pO_2 was not measured but the fetal flow redistribution detected by CPR after each injection leads us to suspect that repeated injections of this drug may induce repeated hypoxic stresses for the fetus, and the question is to evaluate the beneficial effect of any drug (for the mother), and its deleterious effects (hypoxia?) on the fetus.

The fetal cerebral and umbilical flows were monitored during *maternal anesthesia* of 7 hr duration, the objective being to detect any fetal hemodynamic change (hypoxia) in relation to the different drugs used during this period (phenoperidine 7.5 mg, thiopental 500 mg, γ-OH 6 g, and forane 0.3–0.5% at +1 hr 30 min after the beginning of the anesthesia). The patient was operated at 21 weeks gestation for angioma of the posterior cranial fossa. Doppler recordings of the umbilical arteries and the fetal anterior cerebral arteries were performed before anesthesia, during anesthesia (+10 min, +45 min, +1 hr, +1 hr 30 min, +3 hr, +7 hr) and postanesthesia (+2 hr, +7 days, +5 months). The fetal heart rate decreased progressively since +2 hr after the beginning of the anesthesia (from 150/min to 110/min at +3 hr), and recovered partially at +2 hr after the end of the anesthesia. Seven days and 5 months later, fetal heart rate was normal for the gestational age (145/min). At the same time, the cerebral (R_c) and placental (R_p) resistance indices decreased together moderately; however, the CPR oscillated around its basal value. These three parameters stayed within the normal range for the gestational age all during the anesthesia. After the anesthesia, the cerebral and placental indices decreased normally from 22 to 40 weeks, and the CPR remained stable. The evolution of the fetal vascular parameters shows the effects of the drugs on the fetal heart rate (significant decrease) but also the good stability of the fetal flow distribution (cerebral and placental), despite the strong hemodynamic changes on the mother.

These results confirm that the CPR can detect and follow the development of fetal hypoxia with good accuracy. Nevertheless, the variations of CPR are not of the same amplitude in the cord and in the aorta compression tests. This may be explained by the fact that the cord compression induces both hypoxia and hypovolemia,

and that CPR is influenced by these two phenomena. Conversely, on the other "induced hypoxia" tests (aorta compression, drugs) the venous return is not mechanically reduced and volemia remains stable all during the test. Finally, CPR looks to be well adapted to the assessment of fetal hypoxia; the remaining objective will be to use it for the quantification of the degree of fetal hypoxia *in utero*.

Renal Circulation

Hypoxia doesn't affect only the brain circulation. The change in pO_2, pH, and O_2 content may affect several vascular systems such as the renal or the splanchnic circulation. In order to make the Doppler method more sensitive in the evaluation of fetal hypoxia, several groups have conducted studies on the fetal renal circulation (45,46). Some studies concerning severe IUGR and hypoxic fetuses have demonstrated a reduction in renal perfusion, which is expressed as an increase in the pulsatility index (46).

Conversely, the study carried out by our group, on a population with moderate IUGR, with no sign of severe hypoxia or fetal distress, has shown that the renal response could be a vasoconstriction or a vasodilation. The population is presented in the section "Cerebroplacental Ratio and IUGR." In the IUGR group (abnormal CPR in 88% of the cases) the renal index was normal in 33% of the cases, or elevated (27%), or decreased (40%). In the normal group (normal CPR in 97% of the cases) the renal index was normal (73%), or increased (15.5%), or decreased (11.5%) (Fig. 9) (41).

These contradictory findings may be explained by the fact that the renal flow is sensitive to many factors other than hypoxia (45). One can suggest that in the case of severe IUGR, and hypoxia or acidemia, the fetal adaptation consists of cerebral vasodilation along with vasoconstriction of the rest of the vascular bed. Conversely, at the early phase of development of the pathology, the renal vasculature still adapts, like the cerebral, to fetal pO_2 changes. Moreover, in the case of oligohydramnios or polyhydramnios, for instance, the renal resistance increases or decreases and probably the renal flow is also affected by any change in fetal volemia. During ischemic hypoxia in animals and human beings, both polyuria and oliguria have been reported, depending on the experimental conditions and the degree of the insult (47). In severe or prolonged hypoxia, renal blood flow and eventually the glomerular filtration rate are reduced, leading to oliguria. Conversely, mild hypoxia, both in the adult and in the newborn, leads to a rise in renal blood flow and urinary excretion.

Therefore, it seems that presently the renal index needs to be evaluated in larger populations and in several

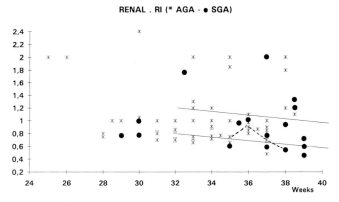

FIG. 9. Renal resistance index $R_r = [(S - D)/S] \times (T/t)$ on hypertensive pregnants: 90 pregnants, with 17 IUGR fetuses (*dark circles*) − 7 with decreased R_r − 4 with increased R_r and 7 with normal R_r. On this population of moderate growth-retarded fetuses, we observe three different renal vascular responses.

pathologies in order to establish if it is a reliable parameter for the evaluation and follow-up of fetal hypoxia.

Aortic Circulation

In the situation of highly impaired blood flow in a vessel, the diastolic velocities might disappear. This finding in umbilical artery and/or fetal descending aorta has been shown to correlate well with an unfavorable pregnancy outcome (48,49). A semiquantitative method of assessing the waveform, "four blood flow classes (BFC)," was defined to describe the appearance of the waveform, with emphasis on its diastolic part (50). These classes are as follows: BFC 0 (normal), positive flow throughout the heart cycle and a normal PI; BFC I, positive flow throughout the cycle and a PI > mean ± 2 SD of normal; BFC II, nondetectable end-diastolic velocity; BFC III, absence of positive flow throughout the major part of the diastole and/or reverse flow in diastole. Another approach to the description of the aortic or umbilical velocity waveform that has also been adopted in a clinical context is a simple qualitative evaluation of the presence or absence of end-diastolic aortic velocity.

The degree of intrauterine and neonatal morbidity was found to be reflected in pathologic changes in the fetal aortic blood velocity (50–52). Furthermore, a relationship has been found to exist between the mean fetal aortic velocity and the degree of fetal hypoxia, hypercapnia, acidosis, and hyperlactemia, as diagnosed in blood samples obtained by cordocentesis in growth-retarded fetuses (53). The BFC was abnormal (BFC I–III) in 57% of the IUGR fetuses and in 93% of those IUGR fetuses that subsequently developed signs of fetal distress requiring operative delivery. The sensitivity in predicting IUGR

was 41% for the aortic PI and 57% for the aortic BFC. In predicting delivery for fetal distress, the corresponding values were 76 and 87%, respectively.

DISCUSSION

The objective of fetal Doppler is to detect as soon as possible any hemodynamic change that could allow the identification and quantification of a placental dysfunction (with fetal malnutrition and low oxygenation), or the consequences of this abnormality on fetal growth and well being.

The umbilical resistance index has been used to confirm the existence of placental hemodynamic disorders in the case of IUGR, but the sensitivity of this parameter for the follow-up of fetal growth remains close to 60%. Nevertheless, the absence of end-diastolic flow on the umbilical or aortic Doppler waveform is an indicator of severe fetal distress and neonatal cerebral complications.

The cerebral flow changes in relation to hypoxia and fetal distress remains one of the most interesting areas to be investigated. Even though many studies have already demonstrated good correlations between cerebral Doppler data and fetal hypoxia, or fetal well-being, it is too early to make conclusion about how to use this cerebral Doppler in routine practice for the management of fetal distress and to make the decision to interrupt a gestation.

The cerebroplacental index that measures the proportion of flow supplying the brain and the placenta is now the most widely used parameter for the assessment of IUGR and hypoxia. One reason is that it takes into account the causes and the consequences of the placental insufficiency responsible for IUGR and hypoxia. The second reason is that this parameter is not heart rate–dependent, and has a single cutoff value (CPR normal if >1, or 1.1), at least during the second half of the pregnancy. On the other hand, because IUGR is most of the time associated with brain metabolism disturbances and delayed brain development, the CPR, already an indicator of IUGR, is also an accurate parameter for the prediction of poor perinatal outcome.

It is also clear that, because the resistance indices are heart rate–dependent, it is hazardous to make any conclusion from one absolute value of any of these parameters. Only several successive daily measures of the Doppler indices may lead to a more realistic evaluation of fetal hemodynamics. Moreover, any increase in the umbilical index or decrease in the cerebral or CPR index, even inside the normal range, will have to be considered as pathologic. Conversely, the progressive decrease in the umbilical index, the progressive decrease in the cerebral index, or the stability of the CPR, even out of the normal limits on the diagram, will be considered as normal. Figure 10 shows the fluctuations of both the umbilical and

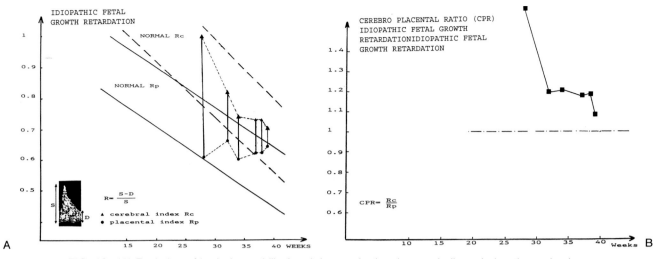

FIG. 10. (A) Evolution of both the umbilical and the cerebral resistance indices during the early phase of development of a moderate IUGR (normal delivery, fetal weight 10th centile). **(B)** Evolution of the cerebroplacental ratio. One can note that these two resistance indices show large fluctuations even within their normal range or at the limit; however, the CPR decreases regularly toward its cutoff line of normality.

cerebral resistance indices; however, the CPR decreases regularly during the early phase of development of moderate IUGR (normal delivery, fetal weight 10th centile). One can note that all these indices stay within their normal range or at the limit.

Finally, even if the Doppler measurements increasingly help the obstetrician, the objectives for the near future must be first to test in routine practice the true possibilities of Doppler indices in large randomized studies, and second to point out the physiopathologic phenomena responsible for fetal flow disturbances. For those aims the animal experimentation will be of great interest.

REFERENCES

1. Adamson SL, Morrow RJ, Langille BL, et al. Site-dependent effects of increases in placental vascular resistance on the umbilical arterial velocity waveform in fetal sheep. *Ultrasound Med Biol* 1990;16:19–27.
2. Gosling RG, King DH. Ultrasonic angiology. In: Harius AW, Adamsson SL, eds. *Arteries and veins,* Edinburg: Churchill-Livingstone; 1975;61–98.
3. Maulik D, Yarlagadda P, Nathanielsz P, et al. Hemodynamic validation of doppler assessment of fetoplacental circulation in a sheep model system. *J Ultrasound Med* 1989;8:177–181.
4. Pourcelot L. Applications cliniques de l'examen Doppler transcutané: vélocimétrie ultrasonore doppler. *Semin. INSERM* 1974;34: 213–240.
5. Stuart B, Drumm J, Fitzgerald De, Duignan NM. Fetal blood velocity waveforms in normal pregnancies. *Br J Obstet Gynaecol* 1980;87:780–786.
6. Arbeille Ph, Tranquart F, Body G, et al. *Evolution de la circulation artérielle ombilicale et cérébrale du foetus au cours de la grossesse. Progrès en néonatologie.* Karger Edit. 1986;6:30–37.
7. Arbeille Ph, Roncin A, Berson M, et al. Exploration of the fetal cerebral blood flow by Doppler ultrasound in normal and pathological pregnancies. *Ultrasound Med Biol* 1987;13:329–337.
8. Wladimiroff JW, van de Wijngaard JA, Degani S, Noordam MJ,

Eyck J, Tonge HM. Cerebral and umbilical arterial blood flow velocity wave form in normal and growth retarded pregnancies. *Obstet Gynaecol* 1987;69:705–709.
9. Arbeille Ph, Asquier E, Moxhon E, et al. Nouvelle technique dans la surveillance de la grossesse: l'Etude de la circulation foetale et placentaire par les ultrasons. *J Gynécol Obst Biol Repr* 1983;12: 851–859.
10. Cameron AD, Nicholson SF, Nimrod CA, Harder JR, Davies DM. Doppler waveforms in the fetal aorta and umbilical artery in patients with hypertension in pregnancy. *Am J Obstet Gynecol* 1988;158:339–345.
11. Eik-Nes SH, Marsal K, Kristoffersen K. Methodology and basic problems related to blood flow studies in the human fetus. *Ultrasound Med Biol* 1984;10:329–337.
12. Erskine RLA, Ritchie JWK. Quantitative measurement of fetal blood flow using Doppler ultrasound. *Br J Obstet Gynaecol* 1985;92:600–604.
13. Fleischer A, Schulman M, Farmakides G, et al. Umbilical artery velocity waveform and intrauterine growth retardation. *Am J Obstet Gynecol* 1985;151:502–505.
14. Gudmundsson S, Marsal K. Umbilical artery and uteroplacental blood flow velocity waveforms in normal pregnancy: A cross-sectional study. *Acta Obstet Gynecol Scand* 1988;67:347–354.
15. McCallum WD, Williams CS, Daigle RE. Fetal blood velocity waveforms. *Am J Obstet Gynecol* 1978;132:425–429.
16. Maulik D, Arbeille P, Kadado T. Hemodynamic foundation of umbilical arterial Doppler waveform analysis. *Biol Neonate* 1992;62:280–289.
17. Reuwer PJHM, Nuyen WC, Beijer HJM, et al. Characteristics of flow velocities in the umbilical arteries, assessed by Doppler ultrasound. *Eur J Obstet Gynecol Repr Biol* 1984;17:397–408.
18. Schulman H, Fleischer A, Stern W, Farmakides G, Jagani N, Blattner P. Umbilical velocity wave ratios in human pregnancy. *Am J Obstet Gynecol* 1984;148:985–990.
19. Trudinger BJ, Giles WB, Cook CM, et al. Fetal umbilical artery flow velocity waveforms and placental resistance: Clinical significance. *Br J Obstet Gynaecol.* 1985a;92:23–20.
20. Trudinger BJ, Cook CM, Giles WB, Connelly A, Thompson RS. Umbilical artery flow velocity waveforms in high-risk pregnancies. *Lancet* 1987;188–190.
21. Brar HS, Platt LD. Reverse end-diastolic flow on umbilical artery velocimetry in high-risk pregnancies: An ominous finding with adverse pregnancy outcome. *Am J Obstet Gynecol* 1988;159:559–561.

22. Divon MY, Girz BA, Lieblich R, Langer O. Clinical management of the fetus with markedly diminished umbilical artery end-diastolic flow. *Am J Obstet Gynecol* 1989;161:1523–1527.

23. Nicolaides KH, Bilardo CM, Soothill PW, Campbell S. Absence of end diastolic frequencies in umbilical artery: A sign of fetal hypoxia and acidosis. *Br Med J* 1988;297:1026–1027.

24. Rochelson B, Schulman H, Farmakides G, et al. The significance of absent end-diastolic velocity in umbilical artery velocity waveforms. *Am J Obstet Gynecol* 1987;156:1213–1218.

25. Woo JSK, Liang ST, Lo RLS, Chang FY. Middle cerebral artery doppler flow velocity waveform. *Obstet Gynecol* 1987;70:613–616.

26. Wladimiroff JW, Tonge HM, Stewart PA. Doppler ultrasound assessment of cerebral blood flow in the human fetus. *Br J Obstet Gynaecol* 1986;93:471–475.

27. Archer L, Levene MI, Evans DH. Cerebral artery Doppler ultrasonography and prediction of outcome after perinatal asphyxia. *Lancet* 1986;2:1116–1118.

28. Laurin J, Marsal K, Persson Ph, et al. Ultrasound measurement of fetal blood flow in predicting fetal outcome. *Br J Obstet Gyn* 1987;94:940.

29. Bilardo CM, Nicolaides KH, Campbell S. Doppler measurements of fetal & uteroplacental circulations: Relationship with umbilical venous blood gases measured at cordocentesis. *Am J Obstet Gynecol* 1990;162:115–120.

30. Bonnin Ph, Guyot O, Blot Ph, et al. Relationship between umbilical and fetal cerebral flow velocity waveforms and umbilical venous blood gases. *Ultrasound Obstet Gynecol* 1992;2:18–22.

31. Rizzo G, Arduini D, Luciano R, et al. Prenatal cerebral doppler ultra sonography and neonatal neurologic outcome. *J Ultrasound Med* 1989;8:237–240.

32. Arbeille Ph, Collet M, Fignon A, et al. Cerebral flow assessment by conventional and color-coded doppler in human fetuses during pregnancies with hypertension. *Echocardiogr J* 1989;6:265–270.

33. Arduini D, Rizzo G, Romanini C, Mancuso S. Hemodynamic changes in growth retarded fetuses during maternal oxygen administration as predictors of fetal outcome. *J Ultrasound Med* 1989;8:193–196.

34. Edelstone DI, Peticca BB, Goldblum LJ. Effects of maternal oxygen administration on fetal oxygenation during reductions in umbilical blood flow in fetal lambs. *Am J Obstet Gynecol* 1985;152:351–358.

35. Nicolaides KH, Bradley RJ, Soothill PW, et al. Maternal oxygen therapy for intrauterine growth retardation. *Lancet* 1987;1:942.

36. Richardson B, Potts P, Connors G, et al. The effect of carbon dioxide on cerebral flow velocity waveforms in the human fetus. *Proceedings of IIIrd International Perinatal Doppler Society,* Los Angeles, Sept. 26–28, 1990:56.

37. Arbeille Ph, Bosc M, Vaillant M, et al. Nicotine-induced changes in the cerebral circulation in ovine fetuses. *Am J Perinatol* 1992;8:268–272.

38. Brar HS, Horenstein J, Medearis AL, Platt LD, Phelan JP, Paul RH. Cerebral, umbilical and uterine resistance using Doppler velocimetry in postterm pregnancy. *J Ultrasound Med* 1989;8:187–191.

39. Gramellini D, Folli MC, Raboni S, Vadora E, Merialdi M. Cerebral-umbilical Doppler ratio as predictor of adverse outcome. *Obstet Gynecol* 1992;79:416–420.

40. Arbeille Ph, Henrion CH, Paillet CH, et al. *Hemodynamique cerebrale et placentaire dans les grossesses gemellaires.* Progrès en néonatologie. Karger Edit., 1988;7:223–229.

41. Arbeille Ph, Leguyader P. Cerebral, renal, and umbilical Doppler in the evaluation of IUGR and fetal well being on hypertensive pregnancies. *J Ultrasound Med* 1992;11:31.

42. Kjellmer I, Thordstein M, Wennergren M. Cerebral function in the growth-retarded fetus and neonate. *Biol Neonate* 1992;62:265–270.

43. Fouron JC, Teyssier G, Maroto E, Lessart M, Marquette G. Diastolic circulatory dynamics in the presence of elevated placental resistance and retrograde diastolic flow in the umbilical artery: Doppler echographic study in lambs. *Am J Obstet Gynecol* 1991;164:195–203.

44. Arbeille Ph, Berson M, Maulik D, et al. New implanted Doppler sensors for the assessment of the main fetal hemodynamics. *Ultrasound Med Biol* 1992;18:97–103.

45. Moretti M, Mercer B, Cartier M, et al. Pulsatility index of the fetal renal artery in postdates pregnancies and relation to amniotic fluid. *Proceedings IIIrd International Perinatal Doppler Society,* Los Angeles, Sept. 26–28, 1990:48.

46. Vyas S, Nicolaides KH, Campbell S. Renal artery flow velocity waveforms in normal and hypoxemic fetuses. *Am J Obstet Gynecol* 1989;161:168–172.

47. Daniel SS, Yeh MN, Bowe ET, Fukunaga A, James LS. Renal response of the lamb fetus to partial occlusion of the umbilical cord. *J Pediatrics* 1975;87(5):788–794.

48. Jouppila P, Kirkinen P. Increased vascular resistance in the descending aorta of the human fetus in hypoxia. *Br J Obstet Gynaecol* 1984;91:853–856.

49. Lingman G, Laurin J, Marsal K. Circulatory changes in fetuses with imminent asphyxia. *Biol Neonate* 1986;49:66–73.

50. Laurin J, Lingman G, Marsal K, Persson Ph. Fetal blood flow in pregnancies complicated by intrauterine growth retardation. *Obstet Gynecol* 1987;69:895–902.

51. Hackett GA, Campbell S, Gamsu H, Cohen-Overbeek T, Pierce JMF. Doppler studies in the growth retarded fetus and prediction of neonatal necrotising enterocolitis, haemorrhage, and neonatal morbidity. *Br Med J* 1987;294:13–16.

52. Griffin D, Bilardo K, Masini L, Diaz-Recasen J, Pierce JM, Willson K, Campbell S. Doppler blood flow waveforms in the descending thoracis aorta of the human fetus. *Br J Obstet Gynaecol* 1984;91:997–1006.

53. Soothill PW, Nicolaides KH, Bilardo CM, Campbell S. Relation of fetal hypoxia in growth retardation to mean blood velocity in the fetal aorta. *Lancet* 1986;2:1118–1120.

Doppler Ultrasound in Obstetrics and Gynecology,
edited by Joshua A. Copel and Kathryn L. Reed.
Raven Press, Ltd., New York © 1995.

CHAPTER 3

Ultrasonic Physics and Ultrasonic Imaging

Kirk W. Beach

The topic of ultrasound physics applied to imaging can be divided into three categories: (1) effects used in imaging, (2) compensated effects, and (3) unmanageable problems. The last group leads to "artifacts." Such artifactual problems must be recognized and should be avoided. This chapter will be organized around these effects. The effects used in imaging are (1a) linear, uniform, directed propagation, (1b) ultrasound back reflection and backscattering, and (1c) Doppler and phase effects. The compensated effects are (2a) attenuation and (2b) resolution. The unmanageable problems are (3a) nonuniform wave propagation velocity and (3b) ultrasound beam deflection. Preceding the discussion of imaging effects, a historic background will place the discussion of ultrasound in context; following the discussion of imaging effects, the issue of ultrasound safety will be addressed.

BACKGROUND

Three centuries ago, Sir Isaac Newton used his expression of the basic laws of motion:

$$\text{Force} = \text{mass} \times \text{acceleration} \qquad [1]$$

and of elasticity:

$$\text{Force} = \text{stiffness} \times \text{compression} \qquad [2]$$

to predict the propagation of sound. The equations were applied to each tiny volume, or "voxel," of tissue (Fig. 1). Therefore, instead of mass, the first equation used density (mass/volume). With a little calculus, two ex-

K. W. Beach: Department of Surgery RF-25, University of Washington, Seattle, Washington 98195.

pressions result from solving the above equations together:

$$(\text{Wave speed})^2 = \frac{\text{stiffness}}{\text{density}} \qquad [3]$$

and

$$(\text{Impedance})^2 = \text{stiffness} \times \text{density} \qquad [4]$$

The meaning of wave speed can be understood by watching waves travel on the surface of water or on a rope. At one time the wave shape is in one location, at another time it is in another location. Although the location has changed, the wave shape remains the same. The wave speed is the change in position of the wave divided by the change in time. Wave speed is used so frequently in ultrasound discussions that it is abbreviated as the letter C. Material does not travel along with the wave, but the wave carries information and energy in its shape and size.

Understanding the meaning of impedance is a little more difficult than that of wave speed. As ultrasound, a compressional longitudinal wave, travels through tissue, the molecules oscillate in the direction of wave travel, like little pendulums. The positional oscillations are associated with oscillations in molecular velocity, in molecular acceleration, and in local pressure fluctuations. Based on the solution of Newton's equations, two of these oscillations are in a fixed ratio: the local pressure fluctuations and the molecular velocity. This ratio is called the *impedance*. Impedance (like wave velocity) is a property of the tissue through which the ultrasound passes. Impedance is abbreviated by the letter Z.

Impedance has two uses in our understanding of ultrasound. (a) If ultrasound passes from a tissue with one impedance to a tissue with another impedance, part of the ultrasound energy is reflected at the interface (boundary) between the tissues. (b) The relationship between the

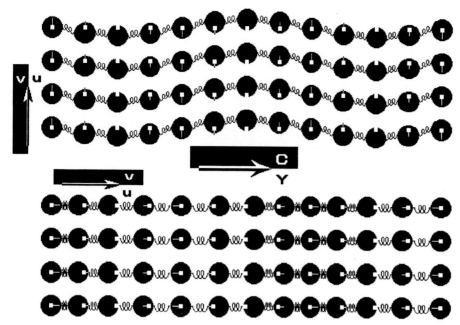

FIG. 1. Molecular model of tissue, masses and springs. Above: Transverse wave passing through a model of tissue. Molecular velocity (v) and molecular displacement (u) is in a direction perpendicular to the direction of wave propagation (Y with velocity C). Transverse waves are easy to visualize. Below: Longitudinal wave passing through a model of tissue. Molecular velocity (v) and molecular displacement (u) are in a direction parallel to the direction of wave propagation (Y with velocity C).

pressure fluctuations of ultrasound and the intensity of the wave is determined by impedance.

In a continuously oscillating wave, the number of oscillations per second is called the frequency (F). The units of measurement are cycles per second (c/sec), which are called Hertz (Hz) in modern texts. Sometimes it is more convenient to talk about wave period than frequency. The wave period (T) is the time between oscillations (sec/c). Medical diagnostic ultrasound systems usually use frequencies of millions of cycles per second or megahertz (MHz), which means that the period is in fractions of a microsecond (μsec).

The distance between two adjacent peaks in a wave is easily observed on water surface waves. This distance is called the wavelength (λ). Wavelength is the most important property of a wave because it determines the size of objects that can be seen using the wave. Wavelength and frequency are related by the wave speed.

$$\lambda = \frac{C}{F} = CT \quad cm/c = \frac{cm/sec}{c/sec\ (Hz)} = cm/sec \times sec/c \quad [5]$$

Typical ultrasound wavelengths range from 1 mm (1.5 MHz) to 0.15 mm (10 MHz). Most abdominal ultrasound is done with 0.5 mm (3 MHz) ultrasound.

ULTRASOUND EFFECTS USED IN IMAGING

There are two problems that must be solved to form an ultrasound image. First is to determine the location of each voxel of tissue which will appear in the image. Second is to characterize the tissue in the voxel, either by echogenicity or by velocity. These are discussed in the following sections.

Linear, Uniform, Directed Propagation

During ultrasound imaging, the ultrasound transmit pulse is directed into tissue along a line. Ten or a hundred microseconds later, echoes are received from tissue voxels along that line. Echoes from tissues at a depth of 1 cm return 13.4 μsec after the pulse is transmitted; echoes from a tissue voxel at a depth of 3 cm return 40.2 μsec after the pulse is transmitted. Thus, based on the time for an echo to return after the transmit pulse, the depth can be determined.

$$Depth = \frac{echo\ time \times C}{2} \quad [6]$$

The values given above were computed using the wave speed of ultrasound in tissue (C = 154,000 cm/sec). The location of each tissue voxel studied can be determined by knowing the direction of pulse transmission and echo reception and the time for the echo. Typical values are listed in Table 1.

TABLE 1. *Voxel depth, ultrasound echo time, and pulse repetition frequency*[a]

Depth (cm)	Time for echo (μsec)	PRF if depth is maximum (kHz)
2	26.8	37
3	40.2	24.7
5	67	14.8
10	134	7.4
15	201	4.9
20	268	3.7

[a] Assuming an ultrasound wave speed of 154,000 cm/sec.

TABLE 2. *Strength of ultrasound reflection (%)*

Tissue	Impedance[a]	Air 0.4	Fat 138	AF 150	Blood 161	M 170	Lens 184	Bone 780
Air	0.4	0	98.8	98.9	99.0	99.1	99.1	99.8
Fat	138	98.8	0	0.2	0.6	1.1	2.0	48.9
AmnioticFluid(AF)	150	98.9	0.2	0	0.1	0.4	1.0	45.9
Blood	161	99.0	0.6	0.1	0	0.1	0.4	43.3
Muscle(M)	170	99.1	1.1	0.4	0.1	0	0.2	41.2
Lens(Eye)	184	99.1	2.0	1.0	0.4	0.2	0	38.2
Bone	780	99.8	48.9	45.9	43.3	41.2	38.2	0

[a] Impedance units are kilodynes·sec/cm³.

Ultrasound Backscattering and Reflection

As ultrasound passes from tissue with one impedance to tissue of another impedance, two boundary conditions must be satisfied at the interface: the pressure in the two tissues must be equal and the molecular velocities in each tissue must be equal. Since the impedance in the first tissue is different from the impedance in the second, the ratio of pressure to molecular velocity in one must be different than the ratio in the other. The boundary condition of equal pressures and velocities cannot be satisfied by one wave coming in and one wave going out. The boundary condition can be satisfied if the incident sound wave results in two outbound sound waves, one reflected and one transmitted. The pressures in the incoming and reflected waves are added together, but the molecular velocities are subtracted. A little algebra will show that the fraction of the incident wave that is reflected is equal to the fractional difference between the two impedances. Thus a boundary between materials that have a great difference in impedance will cause a great reflection (Table 2).

If the interface is large and flat like the pleura around the lung or the luminal boundary of an artery, the reflection is specular (mirror-like, "glare"). Echoes from such interfaces will be seen on an ultrasound image only if the reflector is exactly perpendicular to the transmitted ultrasound beam so that the ultrasound returns to the ultrasound receiver. Otherwise, like a mirror, a specular boundary is never "seen" on the image but images of tissue may be seen in "reflection" (Fig. 2).

The great majority of tissues in ultrasound images are seen because of diffuse reflection rather than specular reflection. Diffuse reflection occurs when the surface between tissues is rough compared to the wavelength of sound. In that case, incident ultrasound is scattered in all directions (Fig. 3). Thus, no matter what the angle of view, the tissue returns some ultrasound echoes to the receiving transducer. In such a case, the strength of the echo represents the echogenicity of the tissue in the voxel under study. Echogenicity is the characteristic of the tissue that is used for identification; echogenicity provides the "contrast" in the image that permits tissues to be seen.

Doppler and Phase Effects

In addition to the strength of the echo (Fig. 4), the phase of the echo can also be used to identify a characteristic of the tissue, i.e., the tissue velocity. The strengths of the echoes from a line of tissue voxels can be determined by measuring the echoes from a single transmission pulse; the phase or timing of the echo oscillations from a single transmit pulse can be measured but has not yielded useful information.

Phase or timing information can be used to measure tissue velocity. The tissue velocity in each voxel can be displayed as the contrast method to identify tissues. To use phase or timing information for velocity measurement, the phase or timing of one echo from a tissue voxel

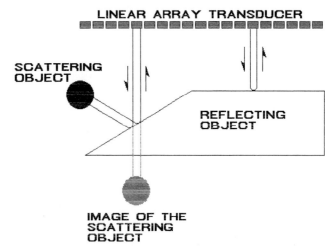

FIG. 2. Reflected image. Right: When a totally reflecting surface is perpendicular to the ultrasound beam, a strong echo is returned to the transducer causing a bright line on the image. Left: When a totally reflecting surface is angled to the beam, ultrasound can reflect and scatter from a secondary object. Using the original direction of the ultrasound beam at the transducer and the time for echo return, the image of the object appears on the line of the ultrasound beam at a great depth associated with the expected ultrasound path.

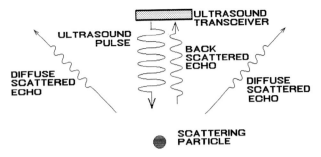

FIG. 3. Diffuse scattering of ultrasound waves. Ultrasound transmitted into tissue scatters in all directions from particles in tissue. Scattering contributes to the attenuation of the ultrasound pulse. Only a portion of the scattered ultrasound is "backscattered" to the ultrasound receiving transducer.

must be compared to the phase or timing of a second echo from the same voxel. If the phase or timing does not change, then the tissue in the voxel is stationary; if the phase or timing of the oscillations in the echo changes, then the tissue in the voxel has moved. Both time domain and Doppler methods are used to measure the amount of phase or timing change, and thus to measure velocity.

A phase measurement system measures the time between pulse transmission and the time of the pressure upsweep of the echo from within the tissue voxel. If the pressure upsweep occurs 0.03 μsec earlier in the second echo than in the first, then the round-trip distance between the ultrasound transducer and a cluster of cells in the voxel has shortened by

$$2d = Ct = 1.57 \text{ mm/μsec} \times 0.03 \text{ μsec} = 0.0471 \text{ mm} \quad [7]$$

The wave speed of ultrasound used here is the speed of ultrasound in blood since the moving cells are assumed to be in blood. The time between pulses is called the pulse period (T). The inverse is called the pulse repetition frequency (PRF). If the time between pulses is 0.1 msec, the speed at which the tissue approaches the ultrasound transducer (S) can be computed:

$$S = \frac{d}{T} = \frac{Ct/2}{0.1 \text{ msec}} = 0.02355 \text{ mm/msec}$$

$$= 2.355 \text{ cm/sec} \quad [8]$$

If the angle (θ) between the blood velocity vector and the ultrasound transmit beam is known, the speed of approach (S) can be related to the velocity (V) by trigonometry:

$$S = V \cos \theta \quad [9]$$

This can all be combined into the velocity equation:

$$V = \frac{tC}{2T \cos \theta} \quad [10]$$

This equation can be converted to the familiar Doppler equation by recognizing that $t/T = f/F$ where F is the

transmitted ultrasound frequency and f is the audible Doppler frequency.

$$V = \frac{fC}{2F \cos \theta} \quad [11]$$

So time domain velocimetry and Doppler velocimetry are equivalent.

There are three features of blood flow that make the velocity measurement more difficult. (1) The echoes from blood are often mixed with echoes from surrounding tissues. (2) The blood flow is often complex, containing many velocities of different magnitude and direction. (3) Blood velocities may be very high causing confusion in the measurement of the Doppler frequency (f). The first two effects will be described briefly. The last, called *aliasing,* will be left for another time.

The development of the equations suggests that velocity measurements can be made with just two pulse–echo cycles, permitting the measurement of the echo phase or timing change in the interval between pulses. If the signals were clean, this would be true. The echoes always contain a combination of weak reflections from moving blood in the voxel and stronger echoes from nearby solid tissues. To extract the weak blood echoes from the strong stationary echoes requires several pulse–echo cycles. Some instruments have limitations in velocity resolution that can be surmounted by combining even more echoes. Commercial instruments use between 4 and 32 pulse–echo cycles for the processing of echo data for color flow images. The number of pulse–echo cycles used

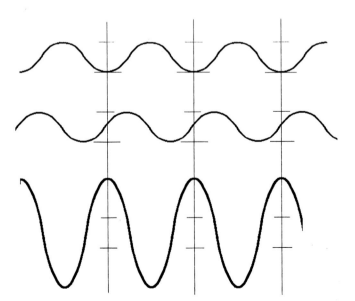

FIG. 4. Phase and amplitude. Two kinds of information can be carried in a wave: phase or timing information and amplitude information. Top: Reference wave. Middle: Wave of the same amplitude as the reference wave and phase shifted $\frac{1}{4}$ cycle or 90 degrees (of 360) to the left. Bottom: Wave of the same phase as the reference wave with a higher amplitude.

for velocity measurement is called the ensemble length, or packet length.

Often blood flow is complex, having many velocities present in the same voxel or sample volume at the same time. To measure all of these takes even more pulse–echo cycles. Fast Fourier transform (FFT) Doppler systems are well suited for this task. Such systems use 128 pulse–echo cycles to compute all of the velocities that are present. Color flow images, which are generated with fewer pulse–echo cycles, show only one of the many velocities present when complex flow is present.

COMPENSATED EFFECTS

In principle, ultrasound images are easy to acquire. However, as always, in practice, there are some solvable problems. The two major solvable problems are ultrasound attenuation and resolution limitations.

Ultrasound Attenuation

As an ultrasound pulse passes through tissue along a line, some of the energy is scattered by diffuse reflection into other directions; some of the energy is absorbed by the tissue and converted to heat. Both effects result in the ultrasound pulse becoming weaker with depth. The echo experiences a similar attenuation on return to the transducer. For B-mode imaging, where the amplitude or strength of the echo is used as an indication of echogenicity to identify the tissue, the attenuation loss confounds the relationship between echo strength and echogenicity of the tissue in a voxel.

To compensate for that, the echoes are amplified by the time gain compensation (TGC) system. The adjustment of the TGC by the examiner is based on the depth of the voxel and the examiner's impression of the attenuation of the tissue (Table 3).

Modern gray scale ultrasound instruments can only process echoes in a range of about 100 dB even with time gain compensation. Typical displays show a range of 40–60 dB. At an attenuation rate of 5 dB/cm used in Table 3 the maximum depth of the image is limited to less than 10 cm. Use of a longer ultrasound wavelength (lower ultrasound frequency) results in less attenuation per centimeter. If the tissue echogenicity is not strongly dependent on ultrasound wavelength, then deep tissues can be seen more easily.

In addition to the effect of the changes in tissue impedance, tissue echogenicity is related to the ratio of tissue size to ultrasound wavelength. The relationship is not linear. Wavelength (0.5 mm) is much greater than erythrocyte size (0.007 mm); wavelength is smaller than the lens of the eye. Echogenicity of erythrocytes increases 16 times as the frequency is doubled (the wavelength is cut in half); echogenicity from the lens of the eye increases little as frequency increases.

To receive a strong ultrasound echo from the tissue in the voxel of interest, the choice of ultrasound frequency must balance between a low frequency to penetrate to that depth and a high frequency to achieve strong echoes.

Resolution Aspect

Depth resolution in an ultrasound image is limited by the length of the ultrasound transmit pulse: a short transmit pulse gives fine (good) depth resolution. This requires a well-damped, high-bandwidth, inefficient high-frequency, ultrasound transducer. Lateral resolution is determined by the diameter of the ultrasound transducer and the focal character. Depth resolution is always better than lateral resolution. Table 4 summarizes the relationship between the ultrasound transducer and resolution. Like a golf score, better resolution is smaller.

There are actually four dimensions of image resolution: depth, lateral, thickness, and time. Depth and lateral appear on the image as the vertical and horizontal

TABLE 3. *Time gain compensation*

Depth (cm)	Time for echo[a] (μsec)	Typical echo strength after attenuation[b]		
		Decimal	Exponent	dB
1	13.4	0.1	$0.1^{10/10}$	10
2	26.8	0.01	$0.1^{20/10}$	20
3	40.2	0.001	$0.1^{30/10}$	30
5	67	0.00001	$0.1^{50/10}$	50
10	134	0.0000000001	$0.1^{100/10}$	100

[a] Assuming an ultrasound wave speed of 154,000 cm/sec.
[b] Assuming an attenuation rate of 5 dB/cm and round trip travel to the depth and back (4 cm travel for a 2 cm depth).

TABLE 4. *Transducer characteristics and resolution*

Transducer	Lateral	Depth
Short-wavelength (high-frequency)[a]	Better	Better
Well-damped (high-bandwidth) (low Q)	—	Better
Large-diameter focused	Better only at focal depth	—
Shallow focus (large numeric aperture)	Better only at focal depth	—

[a] Synonyms are in parentheses.

dimensions. Thickness resolution indicates how much will be included in the image plane. Time resolution is related to the detail that will be seen in moving structures. Modern electronic array scanheads all have much better lateral resolution than thickness resolution. This is because larger apertures and adjustable electronic focusing are possible in the lateral direction. In the thickness direction, the focusing is not adjustable. There is a focal zone in the thickness direction that is determined by the shape of the material covering the transducers.

UNMANAGEABLE PROBLEMS

Artifacts in ultrasound images often result from one of two major factors, both related to errors in correctly identifying the location of the tissue voxel under study. In most images these errors are not serious enough to impede diagnosis, but caution must be exercised. The smaller of the two problems is variation in wave propagation velocity; the greater problem is deflection of the ultrasound beam as it passes through tissue.

Nonuniform Wave Propagation Velocity

As a pulse of ultrasound passes along the ultrasound beam direction, the wave velocity is determined by the material through which it passes. The ultrasound instrument determines the depth of a voxel by measuring the time for the ultrasound to make a round trip to the voxel and a guess at the speed of the ultrasound wave in tissue. Unfortunately, the speed is different in different tissues (Table 5).

TABLE 5. *Ultrasound speed and depth errors in tissue[a]*

Tissue	Speed (cm/sec)	Depth error (%)
Fat	145,000	+6[b]
Urine	148,000	+4
Amniotic fluid	151,000	+2
Brain	154,000	0
Liver	155,000	−1
Blood	157,000[a]	−2
Muscle	158,000	−3
Cartilage	166,000	−8
Bone	350,000	−56

[a] Instruments often assume a speed of 154,000 cm/sec in blood.

[b] + Objects appear thicker on the image than they really are; − objects appear thinner.

When measurements are made in the depth direction, these errors will appear. They may also have importance when using ultrasound in combination with another technique such as ultrasound-guided biopsy. Cursors on the screen may not correctly show where the needle will go. Of course, the image of the needle, once inserted, will appear in the ultrasound image in the correct relationship to the surrounding tissues.

Ultrasound Beam Deflection

The largest problem in ultrasound imaging is deflection of the ultrasound beam. The ultrasound image is formed assuming that the ultrasound pulse travels along straight lines into tissue. When the ultrasound deviates from that line, the information from an echo that is re-

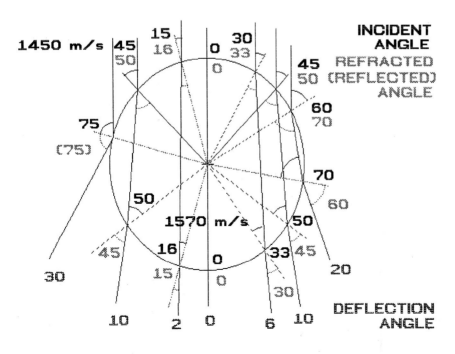

FIG. 5. Refraction and reflection of ultrasound. Exterior ultrasound velocity 145,000 cm/s is C in fat. Interior ultrasound velocity 157,000 cm/s is C in blood. Ultrasound incident on a surface at an angle less than 67 degrees to the perpendicular is refracted away from the center of the circle and refracted again on exit to double the deflection angle. Reflection also doubles the deflection angle. Structures on a deflected ultrasound beam appear on ultrasound images in the wrong lateral location.

TABLE 6. *Maximum angle of deflection between tissues[a]*

vv Fat	145,000 cm/sec							
−12	≪vv Urine	148,000 cm/sec						
−16	−11	≪vv Amniotic Fd	151,000 cm/sec					
−20	−16	−11	≪vv Brain	154,000 cm/sec				
−21	−17	−13	−7	≪vv Liver	155,000 cm/sec			
−23	−19	−16	−11	−9	≪vv Blood	157,000 cm/sec		
−23	−20	−17	−13	−11	−6	≪vv Muscle	158,000 cm/sec	
−29	−27	−25	−22	−21	−19	−18	≪Cartilage	166,000 cm/sec

[a] Angles in degrees, based on ultrasound speeds listed.

turned is displayed at the wrong location in the image. This can result in severe image distortion. If the ultrasound beam is dispersed as it deviates, then the echo information may be additionally distorted.

Deflection of the ultrasound beam results from two processes: reflection and refraction. Refraction occurs as ultrasound passes through an interface from one material to another at an acute angle. The ultrasound beam refraction can be computed using Snell's law.

$$\frac{C_1}{\sin \theta_1} = \frac{C_2}{\sin \theta_2} \qquad [12]$$

Deflection is the difference between the incoming angle and the outgoing refracted transmission angle. Reflection occurs when Snell's law cannot be satisfied, when the incoming angle is too far from perpendicular. When ultrasound passes through a circular object with higher ultrasound speed inside (Fig. 5), refraction occurs when the ultrasound beam is near the diameter and reflection occurs when the ultrasound beam is nearly tangent to the object. Both reflection and refraction cause beam deflection and image distortion; the greatest deflection occurs at the *critical angle* where reflection changes to refraction. Deflection angles may appear quite large (Table 6). However, even small changes in ultrasound speed can deflect the beam markedly; a difference as little as 2% causes a 12° refraction if the interface is intersected near 80°. If the angle is increased above that, total reflection occurs and the resultant deflection angle is double that listed in Table 6. These reflections are responsible for the "shadowing" that occurs at the edge of structures.

In an ultrasound image, everything that appears along an ultrasound scan line, deeper than the point of beam deflection, appears in the wrong lateral location in the image. All lateral measurements in that region are incorrect. In that region, objects may be missing, may be duplicated, and may appear to be adjacent to distant objects or far from adjacent objects.

Sometimes, when considering ultrasound beam deflection, it seems a wonder that ultrasound imaging works at all. Ultrasound imaging works because only a small fraction of the ultrasound lines strike interfaces at such acute angles in most images.

BIOEFFECTS OF ULTRASOUND

Everyone expresses concern about the biologic effects of ultrasound; at the same time, they assure us that ultrasound is safe. The reason for this dichotomy is that the application of ultrasound has been much more rapid than the theoretical understanding. Experience has supported the idea that ultrasound is safe; theory sometimes suggests that it might not be safe. There are two related issues in ultrasound bioeffects: exposure level and exposure time. There are two mechanisms of bioeffects that are usually discussed: (a) heating and (b) nonlinear effects and cavitation. These topics are interwoven in such a way that it is difficult to separate one from the other.

In this discussion, only two aspects of the issues will be mentioned: the effect of automatic two-dimensional scanning and the effect of nonlinear propagation of ultrasound. Finally, the assurance that diagnostic ultrasound is safe will be made.

Automatic Two-Dimensional Scanning and Tissue Exposure

Biologic effects on tissue depend on the intensity and duration of exposure of each voxel of tissue to ultrasound. The instantaneous maximum (temporal peak) intensity of exposure is the same for two-dimensional B-mode imaging as for M-mode examination, and is similar to time–domain color velocity imaging, as all the imaging transmit pulses are similar in duration. The instantaneous maximum (temporal peak) intensity of exposure is the same for color Doppler imaging as for single-gate pulsed Doppler examination, as all the Doppler transmit pulses are similar in duration. The transmit pulse in imaging is shorter than in Doppler, so that the temporal peak intensities are usually higher in imaging.

The two-dimensional techniques sweep the transmit beam across tissue exposing a single tissue element for only a short time during image formation. Therefore, M-mode and single-gate pulsed Doppler always expose individual tissue voxels to more pulses of ultrasound over time than do the two-dimensional imaging methods (Ta-

TABLE 7. *Number of ultrasound pulses per second to a tissue voxel*

Method	Pulses/sec
Single-gate pulsed Doppler	10,000
M-mode	1,000
2-D color Doppler	120
2-D time–domain	60
2-D B-mode	30

ble 7). Each pulse contains about 1 µJ of energy no matter what method of imaging is used. Therefore, during an ultrasound examination, if the examiner can choose between a two-dimensional modality and a single-line modality, the two-dimensional method should be chosen.

Nonlinear Effects and Cavitation

The solution to Newton's equations results in an impossible finding: in any material with the acoustic impedance of tissue, when the spatial peak temporal peak (SPTP, Table 8) intensity equals 320 mW/cm² , the pressure fluctuations equal the atmospheric pressure. Therefore, the pressure in the tissue oscillates, in theory between twice the atmospheric pressure and zero. If the intensity is increased, the highest pressure exceeds twice atmospheric pressure and, in theory, the minimum pressure becomes negative. Negative pressure, according to other theories, is impossible. Therefore, at those intensities, Newton's linear equations must be wrong. Specifically, it is Eq. 2 that is wrong under these conditions. This is *nonlinear* ultrasound wave propagation. The wave, which at lower intensities looks sinusoidal (Fig. 6), now looks flattened on the bottom and peaked at the top like surf breaking on the ocean beach. This condition begins near the transducer, where the beam begins to converge toward the focal zone causing an increase in intensity. When nonlinear propagation occurs, the conversion of the pulse energy to heat is accelerated. With lower en-

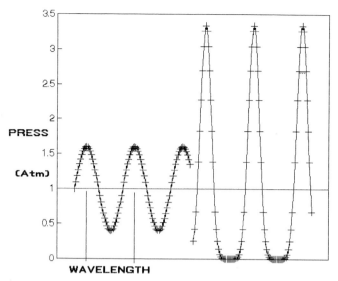

FIG. 6. Nonlinear effects of ultrasound in water Z = 148 Kd − s/cm³. Left: Continuous wave ultrasound with linear propagation. The intensity is less than 320 mW/cm². Right: Continuous wave ultrasound with nonlinear propagation. The intensity is greater than 320 mW/cm² so that the pressure amplitude is expected to be greater than 1 atmosphere. The negative pressure expected theoretically is impossible, so the ''valleys'' of the wave are flattened.

ergy in the pulse, the high intensities predicted by some theories at the focal zone are never reached. Thus, because of high nonlinear losses in tissue, it is probably impossible to achieve SPTP intensities over 500 or 1000 mW/cm². The temporal average intensity (SPTA) seen by an individual tissue voxel is less than 1% of that.

Ultrasound Safety

As long as ultrasound does not raise the temperature of tissue by more than 1°C in an afebrile patient, no hazard should result. Using single-gate pulsed Doppler, the expected achievable SPTA tissue levels are about 10 mW/cm², accounting for the protective effects of nonlinear attenuation. The soft tissue that heats the fastest is fat. Using 3 MHz ultrasound in fat at 10 mW/cm², a temperature rise of 1°C is expected in 8 sec of exposure. Therefore, caution should be used when doing a pulsed Doppler examination: continuous sampling along a single Doppler line should be limited to a few cardiac cycles.

All other forms of ultrasound are expected to have less severe effects than pulsed Doppler.

REFERENCES

1. Gross SA, Johnston RL, Dunn F. Comprehensive compilation of empirical ultrasonic properties of mammalian tissues, *J Acoust Soc Am* 1978; 64(2).

TABLE 8. *Measures of ultrasound intensity*

Label	Meaning	Relative size[a] (mW/cm²)
SATA	Spatial average temporal average	1
SPTA	Spatial peak temporal average	2[b]
SAPA	Spatial average pulse average	1000
SPPA	Spatial peak pulse average	2000
SATP	Spatial average temporal peak	3000
SPTP	Spatial peak temporal peak	6000[c]

[a] Size for the same M-mode imaging ultrasound beam.
[b] Related to tissue heating.
[c] Related to nonlinear effects.

2. Haney MJ, O'Brien WD. Temperature dependency of ultrasonic propagation properties in biological materials. In: Greenleaf JF, ed. *Tissue characterization with ultrasound.* Boca Raton: CRC Press; 1986.

3. Hykes DL, Hedrick WR, Starchman DE. *Ultrasound physics and instrumentation.* 2nd Ed. Chicago: Mosby Year Book; 1992.

4. Kremkau FW. *Diagnostic ultrasound: Principles, instruments and exercises.* 3rd Ed. Philadelphia: WB Saunders; 1989.

5. McDicken WN. *Diagnostic ultrasonics: Principles and use of instruments.* 3rd Ed. New York: Churchill-Livingstone; 1991.

6. National Council on Radiation Protection and Measurements. Biological effects of ultrasound: Mechanisms and clinical complications, NCRP REPORT No. 74, 1983.

Doppler Ultrasound in Obstetrics and Gynecology,
edited by Joshua A. Copel and Kathryn L. Reed.
Raven Press, Ltd., New York © 1995.

CHAPTER 4

Ectopic Pregnancy

John S. Pellerito and Kenneth J. W. Taylor

Suspected ectopic pregnancy is one of the most common indications for pelvic sonography in the first trimester. Although recent improvements in technology allow earlier diagnosis, ectopic pregnancy remains an important clinical problem. The incidence of ectopic pregnancy continues to rise due to pelvic inflammatory disease, newer microsurgical techniques such as gamete intrafallopian transfer (GIFT), and an increase in the use of fertility drugs. There are approximately 75,000 cases of ectopic pregnancy per year in the United States (1). The risk of maternal death is approximately ten times greater than that due to natural childbirth (2,3).

Ectopic pregnancy represents approximately 1.4% of all reported pregnancies (1). Such pregnancies most commonly arise in the Fallopian tube, usually the ampullary portion. Tubal pregnancies account for approximately 98% of all ectopic pregnancies (4). Less common locations for ectopic pregnancy are in the abdomen, uterine cornua, cervix, and within the ovary. It is important to note that intraovarian ectopic pregnancies account for less than 1% of all ectopics (4,5). Hepatic, splenic, and vaginal ectopic pregnancies have been reported but are exceedingly rare occurrences (6).

Pelvic inflammatory disease and endometriosis are considered significant risk factors for occurrence of ectopic pregnancy. This is probably related to mechanical obstruction of the Fallopian tube. An increase in ectopic pregnancy is also seen following tubal surgery or prior ectopic pregnancy for similar reasons. There is also an increased incidence of ectopic pregnancy associated with an intrauterine device in place (Fig. 1).

There is an increased incidence of ectopic pregnancy in infertile patients. *In vitro* fertilization and embryo transfer are recognized as risk factors for ectopic preg-

nancy. This may be related to tubal obstruction or decreased tubal motility. Salpingitis isthmica nodosa is found in 57% of surgically removed tubal pregnancies (7). Besides tubal disease, ovulation induction with gonadotropins is associated with 3% incidence of ectopic pregnancy (8,9). This may be related to changes in tubal transport, which decreases the chance for normal implantation. The increase in the number of embryos also increases the risk for extrauterine gestation.

The classic presentation for a patient with ectopic pregnancy includes pelvic pain, an adnexal mass, and vaginal bleeding. Unfortunately, this triad of findings is found in less than 50% of patients (8,10,11). Since these signs, when present, are nonspecific, endovaginal sonography is indicated. A positive pregnancy test will increase suspicion for ectopic pregnancy. The differential diagnosis will include a threatened abortion and gestational trophoblastic neoplasia.

Since endovaginal sonography can diagnose both intrauterine and ectopic pregnancies earlier than transabdominal sonography, prompt examination should be performed to avoid life-threatening hemorrhage from tubal rupture. Culdocentesis, once considered the most useful test for the diagnosis of ectopic pregnancy, should not be considered the first-line diagnostic examination, as a negative culdocentesis does not exclude ectopic pregnancy. Uterine curettage and laparoscopy are useful, but invasive tests, which should be delayed pending the sonographic results.

The quantitative level of the serum β subunit of human chorionic gonadotropin (hCG) is an indispensable aid in the diagnosis of ectopic pregnancy. The serum hCG titer is a very sensitive and specific indicator of pregnancy. A negative serum hCG virtually excludes the possibility of pregnancy. Quantitative serum hCG assays allow accurate determination of gestational age in normal intrauterine pregnancies.

Bree et al. (12) described serum hCG discriminatory

J. S. Pellerito, and K. J. W. Taylor: Department of Diagnostic Imaging, Division of Ultrasound, Yale University School of Medicine, 333 Cedar Street, New Haven, CT 06510.

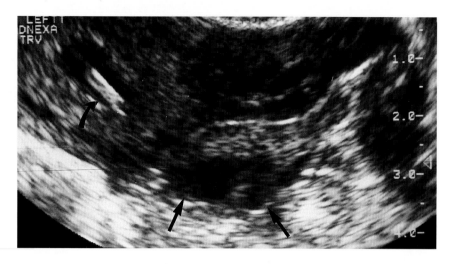

FIG. 1. Ectopic pregnancy with IUD. A well-circumscribed complex mass (*straight arrows*) is seen in the cul-de-sac on the sagittal image. In addition to this ectopic pregnancy, an IUD (*curved arrow*) is seen in the uterus.

levels for the diagnosis of normal early pregnancy with endovaginal ultrasound. They showed that a serum hCG titer greater than 1000 mIU/ml (FIRP) is usually associated with a visible intrauterine gestational sac on endovaginal ultrasound. When the serum hCG level was greater than 7200 mIU/ml, a yolk sac was usually seen. An embryo with a fetal heartbeat was reliably identified when the serum hCG titer was greater than 10,800 mIU/ml. Thus, discrepancy between the serum hCG titer and endovaginal sonogram increases the suspicion for an abnormal pregnancy. It is well known that ectopic pregnancies produce lower levels of hCG than normal pregnancies. Thus, serial serum hCG measurements are extremely valuable in the assessment of ectopic pregnancy when an extrauterine embryo is not readily found. A slowly rising hCG titer or a plateaued level demands repeat ultrasound evaluation to search for an occult ectopic pregnancy. In practice, many of our patients who prove to have an ectopic pregnancy present without symptoms, but with suboptimal hCG increases. In combination, pelvic sonography and hCG assays increase the accuracy for the diagnosis of ectopic pregnancy. Although the serum hCG titers are not always available at the time of sonographic evaluation, endovaginal sonography can provide a specific diagnosis of ectopic pregnancy.

Since its introduction several years ago, endovaginal sonography has had a profound impact on the evaluation of early pregnancy and in particular the diagnosis of ectopic pregnancy. This is due to its ability to define the features of both intra- and extrauterine gestations at an earlier stage. The improved resolution is related to several factors. High-frequency transducers in the 5- to 7.5-MHz range are employed in the endovaginal probe. The probe is placed in the vaginal vault, closer to adnexal structures. In addition, there is avoidance of subcutaneous fat that produces scatter and attenuation of the ultrasound beam. As opposed to transabdominal sonography, the patient is scanned with an empty bladder. A full blad-

der can displace and compress pelvic structures. The patient is also more comfortable with an empty bladder, which allows a more relaxed examination.

Although almost completely replaced by endovaginal sonography as the initial examination, the transabdominal scan remains potentially important in the evaluation of ectopic pregnancy. Transabdominal sonography should be performed in cases when a strong clinical suspicion of ectopic pregnancy exists and findings are inconclusive on endovaginal sonography. The absence of an intrauterine pregnancy with free pelvic fluid in a pregnant patient is strongly suggestive of an occult ectopic pregnancy. Transabdominal sonography may reveal an ectopic pregnancy that is beyond the 8-cm field of view of most endovaginal transducers (Fig. 2).

In addition, transabdominal sonography may identify a normal intrauterine pregnancy in patients presenting with a full bladder. The presence of an intrauterine pregnancy and normal adnexae on transabdominal sonography renders endovaginal sonography unnecessary. Transabdominal sonography is also useful for cases in which large pelvic masses may distort normal anatomy causing confusion on endovaginal sonography. A transabdominal sonogram may assist in the orientation of normal and abnormal structures, facilitating interpretation of the endovaginal scan.

In preparation for the endovaginal scan, the patient should be placed on a lithotomy table in Trendelenburg position. If a dedicated table is not available, the scan can be performed on a standard bed with the patient's knees bent and feet flat on the table top. Pillows or towels should be placed under the buttocks to promote ease of probe angulation.

The patient should empty the bladder just prior to the endovaginal scan. Explanation of the procedure should be given to every patient. This is particularly important for the patient who has not undergone a prior endovaginal scan. Reassurance that the exam should not be painful and lasts approximately 20 min should also be given.

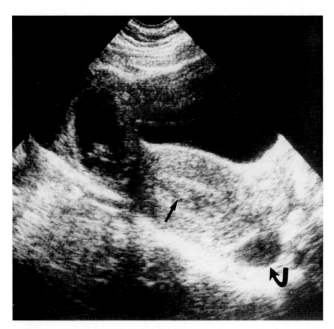

FIG. 2. A large ectopic pregnancy is identified superior to the uterus on this sagittal transabdominal scan that was not visualized on the endovaginal scan. Also note the pseudogestational sac in the endometrial canal (*straight arrow*) and the free fluid in the cul-de-sac (*curved arrow*).

Ultrasound gel should be placed directly on the face of the transducer, which is then covered with a condom. The condom should be secured with an elastic band. Coupling gel is also applied to the condom except in the evaluation of patients undergoing fertility workups as gel can retard sperm motility. The probe can be inserted by the patient or the physician.

Disinfection of the endovaginal probe should be performed after every examination. Most manufacturers recommend at least 20 min in a commercial disinfectant such as Cidex. Prolonged immersion in the disinfectant is discouraged, as damage to the transducer may occur. The transducer should be rinsed with tap water prior to examination.

Upon insertion of the probe, the transducer should be aligned in a transverse projection to identify the uterine body. Once the uterus is found, the transducer should be realigned to view the uterus and, in particular, the endometrial canal in the sagittal plane. The endometrial canal can then be assessed in its entirety for the presence or absence of an intrauterine pregnancy. Color Doppler examination of the intrauterine contents can also be performed at this time.

The uterus may assume a markedly retroverted or anteverted configuration when the bladder is empty. It may be necessary to angle the transducer anteriorally or posteriorly to visualize the uterus. It is important to examine the cul-de-sac for fluid or mass.

The main uterine arteries are best visualized at the level of the lower uterine segment. Small arcuate branches can be seen coursing from the uterine arteries into the myometrium (Fig. 3A). In the nongravid state, a high-impedance flow pattern will be seen during pulsed Doppler examination (Fig. 3B). This is also seen during the first trimester of pregnancy. During the second and third trimesters, the high-impedance uterine waveform changes to low-impedance flow. This is due to the destruction of the elastic lamina of the maternal spiral arteries that occurs as a result of a secondary trophoblastic invasion.

Following examination of the uterus, the transducer is angled laterally to view the adnexa. The ovary is identified as an almond-shaped structure with peripheral follicles. If not immediately found, the internal iliac vessels

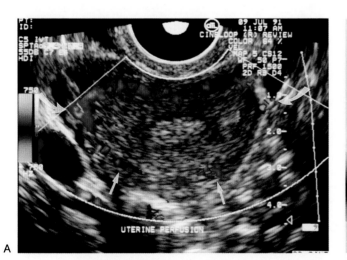

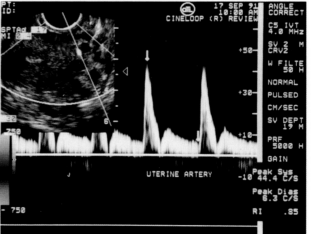

FIG. 3. Nongravid uterus. **A:** Note the uterine arteries (*curved arrows*) at the level of the lower uterine segment. Small arcuate branches (*straight arrows*) are seen within the myometrium. **B:** Pulsed Doppler examination demonstrates a high-impedance waveform with a diastolic notch, which is characteristic of the uterine artery.

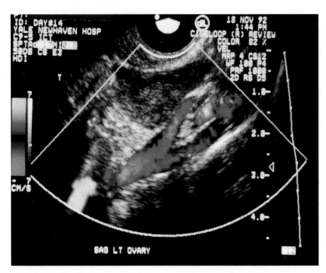

FIG. 4. Normal ovary. Note the peripheral follicles and location of the ovary adjacent to the iliac vessels.

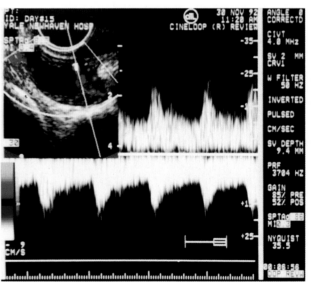

FIG. 5. Resting ovary. A low-velocity, high-impedance waveform is identified from the resting ovary.

should be located. The ovaries typically lie adjacent to the iliac artery and vein (Fig. 4). The ovaries receive a dual blood supply. The ovarian artery, a branch of the abdominal aorta, may be seen entering the ovary. The uterine artery also sends branches to supply the ovary via the Fallopian tube. Doppler interrogation of the ovary shows a high-impedance pattern in the resting state (Fig. 5). During the formation of the corpus luteum, a low-impedance waveform is seen. This is identified on color flow examination as a region of persistent or continuous "glowing" color (Fig. 6). This pattern is seen around day 8 of the menstrual cycle and continues through day 21. A cyst may or may not be present.

Luteal flow is usually confined to one ovary. If the ovaries have been stimulated with fertility drugs such as Clomid or Pergonal, bilateral corpora lutea may be present. Luteal flow can usually be easily demonstrated through the first trimester of pregnancy. This is important to bear in mind during the evaluation for ectopic pregnancy since placental flow may have a similar Doppler appearance. Ectopic placental flow is almost always found separate from the ovary.

Taylor et al. (13) previously described placental flow as a relatively high-velocity, low-impedance signal localized to the site of placentation by duplex Doppler examination. This has been detected in pregnancies within the

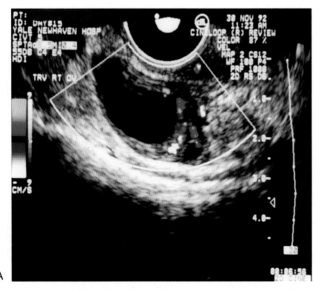

A

B

FIG. 6. Corpus luteum. **A:** Endovaginal color flow imaging demonstrates an area of increased vascularity at the site of the corpus luteum. **B:** A high-velocity, low-impedance waveform is obtained from the luteal cyst.

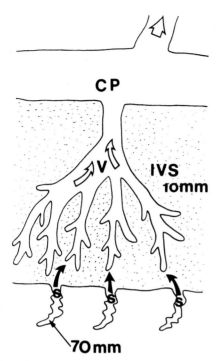

FIG. 7. Invasion of the myometrium by the developing trophoblast allows shunting of blood from the maternal spiral arteries (S) into the intervillous space (IVS) and chorionic villi (V) across a pressure gradient of approximately 60 mm Hg. CP, chorionic plate. From Taylor et al. (13).

the intervillous space accounts for the observed low-impedance waveform.

Endovaginal color flow imaging depicts this signal as an area of increased vascularity around the periphery of the gestational sac (Fig. 8). This flow pattern is difficult to distinguish from luteal flow, as the waveform characteristics are similar. This distinction can be made by the identification of specific ovarian morphology.

In their study, Taylor et al. (13) defined a cutoff value of 2.1 KHz for extrauterine placental flow utilizing a transabdominal approach. Utilizing the endovaginal technique, we have since identified lower systolic velocities and frequencies in early or involuting ectopic pregnancies. These velocities overlap considerably with those obtained from the corpus luteum. Thus, precise cutoff values for peak systolic velocity or resistive index are not desirable to define placental flow. The presence of low-impedance flow, separate from the ovary, is sufficient for the recognition of placental flow.

The definitive diagnosis of ectopic pregnancy relies on the observation of an extrauterine embryo or fetal cardiac pulsations (Fig. 9). In a recent study of 155 patients, this observation was made in 14% of cases (14). In the absence of this observation, we rely on a combination of direct and indirect findings. The uterus, adnexa and cul-de-sac are examined for evidence of ectopic pregnancy.

The uterus should be evaluated first for evidence of an intrauterine gestation. If a normal intrauterine pregnancy is found, the likelihood of an ectopic pregnancy is low, unless the patient is at risk for a heterotopic pregnancy. In the general population, simultaneous intra- and extrauterine gestations occurs in one of 30,000 spontaneous pregnancies (15) (Fig. 10). The risk factors for heterotopic pregnancy include ovulation induction with

uterus or in the adnexa. Taylor theorized that placental flow is related to invasion of maternal tissues by trophoblastic villi. As the developing trophoblast invades the myometrium, the spiral arteries shunt blood to the intervillous space across a pressure gradient of approximately 60 mm Hg (Fig. 7). The low resistance to blood flow into

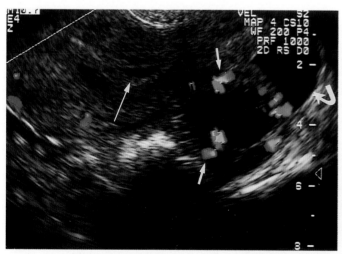
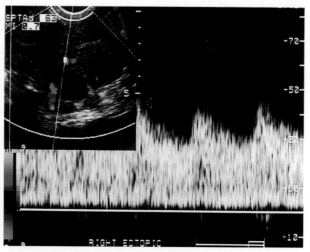

FIG. 8. Placental flow. **A:** Areas of increased vascularity (*small arrows*) are identified around the ectopic gestational sac. Note the pseudogestational sac (*large arrow*) and free fluid in the cul-de-sac (*curved arrow*). **B:** Doppler interrogation of the ectopic pregnancy demonstrates a high-velocity, low-impedance waveform characteristic of placental flow.

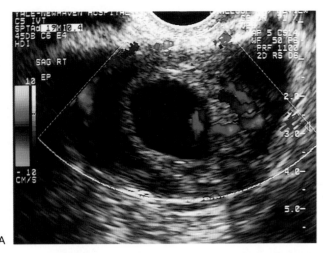

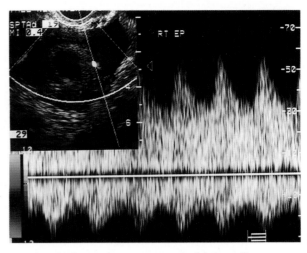

FIG. 9. Live ectopic pregnancy. **A:** Color flow within the developing embryo represents fetal cardiac activity. Increased vascularity is also identified within the gestational sac and early umbilical cord. **B:** Pulsed Doppler interrogation of the sac demonstrates high-velocity, low-impedance blood flow characteristic of placental flow.

Pergonal or Clomid and prior tubal surgery. The frequency in this group may be as high as one of 6000 (16–22).

If the uterus is empty, the adnexa should be carefully evaluated for evidence of ectopic pregnancy. Other possibilities include an early intrauterine pregnancy or complete abortion. Correlation with menstrual data and serial serum hCG titers is helpful in distinguishing among these possibilities.

Thickening of the endometrial canal may be seen due to decidual reaction in the presence of an ectopic pregnancy. In addition, an irregular sac-like structure may be identified in the endometrial canal. This is termed a pseudogestational sac and should be readily distinguishable from a normal intrauterine pregnancy (Fig. 11). Un-

like a normal gestational sac, the pseudosac does not demonstrate a double decidual lining. The pseudosac may demonstrate a crenated appearance without a yolk sac or fetal pole. Serial hCG titers are helpful in distinguishing a pseudosac from an intrauterine pregnancy. A subnormal rise or plateau in the serum hCG levels suggests a diagnosis of ectopic pregnancy.

Duplex and color Doppler examination of the uterus may distinguish the pseudosac from an abnormal intrauterine pregnancy. The identification of placental flow within the sac confirms the presence of an intrauterine pregnancy. Placental flow is never associated with a pseudogestational sac (Fig. 12). Dillon et al. (23) showed that placental flow can be seen in an intrauterine pregnancy approximately 36 days following the last men-

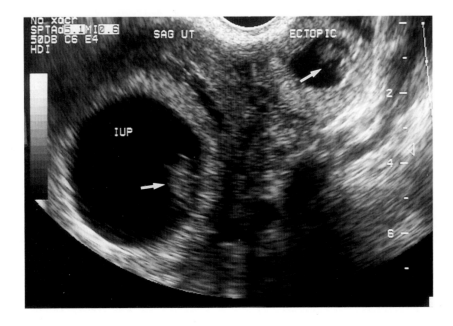

FIG. 10. Heterotopic pregnancy. Intrauterine and extrauterine gestational sacs are identified. Both sacs contain embryos (*arrows*). Courtesy of Maria Straub, MD, Yale University School of Medicine.

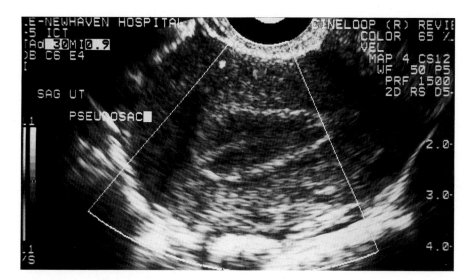

FIG. 11. Pseudogestational sac. A well-defined sac-like structure is identified within the endometrial canal on the sagittal view. Distinction between an abnormal intrauterine pregnancy and a pseudosac associated with an ectopic pregnancy is difficult from grey scale imaging alone.

strual period. A velocity cutoff value of 21 cm/sec was proposed to distinguish an intrauterine pregnancy from a pseudogestational sac associated with ectopic pregnancy. A sensitivity of 84% for the detection of intrauterine pregnancy was achieved utilizing this criterion. The presence of an abnormal sac-like structure in the uterus without evidence of a yolk sac, fetal pole, or placental flow should increase the suspicion for ectopic pregnancy.

Free pelvic fluid is a common finding associated with ectopic pregnancy. Utilizing endovaginal sonography, several studies have shown a range of 40–83% for the presence of free intraperitoneal fluid (24–28). Small amounts of fluid may be seen with a normal intrauterine pregnancy and may be related to leakage from a corpus luteum cyst. Moderate to large amounts of fluid should raise suspicion for ectopic pregnancy in the correct clinical setting (Fig. 13). The absence of fluid, however, does not exclude the possibility of ectopic pregnancy.

Several studies have shown that the presence of echogenic pelvic fluid correlates strongly with ectopic pregnancy (24,29). Echogenic fluid, which represents hemoperitoneum, may result from tubal rupture or leakage of blood from the fimbriated end of the Fallopian tube (Fig. 14). Nyberg et al. (30) showed that echogenic fluid was associated with a high risk (93% positive predictive value) for ectopic pregnancy. Moreover, they found that echogenic fluid was the only finding in 15% of patients with ectopic pregnancy. There is great variability in the detection of echogenic fluid in patients with ectopic pregnancy, ranging from 11% to 56% in recent studies (14,24,29,30).

Apart from free fluid, the adnexa should be examined for the presence of abnormal mass. The ovaries should be identified first for the presence of the corpus luteum. Pellerito et al. (14) found that an ectopic pregnancy was seen on the same side as the corpus luteum in 86% of

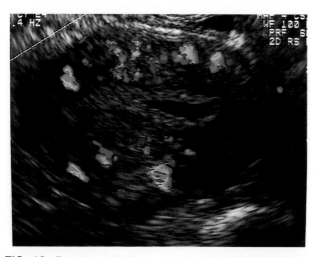

FIG. 12. Doppler color flow examination demonstrates an absence of vascularity around the pseudogestational sac. Note normal vascularity in the surrounding myometrium.

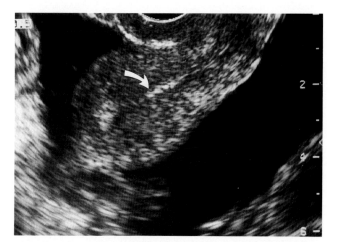

FIG. 13. Free fluid. A large amount of free fluid is seen in this pregnant patient with concomitant ectopic pregnancy. Note the normal endometrial canal echo (*curved arrow*) and the absence of an intrauterine pregnancy.

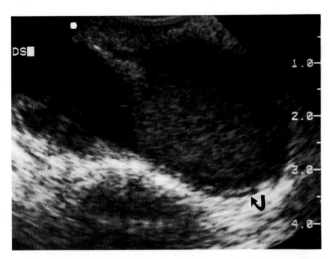

FIG. 14. Echogenic fluid. A collection of echogenic fluid (*curved arrow*) is seen in this patient with known ruptured ectopic pregnancy.

cases. This follows as the fertilized egg is usually derived from the ipsilateral ovary.

Extrauterine sac-like masses comprise the most common sonographic appearance for ectopic pregnancy (Fig. 15). This finding has been found in 46–71% of cases and has a high predictive value for the diagnosis of ectopic pregnancy (24,26,29,31–37). These masses usually demonstrate a thick echogenic ring and occasionally contain a yolk sac or fetal pole. The mass should have a definite plane of separation from the ovary in order to distinguish it confidently from a luteal cyst. If the mass cannot be separated from the ovary, reliance on other findings such as an empty uterus, free fluid, hCG titers, and, if necessary, follow-up endovaginal scanning is required to increase diagnostic confidence.

Solid or complex adnexal masses are also associated with a high risk of ectopic pregnancy in conjunction with an empty uterus and a positive serum hCG titer (38–40). These masses probably represent hemorrhage into the ectopic gestational sac or a ruptured ectopic pregnancy confined within the tube (Fig. 16). Less commonly, they may result from free intraperitoneal hematoma.

Endovaginal color flow imaging aids in the differentiation of ectopic pregnancy from other complex adnexal masses. As discussed earlier, detection of placental flow in a mass separate from the ovary is sufficient for a diagnosis of ectopic pregnancy. In a recent study evaluating endovaginal color flow imaging, Pellerito et al. (14) demonstrated a sensitivity of 95% and a specificity of 98% for the diagnosis of ectopic pregnancy. Placental flow was identified in 55 (85%) of 65 ectopic pregnancies.

All avascular ectopic pregnancies in this study demonstrated serum hCG titers of 6000 mIU/ml (FIRP) or less. This was also described by Myers et al. (41) who found no detectable Doppler flow in ectopic pregnancies with serum hCG levels of less than 5362 mIU/ml. This is con-

sistent with early or nonviable ectopic pregnancies. Thus, the absence of placental flow does not exclude an ectopic pregnancy.

Ectopic pregnancies may be identified on the basis of placental flow alone even in the absence of a well-defined mass (14). Ectopic pregnancies in the uterine cornua and cul-de-sac have been identified with endovaginal color flow imaging that were not seen on endovaginal sonography alone. The detection of low-impedance arterial flow in the adnexa, even in the absence of a well-defined mass, should suggest placental flow (Fig. 17).

In addition to aiding in the detection of ectopic pregnancy, endovaginal color flow imaging also allows a specific diagnosis of spontaneous or incomplete abortion. In the absence of a normal intrauterine pregnancy and adnexal mass, the determination of an intra- or extrauterine gestation can be extremely difficult. By detecting intrauterine placental flow, a confident diagnosis of a failed intrauterine pregnancy can be made regardless of the appearance of the adnexa (23) (Fig. 18). Since luteal cysts often appear complex and may simulate ectopic pregnancies, the determination of intrauterine placental flow can explain bleeding in a pregnant patient and defer unnecessary laparoscopic surgery.

Conversely pulsed Doppler examination of an irregular intrauterine sac can distinguish between an abnormal intrauterine pregnancy and a pseudogestational sac. The absence of placental flow adjacent to an intrauterine sac increases the likelihood of a pseudogestational sac. This should increase the suspicion for an ectopic pregnancy and direct a thorough examination of the adnexa.

Endovaginal color flow imaging should not be considered as a substitute for grey scale endovaginal scanning in the diagnosis of ectopic pregnancy. It is a complementary tool that provides physiologic as well as anatomic information. The combination of morphologic and color flow information in the characterization of adnexal masses should result in higher diagnostic accuracy. In the

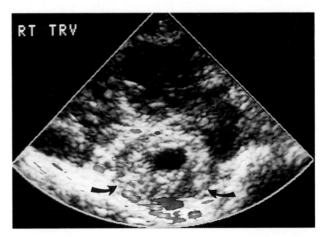

FIG. 15. Extrauterine gestational sac. Note the ring-shaped ectopic pregnancy with peripheral vascularity (*curved arrow*).

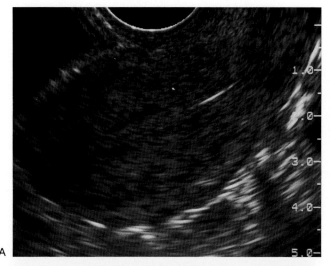

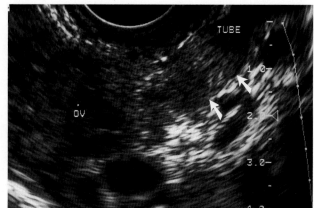

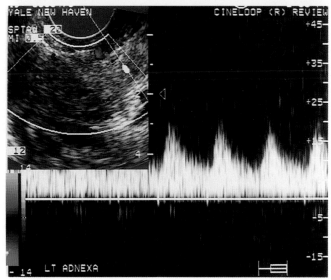

FIG. 16. Solid ectopic pregnancy. This patient presented with left adnexal pain and bleeding. **A:** Sagittal view of the uterus demonstrates a normal endometrial canal echo with no evidence of intrauterine pregnancy. **B:** Examination of the left adnexa demonstrates a linear, solid mass inferior to the ovary compatible with a hematosalpinx (*curved arrow*). **C:** Doppler interrogation of the solid mass demonstrates a low-impedance waveform compatible with placental flow.

setting of suspected ectopic pregnancy, endovaginal color flow imaging can be used to confirm the presence of an intrauterine pregnancy, define a pseudogestational sac, identify placental flow in an adnexal mass, and visualize ectopic flow in the absence of mass.

Several entities may masquerade as an ectopic pregnancy on endovaginal color flow imaging. A luteal cyst and cystic ovarian malignancy may appear as adnexal sac-like masses with low-impedance flow. Their origin from the ovary make them much less likely to represent an ectopic pregnancy since only 1% or fewer ectopics are intraovarian.

Pelvic inflammatory disease represents another potential source of error. Low-impedance blood flow may be detected from a tuboovarian abscess. The clinical history and negative serum hCG titer should distinguish this entity from an ectopic pregnancy.

Pedunculated uterine fibroids have also demonstrated high-velocity, low-impedance vascularity. Their connec-

tion to the uterus and presence on prior scans can aid in their diagnosis. Other vascular pelvic masses, including tumors, may rarely mimic ectopic pregnancy.

Although it has generally been accepted that obstetric ultrasound is safe, several recent changes in the practice of diagnostic ultrasound suggest that continued caution is prudent (42). First, there is the development of endovaginal ultrasound in which improved imaging is obtained by the use of higher frequencies and closer proximity to the target. The use of higher frequencies would decrease the chance of cavitation but increases the heating in the exposed tissues. Second, there has been an increase in the intensity that is employed in ultrasound imaging, partly due to focusing but also in a deliberate attempt to increase signal-to-noise ratio and hence improve image quality. At one stage, the U.S. Food and Drug Administration limited output for obstetric use to the spatial peak temporal average (SPTA) intensities utilized "preenactment" in 1976 (43). The output intensity

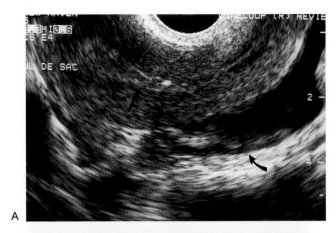

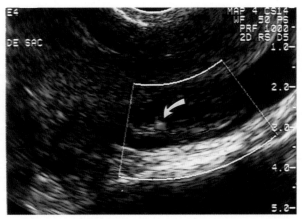

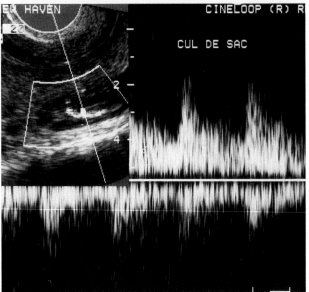

FIG. 17. A: Color flow diagnosis of ectopic pregnancy. This patient presented with pelvic pain and a positive pregnancy test. The sagittal grey scale image demonstrates an ill-defined mass in the cul-de-sac with surrounding fluid (*curved arrow*). This finding was thought to represent hematoma. A normal endometrial canal echo (*straight arrow*) is seen without evidence of intrauterine pregnancy. **B:** Doppler color flow imaging demonstrates increased vascularity within the cul-de-sac mass (*curved arrow*). This finding established the location of the ectopic pregnancy. **C:** Pulsed Doppler examination confirms this diagnosis through demonstration of placental flow. Reprinted with permission from Pellerito, JS and Taylor KJW. Ectopic Pregnancy: evaluation with endovaginal color doppler flow imaging-response. *Radiology,* April 1993; 187:21–22 (Figure 1).

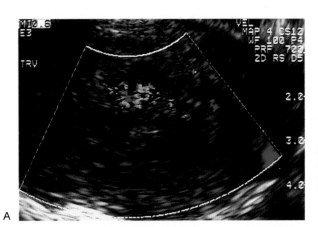

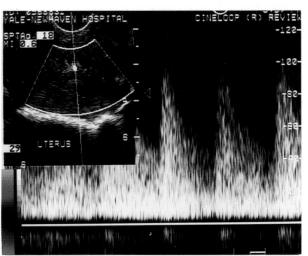

FIG. 18. Incomplete abortion. **A:** Color flow Doppler imaging demonstrates vascularity within a thickened endometrial canal in this pregnant patient with vaginal bleeding. **B:** Pulsed Doppler interrogation demonstrates high-velocity, low-impedance placental flow, which confirms the diagnosis of incomplete abortion.

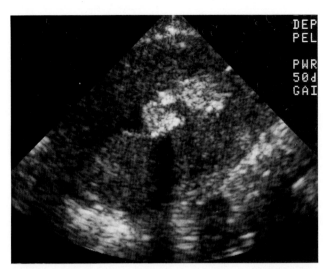

FIG. 19. Retained products of conception. Sagittal grey scale image demonstrates irregular, echogenic debris and fluid within the endometrial canal following therapeutic abortion.

varies greatly between different machines, different transducers, and different modes of usage. High peak intensities occur particularly with the use of pulsed Doppler when intensities (SPTA) in the range of 1 W/cm^2 are available. Third, there is an increase in the use of ultrasound around the time of conception and during the period of organogenesis. Prior to the development of artificial techniques for achieving fertilization, ultrasound examination before 6 weeks gestation was generally not required and usually the first examination was obtained during the second trimester after the completion of organogenesis. In contrast, women now have endovaginal ultrasound on numerous occasions to monitor the devel-

opment of follicles and may have several further examinations to document the earliest evidence of successful conception and implantation.

These points should be kept in mind by the prudent physician and the potential risks carefully weighed against the benefits of diagnostic ultrasound. General early obstetric ultrasound should only be performed for established indications such as locating the site of gestation and measuring maturity and viability. In particular, we do not use pulsed Doppler unless indicated. In a patient with a suspected ectopic pregnancy and in the presence of an abnormal sac within the uterus, Doppler is entirely justified to confirm the presence of placental flow to differentiate between a pseudosac and an abnormal intrauterine gestation. The use of pulsed Doppler, however, would not be justified merely to demonstrate a normal fetal heart, which can be documented equally well by the use of an M-mode at low insonating intensity. It should be appreciated that the use of color involves similar output intensities to grey scale ultrasound. However, color can be very misleading unless it is supplemented by the quantitative aspects only available through pulsed Doppler and it is the use of pulsed Doppler that must be minimized to avoid unnecessary fetal exposure.

Duplex and color flow Doppler studies are also utilized to diagnose retained products of conception. Sonographic findings associated with retained products of conception include an irregular gestational sac or endometrial thickening, and fluid and debris in the endometrial canal (44,45) (Fig. 19). Endovaginal color flow imaging may aid in the diagnosis of retained products of conception by identifying residual placental tissue with its characteristic flow pattern (Fig. 20). Placental flow may be identified in the endometrial canal even in the

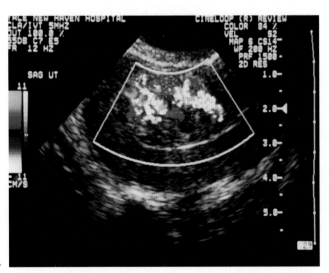

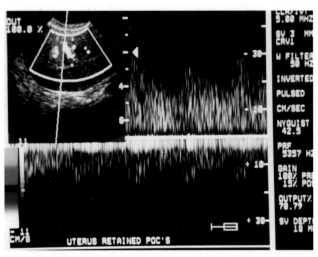

A   B

FIG. 20. Retained products of conception. **A:** Color flow Doppler imaging demonstrates marked vascularity associated with a thickened endometrial canal. **B:** Placental flow is identified confirming the diagnosis of retained products of conception.

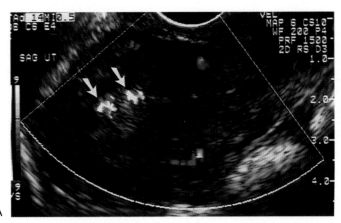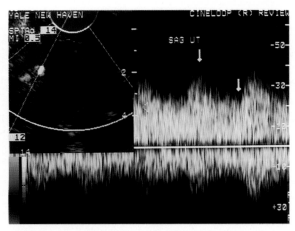

A B

FIG. 21. Retained products of conception. Endovaginal color flow Doppler examination was performed in this patient with persistently elevated β-hCG titer (5000 mIU/ml) and left lower quadrant pain two weeks following therapeutic abortion. **A:** Focal areas of increased vascularity are identified within the endometrium (*arrows*). **B:** Low-impedance placental flow at this site confirms the location of the retained products.

absence of appreciable mass or tissue (Fig. 21). Utilizing a velocity cutoff of 21 cm/sec, Dillon et al. (23) demonstrated a sensitivity of 84% and a specificity of 100% for the detection of intrauterine pregnancy. Endovaginal color flow imaging can differentiate retained products of conception from residual blood clot or complete abortion.

In conclusion, endovaginal sonography allows earlier diagnosis of ectopic pregnancy compared to transabdominal imaging. The addition of color Doppler flow imaging enables increased sensitivity in the detection of ectopic pregnancy. Endovaginal color flow imaging can be utilized to diagnose normal and abnormal intrauterine pregnancies, determine the location of ectopic pregnancies, and distinguish pseudogestational sacs from intrauterine gestations.

REFERENCES

1. Centers for Disease Control. Ectopic pregnancy: United States, 1986. *MMWR* 1989;38:481–484.
2. Filly RA. Ectopic pregnancy: The role of sonography. *Radiology* 1987;162:661–668.
3. Atrash HK, MacKay T, Binkin NJ, Hogue CJR. Legal abortion in the United States: 1972 to 1982. *Am J Obstet Gynecol* 1987;156:605–612.
4. Chow TT, Lindahl S. Ectopic pregnancy. *J Clin Ultrasound* 1979;7:217–218.
5. Breen JL. A 21-year survey of 654 ectopic pregnancies. *Am J Obstet Gynecol* 1970;106:1004–1019.
6. Peterson HB. Extratubal ectopic pregnancies, diagnosis and treatment. *J Reprod Med* 1986;31:108–115.
7. Majmudar B, Henderson PH, Semple E. Salpingitis isthmica nodosa: A high-risk factor for tubal pregnancy. *Obstet Gynecol* 1983;62:73–78.
8. Stabile I, Grudzinskas JG. Ectopic pregnancy: A review of incidence, etiology, and diagnostic aspects. *Obstet Gynecol Surv* 1990;45:335–347.
9. Steptoe PC, Edwards RG. Reimplantation of human embryo with subsequent tubal pregnancy. *Lancet* 1976;1:880.
10. Weckstein LN. Clinical diagnosis of ectopic pregnancy. *Clin Obstet Gynecol* 1987;30:236–244.
11. Halpin TF. Ectopic pregnancy: The problem of diagnosis. *Am J Obstet Gynecol* 1970;106:227–236.
12. Bree RL, Edwards M, Bohm-Velez M, Beyler S, Roberts J, Mendelson EB. Transvaginal sonography in the evaluation of normal early pregnancy: Correlation with hCG level. *AJR* 1989;153:75–79.
13. Taylor KJW, Ramos IM, Feyock AL, et al. Ectopic pregnancy: Duplex Doppler evaluation. *Radiology* 1989;173:93–97.
14. Pellerito JS, Taylor KJW, Quedens-Case C, et al. Ectopic pregnancy: Evaluation with endovaginal color flow imaging. *Radiology* 1992;183:407–411.
15. DeVoe RW, Pratt JH. Simultaneous intrauterine and extrauterine pregnancy. *Am J Obstet Gynecol* 1948;56:1119–1126.
16. Simpson EL, Coleman BG, Sondheimer SJ, Arger PH, Mintz MC. *In vitro* fertilization and embryo transfer complicated by simultaneous ectopic and intrauterine twin gestation. *J Ultrasound Med* 1986;5:49–51.
17. Dimitry ES, Subak-Sharpe R, Mills M, Margara R, Winston R. Nine cases of heterotopic pregnancies in 4 years of *in vitro* fertilization. *Fertil Steril* 1990;53:107–110.
18. Richards SR, Stempel LE, Carlton BD. Heterotopic pregnancy: Reappraisal of incidence. *Am J Obstet Gynecol* 1982;142:928.
19. Gamberdella FR, Marrs RP. Heterotopic pregnancy associated with assisted reproductive technology. *Am J Obstet Gynecol* 1989;160:1520–1524.
20. Kivikoski AI. Combined pregnancy: How common is it? *Int J Gynaecol Obstet* 1989;30:271–277.
21. Hann LE, Bachman DB, McArdle CR. Co-existent intrauterine and ectopic pregnancy: A reevaluation. *Radiology* 1984;152:151–154.
22. Bello GV, Schonholz D, Moshirpur J, Jeng D-Y, Berkowitz RL. Combined pregnancy: The Mount Sinai experience. *Obstet Gynecol Surv* 1986;41:603–613.
23. Dillon EH, Feyock AL, Taylor KJW. Pseudogestational sacs: Doppler US differentiation from normal or abnormal intrauterine pregnancies. *Radiology* 1990;176:359–364.
24. Fleischer AC, Pennell RG, McKee MS, et al. Ectopic pregnancy: Features at transvaginal sonography. *Radiology* 1990;174:375–378.
25. Romero R, Copel JA, Kadar N, et al. Value of culdocentesis in the diagnosis of ectopic pregnancy. *Obstet Gynecol* 1985;65:519–522.
26. Stiller RJ, de Regt RH, Blair E. Transvaginal ultrasonography in patients at risk for ectopic pregnancy. *Am J Obstet Gynecol* 1989;161:930–933.
27. Coleman BG, Baron RL, Arger PH, et al. Ectopic embryo detec-

tion using real-time sonography. *J Clin Ultrasound* 1985; 13:545–554.

28. Kivikoski AI, Martin CM, Smeltzer JS. Transabdominal and transvaginal ultrasonography in the diagnosis of ectopic pregnancy: a comparative study. *Am J Obstet Gynecol* 1990; 163:123–128.

29. Cacciatore B. Can the status of tubal pregnancy be predicted with transvaginal sonography? A prospective comparison of sonographic, surgical, and serum hCG findings. *Radiology* 1990; 177:481–484.

30. Nyberg DA, Hughes M, Mack LA, Wang K. Extrauterine findings of ectopic pregnancy at transvaginal US: Importance of echogenic fluid. *Radiology* 1991; 178:823–826.

31. de Crespigny LC. Demonstration of ectopic pregnancy by transvaginal ultrasound. *Br J Obstet Gynaecol* 1988; 95:1253–1256.

32. Nyberg DA, Mack LA, Jeffrey RB, Laing FC. Endovaginal sonographic evaluation of ectopic pregnancy: A prospective study. *AJR* 1987; 149:1181–1186.

33. Dashefsky SM, Lyons EA, Levi CS, et al. Suspected ectopic pregnancy: Endovaginal and transvesical US. *Radiology* 1988; 169:181–184.

34. Rempen A. Vaginal sonography in ectopic pregnancy: A prospective evaluation. *J Ultrasound Med* 1988; 7:381–387.

35. Cacciatore B, Stenman U-H, Ylostalo P. Comparison of abdominal and vaginal sonography in suspected ectopic pregnancy. *Obstet Gynecol* 1989; 73:770–774.

36. Timor-Tritsch IE, Yeh MN, Peisner DB, Lesser KB, Slavik TA. The use of transvaginal ultrasonography in the diagnosis of ectopic pregnancy. *Am J Obstet Gynecol* 1989; 161:157–161.

37. Bateman BG, Nunley WC, Kolp LA, Kitchin JD III, Felder R. Vaginal sonography findings and hCG dynamics of early intrauterine and tubal pregnancies. *Obstet Gynecol* 1990; 75:421–427.

38. Mahony BS, Filly RA, Nyberg DA, et al. Sonographic evaluation of ectopic pregnancy. *J Ultrasound Med* 1985; 4:221–228.

39. Romero R, Kadar N, Castro D, et al. The value of adnexal sonographic findings in the diagnosis of ectopic pregnancy. *Am J Obstet Gynecol* 1988; 158:52–55.

40. Subramanyam BR, Raghavendra BN, Balthazar EJ, et al. Hematosalpinx in tubal pregnancy: Sonographic-pathologic correlation. *AJR* 1983; 141:361–365.

41. Myers MT. Duplex Doppler and transvaginal sonography for the evaluation of ectopic pregnancy. Thesis, Yale University, 1989.

42. Taylor KJW. A prudent approach to Doppler ultrasound. *Radiology* 1987; 165:283–284.

43. Food and Drug Administration. 510(k) guide for measuring and reporting acoustic output of diagnostic medical devices. Rockville, MD: 1985.

44. Kurtz AB, Shlansky-Goldberg RD, Choi HY, Needleman L, Wapner RJ, Goldberg BB. Detection of retained products of conception following spontaneous abortion in the first trimester. *J Ultrasound Med* 1991; 10:387–395.

45. Hertzberg BS, Bowie JD. Ultrasound of the postpartum uterus: Prediction of retained placental tissue. *J Ultrasound Med* 1991; 10:451–456.

Doppler Ultrasound in Obstetrics and Gynecology,
edited by Joshua A. Copel and Kathryn L. Reed.
Raven Press, Ltd., New York © 1995.

CHAPTER 5

Strategies for Ovarian Cancer Screening

Gordan Crvenkovic, Cindy Smrt, Lawrence D. Platt, and Beth Y. Karlan

EPIDEMIOLOGY OF OVARIAN CANCER

Ovarian cancer remains the leading cause of gynecologic cancer mortality. The highest incidence rates are reported among white females in northwestern Europe and the United States. The mortality for ovarian cancer in these countries is 7.3–13 per 100,000, making ovarian cancer the fifth leading cause of cancer-related death in women. The age-specific incidence rate increases from 2/100,000 for women in their twenties to 55/100,000 for women in their seventies (1).

Although there have been a number of advances in ovarian cancer treatment during the last three decades, the overall survival rate for patients with ovarian cancer has changed little. According to data from the Surveillance, Epidemiology, and End Results (SEER) program, the 5-year survival rate of patients with ovarian cancer has only increased from 36% in 1975 to 39% in 1990 (2). These survival figures are even more disturbing when over 90% of patients with stage I ovarian disease can be cured by a combination of surgery and chemotherapy (3,4).

Consequently, the greatest impact on survival from ovarian cancer can be made by earlier detection and prevention. Early stage ovarian cancer rarely produces symptoms, and screening efforts would necessarily involve apparently healthy, asymptomatic women. The goal would be to detect ovarian tumors before they have metastasized or while they are at potentially curable stages. Routine pelvic examination is imprecise and cannot detect early ovarian cancer with any significant sensitivity or specificity. No reliable test or combination of tests has been available as an effective screening mod-

ality. This is indeed unfortunate since ovarian cancer probably fulfills the conditions for diseases worthy of screening in an at-risk population. (a) It is a major cause of death in the screened population. (b) It has a preclinical phase during which screening could detect the disease while still curable. (c) It has a reasonably high prevalence in the screened population. (d) It is amenable to therapy such that the survival rate of patients with stage I disease is significantly higher than that of patients with advanced disease (5,6). Although unproven, ovarian cancer screening could potentially have a significant impact on disease survival.

Several investigators have shown that selected cases of epithelial ovarian cancer may originate by transformation of benign ovarian tumors (serous cystadenoma, endometriomas, etc.) (7,8). A useful screening test would be inexpensive, easy to administer, and acceptable to patients. Accuracy as determined by sensitivity, specificity, and positive predictive value (PPV) is one of the most important characteristics of an effective screening test (5). To reliably calculate sensitivity and specificity, the screening test must give consistent results when performed by different examiners. Fulfilling these requirements is an important factor when planning a screening strategy for ovarian cancer (9).

The high incidence of ovarian cancer in the industrialized countries has stimulated the hypothesis that environmental agents may be important etiologic factors (10,11). Environmental factors suspected of playing a role in the pathogenesis of ovarian cancer include fat consumption, obesity, and patterns of fat distribution. A strong relationship between a high Quetelet index [defined as weight (kg) divided by height (m) squared] and risk for ovarian cancer has been reported by many authors (12).

However, these findings remain controversial (13,14). Cramer et al. (15) found that women above the highest quartile of animal fat consumption had a twofold increase in risk for ovarian cancer compared with those

G. Crvenkovic, C. Smrt, L. D. Platt, and B. Y. Karlan: Department of Obstetrics and Gynecology, Cedars-Sinai Medical Center, University of California Los Angeles, School of Medicine, Los Angeles, CA 90048.

with the lowest quartile. The mechanism by which animal fat could contribute to the genesis of ovarian cancer might be direct, via carcinogenic contaminants in the fat, or indirect via their contribution to extragenital estrogen production (15). A relationship between alcohol consumption and/or smoking and ovarian cancer has not been found (14,15). Also, at this time there is no conclusive evidence for a causal relationship between caffeine consumption and ovarian cancer.

The role of pregnancy, breastfeeding, and hormonal therapy on the pathogenesis of ovarian cancer has been widely discussed in the literature (16–18). The most consistent finding among case-control studies of ovarian cancer has been a relative deficit of pregnancies among cases. Several case-control studies have found a decrease in risk of the epithelial ovarian cancer associated with pregnancy, breastfeeding, and the use of oral contraceptives (OCs). This prompted the hypothesis of incessant ovulation, which proposes that factors that suppress ovulation may reduce the risk of developing ovarian cancer due to multiple injuries to the surface epithelium of the ovary and the subsequent growth factor–mediated repair mechanism (19,20).

The risk of ovarian cancer seems to continue to decrease with increasing duration of OC use. The protective effect of OCs was even noticed in former users (for at least 15 years following OC discontinuation) (21). The most impressive study was reported by the Centers for Disease Control Cancer and Steroid Hormone Study (22). They estimated that the incidence of ovarian cancer among women between 20 and 54 years of age in the United States might be 30% higher if OCs had not been used. Another interesting finding in the study was that the use of OCs by nulliparous women decreased their relative risk below that for parous women. Most recently, Hankinson et al. concluded that the protective effect of OC against ovarian cancer risk should be considered in a woman's decision to use the pills (21).

Similarly, the risk of ovarian cancer was significantly decreased in women reporting lifelong menstrual irregularities (17). The explanation for these correlations is probably multifactorial, including effects of anovulatory cycles and an altered hormonal milieu (23).

Ovarian cancer has been studied most in connection with mumps virus. It has been suggested that ovarian cancer patients have a decreased incidence of clinical mumps in their history when compared with control subjects (24). The mumps virus has many affinities including the gonads. Mumps orchitis is known to occur in about 20% of affected males. The incidence of similar involvement of the ovaries is lower and is estimated to be 5% (25). The Royal College of General Practitioners and the Association for the Study of Infectious Diseases, however, published an incidence rate of mumps in Great Britain of 6.0 per 1000 and an incidence of mumps oophoritis of only 0.1–0.2% (26). This means that with

an incidence of mumps of 6.0 per 1000 a year, the incidence of oophoritis must be about 1.2 per 100,000. Although some studies provide data suggestive of a relationship between ovarian cancer and exposure to mumps virus, more recent data do not support this.

Although another possible reason for premature oocyte loss and ovarian failure is irradiation of pelvic organs, no increased incidence of ovarian carcinoma has been reported in women who have undergone this therapeutic pelvic radiation (27).

GENETIC CONSIDERATIONS IN OVARIAN CANCER

A positive family history for ovarian cancer is the best risk factor for getting the disease. Many epidemiologic studies support this findings (28–32) as well as many cases and series reports (33–36). The most recent report from the Familial Ovarian Cancer Registry, established in 1981, notes that 435 families (1020 patients) have been accessed and studied (37).

First, there are several features that are noteworthy in this family data. Although there are rare genetic syndromes associated with ovarian neoplasms (38), our focus here is on epithelial ovarian malignancies. While these epithelial familial ovarian carcinoma syndromes make up less than 10% of all ovarian cancers, three distinct pedigree patterns have been described: (a) "site-specific" ovarian cancer, (b) familial ovarian cancer associated with breast cancer in the family; and (c) familial ovarian cancer as part of the cancer family syndrome (or Lynch syndrome II), which is characterized by inherited nonpolyposis colon cancer and/or endometrial cancer in family members (39).

Extended pedigrees have been reported for each of these three familial aggregations. These data strongly suggest that in some families the genetic susceptibility to ovarian cancer is inherited in an autosomal dominant fashion, thereby making the paternal family history equally as significant as the maternal family history with regard to ovarian cancer risk. The diversity in the phenotypic expression and the patterns of inheritance most likely represents the presence of genetic heterogeneity (different inherited gene defects leading the disease). This might be due to locus heterogeneity (the involvement of entirely different genes) or allelic heterogeneity (different mutations at the same locus giving rise to different phenotypes).

Third, the case-control studies demonstrate that of all ovarian cancer patients, there is an increased risk of epithelial ovarian cancer in first-degree relatives as well. An increased family risk is seen even when one examines random series of consecutive ovarian cancer patients, without any prior selection for family history (28–31). This increased risk factor includes breast and colon cancer, and can occur on either the maternal or paternal side of the family (40).

The estimated magnitude of this risk to first-degree relatives ranges from approximately fourfold to eightfold when compared to general population frequencies. Given the 1-in-70 estimated lifetime risk of ovarian cancer, a working estimate of a 5% risk to first-degree relatives seems appropriate. This could have a number of genetic interpretations. At one end of the spectrum, all the familial cases could be due to dominant susceptibility (presumably in each case one of the three different dominant inheritance patterns reviewed above). Given the 50% transmission rate for an autosomal dominant disorder, this would mean that up to 20% of all ovarian cancers are due to dominant susceptibilities. At the other end of the spectrum, the dominant ovarian cancer syndromes would comprise an ill-defined but small proportion of the total cases, and the general increased empiric risk to relatives would be due to more complex genetic mechanisms. We will need to distinguish between these possibilities in order to provide the best counseling for our patients.

Piver and coworkers recommend prophylactic oophorectomy in women with family histories that include two or more first-degree relatives with the disease before the age of 35. Their ovarian cancer registry's data support an earlier age of disease onset in the offspring as compared to their mothers (41). Other studies have not confirmed this finding, however. At this time, we believe that genetic susceptibility to epithelial ovarian cancer is a significant risk factor. It appears to be heterogeneous (i.e., involves more than one gene defect), and it is most likely complex. None of the actual genes, genetic linkage markers, or other genetically determined preclinical markers are currently available. Improved definitions of empiric risks and markers are needed. A major goal of the work is to identify specific susceptibility genes that predispose women to ovarian cancer. We will then have the ability to identify and effectively counsel individuals in cancer families or in the general population who might be at the highest risk for this deadly disease.

Until the actual genes are identified, there is an urgent need for well-designed family-based genetic counseling and screening protocols. These protocols can take advantage of the latest epidemiologic and genetic observations: (a) the high risk when two first-degree relatives are affected; (b) the substantial risk, on the order of 6–10%, when even one first-degree relative is affected; (c) the data demonstrating that a family or personal history of breast and/or endometrial and/or colon cancer is also a genetically mediated risk factor; (d) the observation that although many of the familial cases have a younger age of onset, the older onset cases can also be familial as well; and (e) the genetic risk transmissible by fathers (as well as mothers) even though the men do not manifest the disease clinically. This genetic information can be used

for counseling patients and their family members. In addition, it will play an integral role in delineating the frequency of ovarian cancer screening using the modalities described below and in making recommendations for ovulation control, family planning, and prophylactic oophorectomy.

DIAGNOSTIC METHODS IN A SCREENING FOR OVARIAN CANCER

The two screening methods for ovarian cancer that lately have been most extensively evaluated are ultrasound and serum tumor marker determinations.

Tumor Biomarkers

CA-125 is an antigenic determinant on a high molecular weight glycoprotein that is recognized by the monoclonal antibody OC-125. Serum levels of CA-125 have been shown to be elevated in more than 80% of epithelial ovarian cancer patients and the frequency of marker elevation varies directly with stage of disease. However, it is important to recognize limitations of CA-125. Although the majority (80%) of patients with advanced epithelial ovarian carcinoma have preoperative CA-125 levels above 35 U/ml, only 23–50% of stage I ovarian cancers are associated with CA-125 elevations (42,43).

In addition, CA-125 elevations are associated with a wide range of other conditions both benign (endometriosis, pelvic inflammatory disease, uterine fibroids, pregnancy, cirrhosis) and malignant (pancreatic, breast, lung, and endometrial) cancers (44–46). Thus, this tumor marker has not demonstrated adequate sensitivity or specificity to be an effective screening test for ovarian cancer.

With these limitations in mind, a normal CA-125 level is reassuring in a woman with a mass with no sonographic characteristics of malignancy, i.e., a unilocular cystic mass with a diameter less than 5 cm, thin walls, presence of septae less than 3 mm thick or complex predominantly cystic ovarian mass (47). However, a suspicious lesion should not be ignored based on a normal serum CA-125.

At this time, no single marker has been an effective screening tool for ovarian cancer. Combining marker data and longitudinal monitoring of patients, however, may play an integral role in directing appropriate clinical intervention.

Transvaginal Sonography and Pulsed Color Doppler Flow Imaging

Transvaginal sonography (TVS) as a screening method for ovarian cancer has been performed increasingly since 1987. This method has been shown to be safe and well-accepted by patients. It has a high sensitivity, but it lacks specificity in distinguishing benign from malignant ovarian lesions.

The introduction of the transvaginal ultrasound transducer has improved the ease and resolution of ovarian imaging. Tissue differentiation has been improved by transvaginal sonography as well. Ninety-five percent of premenopausal and 85% of postmenopausal ovaries can accurately be visualized by the transvaginal approach (48,49–51). Difficulties have remained, however, in predicting significant ovarian pathology based solely on ultrasound findings (49,52).

In an attempt to increase the sensitivity and specificity, transvaginal sonography has been evaluated in several studies. In a recent screening study of 1300 asymptomatic postmenopausal women, 27 (2.1%) were found to have a persisting ovarian abnormality on TVS (50). Only 30% of these tumors were palpable on clinical examination. Fourteen of these patients had ovarian serous cystadenomas and three had primary ovarian carcinomas, two of which were stage I. These two women had normal pelvic examinations and normal serum CA-125 values. The sensitivity of TVS in this screening study was 1.000 and its specificity was 0.981. One of the concerns about TVS has been that it might cause unnecessary surgery. Based on the results of this preliminary study, the authors concluded that a multiinstitutional trial comparing the efficacy of TVS and serum CA-125 versus pelvic examination in asymptomatic postmenopausal women is warranted.

TVS screening is optimal in postmenopausal women where ovarian volume does not vary throughout the menstrual cycle. When applied to the premenopausal age group, 60% of ovarian abnormalities detected primarily on sonography disappeared spontaneously and no cancers were detected. In postmenopausal patients, however, more than 90% of initial ovarian abnormalities were present at the time of repeat sonography in 4 weeks, and all patients with persisting abnormalities had ovarian tumors at laparotomy (53).

Adjunctive methods proposed to improve the specificity of TVS include the use of a morphology index (47) and Doppler flow sonography (54). The combination of high-quality B-mode image, pulsed wave, and color Doppler in the same vaginal probe allows simultaneous visualization of structure and blood flow characteristics of the ovaries. This new technique displays flow as multiple points in a two-dimensional plane, superimposed on a two-dimensional ultrasound image. Flow velocity is proportional to the color brightness. Preliminary data suggest that it may be possible to detect the vascular changes associated with early ovarian cancers using color Doppler ultrasound modality (55).

In malignant lesions, blood flow can be demonstrated throughout diastole, probably reflecting a decrease in impedance to flow distal to the point of sampling. A possible explanation for this is that the new vessels associated with carcinoma (tumor angiogenesis) have limited vascular tone due to the absence of the tunica media (56). As a result of this, low-impedance shunts are formed.

In a pilot study using color Doppler flow imaging and vaginal sonography, benign and malignant ovarian pathology could be differentiated (57). No neovascularization was seen in 30 morphologically normal ovaries. Benign and malignant ovarian masses could be differentiated by Doppler flow in the 20 women with abnormal ovarian morphology demonstrating a high degree of accuracy.

Kurjak and colleagues examined 1753 women with adnexal masses by vaginal sonography and color Doppler imaging (58). Pathologic data are available for the 680 patients who underwent surgical exploration: there were 624 benign and 56 malignant adnexal masses. The presence of color flow and a resistance index < 0.40 enabled the prediction of histopathology with a sensitivity, specificity, and positive predictive value of 96.4, 98.8, and 98.2%, respectively.

In their other study, Kurjak et al. evaluated 14,317 asymptomatic women for ovarian carcinoma. Neovascularization was found in six of seven stage I carcinomas as demonstrated as RI < 0.40 (59). These authors concluded that color flow Doppler enhances the value of sonography in screening for ovarian cancer.

Bourne et al. applied vaginal ultrasound screening to a patient cohort with at least one family member with ovarian cancer (60). Three stage Ia epithelial ovarian carcinomas were found in the 776 women screened. One woman who screened negative subsequently developed peritoneal carcinomatosis 11 months later. The prevalence of ovarian cancer in this high-risk group of patients (0.4%) was ten times that of the general population.

We have been involved in a comprehensive study to evaluate a multidisciplinary approach to the diagnosis of ovarian cancer in the Gilda Radner Ovarian Cancer Detection Study at Cedars-Sinai Medical Center (50). Patients with a family history of ovarian, breast, colon, or endometrial carcinomas undergo detailed genetic counseling, venipuncture for five tumor biomarker measurements, and a transvaginal color Doppler ultrasound examination (Fig. 1).

A total of 597 asymptomatic patients were seen between 7/91 and 7/92. Repeat studies were performed on 115 of the patients due to abnormal test results. Nineteen participants have undergone oophorectomy at this time. One tumor of low malignant potential was discovered based on TVS morphologic characteristics (complexity and multiple septations), as well as one case of early endometrial carcinoma. Among the patients in whom oophorectomy was suggested based on persistently abnormal color Doppler ultrasound findings ($N = 7$), no

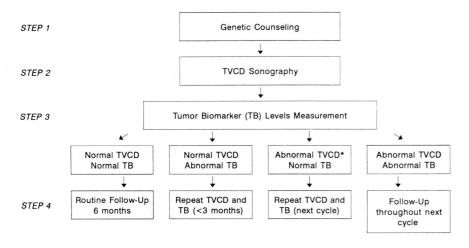

STEP 1 — Genetic Counseling

STEP 2 — TVCD Sonography

STEP 3 — Tumor Biomarker (TB) Levels Measurement

| Normal TVCD Normal TB | Normal TVCD Abnormal TB | Abnormal TVCD* Normal TB | Abnormal TVCD Abnormal TB |

STEP 4 —

| Routine Follow-Up 6 months | Repeat TVCD and TB (<3 months) | Repeat TVCD and TB (next cycle) | Follow-Up throughout next cycle |

FIG. 1. Screening for ovarian carcinoma of women (>35 years of age) with positive family history of ovarian, breast, and/or colon cancers, Cedars-Sinai Medical Center, Los Angeles. TVCD, transvaginal color Doppler; TB, tumor biomarker. *Abnormal TVCD includes abnormal ovarian morphology, RI ≤ 0.4, and/or ascites.

ovarian cancers were detected. No cancer was found in a group of patients with persistently increasing serum tumor biomarker levels.

Although the hierarchy of screening modalities remains controversial, it seems that a combination of diagnostic methods will significantly improve the detection of early ovarian cancer. Subsequent analysis and follow-up are still required to determine if there will be an impact of this testing on the long-term survival from the disease. At this time, performing cost–benefit analysis of this multidisciplinary ovarian cancer screening program is still premature. In the future, our efforts should focus on the biologic, economic, and psychologic costs and benefits that patients experience in screening for ovarian carcinoma.

REFERENCES

1. Cutler SJ, Young JL. Third National Cancer Survey: Incidence data. DHEW Publication (NIH) 1975:75–787.
2. Boring C, Squires T, Tong T. Cancer statistics—1991. *Cancer* 1991;41:19–36.
3. Gallion H, van Nagell JR, Donaldson ES. Adjuvant oral alkylating agent chemotherapy in patients with stage I epithelial ovarian cancer. *Cancer* 1989;63:1070–1073.
4. Young RC, Walton LA, Ellenberg SS, et al. Adjuvant therapy in stage I and stage II epithelial ovarian cancer. *N Engl J Med* 1990;322:1021–1027.
5. Hulka BS. Cancer screening: Degrees of proof and practical application. *Cancer* 1988;62:1776–1780.
6. Van Nagell JR. Editorial. *Gynecol Oncol* 1991;43:89–91.
7. Stenback F. Benign, borderline and malignant serous cystadenomas of the ovary. *Pathol Res Pract* 1981;172:58–72.
8. Aure JC, Kolstad P. Carcinoma of the ovary and endometriosis. *Acta Obstet Gynecol Scand* 1971;50:63–67.
9. Higgins RV, van Nagell JR, Woods CH, Thompson EA, Kryscio RJ. Interobserver variation in ovarian measurements using transvaginal sonography. *Gynecol Oncol* 1990;39:69–71.
10. Haenszel W, Kurihara M. Studies of Japanese migrants. *J Natl Cancer Inst* 1986;40:43–68.
11. Kolnel LN, Hinds MW, Hankin JH. Cancer patterns among migrants and native-born Japanese in Hawaii in relation to smoking, drinking and dietary habits. In: Gelboln HV, ed. *Genetic and environmental factors in experimental and human cancer.* Tokyo: Japan Sci Soc Press; 1980.
12. Farrow DC, Weiss NS, Daling JR. Association of obesity and ovarian cancer in a case control study. *Am J Epidemiol* 1989;6:1330–1334.
13. Lingeman CM. Environmental factors in the etiology of carcinoma of the human ovary. *Am J Ind Med* 1983;4:365–370.
14. Byers T, Marshall J, Graham S, Mettlin C, Swanson M. A case-control study of dietary and nondietary factors in ovarian cancer. *J Natl Cancer Inst* 1983;71:681–686.
15. Cramer DW, Welch RW, Hutchinson GB, Willett W, Scully RE. Dietary animal fat in relation to ovarian cancer risk. *Obstet Gynecol* 1984;63:833–838.
16. Franceschi S. Reproductive factors and cancers of the breast, ovary and endometrium. *Eur J Cancer Clin Oncol* 1989;25:1933–1934.
17. Parazzini F, La Vecchia C, Negri E, Gentile A. Menstrual factors and the risk of epithelial ovarian cancer. *J Clin Epidemiol* 1989;42:443–448.
18. Harding M, Cowan S, Hole D, et al. Estrogen and progesterone receptors in ovarian cancer. *Cancer* 1990;65:486–491.
19. Wu ML, Whittemore AS, Paffenbarger RS, et al. Personal and environmental characteristics related to epithelial ovarian cancer. Reproductive and menstrual events and oral contraceptive use. *Am J Epidemiol* 1988;128:1216–1227.
20. Gwinn ML, Lee N, Rhodes PH, Layde PM, Rubin GL. Pregnancy, breast feeding, and oral contraceptives and the risk of epithelial ovarian cancer. *J Clin Epidemiol* 1990;43:559–568.
21. Hankinson SE, Colditz GA, Hunter DJ, Spencer TL, Rosner B, Stampfer MJ. A quantitative assessment of oral contraceptive use and risk of ovarian cancer. *Obstet Gynecol* 1992;80:708–714.
22. Centers for Disease Control Cancer and Steroid Hormone Study. Oral contraceptive use and the risk of ovarian cancer. *JAMA* 1983;249:1596–1599.
23. Risch HA, Weiss NH, Lyon JL. Events of reproductive life and the incidence of epithelial ovarian cancer. *Am J Epidemiol* 1983;117:1128–1139.
24. West RO. Epidemiologic study of malignancies of the ovary. *Cancer* 1966;19:1001–1019.
25. Marcy SM, Kilbrick S. In: Hoperich PD, ed. *Mumps in infectious diseases.* Philadelphia: Harper & Row; 1983:228–236.
26. Research Unit of the Royal College of General Practitioners. The incidence and complications of mumps. *J R Coll Gen Prac* 1974;245:45–55.
27. Lingeman CM. Etiology of cancer of the human ovary: A review. *J Natl Cancer Inst* 1974;53:1603–1608.
28. Casagrande JT, Pike MC, Ross RK, Louie EW, Roy S, Henderson BE. "Incessant ovulation" and ovarian cancer. *Lancet* 1979;2:170–172.
29. Hildreth NG, Kelsey JL, LiVolsi VA, et al. An epidemiologic study of epithelial carcinoma of the ovary. *Am J Epidemiol* 1981;114:398–405.
30. Cramer DW, Hutchinson GB, Welch WR, Scully RE, Ryan KJ. Determinants of ovarian cancer risk. I. Reproductive experiences and family history. *J Natl Cancer Inst* 1983;71:711–716.

31. Schildkraut JM, Thompson WD. Familial ovarian cancer. A population-based case-control study. *Am J Epidemiol* 1988;128:456–466.

32. Mori M, Harabuchi I, Miyake H, Casagrande JT, Henderson BE, Ross RK. Reproductive, genetic, and dietary risk factors for ovarian cancer. *Am J Epidemiol* 1988;128:771–777.

33. Fraumeni JF, Grundy CW, Creagan ET, Everson RB. Six families prone to ovarian cancer. *Cancer* 1975;36:364–369.

34. Lynch HT, Albano WA, Lynch JF, Lynch PM, Campbell A. Surveillance and management of patients at high genetic risk for ovarian carcinoma. *Obstet Gynecol* 1982;59:589–596.

35. Lynch HT, Schuelke GS, Wells IC, et al. Hereditary ovarian carcinoma: Biomarker study. *Cancer* 1985;55:410–415.

36. Lynch HT, Wells IC, Bewtra C, et al. Clinical and biomarker findings in familial ovarian carcinoma. In: Lynch HT, Kullander S, eds. *Cancer genetics in women.* Boca Raton: CRC Press; 1987:49–61.

37. Piver MS, Nasea P, Baker TR, et al. *Familial Ovarian Cancer Registry Newsletter,* 1989.

38. Heintz APM, Hacker NF, Lagasse LD. Epidemiology and etiology of ovarian cancer: A review. *Obstet Gynecol* 1985;66:127–135.

39. Lynch HT, Harris RE, Guirgis HA, Maloney K, Carmody LL, Lynch JF. Familial association of breast/ovarian carcinoma. *Cancer* 1978;41:1543–1549.

40. Schildkraut JM, Risch N, Thompson WD. Evaluating genetic association among ovarian, breast, and endometrial cancer: Evidence for breast/ovarian cancer relationship. *Am J Hum Genet* 1989;45:521–529.

41. Piver MS, Baker TR, Piedmonte M, Sandecki AM. Epidemiology and etiology of ovarian cancer. *Semin Oncol* 1991;18:177–185.

42. Bast RC, Klug TL, St John E, et al. A radioimmunoassay using monoclonal antibody to monitor the course of epithelial ovarian cancer. *N Engl J Med* 1983;309:883–887.

43. Mann WJ, Pastner B, Cohen H, Loesch M. Preoperative serum CA-125 levels in patients with surgical stage I invasive ovarian adenocarcinomas. *J Natl Cancer Inst* 1988;80:208–209.

44. Pittaway DE, Douglas JW. Serum CA-125 in women with endometriosis and chronic pelvic pain. *Fertil Steril* 1989;51:68–73.

45. Jaeger W, Meier C, Wildt L, Sauerbrei W, Lang N. CA-125 serum concentrations during the menstrual cycle. *Fertil Steril* 1988;50:223–227.

46. Niloff JM, Klug TL, Schaetzl E, Zurawski VR, Knapp RC, Bast RC. Elevation of serum CA-125 in carcinomas of the fallopian tube, endometrium and endocervix. *Am J Obstet Gynecol* 1984;148:1057–1059.

47. Sassone AM, Timor-Tritsch IE, Artner A, Westhoff C, Warren WB. Transvaginal sonographic characterization of ovarian disease: Evaluation of a new scoring system to predict ovarian malignancy. *Obstet Gynecol* 1991;78:70–77.

48. Rodriguez MH, Platt LD, Medearis AL, Lacarra M, Lobo RA. The use of transvaginal sonography for evaluation of postmenopausal ovarian size and morphology. *Am J Obstet Gynecol* 1988;159:810–814.

49. Higgins RV, van Nagell JR, Donaldson ES, et al. Transvaginal sonography as a screening method for ovarian cancer. *Gynecol Oncol* 1989;34:402–406.

50. Karlan BY, Raffel LJ, Crvenkovic G, et al. A multidisciplinary approach to the early detection of ovarian carcinoma: rationale, protocol design, and early results. *Am J Obstet Gynecol* 1993;169:494–501.

51. Van Nagell JR, DePriest P, Puls L, et al. Ovarian cancer screening in asymptomatic postmenopausal women by transvaginal sonography. *Cancer* 1991;68:458–462.

52. Benacerraf BR, Finkler NJ, Wojciechowski C, Knapp RC. Sonographic accuracy in the diagnosis of ovarian masses. *J Reprod Med* 1990;35:491–495.

53. Van Nagell JR. Ovarian cancer screening. *Cancer* 1991;68:679–680.

54. Taylor KJW, Burns PN, Wells PNT, Conway DI, Hull MGR. Ultrasound Doppler flow studies of the ovarian and uterine arteries. *Br J Obstet Gynaecol* 1985;92:240–246.

55. Kurjak A, Zalud I, Jurkovic D, et al. Transvaginal color flow Doppler for the assessment of pelvic circulation. *Acta Obstet Gynecol Scand* 1989;68:131–135.

56. Folkman J, Watson K, Ingber D, Hanahan D. Induction of angiogenesis during the transition from hyperplasia to neoplasia. *Nature* 1989;339:58–61.

57. Bourne TH, Campbell S, Steer C, Whitehead MI, Collins WP. Transvaginal colour flow imaging: A possible new screening technique for ovarian cancers. *Br Med J* 1989;299:1367–1370.

58. Kurjak A, Zalud I. International Perinatal Doppler Society Meeting. Book of Abstracts, 1990, Los Angeles.

59. Kurjak A, Zalud I, Alfirevic Z. Evaluation of adnexal masses with transvaginal color ultrasound. *J Ultrasound Med* 1991;10:295–297.

60. Bourne TH, Whitehead MI, Campbell S, Royston P, Bhan V, Collins WP. Ultrasound screening for familial ovarian cancer. *Gynecol Oncol* 1991;43:92–97.

Doppler Ultrasound in Obstetrics and Gynecology,
edited by Joshua A. Copel and Kathryn L. Reed.
Raven Press, Ltd., New York © 1995.

CHAPTER 6

Pelvic Masses

Arthur C. Fleischer and Jeanne Anne Cullinan

The ability to assess the flow to and within pelvic masses expands the capability of diagnostic sonography from anatomic information to include pathophysiologic data. Although the differential diagnosis of pelvic masses by morphology can achieve accuracies in the 80–90% range, a secondary test such as transvaginal color Doppler sonography (TV-CDS) is occasionally needed to further characterize masses that have nonspecific morphologic sonographic features (1). By depiction of their vascular supplies, ovarian masses can be distinguished from uterine. In addition, areas of abnormal vascularity (tumor neovascularity) can be used to distinguish benign from malignant masses.

As greater experience with color Doppler sonography (CDS) is obtained, its role in the evaluation of pelvic masses is becoming clearer. Its practical role as an adjunct to morphologic assessment by traditional transvaginal imaging (TVS) in the evaluation of pelvic masses has been suggested in several published studies (2–7). However, a double-blind study that evaluates the relative accuracy of CDS versus TVS is needed in order to assess the added specificity or sensitivity of CDS over TVS accurately.

The information obtained from color Doppler sonography can potentially add to the clinical management of patients in a variety of areas:

1. Adding confidence in the observation of masses that may represent hemorrhagic masses, which may spontaneously regress
2. Confirming the diagnosis of ovarian torsion, which requires immediate surgical intervention

3. Differentiating those patients whose masses may be treated with a minimally invasive approach (such as pelviscopic surgery) from those needing standard laparotomy and extensive cancer surgery

This chapter will emphasize those areas in which Doppler sonography can significantly assist in the differential diagnosis of pelvic masses beyond that information obtained with conventional transabdominal or transvaginal sonography.

INSTRUMENTATION AND TECHNIQUE

Doppler sonography can be obtained with either transabdominal or transvaginal transducer/probes. Once a line of sight is established, the sample volume should be tailored to the size of the vessel examined. Large feeding vessels should have their entire volume sampled whereas small intraparenchymal vessels need only the smallest sample volume that encompasses the entire vessel. The waveform shape gives a rough indication of the type of flow within the vessel. With major feeding vessels, the flow is of more uniform velocity, thus giving a thinner frequency envelope rather than the turbulent flow of smaller intraparenchymal vessels, which give a larger range of velocities as evidenced by the width of the waveform. Resistance is typically higher the further into the parenchymal bed the blood flows.

Maximum systolic velocity can be estimated if the Doppler angle is kept between 20° and 60° of the actual course of the vessel. When the vessel is visualized, angle correction is recommended. Wall filters should be set at a minimum so that even the lowest velocities can be determined.

Analysis of waveforms can be accomplished using standard indices such as the resistance index or pulsatility index. Although there is some debate as to which

A. C. Fleischer and J. A. Cullinan: Departments of Radiology and Radiological Sciences, and Obstetrics and Gynecology, Vanderbilt University Medical Center, Nashville, TN 37232-2675.

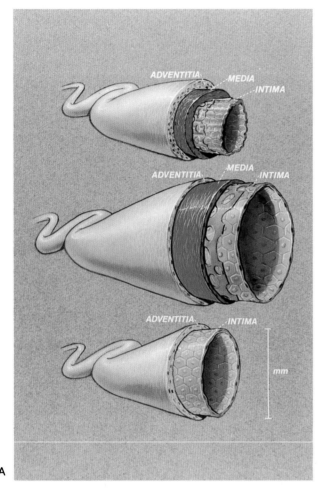

A

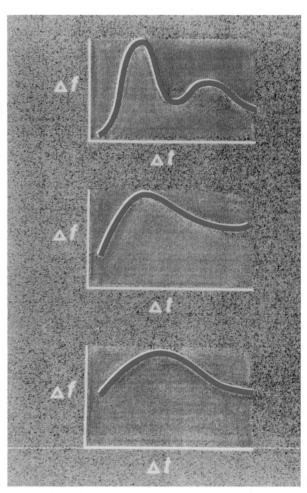

B

FIG. 1. Typical Doppler waveforms in normal vasodilated and neoplastic vessels. **A:** Normal arteriole with muscular media (*top*); vasodilated normal vessel (*middle*) and tumor arteriole without muscular media (*bottom*). **B:** Corresponding Doppler waveform for these vessels. The normal arteriole (*top*) demonstrates high pulsatility (difference between maximum systoles velocity and end-diastolic velocity) and a diastolic notch whereas the arteriole within the tumor has low pulsatility and lacks a notch. The vasodilated vessels have a waveform similar to that of the tumor vessel.

of these indices is more accurate, either is sufficient if diastolic flow is present. If diastolic flow is absent or reversed, the resistance index cannot be used and the pulsatility index is needed. We prefer the pulsatility index because it takes into account more of the shape of the waveform. Another index that can be used is the perfusion index, which is the area under the curve in systole divided by the area under the curve in diastole. Future systems may allow assessment of the relative perfusion similar to that on a scintigraphic camera with quantification of the number of excited pixel elements per unit time.

A transvaginal approach is recommended if the lesion is within 5–10 cm of the cul-de-sac. Transabdominal scanning is needed if the lesion is over 10 cm in size or superior to the uterine fundus. Gentle pressure can be applied to the mass in an attempt to determine whether the mass is intra- or extrauterine, adherent or freely mobile.

BASIC DIAGNOSTIC PRINCIPLES

The waveform obtained from Doppler assessment of flow indicates the relative resistance to flow within an

TABLE 1. *Typical TV-CDS parameters*

Benign	Pulsatility index greater than 1.0 (high-impedance flow)
	Flow in periphery, not in center
	Diastolic "notch"
Malignant	Pulsatility index less than 1.0 (low-impedance flow)
	Flow in center, not in periphery
	Absent diastolic "notch"

TABLE 2. *Typical Doppler findings*

Peripheral vascularity, low maximum systolic velocity, high
    impedance, present notch:
  Simple cyst
  Dermoid cyst
  Endometrioma
Central vascularity, high maximum systolic velocity, low
    impedance, absent notch:
  Ovarian neoplasms
  Tuboovarian abscesses
  Hemorrhagic mass

TABLE 3. *Typical impedance of ovarian masses*

High (pulsatility index greater than 1.5)
  Cystadenomas
  Hemorrhagic cysts
Intermediate and/or variable (pulsatility index between 1.0
    and 1.5)
  Dermoid cyst
  Endometrioma[a]
Low (pulsatility index less than 1.0)
  Ovarian malignancies
  Inflammatory masses
  Metabolically "active" masses
  Corpus luteum

[a] May vary with menstrual cycle.

organ or area within a particular structure. Waveforms can be analyzed by their resistance index or pulsatility index, the location and distribution of vessels, maximum systolic velocity, and the presence or absence of a diastolic notch.

Figure 1 demonstrates the microscopic appearance of normal vessels and those that are within tumors. Normal arterioles have a layer of muscular lining that is not present in tumors. This muscular lining has a role in regulating parenchymal perfusion and thereby is typically associated with a flow pattern that has relatively high pulsatility. With a paucity of this muscular lining seen in tumor vessels, there is continuous diastolic flow and less of a difference in systolic and diastolic peaks and low pulsatility. There usually is a lack of a diastolic notch as well. When a vessel is dilated, the pulsatility is reduced as a reflection of decreased resistance to forward flow. This pattern simulates that of a tumor vessel, although a diastolic notch is often present.

Tumor vessels typically have high diastolic flow related to the multiple areas of stenosis and vasodilation within the network of tumor vessels. The velocities may also be increased related to the requirements of tumor perfusion and arteriovenous communications within the network of tumor vessels.

A clear understanding of these principles is needed in the analysis of pelvic masses with Doppler sonography. With this basis for understanding, it is clear that some

nonneoplastic tumors may demonstrate blood flow characteristics of truly malignant masses (Tables 1–3). Future developments may include more precise determination of the blood flow characteristics of these vessels as depicted by their Doppler waveforms.

CDS: ACCURACY AND SPECIFICITY

Diagnostic accuracies over 90% have been reported in several series in differentiating benign from malignant ovarian lesions using these diagnostic principles (3,4) (Fig. 2). In general, the true positive rate (% of malignant masses with low impedance) is 90–95% whereas the false-positive rate (% of benign lesions with low pulsatility index) ranges from 2% to 5%. Even though TV-CDS may not improve the actual detection of a mass, it seems to improve specificity in differentiating benign from malignant masses. The figures from these studies substantiate the use of TV-CDS in selected cases as a means to differentiate benign from malignant masses.

Using a pulsatility index value less than 1.0 as indicative of malignancy, we documented a very high negative predictive value of 98% and nearly as high a positive predictive value of 85% (Table 4). Thus, TV-CDS seems to exclude the possibility of malignancy accurately thereby allowing for less invasive approaches, such as pelviscopic

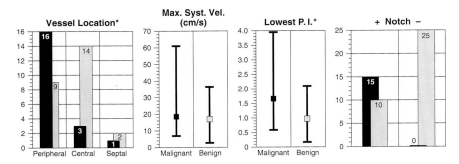

FIG. 2. Multi-parameter analysis. n = 25 benign, 25 malignant ovarian masses.

TABLE 4. *TV-CDS reported series*

Author (date)	n	True positive (% malignancies with low impedance)	False positive (% benign with low impedance)	No. stage I CaO
Bourne 1989	50	7/8 (88%)	1/11 (12%)	3
Fleischer 1991	63	13/15 (87%)	3/42 (7%)	7
Weiner 1992	24	15/16 (94%)	1/36 (3%)	5
Kawai 1992	24	5/5 (100%)	0/19 (0%)	4
Kurjak 1992	628	55/56 (98%)	1/572 (0.2%)	6
Natori 1992	30	12/15 (80%)	3/15 (20%)	?

surgery, to be considered. Analysis of multiple parameters such as vessel location, maximum systolic velocity, and the presence or absence of a notch may also enhance specificity (4) (Table 5).

Retrospective analysis of 66 patients who underwent surgery and pathologic evaluation of the excised tissue after TVS and CDS indicates that in approximately 40% of cases studied, CDS provided enhanced specificity concerning organ of origin and histologic type of mass over those obtained with TVS alone (9). In particular, the enhanced specificity of CDS was most evident in the detection of ovarian malignancy, adnexal torsion, and ectopic pregnancy. In 40% of the cases, the specificity of CDS and TVS were considered equal whereas in 6% of cases TVS was more specific than CDS. In 14% of cases, however, neither CDS or TVS was histologically specific. These cases included a patient in whom a 2-cm metastatic ovarian cancer was not diagnosed, and another in whom a necrotic leiomyosarcoma was misdiagnosed as an ovarian neoplasm.

The true sensitivity of CDS awaits studies which compare preoperative to postoperative findings in women undergoing surgery for conditions not related to the ovary. This will require studies similar to those done with conventional transvaginal sonography in women undergoing urologic surgery or hysterectomy and oophorectomy secondary to endometrial carcinoma (10,11). In general, it is felt that the added specificity afforded by CDS supports its use in selected cases in which TVS is equivocal or nondiagnostic.

OVARIAN MASSES

The ovary is the source of a variety of pelvic masses ranging from benign cysts to solid neoplasms. It can also

TABLE 5. *TV-CDS*

Pathology	Benign	Malignant
Benign	41	3
Malignant	1	17

Sensitivity = 85% positive predictive value = 85%.

Specificity = 93% negative predictive value = 98%.

be the site of metastases, usually from gastrointestinal tract primaries. Some pelvic masses may also simulate the appearance of an ovarian mass. These include endometriomas and parovarian cysts that are adjacent to, but not within, the substance of the ovary.

The waveforms seen in the ovary vary in women of reproductive age according to the phase of the menstrual cycle. During the menstrual and follicular phase, there is high-resistance flow (Fig. 3A). With formation of the corpus luteum, low-resistance waveforms are seen as the result of newly formed vessels within the walls of the corpus luteum (Fig. 3B).

Although the morphology as depicted by conventional TVS can be used in the majority of cases to determine their probable histologic composition, there clearly are times that an adjunctive test such as Doppler sonography can be helpful in further clarifying the etiology of some pelvic masses. For example, complex masses containing cystic and solid areas may represent either benign hemorrhagic corpora lutea or ovarian tumors (Fig. 3). Some irregularities in the wall of a mass may be due to benign causes such as dermoid cysts or a sign of malignant change. Thus, Doppler sonography is most useful in cases that have nonspecific morphologic features as well as in cases where torsion is suspected.

The waveforms obtained from vessels using Doppler sonography give a general impression on the distribution and characterization of blood flow to and within ovarian masses. The feeding arteries, mainly the adnexal branch of the uterine artery and the main ovarian artery, have a muscular coating that is present in both benign and malignant lesions. However, vessels located within the mass typically are low-flow high-impedance with the important exception of the corpus luteum. In the corpus luteum, there are vessels along the wall that have a paucity of muscular lining and high diastolic flow, which is clearly suggestive of tumor neovascularity.

In patients in whom a corpus luteum is suspected clinically, it is highly recommended that a repeat scan be performed in the late menstrual phase of the next cycle in order to exclude the possibility of a corpus luteum. If low-impedance flow persists after repeat scan or cessation of hormone replacement medications, an abnormal mass is probably present and surgery indicated.

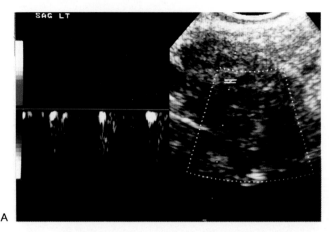 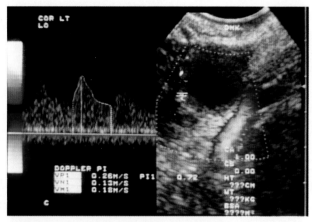

FIG. 3. Normal variations in ovarian waveform. **A:** TV-CDS of the ovary during menstrual phase, showing high resistance flow. **B:** With formation of the corpus luteum, a low-impedance waveform is seen as a reflection of the newly formed vessels within the luteal wall.

There are a variety of lesions that may demonstrate low-impedance high-diastolic flow. These include inflammatory masses such as tuboovarian abscesses, actively hemorrhaging luteal cysts, and some dermoid cysts. These masses have in common enlarged and vasodilated normal vessels that can simulate the flow pattern seen in some ovarian tumors (Figs. 4, 5). It is important to determine whether or not the waveform has a diastolic notch since this is an indication that there is initial resistance to forward flow offered by the muscular lining of the arteriole. Since resistance typically is greater as the vessel courses toward the center of an organ, the absence of a notch in a feeder vessel probably suggests malignancy with higher predictive value than if it was obtained on an intraparenchymal branch.

Malignancies tend to demonstrate color Doppler flow in the solid areas in the center portion of the mass, in papillary excrescences, or in irregular areas of the wall (Fig. 6). This flow typically has low pulsatility (pulsatility index less than 1.0) that lacks a diastolic notch. Some metabolically active tumors and germ cell tumors demonstrate this pattern as well.

There are a group of lesions that demonstrate a range of Doppler flow from high resistance to low resistance (Fig. 7). These include dermoid cysts and endometriomas. Dermoid cysts may have low-impedance flow when there are actively dividing cells within the dermoid cysts as opposed to relatively stagnant growth in established masses. Endometriomas may demonstrate low-impedance flow when there is hemorrhage in the menstrual phase of the cycle.

Although there are only approximately 40 stage I cancers reported in the literature as detected by color Doppler sonography at this time, it is clear that most of these are recognizable by their characteristic low-pulsatility flow patterns (Table 2). In one study, 16 of 17 malignan-

cies had a pulsatility index less than 1 whereas benign lesions had a pulsatility index greater than 1 in 35 of 36 examples (5). The overall accuracy of color Doppler sonography appears to be better than that of CA-125 and probably is greatest in rapidly growing tumors that require significant blood flow, such as in some aggressive stage I and II lesions.

EXTRAOVARIAN MASSES

There are a variety of lesions that may mimic the morphologic and Doppler features of ovarian masses. These include pedunculated uterine fibroids, some tubal masses, paraovarian cysts, and, rarely, bowel lesions (Fig. 8). Gentle pressure may be used between the uterus and the mass to differentiate pedunculated uterine lesions from those arising in the adnexa. It should be realized that vascular fibroids tend to have low pulsatility characteristics similar to ovarian neoplasms. Tubal cancers, although extremely rare, may also demonstrate low pulsatility. Paraovarian lesions tend to be cystic and have low pulsatility when infected. Some bowel lesions may simulate the appearance of adnexal pathology due to their multiloculated appearance if matted. Diverticular abscesses and inflammatory bowel lesions may also have low-impedance flow.

ADNEXAL OVARIAN TORSION

One of the major applications of color Doppler sonography is in the diagnosis of ovarian torsion. Although the ovary has a dual blood supply, torsion typically affects flow both from the ovarian artery and from the adnexal branch of the uterine artery. Typically, there is absent arterial flow within an enlarged ovary that may demon-

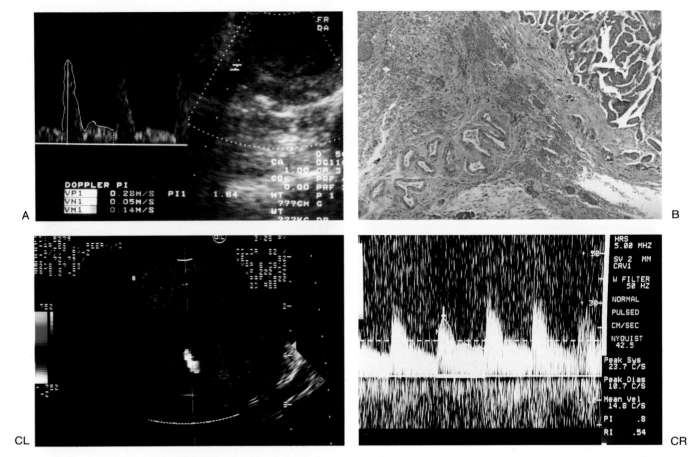

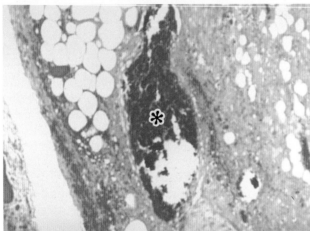

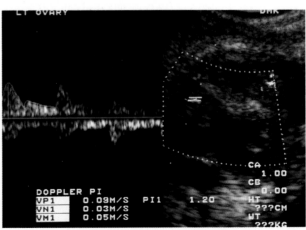

FIG. 4. Hemorrhagic masses. A: Hemorrhagic mass within an enlarged left ovary. B: Low-power photomicrograph of 3A showing hemorrhagic area (∗). C: Hemorrhagic mass with low impedance (PI = 0.5) flow. Courtesy of C. Peery, MD. D: Low-power photomicrograph showing large arteriole (∗) and surrounding hemorrhage within wall.

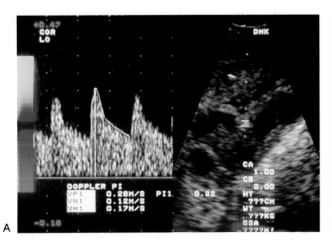

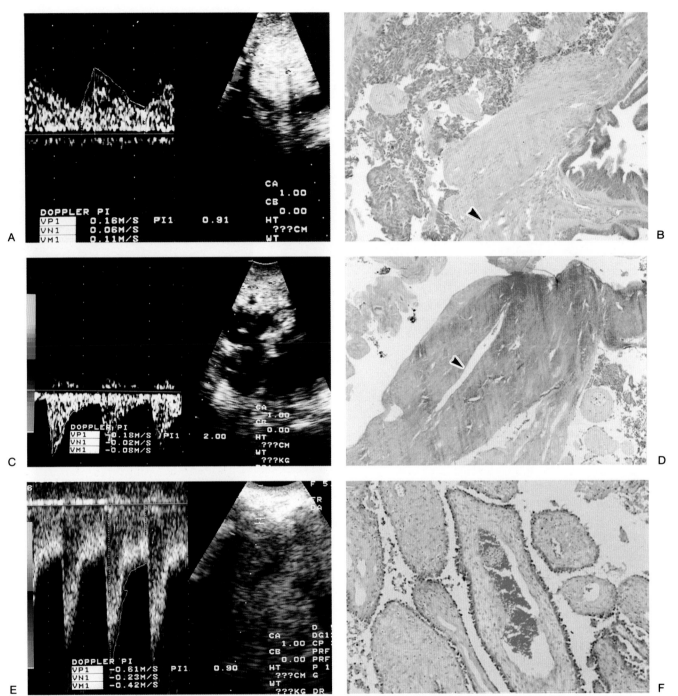

FIG. 6. Ovarian neoplasms. **A:** TV-CDS of a complex mass showing low impedance in centrally located vessel. **B:** High-power (20×) photomicrograph showing tumor vessels (*arrow*) in central portion of mass. **C:** TV-CDS showing high-impedance flow area of papillary excrescence in the same mass as 5A. **D:** Low-power (10×) photomicrograph of a normal vessel near a papillary excrescence (*arrowhead*). **E:** TV-CDS of solid mass with low-impedance flow that lacks a diastolic notch. **F:** High-power (20×) photomicrograph showing an abnormal vessel within a tumor excrescence without a muscular media.

FIG. 5. Inflammatory masses. **A:** TV-CDS of left ovary showing high-velocity, low-impedance flow within the wall of a tuboovarian abscess. **B:** TV-CDS of the left ovary showing low-velocity, low-pulsatility waveform in solid area. A notch is present in diastole suggesting a benign process. This is another example of tuboovarian abscess.

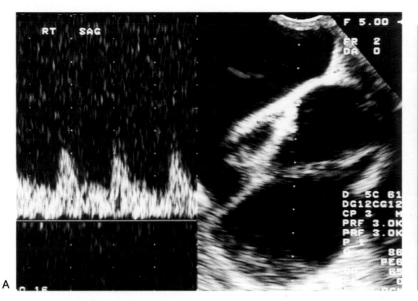
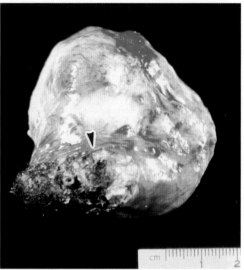

FIG. 7. Masses with variable impedance. **A:** TV-CDS of a dermoid cyst with multiple septae and solid areas showing intermediate-impedance flow. **B:** Excised gross specimen showing vessels adjacent to a locus of hair and teeth.

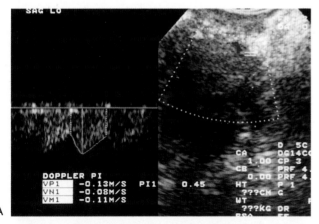
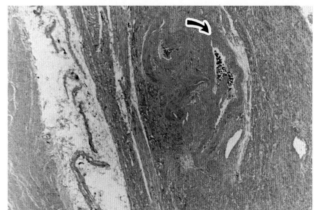
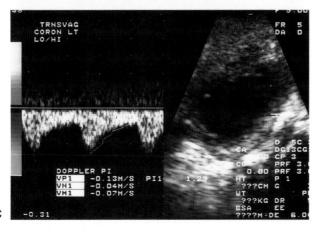

FIG. 8. Extraovarian masses. **A:** TV-CDS of an interligamentous fibroid with low-impedance flow. **B:** Low-power (10×) photomicrograph showing dilated vessels (*curved arrow*) in the rim of the fibroid. **C:** TV-CDS of diverticular abscess showing low-impedance flow. **D:** TV-CDS of an omental/peritoneal metastasis from a uterine sarcoma with low-impedance flow. **E:** Low-power photomicrograph showing extensive vascularity within a metastatic deposit.

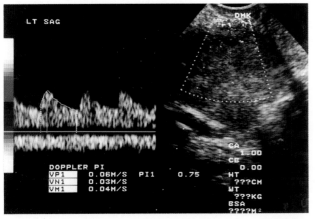

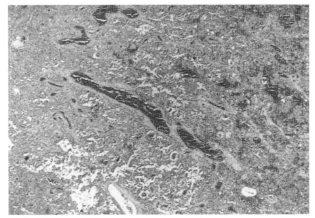

FIG. 8. *Continued*.

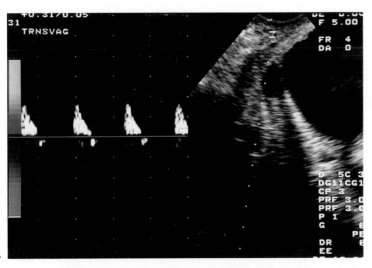

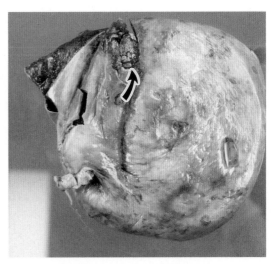

FIG. 9. Adnexal torsion. **A:** TV-CDS of a peripheral arteriole within a hemorrhagic mass showing high-resistance flow as evidenced by reversed diastolic flow. **B:** Excised specimen showing a torsed gangrenous ovary with partially perfused tube (*curved arrow*).

strate irregular solid areas related to hemorrhage, which may precipitate the torsion initially (Fig. 9). There may be high-resistance flow in the hilar vessels and, in some cases, venous flow in the capsular vessels as well.

The optimal time for diagnosing ovarian torsion is prior to development of gangrenous changes. This may require some hypoperfused lesions to be overdiagnosed as torsion, but these lesions may be amenable to early surgical intervention anyway.

SUMMARY

Color Doppler sonography is most useful in differentiating morphologically similar masses such as hemorrhagic corpora lutea from ovarian neoplasms. It has a primary role in evaluating ovarian torsion. It is impor-

tant to realize that the areas of overlap in benign vs. malignant lesions tend to involve masses that contain vasodilated vessels or those that are actively hemorrhaging.

ACKNOWLEDGMENT

Many tables and figures in this chapter are reprinted with permission from Fleischer, AC and Jones, HW. *Early detection of ovarian carcinoma with transvaginal sonography: potentials and limitations.* New York: Raven Press; 1993.

REFERENCES

1. Granberg S, Wikland M, Jansson I. Macroscopic characterization of ovarian tumors and the relation to the histological diagnosis:

Criteria to be used for ultrasound evaluation. *Gynecol Oncol* 1989;35:139–144.

2. Bourne T, Campbell S, Steer C, Whitehead MI, Collins WP. Transvaginal color flow imaging: A possible new screening technique for ovarian cancer. *Br Med J* 1989;299:1367–1370.

3. Kurjak A, Zalud I, Alfirevic Z. Evaluation of adnexal masses with transvaginal color ultrasound. *J Ultrasound Med* 1991;10:295–297.

4. Fleischer AC, Rodgers WH, Rao BK, et al. Assessment of ovarian tumor vascularity with transvaginal color Doppler sonography. *J Ultrasound Med* 1991;10:563–568.

5. Weiner Z, Thaler I, Beck D, Rottem S, Deutsch M, Brandes JM. Differentiating malignant from benign ovarian tumors with transvaginal color flow imaging. *Obstet Gynecol* 1992;79:159–162.

6. Kawai M, Kano T, Kikkawa F, Maeda O, Oguchi H, Tomoda Y. Transvaginal Doppler ultrasound with color flow imaging in the diagnosis of ovarian cancer. *Obstet Gynecol* 1992;79:163–167.

7. Natori M, Kouno H, Nozawa S. Flow velocity waveform analysis for the detection of ovarian cancer. *Med Rev* 1992;40:45–50.

8. Fleischer AC, Kepple DM, Rodgers W. Color Doppler sonography of ovarian masses: A multiparameter analysis. *J Ultrasound Med* 1993;12:41–48.

9. Fleischer AC, Cullinan JA, Kepple DM. Color Doppler sonography vs. transvaginal sonography of pelvic masses: Comparative specificity. *J Ultrasound Med* 1993;12:705–712.

10. Rodriques MH, Platt LD, Medearis AL, Lacarra M, Lobo RA. The use of transvaginal sonography for evaluation of postmenopausal ovarian size and morphology. *Am J Obstet Gynecol* 1988;159:810–814.

11. Fleischer AC, McKee MS, Gordon AN, et al. Transvaginal sonography of postmenopausal ovaries with pathologic correlation. *J Ultrasound Med* 1990;9:637.

Doppler Ultrasound in Obstetrics and Gynecology,
edited by Joshua A. Copel and Kathryn L. Reed.
Raven Press, Ltd., New York © 1995.

CHAPTER 7

The Menstrual Cycle, Menopause, Ovulation Induction, and *In Vitro* Fertilization

Michael Applebaum

For one practicing diagnostic ultrasound, examination of the female pelvis presents a unique challenge. Virtually no other area within the human body undergoes transformations as frequently as the reproductive tract of a woman during her fertile years. Its organs are not static and change on a daily basis. Familiarity with the diverse presentations of the various structures during different times of the menstrual cycle is important. This allows the experienced sonologist or sonographer to picture, in the "mind's eye," the expected normal appearance prior to performing an ultrasound study. Knowing what to anticipate anatomically, together with the clinical history, makes detection of abnormalities more likely.

Chance favors the prepared mind.

For a woman past her reproductive years, changes still occur, albeit more slowly and less dramatically.

EXAMINATION TECHNIQUE

Sonographic examination of the female pelvic organs is most commonly performed using two different approaches. The first and older is transabdominal; the second and more recent is transvaginal (1–3). A third method, transperineal, is also employed though less frequently (4–6). A thorough ultrasound examination of the pelvis should include both complete transabdominal and transvaginal studies, unless either limited information is needed (e.g., follicle size) or extenuating circumstances dictate otherwise (e.g., patient refusal). The techniques are complementary, not mutually exclusive. The person performing the ultrasound examination can vary

certain parameters to optimize the quality of the study. These include bladder distention, manual manipulation of the anatomy, and patient positioning.

Bladder Filling

Transabdominal ultrasound of the female pelvis should be performed with the bladder optimally distended. The operative phrase is "optimally distended." If too full, the patient may experience excessive discomfort, which might result in guarding. Also, the overdistended bladder may push the target structures so far from the transducer that image quality suffers. Optimal distention of the bladder can be achieved by having the patient void incrementally. If too empty, near-field artifacting and overlying bowel gas may degrade image quality. Optimal distention of the bladder can be achieved either by waiting for the bladder to fill more completely or having the patient ingest additional fluid and then waiting.

Unequivocally, there are occasions in which the empty bladder transabdominal examination may yield better results than either the transvaginal or filled bladder approaches. This is particularly true when relatively large, especially fundal, fibroids are present.

Transvaginal (or endovaginal) ultrasound is generally performed with the bladder empty. The operative phrase is "generally performed." If too full, the patient may experience excessive discomfort. Also, the distended bladder may push the target structures so far from the transducer that image quality suffers. Optimal distention of the bladder may be achieved by having the patient void, perhaps incrementally.

Unequivocally, there are occasions in which the transvaginal examination may yield better results with a filled or filling bladder than with an empty bladder. If a struc-

M. Applebaum: Finch University of Health Sciences/The Chicago Medical School, North Chicago, IL 60064.

ture of interest either is not apparent or is suboptimally seen, patience and bladder filling may result in better visualization.

Manipulation

Manual manipulation of the anatomy using the transducer and/or the nonexamining free hand can significantly improve the quality of the study. All manipulations are performed to move target structures into more favorable scanning circumstances (e.g., location). When employing a two-handed technique, one hand is placed generally between the pubis and umbilicus to shift the pelvic and abdominal structures while the other is maneuvering the transducer.

Positioning

Proper patient positioning can also improve examination quality. When performing endovaginal ultrasounds, elevating the patient's hips or placing the patient at the end of the examining table facilitates greater downward excursion of the probe handle. Occasionally, placing the patient's leg on the examiner's shoulder allows for increased lateral range of motion of the transducer. Further, some findings are more apparent when the examination is performed with the patient placed in a position similar to the one employed during a proctoscopy or colonoscopy. To assist in characterizing findings, having the patient move or roll from side to side may demonstrate motion in structures that would otherwise appear static (e.g., swirling within endometriomas; endovaginally, palpation with the probe may produce similar results). Moving the patient can also place target structures in more accessible locations.

Conclusion

In conclusion, after positioning the patient properly, the technique of the ultrasound study can be remembered by the mnemonic KID CAN, where:

K = *K*now what you expect to see based on the patient's clinical history and presentation prior to the exam
I = *I*ncremental bladder voiding, to achieve . . .
D = optimal bladder *D*istention
C = *C*ompression, with the nonscanning hand and/or the transducer
A = *A*ngulation of the transducer to place target objects an optimal distance from the transducer and use favorable superficial structures as acoustic "windows"
N = be *N*ice to the patient. A relaxed patient is much easier to examine than a tense patient

The most valuable imaging skills we possess are observation, creativity, and technique.

THE OVARIES

The ovaries are generally situated on either side of the uterus, although locations superior or posterior to the uterus are not uncommon. In addition to the techniques described above, if one has difficulty finding the ovaries, a search along the internal iliac artery may prove useful. The ovary is often located anterior to the vascular bifurcation into anterior and posterior branches (7,8). Successful visualization of the ovaries varies among investigators and also depends on the patient's age (9,10).

During the reproductive years of a normal female, the ovaries undergo changes characterized by the cyclical development and resolution of functional cysts. In fact, the identification of an ovary is made by demonstrating follicle cysts surrounded by ovarian parenchyma (8). The normal dimensions of a premenopausal ovary are 2.2–5.5 cm in length, 1.5–2.0 cm in width, and 1.5–3.0 cm in depth (anteroposterior dimension) (11). Others have obtained different measurements (12–14).

The blood supply to the ovaries is derived from two sources. Arising from the abdominal aorta, just caudal to the origins of the renal arteries, the ovarian arteries enter the pelvis through the infundibulopelvic ligament. They reach the ovaries through the hilus via the mesovarium. From each artery originate primary and secondary branches. These branches spiral, perhaps allowing for extension as follicles grow. The ovaries are also supplied by the ovarian branches of the uterine arteries. The ovarian divisions of the uterine arteries anastomose with the ipsilateral ovarian arteries (15).

The gray scale findings of the ovaries during the normal menstrual cycle are predominantly related to the development and resolution of follicular cysts. From Day 1 of a normal menstrual cycle until the midcycle, progressive enlargement of the follicle cysts occurs. The inner dimension of a mature follicle measures between 17 and 25 mm (16). The average diameter of a preovulatory follicle is 20 mm (17,18). Others have obtained different measurements (19,20). Around the midcycle, the dominant follicle cyst ruptures, releasing the egg and fluid it contains (21,22). The ruptured follicle forms the corpus luteum cyst (13) (Fig. 1). This structure either will undergo resolution if no pregnancy occurs or will remain in the event of a normal pregnancy (23).

It should be remembered that the corpus luteum is the great sonographic mimic within the female pelvis. Its appearance can simulate other entities including an endometrioma, an abscess, a neoplasm, or an ectopic pregnancy (24).

Multiple ovulation is an event that occurs in approximately 5% of unstimulated cycles (19). Interestingly, in our experience, a substantial proportion of spontaneous multiple ovulators have a family history (self, mother, grandmother, aunt, cousin) of multiple births.

Concomitant with the gray scale changes, both color and duplex Doppler changes can be demonstrated.

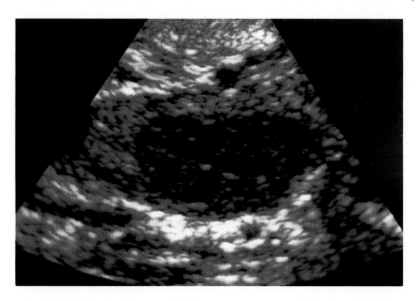

FIG. 1. A corpus luteum. The interior of the corpus luteum is filled with echoes, representing blood (clot). Ovarian parenchyma is seen surrounding the corpus luteum.

The ovarian arterial supply exhibits different flow characteristics during the different phases of a normal menstrual cycle (25–27). These phases are as follows: early follicular (Days 5–7), late follicular (Days 11–13), early luteal (Days 15–17), and late luteal (Days 26–28). In general, the index values for these arteries are relatively high during the early follicular phase. They progressively decrease to the lower values seen in the early luteal phase. During the late luteal phase a rise in values is seen (25–27). The variations are believed to be hormone-related and reflect changes in vascular compliance. Increased compliance leads to the increased blood flow seen during the late follicular and early luteal phases. Other patterns have been described (26).

Kurjak et al. determined that ovarian artery blood flow is detectable when the dominant follicle reaches a size of 12–15 mm (28). The resistance index (RI) is 0.54 ± 0.04 and declines the day before ovulation. The nadir of 0.44 ± 0.04 is reached 4–5 days later and rises to 0.50 ± 0.04 before menstruation.

Differences in flow characteristics between the dominant and nondominant ovaries have been demonstrated (25,27). These differences are significant and appear to develop relatively early during the menstrual cycle (25–27). End-diastolic flow may not be seen until later than Day 7. In the ovary containing the dominant follicle, continuous diastolic flow may be seen from one cardiac cycle to the next by the early luteal phase. In contrast, both diastolic flow and cyclical changes may be absent in the ovary without the corpus luteum (25,27). Multiple ovulators may not demonstrate interovarian differences in flow velocity waveforms and index values when each ovary contains a corpus luteum.

Color Doppler ultrasound can demonstrate the neovascularity within the wall of the corpus luteum (21). Demonstrable color flow surrounding the developing dominant follicle becomes more apparent as the midcycle

approaches and continues around the corpus luteum until the late luteal phase. In the event of a pregnancy, both the low resistance flow and the color flow to the corpus luteum may remain until approximately the eleventh week of amenorrhea (29).

Luteal phase abnormalities may be diagnosed by duplex and color Doppler. The functional status of a corpus luteum may be assessed by detecting its characteristic low-impedance flow and the appearance of the color flow surrounding it (23,30; see section, "Ovulation Induction and IVF").

Is the flow to the corpus luteum different between patients who are pregnant and those who are not? Yes, according to the work of Zalud and Kurjak (29). Comparing RI values, these investigators found significant flow differences between the two groups. The RI for pregnant patients (0.53 ± 0.09) was higher than those who were not pregnant (0.42 ± 0.12).

Is the flow to the corpus luteum different between patients who are pregnant with ectopics from those who have intrauterine pregnancies (IUPs)? According to these same investigators, the answer is yes (29). Patients with ectopic pregnancies were found to have lower RIs (0.48 ± 0.07) than those with IUPs (0.53 ± 0.09), but not lower than nonpregnant patients (0.42 ± 0.12).

During the postmenopausal years of a normal female, the ovaries undergo changes characterized by diminution in size and decreased or absent folliculogenesis (31). In fact, the reliable identification of an ovary can often no longer be made by demonstrating follicle cysts surrounded by ovarian parenchyma. One occasionally must resort to scanning along the route of the internal iliac vessels to discover its location (7,8). Gray scale examination generally reveals an inverse relationship between ovarian size and the time since menopause: ovarian size progressively decreases as the duration of the postmenopausal period increases (9,10,31). However, patients receiving hormone replacement therapy may demonstrate no changes in ovarian volume (31). Reliable identification of the postmenopausal ovary may be noted in only 20% of patients, although some claim better results, even approaching 100% (32–37).

Just how big is a postmenopausal ovary? Apparently, it depends on the investigator. According to Schoenfeld et al., the mean ovarian volume (calculated as [length × width × height]/2) in normal postmenopausal women is 1.3 ± 0.7 cm^3 (34). Aboulghar et al. determined the postmenopausal ovarian volume to be 3.4 ± 1.7 cm^3 (38). Goswamy calculated right ovarian volume at 3.58 ± 1.40 cm^3 (range 1.00–14.01) and left ovarian volume at 3.57 ± 1.37 cm^3 (range 0.88–10.90) (35).

Concomitant with the gray scale changes seen in postmenopausal women, both color and duplex Doppler changes can be demonstrated.

As there is no menstrual cycle, the sequential changes in blood flow to the ovary seen during the reproductive years are generally not demonstrated in the normal postmenopausal patient.

These cyclical changes, however, may be evident if the patient is on hormone replacement therapy. In fact, a premenopausal ovarian blood flow pattern in a postmenopausal patient should prompt the search for a history of hormone replacement therapy (although there are other differential diagnostic possibilities).

In the postmenopausal patient (as with the premenopausal patient), one of the most important uses of ultrasound involves the diagnosis and characterization of adnexal masses.

To diagnose the presence of an adnexal mass, gray scale ultrasound is of substantial importance (7,9,35, 39,40). This is especially true as the postmenopausal ovary may not be reliably palpated (36,38). In one study, 10% of masses less than 10 cm in size were missed on palpation (41). Transvaginal sonography is generally more sensitive than transabdominal sonography (1,7, 42,43). Some investigators feel that the absence of an adnexal mass on gray scale examination may not rule out the presence of a malignancy, whereas others presume that it does (32,44,45).

Interestingly, many postmenopausal women (10–15%) continue to demonstrate cysts within their ovaries (10,40,46–50). Ovarian cancers may manifest their presence as postmenopausal cysts (10,44,51–53). In fact, 80% of ovarian neoplasms occur in women older than 50 years of age and of these as much as 85–90% are of a cystic epithelial type (40,54,55). Also, some patients clinically diagnosed as "postmenopausal" are, in reality, perimenopausal and continue to "cycle," though irregularly. This latter differential diagnostic possibility can generally be confirmed clinically, biochemically, or by follow-up ultrasound examination.

For characterizing a discovered mass, gray scale and Doppler (both duplex and color) ultrasound may be of

significant utility in distinguishing benign from malignant processes (45,48,49,56–58).

Gray scale sonography has been used with varying success to characterize adnexal disease (45,59–62). Findings such as septations, papillary projections, and mural nodules are more likely to be associated with malignant changes than are clear cystic masses (46,56,59,63). Also, size may be important (31,34,40,41,50,59,64–67). Rulin and Preston found that masses less than 5.0 cm were unlikely to be malignant (41). In their series, only one case of cystic ovarian mass in 32 (3%) was malignant. In a study by Goldstein et al., the results of sonographically detected simple cysts (defined as cysts without internal septations or solid components) of the adnexa yielded a 0% incidence of malignancy in patients with cysts less than 5.0 cm in maximum diameter (40). Hall and McCarthy included septated cysts in their definition of "simple cyst." They found an 8% malignancy rate in their series of cysts ranging from 1.5 to 10.0 cm. One malignancy was within a 3.5-cm nonseptated cyst (67).

Some investigators have concluded that both color and duplex Doppler are valuable tools for the diagnosis of ovarian and other malignancies (44,51,53,68–72). These conclusions are based on the unique differences between normal and tumoral vascularity (neovascularity) and the apparent ability of Doppler sonography to distinguish between them (68,73).

Tumor vessels are disorganized. The standard hierarchical organization of normal vessels, in which flow progresses from arteries of decreasing size through capillaries to veins of increasing size, is absent. Instead, tumoral flow may be short-circuited through shunts (30,70). Also, tumor vessels may possess altered architecture (74,75).

Abnormal flow patterns can be demonstrated in vessels surrounding malignant masses (70,76,77). Finding these areas of neovascularity may not be possible on gray scale examination only. Because color Doppler may make these vessels visible, it allows the examiner to survey the anatomy of the target structure for vascular areas of interest (78).

There is substantial data to suggest that the flow characteristics of some malignant diseases of the ovary are different from benign processes (29,44,53,79,80). In general, a low-resistance pattern is unusual in the ovary of a postmenopausal patient, as are low index values, and may be associated with malignancy (52). False positives do occur (44). The absence of neovascularity and the presence of a normal index value has been shown to exclude malignancy, whereas the presence of neovascularity had a high association with malignant change (51,81).

Doppler ultrasound for adnexal masses should be performed within Days 3–10 of the menstrual cycle in menstruating patients; within Days 3–10 in postmenopausal patients on hormone replacement therapy; at anytime in postmenopausal patients not on replacement (78).

THE UTERUS

The uterus is located in the lesser pelvis between the urinary bladder and the rectum. Although generally a midline structure, lateral deviations of the uterus are not uncommon. The broad ligaments extend from the uterus laterally to the pelvic side walls. They contain the fallopian tubes and vessels. The uterosacral ligaments serve to keep the uterus in an anterior position. They arise from the upper cervix posteriorly and extend to the fascia over the second and third sacral vertebrae. The round ligaments arise anterior to and below the fallopian tubes and cross the inguinal canal to end in the upper portion of the labia majora (82).

The normal adult uterus measures approximately 7.0–9.0 cm long, 4.5–6.0 cm wide, and 2.5–3.5 cm deep (anteroposterior dimension) (82). Its corpus-to-cervix ratio is 2:1 (82,83).

The blood supply to the uterus is via the uterine artery, a branch of the internal iliac artery. This vessel enters the uterus at the cervicocorporal junction and ascends along the lateral aspect of the uterine body to the cornua. At the uterine cornua an adnexal branch originates that supplies the ipsilateral ovary and anastomoses with the ipsilateral ovarian artery (84).

From the uterine artery arise perforating branches that extend through the serosa. The uterine arteries anastomose through the anterior and posterior arcuate vessels. These vessels are located in the outer one-third of the myometrium, between the exterior longitudinal muscle fibers and the inner oblique muscle fibers (85).

The blood supply to the endometrium is derived from branches of the uterine arteries. Radiating from the arcuate arteries are the radial arteries. These vessels extend through the myometrium to just outside the endometrium where they form terminal branches of two types: straight and coiled. The straight branches, also called basal arteries, supply the basalis layer of the endometrium. The coiled branches, also called spiral arteries, traverse the endometrium and supply the functionalis layer. The spiral arteries, like the endometrium and unlike the basal arteries, are remarkably responsive to the hormonal changes of the menstrual cycle (86).

During the reproductive years of a normal female, the uterus undergoes sonographically detectable changes characterized by cyclical alterations in the appearance of the endometrium. In fact, it is possible to infer the approximate day of a normal woman's menstrual cycle by the ultrasound appearance of her endometrium (87).

Following menstruation until the midcycle, progressive thickening and layering of the normal endometrium occur (Fig. 2). Past the midcycle, brightening and progressive thinning of the endometrium occur (88). These sonographic endometrial patterns appear to be related to the changes in the glandular and vascular elements of the endometrium during the menstrual cycle (89–91).

Fleischer et al. determined that the endometrium is thickest during the secretory phase (3.6 ± 1.4 mm), less thick during the proliferative phase (2.9 ± 1.0 mm) and thinnest during menstruation (90,91). The values obtained are for half-thickness as measured from the endometrial canal to the endometrial–myometrial interface. Full-thickness measurements ranged from 4 to 12 mm, with an average thickness of 7.5 mm. The endometrium will either slough if no pregnancy occurs or will undergo various changes in the event of a pregnancy.

Concomitant with the gray scale changes, both color and duplex Doppler changes can be demonstrated.

The general pattern of uterine blood flow throughout the menstrual cycle is that perfusion increases in response to rising plasma estrogen and progesterone and

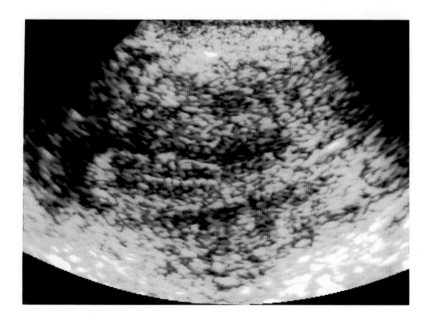

FIG. 2. The typical five-line appearance of the endometrium is seen in sagittal plane. Note the endometrial canal located centrally. On either side are relatively hypoechoic areas. These areas are surrounded by a relatively hyperechoic area immediately adjacent to the myometrium.

decreases with the periovulatory fall in estrogen (29,92–94). The lowest pulsatility index (PI) values are seen around Days 8 and 21, whereas the highest values are seen around Days 1, 14, and 17 (92,94). Significant changes in diastolic blood flow at the different times of the cycle may not be noted (26,95). In general, the index values for the uterine artery ipsilateral to the ovary containing the dominant follicle are lower than the contralateral artery (87).

Other patterns of uterine artery blood flow have been described (87). When the uterine arteries were interrogated at the level of the uterine cornua, the PI reached its peak by Day 11 and remained relatively constant until Day 16. The lowest values were generally seen around Days 1 and 21. At this anatomic level, end-diastolic flow was commonly absent during the early follicular phase but was demonstrable by the luteal phase.

The cyclical changes reflected by the flow velocity waveforms and index values appear to be mediated by the reproductive hormones (96). Patients with inactive ovaries on transdermal estradiol and vaginal progesterone therapy were studied using transvaginal ultrasound technique. These patients received their medications on a 28-day regimen. The baseline evaluation (pretreatment) demonstrated a narrow systolic spectral flow pattern with a mean PI of 5.2 ± 0.4. Evaluations performed on Days 13–14 showed a spectral tracing that was broader with an uninterrupted diastolic component. The mean PI was 1.5 ± 0.2. On Days 26–27, no significant differences were noted (mean PI = 1.7 ± 0.3).

The blood flow to the endometrium undergoes changes that are described below (see section, "Ovulation Induction and IVF").

In the event of a pregnancy, low-resistance flow to the uterus remains. In my experience, the finding of blood flow within the endometrium, on gray scale examination, has been reliably associated with the gravid state (97). I have seen this in both IVF and non-IVF patients. False positives or false negatives have rarely occurred. This flow has been visible as early as day 27 after the last normal menstrual cycle, prior to visualization of the gestational sac and with a β-hCG of 156 (97). The distribution of this finding may not be generalized. This is similar to the pathologic specimens in which endometrial changes induced by the sex hormones demonstrate nonuniform, regional differences (86). In one case, very localized changes were demonstrated. It was in this area that the gestational sac eventually appeared. Histologically, at the time of implantation (the seventh day following ovulation), hypertrophic and proliferative changes of the spiral arterioles occur within the endometrium (86). As the blastocyst implants over these spiral vessels, those beneath the lower pole of the implanting blastocyst hypertrophy further with the capillaries in the surrounding stroma dilating widely and their walls thinning. It is possible that these are the changes that were reflected on ultrasound examination (86). The finding of endometrial blood flow is not specific for intrauterine gestations, as it can be seen in the presence of ectopic pregnancies (97,98). Perhaps this represents a sonographic appearance of the Arias–Stella reaction (99).

During the postmenopausal years of a normal female, the uterus decreases in size and the endometrium atrophies.

As the ovaries undergo involution, there is an associated reduction in the amount of estrogen produced. This leads to the gradual atrophy and involution of the endometrium that characterizes the uterine lining of the postmenopausal patient (100,101). In asymptomatic postmenopausal women, the mean endometrial thickness has been determined to be 3.2 ± 0.7 mm, although other investigators have reached different conclusions (91,101–107).

Gray scale examination generally reveals an inverse relationship between uterine size and the time since menopause: uterine size and volume decrease as the duration of the postmenopausal period increases. The greatest changes occur within the first 10 years after the menopause and more gradually thereafter (108).

Just how big is the postmenopausal uterus? The postmenopausal uterus has been measured at 8.0 ± 1.2 cm long by 5.0 ± 0.8 cm wide by 3.2 ± 0.7 cm deep (anteroposterior dimension). A significant relationship between parity and both uterine volume and weight was not found (108). Others have reached different conclusions (109–111).

As there is no menstrual cycle, successive changes in blood flow to the uterus are generally not demonstrated. However, some similarities between pre- and postmenopausal women may be present. Kurjak and Zalud compared the RI values of the uterine arteries in pre- and postmenopausal women. The RI was noted to be higher in the postmenopausal patients, but apparently not statistically different. Diastolic flow was demonstrated in all subjects (112).

If the patient is on hormone replacement therapy, the above-described findings may not be present (107). Among these patients, both uterine size and cyclical endometrial changes may remain. Even the corpus-to-cervix ratio approximates the premenopausal state (83). In general, estrogen therapy affects the postmenopausal endometrium similarly to estrogens in the normal cycle. The conjugated estrogens have a proliferative effect (100). Progestational therapy may cause the endometrium to respond with a quiescent appearance that is characteristic of the normal secretory endometrium (100). When used together with exogenous estrogens, synthetic progestogens reproduce the characteristic biochemical and morphologic changes seen in the secretory phase of the normal menstrual cycle.

Bourne et al. showed altered blood flow to the uterus in patients receiving hormone replacement therapy

(113). Using endovaginal ultrasound, significant arterial changes were demonstrated. The PI was reduced by 50% within 6–10 weeks of initiating therapy. Also, endometrial thickness almost doubled. Before treatment, the mean thickness was 0.37 ± 0.08 cm. Following treatment, the values were 0.68 ± 0.13 cm. Others have reported a possible 2- to 3-mm increase in endometrial thickness in patients receiving estrogen therapy (105). But some have obtained results different from the above (107). Their data suggest no statistically significant differences between the endometrial thicknesses of patients taking and patients not taking hormones.

Thus, a premenopausal-appearing uterus or uterine blood flow pattern in a postmenopausal woman should prompt the search for a history of hormone replacement therapy (although there are other differential diagnostic possibilities) (114,115).

In the postmenopausal patient, one of the most important uses of ultrasound involves the diagnosis and management of endometrial cancer. In general, endovaginal ultrasound is superior to transabdominal ultrasound for visualization of the myometrium and endometrium (63,116).

Sonographic signs of endometrial cancer in the postmenopausal patient include an obstructed fluid-filled canal, a thickened uterine cavity, an enlarged uterus, and a lobular uterus with a mixed-echo pattern (117). Gray scale ultrasound has accurately demonstrated the presence and extent of myometrial invasion. Cacciatore et al., using transabdominal technique, found that sonographic staging of endometrial cancer by ultrasound was accurate in 91% of cases and myometrial invasion was correctly identified in 80% of cases (118). Transvaginally, Cruickshank et al. demonstrated good agreement between the ultrasound examination and myometrial invasion as determined microscopically (119). These investigators suggested that more accurate preoperative diagnosis may allow for selective therapies, perhaps yielding better results. Granberg et al., using transvaginal technique, demonstrated that with a full-thickness endometrial measurement of 8 mm or less, in patients with postmenopausal bleeding, no endometrial cancer was discovered by curettage (101). In general, the data would seem to indicate that a full-thickness postmenopausal endometrium of 10 mm or greater should be further evaluated, either by biopsy or D&C, to exclude either malignancy or hyperplasia (43,91,102,105,106, 120,121).

Some investigators have demonstrated the utility of Doppler ultrasound in diagnosing endometrial cancer. Bourne et al. demonstrated increased blood flow in the uterine artery and the area of the suspected tumor in patients with malignant disease (114). One group appears to have substantial experience in evaluating pelvic masses and distinguishing benign from malignant disease (53,79,80). It is their conclusion that abnormal blood flow can be identified in virtually all cases of endometrial carcinoma as well as uterine sarcoma. With color Doppler, the abnormal findings include the presence of irregular, thin, and randomly distributed vessels. Abnormal flow velocity waveform patterns have also been described (71).

OVULATION INDUCTION AND IVF

All IVF treatment regimens are designed to maximize the likelihood of a successful implantation (and, hopefully, a take-home baby). To this end, IVF protocols attempt medical hyperstimulation of the ovaries to produce multiple follicles of sufficient size for an egg harvesting procedure (122). The aspirated eggs are exposed to sperm for fertilization. Fertilized eggs are subsequently transferred to the uterus via catheter in the hope that one or more will implant. Other strategies, such as ZIFT (zygote intrafallopian transfer), GIFT (gamete intrafallopian transfer), and transfer of thawed embryos are also employed (123).

Infertility is the end result of numerous causes. These include (this list is not exhaustive):

Mechanical (e.g., fibroids, endometriosis, tubal blockage, endometrial polyps, synechiae, etc.)

Genetic (e.g., Turner's syndrome, premature ovarian failure, etc.)

Developmental (e.g., congenital organ absence, congenital anomalies of the uterus, etc.)

Iatrogenic (e.g., organ removal/ablation)

Vascular (poor uterine perfusion), or

Endocrine (e.g., polycystic ovaries)

Many of these conditions are diagnosable by ultrasound.

Rather than describe each of the myriad causes of infertility, the reader is referred to the available texts on this subject. Instead, some of the more common causes, their associated ultrasound findings, and the potential value of Doppler imaging will be presented.

Fibroids

Uterine leiomyomas may be associated with infertility (124,125). Although fibroids are generally seen on gray scale examination, their borders are not always well demarcated. In this situation, color flow Doppler imaging may be of benefit. Frequently, vascular structures can be seen surrounding the myoma, making localization and measurement more accurate. This can be of significance in patients undergoing medical treatment to decrease fibroid size and blood flow prior to surgical removal or attempted IVF (126,127). Monitoring is thereby made easier. Patients receiving gonadotropin-releasing hormone (GnRH) agonists demonstrate impedance to vascular flow while on treatment. This suggests that any decrease in fibroid size may be related to hypoestrogenic-mediated reduction in blood flow (128). I have investigated pre- and posttreatment flow velocities to fibroids but have yet to define predictors of response to medical therapy with GnRH agonists. Of interest, careful examination using gray scale can also reveal flow differences between fibroids and the surrounding myometrium. Also, color Doppler can help make an otherwise iso-echoic myoma apparent by demonstrating either its blood supply or the vessels it displaces.

Endometriosis

Endometriosis is also associated with infertility. The mechanism by which this occurs is either mechanical or uncertain. Gray scale scanning may detect the classical homogeneously echogenic intraovarian endometrioma. Occasionally, small endometriomas may appear as subtle, mottled areas within the ovary. Again, color Doppler may demonstrate flow around and not within these apparently solid structures, thereby highlighting and confirming their presence and suggesting the diagnosis. Extraovarian endometriosis is usually difficult to visualize.

Tubal Abnormalities

The application of ultrasound to the diagnosis of tubal abnormalities has been broadened through the use of Doppler. By using contrast medium and duplex Doppler, disorders, especially obstructions, can be evaluated with greater accuracy than by gray scale alone (129). To diagnose patency, the addition of color flow Doppler may not provide any advantage over duplex Doppler (130) although in my experience color Doppler is valuable in diagnosing tubal blockage. Fallopian tube masses can be diagnosed and characterized by color and duplex Doppler techniques (131).

Vascular

The possibility that decreased uterine blood flow may be associated with infertility was investigated by Goswamy et al. (132). In their study, the uterine arteries of patients who had been unsuccessful in three attempts at IVF were interrogated using Doppler ultrasound. Almost half demonstrated a poor midsecretory uterine response. Of these, patients demonstrating improved uterine perfusion on oral hormone therapy had a pregnancy rate comparable to or better than that obtained in the first three attempts by other patients. Although the numbers of patients in each group studied were too small for statistical analyses, the trend suggested that improving uterine perfusion may improve the outcome of IVF therapy. Two years later, results from a greater number of patients were reported (133). This confirmed the results

of the earlier work. The data indicated that 20% of all women undergoing IVF therapy would have poor uterine perfusion. This latter work utilized the concept of a perfusion index to analyze the flow velocity waveform. This index is derived from the ratio of the area under the curve of the systolic component of the flow velocity waveform ($*S$) over the area beneath the diastolic component ($*D$) (Perfusion Index = $*S/*D$). This analysis allows for a different approach to the evaluation of the waveform.[1]

In preparation for implantation, the endometrium undergoes transformations influenced by the ovarian hormones produced during the early secretory phase. These modifications include an increased rate of blood flow, an increase in the number of cells in the stroma and epithelium, an increase in uterine oxygen consumption, an increase in oxygen diffusion into the uterine lumen, and a generalized edema (13). The spiral arteries, like the endometrium (and unlike the basal arteries), are remarkably responsive to the hormonal changes of the menstrual cycle and undergo transformations as well (86). These include endothelial proliferation, wall thickening, and coiling. These vessels play an important role in implantation. The chances for a normal implantation may be reduced if the spiral arterioles are inadequately developed (100).

In my experience, changes in endometrial vascularity appear present on color Doppler examination that may reflect the histologic changes described by the pathologists (134,135). Vascular penetration toward the endometrial canal differs among patients. Some investigators appear unable to demonstrate this (136). Perhaps this is due to equipment or technique differences.

If one divides the endometrial and periendometrial areas into the following four Zones (Fig. 3):

Zone 1—a 2-mm-thick area surrounding the hyperechoic outer layer of the endometrium
Zone 2—the hyperechoic outer layer of the endometrium
Zone 3—the hypoechoic inner layer of the endometrium
Zone 4—the endometrial cavity

it is possible to see variations in the depth of vascular penetration before, during, and after the midcycle. In patients with uterine artery PIs of less than 3.0, my prelim-

---

[1] These investigators performed their $*S/*D$ analysis using a new computer program. It has been our practice to perform a similar type of analysis in the following fashion: Once the spectral tracing is obtained, the angle correction is set to the minimum angle (a constant) where both velocity and frequency can be measured. The area beneath the systolic component of the waveform is calculated. Then the area beneath the diastolic component of the waveform is calculated. The ratio between the two is derived. Our experience to date is insufficient to reach a conclusion regarding the usefulness of this approach. However, it is apparent that different-appearing waveforms have yielded similar RI or PI values. A different approach to waveform analysis may assist in distinguishing among such tracings.

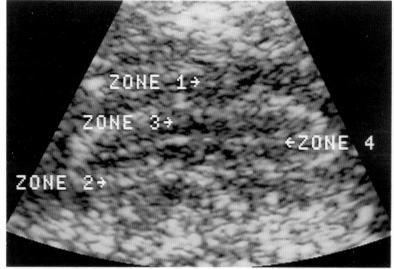

FIG. 3. The typical five-line appearance of the endometrium is seen in coronal plane. Zones 1–4 are indicated.

inary results have not revealed any successful pregnancies in IVF patients unless there is vascularity demonstrated either within Zone 3 or within Zones 3 and 4 prior to transfer. Successful pregnancies with demonstrable blood flow in Zone 4, suggesting the presence of an intracavitary mass, have been noted. I have also been looking at both the thicknesses and the relative thicknesses of these Zones, the spectral tracings obtained from the different Zones, the ratio of the index values, and the ratio of the values obtained from the endometrial vessels and the uterine and ovarian vessels, but have yet to reach a conclusion. Most patients without diagnosed infertility (presumed normal) usually demonstrate flow into Zone 3 by the midcycle (134) (Fig. 4). I have not yet determined if patients without both diagnosed infertility and midcycle flow past Zone 2 are more likely to be infertile. Such a prospective study may prove interesting (Figs. 5–9).

These color Doppler findings in unsuccessful cycles may relate to the histologic findings described by Sterzik et al. (137). In their study of 58 IVF patients, a majority demonstrated an immature endometrium at the time of embryo transfer. The abnormalities included a variety of patterns, all indicating a lack of secretory transformation suggestive of unpreparedness for implantation.

The complete evaluation of the IVF patient may require attention to the gray scale appearance of the endometrium as well. Glissant et al. noted that the thickness of the endometrium was significantly greater in cycles resulting in a pregnancy than those that did not, although it was not possible to predict the probability of a pregnancy based on endometrial thickness (138). In contrast, Welker et al. were unable to relate endometrial thickness to outcome but were able to relate endometrial pattern to outcome. In their experience, the five-line appearance was the most likely to be associated with im-

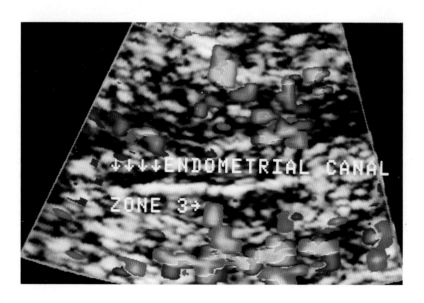

FIG. 4. Normal penetration of Day 14 blood flow within the endometrium. Note the Zone 1 vascularity surrounding the endometrium, seen best at bottom. Projecting from Zone 1 is a vessel extending through Zone 2 into Zone 3.

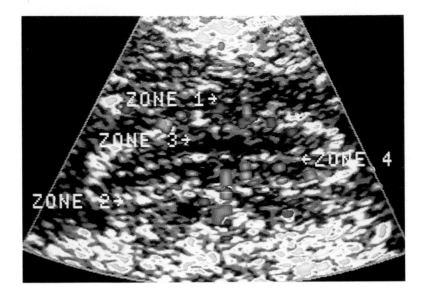

FIG. 5. Blood flow from Zone 1 to Zone 3. The typical five-line appearance of the endometrium is seen in coronal plane. Extending from Zone 1 is a vessel projecting through Zone 2 into Zone 3. Compare this figure with Fig. 4. Note more areas of flow within Zone 3 in this patient. It should be remembered that endometrial flow of this type may not be seen in all areas and may be distributed unevenly within the endometrium. Careful and complete examination of the endometrium is necessary to conclude that flow is absent.

plantation (139). Smith et al. felt that both endometrial thickness and pattern were important (140). Other investigators have also looked at the relationship between endometrial thickness or texture and outcome (141–144).

In a retrospective study of non-IVF medically stimulated cycles, Kepic et al. determined that endometrial thickness and pattern, follicle size, and estradiol levels correlated not only with the likelihood of pregnancy but with subsequent outcome (i.e., miscarriage vs. nonmiscarriage) (145,146).

During ovarian stimulation, the waveform and index value differences normally noted between the two ovaries may be absent. Bilaterally, the ovarian arterial blood supply may demonstrate pulsatility waveforms typical of low impedance (27).

During the stimulation process, ultrasound has its greatest contribution in monitoring follicular development and guiding the oocyte harvesting procedure (147,148).

Different stimulation protocols may produce mature follicles at different size thresholds (149). Also, the gross sonographic morphology of the follicles may be different depending on the medication used. For example, ovaries stimulated with human menopausal gonadotropins tend to have more polygonal cysts and "stacked coin" appearances, whereas clomiphene citrate–induced follicles are generally more spherical. Depending on the stimulation protocol, aspiration may be performed following the ad-

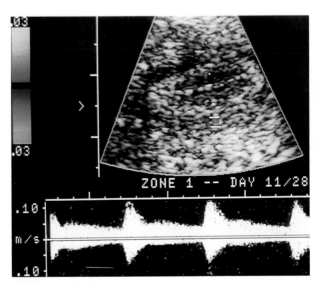

FIG. 6. Zone 1 flow velocity waveform. I have yet to observe a successful pregnancy in an IVF patient when blood flow goes no further than this Zone.

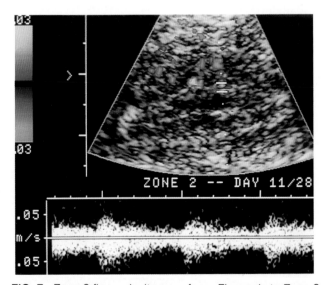

FIG. 7. Zone 2 flow velocity waveform. Flow only to Zone 2 is, in my experience, relatively rare. In IVF patients with flow only to Zone 2, I have not observed a successful pregnancy; however, the number of patients within this category is quite small.

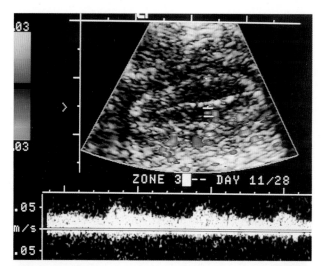

FIG. 8. Zone 3 flow velocity waveform. In my experience, blood flow within Zone 3 has been most reliably associated with successful pregnancies in IVF patients. I have yet to correlate time of Zone 3 blood flow appearance with outcome. It is possible that "late developers" may have outcomes different from "early developers." In patients referred for conditions other than infertility (presumed normals), I have observed Zone 3 blood flow with regularity. I do not know if presumed normal patients in whom this finding may be absent will subsequently have difficulty conceiving. Zone 4 blood flow has also been associated with successful pregnancies. This pattern has been seen with intracavitary masses.

ministration of human chorionic gonadotropin (hCG). The hCG acts as a surrogate luteinizing hormone (LH) surge (122). The timing of the hCG administration may be determined by the size of the follicles (150,151). Gray scale evaluation of ovarian follicles can help distinguish physiologic from insufficient or abnormal cycles. Transvaginal color Doppler can be employed to assess the physiologic development of the follicles through depiction of flow parameters (85,152,153).

Egg aspiration, performed transvaginally under ultrasound guidance, is considered the state of the art. Prior to this method, various laparoscopic techniques were employed (154,155). Obviously, the ultrasound-guided procedure is far less invasive (156).

The application of duplex and color Doppler ultrasound to the aspiration phase of the IVF process is not widespread. This is to be expected because:

1. There is good success in monitoring follicle growth and obtaining eggs using gray scale technique only, and
2. The inherent annoyance in monitoring an aspiration under color Doppler (due to motion artifacting) would be undesirable.

Ovarian hyperstimulation syndrome (OHS) is one of the possible complications of IVF treatment. Various investigators have attempted to predict its occurrence (157,158). Generally, the presence of multiple small or intermediate size follicles prior to stimulation is associated with the development of OHS, while the presence of several large follicles is associated with no OHS development. Color Doppler imaging is most useful for the diagnosis of ovarian torsion, a complication of OHS. In this case, lack of blood flow may be demonstrated. It is important to remember that the ovary possesses a dual blood supply, one of which may be compromised to a greater degree than the other. Duplex Doppler findings include a lack of diastolic flow with a "spike" configuration of the systolic peak or a loss of phasic venous flow (159).

Some IVF programs use ultrasound to guide the transfer catheter to an optimal location by the uterine fundus (156). This is accomplished using gray scale technique. Others use ultrasound to guide GIFT procedures, claiming superiority over hysteroscopically guided tubal cannulation (160).

Doppler ultrasound has been used as a means to predict a negative outcome for a given IVF cycle. Pretransfer, if failure could be predicted, the embryos could be frozen until a more favorable cycle occurs. This could prevent embryo wastage and subsequent patient disappointment. Posttransfer, earlier prediction of failure could help some patients cope better with the setback.

Sterzik et al. examined the ovarian and uterine arteries on the day of follicle aspiration. The conclusion they derived was that in patients who became pregnant after

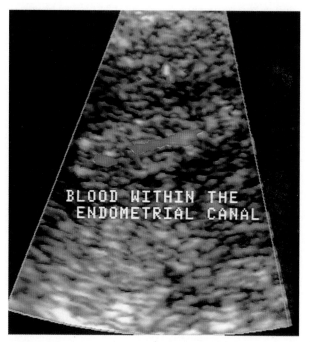

FIG. 9. Blood within the endometrial canal. One should not confuse endometrial vascularity (particularly zone 4) on color Doppler examination with blood flowing within the endometrial canal during menses.

embryo transfer, the RI of the uterine arteries was significantly lower than that of those who did not get pregnant (137).

Steer et al. demonstrated that patients with a low uterine artery PI on the day of embryo transfer were more likely to conceive than those with a high PI. In this series, no one with a PI > 3.0 conceived (161).

In my experience, inadequate vascular penetration of endometrial blood flow (i.e., not within Zone 3) prior to transfer has been associated with an unfavorable outcome (see above).

Taylor et al. showed that the absence of luteal flow could be used to predict an abortion (30). In general, the normal corpa lutea demonstrates relatively bright flow almost completely around its periphery (Fig. 10). In both the IVF and non-IVF settings, I have seen pregnant patients whose corpora lutea demonstrated subjectively decreased color flow—either in intensity or surface area (Fig. 11). This has accompanied both low progesterone levels and subsequent embryonal demise. Whether earlier detection and initiation of treatment would salvage such a pregnancy remains to be seen.

Baber et al. showed that patients with a successful transfer cycle demonstrated RI values for the blood flow to the corpus luteum that were significantly different from those who had unsuccessful transfer cycles. These investigators concluded that no patients who became pregnant had an RI greater than 0.5. Spectral tracings, without color visualization of the vessels, were obtained (162).

Battaglia et al. demonstrated a progressive decrease in the PI of the uterine arteries during the second half of the menstrual cycle in successful IVF pregnancies (163).

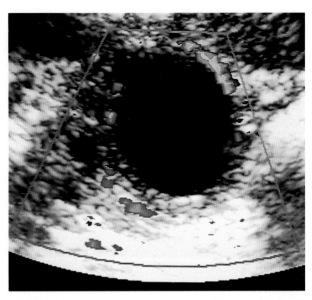

FIG. 11. A corpus luteum of pregnancy. Observe the quality of blood flow demonstrated on color Doppler examination. Appreciate its "anemic" appearance with relatively little flow. This corpus luteum was associated with a pregnancy that subsequently failed. The progesterone levels were low. Compare with Fig. 10.

Of course, one of the consequences of IVF is an increased incidence of ectopic pregnancy. According to Taylor et al., transabdominal duplex Doppler evaluation appears superior to gray scale technique in the diagnosis of extrauterine gestations (30). For Doppler, the positive predictive value (PPD) was 85% and the negative predic-

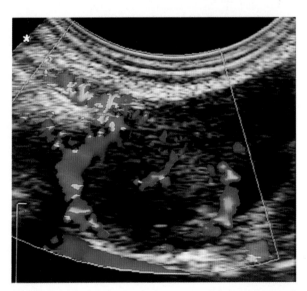

FIG. 10. A corpus luteum of pregnancy. Observe the quality of blood flow demonstrated on color Doppler examination. Appreciate its "robust" appearance and high velocity flow. This corpus luteum was associated with a successful pregnancy and normal progesterone levels. Compare with Fig. 11.

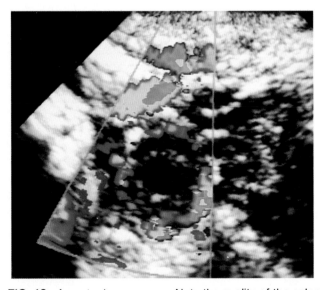

FIG. 12. An ectopic pregnancy. Note the quality of the color surrounding this ectopic gestation. No embryo was present. Compare with Figs. 10 and 11. Observe the similarity in appearance to a corpus luteum. Although this ectopic was apparent without the use of color Doppler, in difficult cases, a survey of the adnexae using color Doppler may reveal the presence of an ectopic gestation.

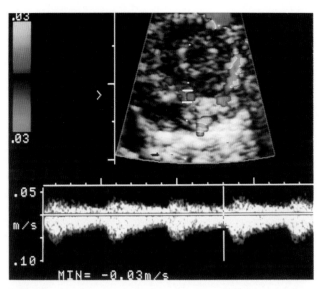

FIG. 13. An ectopic pregnancy. The flow velocity waveform demonstrates low resistance to flow. Although this flow is seen surrounding a well-defined sac, the presence of rupture, bleeding, or clot formation may distort the color pattern. Flow may then appear in scattered areas within the clot.

tive value (NPD) was 81%. For gray scale the PPD was 47% and the NPD was 60%. Color flow Doppler ultrasound evaluation of ectopic pregnancies has been performed (164,165). Transvaginally, ectopics may appear as very colorful areas of low-impedance flow with an RI below 0.40, although others have obtained different values (166) (Figs. 12 and 13). It has been suggested that the behavior of ectopic pregnancies may be predicted based on the duplex and color Doppler findings (30,167,168). This may assist in the making of management decisions and the selection of an appropriate treatment (166,167).

CONCLUSION

Ultrasound imaging of the female pelvis has contributed greatly to the understanding, identification, diagnosis, treatment, and management of numerous conditions. The introduction of endovaginal scanning represented a quantum leap in our ability to image the anatomy. The advent of Doppler imaging, both duplex and color, has enabled us to extend our evaluation much further. We now possess the means to perform a sonographic physiologic assessment of the structures we visualize. How we apply this technology is currently limited only by our imaginations.

REFERENCES

1. Mendelson EB, Bohm-Velez M, Joseph N, Neiman HL. Gynecologic imaging: Comparison of transabdominal and transvaginal sonography. *Radiology* 1988;166:321–324.
2. Coleman BG, Arger PH, Grumbach K, et al. Transvaginal and transabdominal sonography: Prospective comparison. *Radiology* 1988;168:639–643.
3. Tessler FN, Schiller VL, Perrella RR, Sutherlan ML, Grant EG. Transabdominal versus endovaginal pelvic sonography: Prospective study. *Radiology* 1989;170:553–556.
4. Scanlan KA, Pozniak MA, Fagerholm M, Shapiro S. Value of transperineal sonography in the assessment of vaginal atresia. *Am J Roentgenol* 1990;154:545–548.
5. Graham D, Nelson MW. Combined perineal-abdominal sonography in the assessment of vaginal atresia. *J Clin Ultrasound* 1986;14:735–738.
6. Jeanty P, d'Alton M, Romero R, Hobbins JC. Perineal scanning. *Am J Perinatol* 1986;13:289–295.
7. Rodriguez MH, Platt LD, Medearis AL, Lobo RA. The use of transvaginal sonography for evaluation of postmenopausal ovarian size and morphology. *Am J Obstet Gynecol* 1988;159:810–814.
8. Lyons EA, Gratton D, Harrington C. Transvaginal sonography of normal pelvic anatomy. *Radiol Clin North Am* 1992;30:663–675.
9. Fleischer AC, McKee MS, Gordon AN, et al. Transvaginal sonography of postmenopausal ovaries with pathologic correlation. *J Ultrasound Med* 1990;9:637–644.
10. Wolf SI, Gosink BB, Feldesman MR, et al. Prevalence of simple adnexal cysts in postmenopausal women. *Radiology* 1991;180:65–71.
11. International Commission on Radiological Protection. Task Group on Reference Man. Report of the Task Group on Reference Man. Prepared by the Task Group Committee No. 2, International Commission on Radiological Protection, Snyder WS (chairperson). New York: Pergamon Press; 1975.
12. Sample WF, Lippe BM, Gyepes MT. Gray-scale ultrasonography of the normal female pelvis. *Radiology* 1977;125:477–483.
13. Edwards RG. *Conception in the human female.* New York: Academic Press; 1980.
14. Yeh HC, Futterweit W, Thornton JC. Polycystic ovarian disease: US features in 104 patients. *Radiology* 1987;163:111–116.
15. Hackeloer B-J, Nitschke-Dabelstein S. Ovarian imaging by ultrasound: An attempt to define a reference plane. *J Clin Ultrasound* 1980;8:497–500.
16. Fleischer AC, Daniell JF, Rodier J, Lindsay AM, James AE Jr. Sonographic monitoring of ovarian follicular development. *J Clin Ultrasound* 1981;9:275–280.
17. Bomsel-Helmreich O, Gougeon A, Thebault A, et al. Healthy and atretic human follicles in the preovulatory phase: Differences in evolution of follicular morphology and steroid content of the follicular fluid. *J Clin Endocrinol Metab* 1979;48:686–694.
18. Nitschke-Dabelstein S, Hackeloer BJ, Sturm G. Ovulation and corpus luteum formation observed by ultrasonography. *Ultrasound Med Biol* 1981;7:33–39.
19. O'Herlihy C, de Crespigny LJ Ch, Robinson HP. Monitoring ovarian follicular development with real-time ultrasound. *Br J Obstet Gynaecol* 1980;87:613–618.
20. Renaud R, Macler J, Dervain I. Echographic study of follicular maturation and ovulation during the normal menstrual cycle. *Fertil Steril* 1980;33:272–276.
21. Fleischer AC, Kepple DM, Vasquez J. Conventional and color Doppler transvaginal sonography in gynecologic infertility. *Radiol Clin North Am* 1992;30:693–702.
22. Hall DA, Hann LE, Ferrucci JT Jr, et al. Sonographic morphology of the normal menstrual cycle. *Radiology* 1979;133:185–188.
23. Dillon EH, Taylor KJW. Doppler ultrasound in the female pelvis and first trimester pregnancy. *Clin Diagn Ultrasound* 1990;26:93–117.
24. Coleman BG. Transvaginal sonography of adnexal masses. In: Coleman BG, ed. *The radiologic clinics of North America.* Philadelphia: WB Saunders; 1992;30:677–691.
25. Hata K, Hata T, Senoh D, et al. Change in ovarian arterial compliance during the human menstrual cycle assessed by Doppler ultrasound. *Br J Obstet Gynaecol* 1990;97:163–166.
26. Scholtes MCW, Wladimiroff JW, van Rijen HJM, Hop WC. Uterine and ovarian flow velocity waveforms in the normal menstrual cycle: A transvaginal Doppler study. *Fertil Steril* 1989;52:981–985.

27. Taylor KJW, Burns PN, Wells PNT, Conway DI, Hull MGR. Ultrasound Doppler flow studies of the ovarian and uterine arteries. *Br J Obstet Gynaecol* 1985;92:240–246.

28. Kurjak A, Kupesic-Urek S, Schulman H, Zalud I. Transvaginal color flow Doppler in the assessment of ovarian and uterine blood flow in infertile women. *Fert Steril* 1991;56:870–873.

29. Zalud I, Kurjak A. The assessment of luteal blood flow in pregnant and non-pregnant women by transvaginal color Doppler. *J Perinat Med* 1990;118:215–221.

30. Taylor KJW, Ramos IM, Feyock AL, et al. Ectopic pregnancy: Duplex Doppler evaluation. *Radiology* 1989;173:93–97.

31. Andolf E, Jorgensen C, Svalenius E, Sunden B. Ultrasound measurement of the ovarian volume. *Acta Obstet Gynecol Scand* 1987;66:387–389.

32. Fleischer AC. Transvaginal sonography helps find ovarian cancer. *Diagn Imaging* 1988;10:124–128.

33. Arger PH. Transvaginal ultrasonography in postmenopausal patients. In: Coleman BG, ed. *The radiologic clinics of North America.* Philadelphia: WB Saunders; 1992;30:759–767.

34. Schoenfeld A, Levavi H, Hirsch M, Pardo J, Ovadia J. Transvaginal sonography in postmenopausal women. *J Clin Ultrasound* 1990;18:350–358.

35. Goswamy RK, Campbell S, Royston JP, et al. Ovarian size in postmenopausal women. *J Obstet Gynaecol* 1988;95:795–801.

36. Granberg S, Wikland M. A comparison between ultrasound and gynecologic examination for detection of enlarged ovaries in a group of women at risk for ovarian carcinoma. *J Ultrasound Med* 1988;7:59–64.

37. Hall DA, McCarthy KA, Kopans DB. Sonographic visualization of the normal postmenopausal ovary. *J Ultrasound Med* 1985;5:9–11.

38. Aboulghar M, Mansour RT, Serour G, Sattar MA, Awad MM, Amin Y. Transvaginal ultrasonic needle-guided aspiration of pelvic inflammatory septic masses before ovulation induction for in vitro fertilization. *Fertil Steril* 1990;53:311–314.

39. van Nagell JR Jr, DePriest PD, Puls LE, et al. Ovarian cancer screening in asymptomatic postmenopausal women by transvaginal sonography. *Cancer* 1991;68:458–462.

40. Goldstein SR, Subramanyam B, Snyder JR, Beller U, Raghavendra N, Beckman EM. The postmenopausal cystic adnexal mass: The potential role of ultrasound in conservative management. *Obstet Gynecol* 1989;73:8–10.

41. Rulin MC, Preston AL. Adnexal masses in postmenopausal women. *Obstet Gynecol* 1987;70:578–581.

42. Fleischer AC. Transabdominal and transvaginal sonography of ovarian masses. *Clin Obstet Gynecol* 1991;34:433–442.

43. Fleischer AC, Mendelson EB, Bohm-Velez M, Entman SS. Transvaginal and transabdominal sonography of the endometrium. *Semin Ultrasound CT MR* 1988;9:81–101.

44. Kurjak A, Zalud I. Transvaginal colour flow imaging and ovarian cancer. *Br Med J* 1990;300:330.

45. Andolf E, Svalenius E, Anstedt B. Ultrasonography for early detection of ovarian carcinoma. *Br J Obstet Gynaecol* 1986;93:1286–1289.

46. Andolf E, Jorgensen C. Cystic lesions in elderly women diagnosed by ultrasound. *Br J Obstet Gynaecol* 1989;96:1076–1079.

47. Bhan V, Amso N, Whitehead WJ, Campbell S, Royston P, Collins WP. Characteristics of persistent ovarian masses in asymptomatic women. *Br J Obstet Gynaecol* 1989;96:1384–1391.

48. Campbell S, Bhan V, Royston P, Whitehead MI, Collins WP. Transabdominal ultrasound screening for early ovarian cancer. *Br Med J* 1989;299:1363–1367.

49. Goswamy RK, Campbell S, Whitehead MI. Screening for ovarian cancer. *Clin Obstet Gynecol* 1983;10:621–643.

50. Hurwitz A, Yagel S, Zion I, Zakut D, Palti Z, Adoni A. The management of persistent clear pelvic cysts diagnosed by ultrasonography. *Obstet Gynaecol* 1988;72:320–322.

51. Bourne TH, Campbell S, Steer C, Whitehead MI, Collins WP. Transvaginal colour flow imaging: A possible new screening technique for ovarian cancer. *Br Med J* 1989;299:1367–1370.

52. Fleischer AC, Roger WH, Rao BK, et al. Transvaginal color Doppler sonography of ovarian masses with pathologic correlation. *Ultrasound Obstet Gynecol* 1991;1:275–278.

53. Kurjak A, Zalud I, Jurkovic D, Alfirevic Z, Miljan M. Transvaginal color Doppler for the assessment of pelvic circulation. *Acta Obstet Gynecol Scand* 1989;68:131–135.

54. Silverberg E, Boring CC, Squires TS. Cancer statistics 1990. *CA* 1990;40:9–26.

55. Buy J-N, Ghossain MA, Sciot C, et al. Epithelial tumors of the ovary: CT findings and correlation with US. *Radiology* 1991;178:811–818.

56. Fleischer AC, James AE, Millis JB, Julian C. Differential diagnosis of pelvic masses by gray scale sonography. *AJR* 1978;131:469–476.

57. Luxman D, Bergman A, Sagi J, David MP. The postmenopausal adnexal mass: Correlation between ultrasonic and pathologic findings. *Obstet Gynecol* 1991;77:726–728.

58. Kurjak A, Jurkovic D. The value of ultrasound in the initial assessment of gynecological patients. *Ultrasound Med Biol* 1987;13:401–418.

59. Meine HB, Farravt P, Guha T. Distinction of benign from malignant ovarian cysts by ultrasound. *Br J Obstet Gynaecol* 1978;85:893–899.

60. Requard CK, Mettler FA Jr, Wicks JD. Preoperative sonography of malignant ovarian neoplasms. *AJR* 1981;137:79–82.

61. Finkler NJ, Benacerraf B, Lavin PT, Wojciechowski C, Knapp RC. Comparison of CA-125, clinical impression and ultrasound in the preoperative evaluation of ovarian masses. *Obstet Gynecol* 1988;72:659–664.

62. Campbell S, Goessens L, Goswamy RK, Whitehead MI. Real-time ultrasonography for the determination of ovarian morphology and volume. A possible early screening test for ovarian cancer. *Lancet* 1982;1:425–426.

63. Andolf E, Jorgensen C. A prospective comparison of transabdominal and transvaginal ultrasound with surgical findings in gynecologic disease. *J Ultrasound Med* 1990;9:71–75.

64. Barber HRK, Graber EA. The PMPO syndrome. *Obstet Gynecol* 1971;38:921–923.

65. Barber HRK. Ovarian cancer: Diagnosis and management. *Am J Obstet Gynecol* 1984;150:910–916.

66. Deland M, Fried A, van Nagell JR Jr, et al. Ultrasonography in the diagnosis of tumors of the ovary. *Surg Gynecol Obstet* 1979;148:346–348.

67. Hall DA, McCarthy KA. The significance of the postmenopausal simple adnexal cyst. *J Ultrasound Med* 1986;5:503–505.

68. Taylor KJW, Burns PN. Duplex Doppler scanning in the pelvis and abdomen. *Ultrasound Med Biol* 1985;11:643–658.

69. Taylor KJW, Morse SS. Doppler detects vascularity of some malignant tumors. *Diagn Imaging* 1988;10:132–136.

70. Taylor KJW, Ramos I, Carter D, Morse SS, Snower D, Fortune K. Correlation of Doppler ultrasound tumor signals with neovascular morphologic features. *Radiology* 1988;166:57–62.

71. Hata T, Hata K, Senoh D, et al. Doppler ultrasound assessment of tumor vascularity in gynecologic disorders. *J Ultrasound Med* 1989;8:309–314.

72. Farquhar CM, Rae T, Thomas DC, Wadsworth J, Beard RW. Doppler ultrasound in the non-pregnant pelvis. *J Ultrasound Med* 1989;8:451–457.

73. Folkman J. Tumor angiogenesis. *Adv Cancer Res* 1985;43:175–203.

74. Gammill SL, Shipkey FH, Himmelfarb EH, Parvey LS, Rabinowitz JG. Roentgenology–pathology correlation study of neovascularization. *AJR* 1976;126:376–385.

75. Jain RK. Determinants of tumor blood flow: A review. *Cancer Res* 1988;48:2641–2658.

76. Wells PNT, Halliwell M, Skidmore R, Webb AJ, Woodcock JP. Tumor detection by ultrasonic Doppler flow signals. *Ultrasonics* 1977;15:231–236.

77. Burns PN, Halliwell M, Wells PNT, Webb AJ. Ultrasonic Doppler studies of the breast. *Ultrasound Med Biol* 1982;8:127–143.

78. Kurjak A, Zalud I, Schulman H. Adnexal masses. In: Kurjak A, ed. *Transvaginal color Doppler: A comprehensive guide to transvaginal color Doppler sonography in obstetrics and gynecology.* Pearl River, NY: Parthenon; 1991:103–122.

79. Kurjak A, Zalud I, Alfirevic Z, Jurkovic D. The assessment of abnormal pelvic blood flow by transvaginal color and pulsed Doppler. *Ultrasound Med Biol* 1990;16:437–442.

80. Kurjak A, Jurkovic D, Alfirevic Z, Zalud I. Transvaginal color Doppler imaging. *J Clin Ultrasound* 1990;18:227–234.

81. Kurjak A, Zalud I. Tumor neovascularization. In: Kurjak A, ed. *Transvaginal color Doppler: A comprehensive guide to transvaginal color Doppler sonography in obstetrics and gynecology.* Pearl River, NY: Parthenon; 1991:93–102.

82. Demopoulos RI, Mittal KR. Anatomy, histology, and physiology. In: Altchek A, Deligdisch L, eds. *The uterus.* New York: Springer-Verlag; 1991:1–13.

83. Hricak H. MRI of the female pelvis: A review. *AJR* 1986;146:1115–1122.

84. Levi CS, Lyons EA, Lindsay DJ, Ballard G. Normal anatomy of the female pelvis. In: Callen PW, ed. *Ultrasonography in obstetrics and gynecology,* ed 2. Philadelphia: WB Saunders; 1988:375–392.

85. Fleischer AC. Ultrasound imaging—2000: Assessment of utero-ovarian blood flow with transvaginal color Doppler sonography; Potential clinical applications in infertility. *Fertil Steril* 1991;55:684–691.

86. Dallenbach-Hellweg G. *Histopathology of the endometrium.* New York: Springer-Verlag; 1981.

87. Santolaya-Forgas J. Physiology of the menstrual cycle by ultrasonography. *J Ultrasound Med* 1992;11:139–142.

88. Hackeloer B-J. Ultrasound scanning of the ovarian cycle. *J In Vitro Fertil Embryo Trans* 1984;1:217–220.

89. Duffield SE, Picker RH. Ultrasonic evaluation of the uterus in the normal menstrual cycle. *Med Ultrasound* 1981;5:70–74.

90. Fleischer AC, Kalemeris GC, Entman SS. Sonographic depiction of the endometrium during normal cycles. *Ultrasound Med Biol* 1986;12:271–277.

91. Fleischer AC, Kalemeris GC, Machin JE, Entman SS, Everett AE Jr. Sonographic depiction of normal and abnormal endometrium with histopathologic correlation. *J Ultrasound Med* 1986;5:445–452.

92. Goswamy RK, Steptoe PC. Doppler ultrasound studies of the uterine artery in spontaneous cycles. *Hum Reprod* 1988;3:721–726.

93. Kurjak A, Breyer B, Jurkovic D, Alfirevic Z, Miljan M. Color flow mapping in obstetrics. *J Perinat Med* 1987;15:271–281.

94. Steer CV, Campbell S, Pampiglione JS, Kingsland CR, Mason BA, Collins WP. Transvaginal color flow imaging of the uterine arteries during the ovarian and menstrual cycles. *Hum Reprod* 1990;5:391–395.

95. Long MG, Boultbee JE, Hanson ME, Begent RHJ. Doppler time velocity waveform studies of the uterine artery and uterus. *Br J Obstet Gynaecol* 1989;96:588–593.

96. de Ziegler D, Bessis R, Frydman R. Vascular resistance of uterine arteries: Physiologic effects of estradiol and progesterone. *Fertil Steril* 1991;55:775–779.

97. Applebaum M, Cadkin AV. Decidual flow—an early sign of pregnancy. *Ultrasound Obstet Gynecol* 1992;2:65(abstract).

98. Cadkin AV, Applebaum M. Ultrasonographic visualization of endometrial vascularity with ectopic pregnancy. *Am J Obstet Gynecol* 1991;165:236.

99. Robertson WB. *The endometrium.* Boston: Butterworth; 1981.

100. Deligdisch L. Endometrial response to hormonal therapy. In: Altchek A, Deligdisch L, eds. *The uterus.* New York: Springer-Verlag; 1991:102–114.

101. Granberg S, Wikland M, Karlsson B, Norstrom A, Friberg L-G. Endometrial thickness as measured by endovaginal ultrasonography for identifying endometrial abnormality. *Am J Obstet Gynecol* 1991;164:47–52.

102. Malpani A, Singer J, Wolverson MK, Merenda G. Endometrial hyperplasia: Value of endometrial thickness in ultrasonographic diagnosis and clinical significance. *J Clin Ultrasound* 1990;18:173–177.

103. Varner RE, Sparks JM, Cameron CD, Roberts LL, Soong SJ. Transvaginal sonography of the endometrium in postmenopausal women. *Obstet Gynecol* 1991;778:195–199.

104. Osmers R, Volksen M, Schauer A. Vaginosonography for early detection of endometrial carcinoma? *Lancet* 1990;335:1569–1571.

105. Fleischer AC, Gordon AN, Entman SS, Kepple DM. Transvaginal sonography (TVS) of the endometrium: Current and potential clinical applications. *Crit Rev Diagn Imaging* 1990;2:85–110.

106. Rudelstorfer R, Nanz S, Bernaschek G. Vaginosonography and its diagnostic value in patients with postmenopausal bleeding. *Arch Gynecol Obstet* 1990;248:37–44.

107. Lin MC, Gosink BB, Wolf SI, et al. Endometrial thickness after menopause: Effect of hormone replacement. *Radiology* 1991;180:427–432.

108. Platt JF, Bree RL, Davidson D. Ultrasound of the normal nongravid uterus: Correlation with gross and histopathology. *J Clin Ultrasound* 1990;18:15–19.

109. Miller EI, Thomas RH, Lines P. The atrophic postmenopausal uterus. *J Clin Ultrasound* 1977;5:261–263.

110. Zemlyn S. The length of the uterine cervix and its significance. *J Clin Ultrasound* 1981;9:267–269.

111. Flickinger L, D'Ablaing G III, Mishell DR Jr. Size and weight determinations of nongravid enlarged uteri. *Obstet Gynecol* 1986;68:855–858.

112. Kurjak A, Zalud I. Transvaginal color Doppler in the study of uterine perfusion. In: Mashiach S, Ben-Rafael Z, Laufer N, Schenker JG, eds. *Advances in assisted reproductive technologies.* New York: Plenum Press; 1990:541–544.

113. Bourne TH, Hillard TC, Whitehead MI, Crook D, Campbell S. Oestrogens, arterial status and postmenopausal women. *Lancet* 1990;335:1470–1471.

114. Bourne TH, Campbell S, Whitehead MI, Royston P, Steer CV, Collins WP. Detection of endometrial cancer in postmenopausal women by transvaginal ultrasonography and colour flow imaging. *Br Med J* 1990;301:369.

115. Bourne TH, Campbell S, Steer CV, Royston P, Whitehead MI, Collins WP. Detection of endometrial cancer by transvaginal ultrasonography with color flow imaging and blood flow analysis: A preliminary report. *Gynecol Oncol* 1991;40:253–259.

116. Fleischer AC, Gordon AN, Entman SS, Kepple DM. Transvaginal scanning of the endometrium. *J Clin Ultrasound* 1990;18:337–349.

117. Chambers CB, Unis JS. Ultrasonographic evidence of uterine malignancy in the postmenopausal uterus. *Am J Obstet Gynecol* 1986;154:1194–1199.

118. Cacciatore B, Lehtovirta P, Wahlstrom T, Ylostalo P. Preoperative sonographic evaluation of endometrial cancer. *Am J Obstet Gynecol* 1989;160:133–137.

119. Cruickshank DJ, Randall JM, Miller ID. Vaginal endosonography in endometrial cancer. *Lancet* 1989;1:445–446.

120. Goldstein SR, Nachtigall M, Snyder JR, Nachtigall L. Endometrial assessment by vaginal ultrasonography before endometrial sampling in patients with postmenopausal bleeding. *Am J Obstet Gynecol* 1990;163:119–123.

121. Nasri MN, Coast GJ. Correlation of ultrasound findings and endometrial histopathology in postmenopausal women. *Br J Obstet Gynaecol* 1989;96:1333–1338.

122. Kenigsberg D, Hodgen GD. Ovarian physiology and in vitro fertilization. In: Behrman SJ, Kistner RW, Patton GW, eds. *Progress in infertility.* Boston: Little, Brown; 1988:563–580.

123. Henriksen T, Abyholm TH, Magnus O. Pregnancies after intrafallopian transfer of embryos. *J In Vitro Fertil Embryo Trans* 1988;5:296–298.

124. Israel SL, Mutch JC. Myomectomy. *Clin Obstet Gynecol.* 1958;1:455–466.

125. Ingersoll FM. Fertility following myomectomy. *Fertil Steril* 1963;14:596–602.

126. Maheux R, Lemay A, Merat P. Use of intranasal luteinizing hormone-releasing hormone agonist in uterine leiomyomas. *Fertil Steril* 1987;47:229–233.

127. Adamson GD. Treatment of uterine fibroids: Current findings with gonadotropin-releasing hormone agonists. *Am J Obstet Gynecol* 1992;166:746–751.

128. Matta WHM, Stabile I, Shaw RW, Campbell S. Doppler assessment of uterine blood flow changes in patients with fibroids receiving the gonadotropin-releasing hormone agonist Buserelin. *Fertil Steril* 1988;49:1083–1085.

129. Deichert U, Schleif R, van de Sandt M, Juhnke I. Transvaginal hysterosalpingo–contrast sonography (Hy-Co-Sy) compared with conventional tubal diagnostics. *Hum Reprod* 1989;5:418–424.

130. Deichert U, Schleif R, van de Sandt M, Daume E. Transvaginal hysterosalpingo–contrast sonography for the assessment of tubal patency with gray scale imaging and additional use of pulsed wave Doppler. *Fertil Steril* 1992;57:62–67.

131. Shalan H, Sosic A, Kurjak A. Fallopian tube carcinoma: Recent diagnostic approach by color Doppler imaging. *Ultrasound Obstet Gynecol* 1992;2:297–299.

132. Goswamy RK, Williams G, Steptoe PC. Decreased uterine perfusion: A cause of infertility. *Hum Reprod* 1988;3:955–959.

133. Goswamy RK. Doppler ultrasound in infertility. In: Mashiach S, Ben-Rafael Z, Laufer N, Schenker JG, eds. *Advances in assisted reproductive technologies.* New York: Plenum Press; 1990;533–539.

134. Applebaum M. Ultrasound visualization of endometrial vacularity in normal premenopausal women. *The third world congress of ultrasound in obstetrics and gynecology.* Pearl River, NY: Parthenon; 1993;3:11.

135. Applebaum M. Ultrasound visualization of endometrial vacularity in IVF patients and outcome. *The third world congress of ultrasound in obstetrics and gynecology.* Pearl River, NY: Parthenon; 1993;3:10.

136. Schiller VL, Grant EG. Doppler ultrasonography of the pelvis. In: Coleman BG, ed. *The radiologic clinics of North America.* Philadelphia: WB Saunders; 1992;30:735–742.

137. Sterzik K, Dallenbach C, Schneider V, Sasse V, Dallenbach-Hellweg G. In vitro fertilization: The degree of endometrial insufficiency varies with the type of ovarian stimulation. *Fertil Steril* 1988;50:457–462.

138. Glissant A, de Mouzon J, Frydman R. Ultrasound study of the endometrium during in vitro fertilization cycles. *Fertil Steril* 1985;44:786–790.

139. Welker BG, Gembruch U, Diedrich K, Al-Hasani S, Krebs D. Transvaginal sonography of the endometrium during ovum pickup in stimulated cycles for in vitro fertilization. *J Ultrasound Med* 1989;8:549–553.

140. Smith B, Porter R, Ahuja K, Craft I. Ultrasonic assessment of endometrial changes in stimulated cycles in an in vitro fertilization and embryo transfer program. *J In Vitro Fertil Embryo Trans* 1984;1:233–238.

141. Fleischer AC, Herbert CM, Sacks GA, Wentz AC, Entman SS, James AE Jr. Sonography of the endometrium during conception and nonconception cycles of in vitro fertilization and embryo transfer. *Fertil Steril* 1986;46:442–447.

142. Jansen RPS, Anderson JC. Catheterisation of the fallopian tubes from the vagina. *Lancet* 1987;2:309–310.

143. Rabinowitz R, Laufer N, Lewin A, et al. The value of ultrasonographic endometrial measurement in the prediction of pregnancy following in vitro fertilization. *Fertil Steril* 1986;45:824–828.

144. Thickman D, Arger P, Turek R, Biasco L, Mintz M, Coleman B. Sonographic assessment of the endometrium in patients undergoing in vitro fertilization. *J Ultrasound Med* 1986;5:197–210.

145. Kepic T, Applebaum M, Valle J. Preovulatory follicular size, endometrial appearance, and estradiol levels in both conception and nonconception cycles: A retrospective study. 40th Annual Clinical Meeting of the American College of Obstetricians and Gynecologists 1992;April:20 (abstract).

146. Kepic T, Applebaum M, Criscione L, Naemyi-Rad F, Valle JA. Pre-ovulatory follicular size, endometrial appearance and estradiol levels in conception and non-conception cycles: A retrospective study. *The third world congress of ultrasound in obstetrics and gynecology.* Pearl River, NY: Parthenon; 1993;3:12

147. Ritchie WGM. Sonographic evaluation of normal and induced ovulation. *Radiology* 1986;161:1–10.

148. Tarlatzis BC, Laufer N, DeCherney AH. The use of ovarian ultrasonography in monitoring ovulation induction. *J In Vitro Fertil Embryo Trans* 1984;1:226–232.

149. Jones HW Jr. In vitro fertilization. In: Behrman SJ, Kistner RW, Patton GW, eds. *Progress in infertility.* Boston: Little, Brown; 1988:543–561.

150. Nilsson L, Wikland M, Hamberger BJ. Recruitment of an ovulatory follicle in the human following follicle-ectomy and luteectomy. *Fertil Steril* 1982;137:30–34.

151. O'Herlihy C, Pepperell RJ, Robinson HP. Ultrasound timing of human chorionic gonadotropin administration in clomiphene-stimulated cycles. *Obstet Gynecol* 1982;59:40–45.

152. Geisthovel F, Skubsch U, Zabel G, Schillinger H, Breckwoldt M. Ultrasonographic and hormonal studies in physiologic and insufficient menstrual cycles. *Fertil Steril* 1983;339:277–283.

153. McArdle CR, Seibel M, Weinstein F, Hann LE, Nickerson C, Taymor ML. Induction of ovulation monitored by ultrasound. *Radiology* 1983;148:809–812.

154. Jones HW Jr, Acosta AA, Garcia JE. A technique for the aspiration of oocytes from human ovarian follicles. *Fertil Steril* 1982;37:26–29.

155. Renou P, Trounson AO, Wood C, Leeton JF. The collection of human oocytes for in vitro fertilization. I. An instrument for maximizing oocyte recovery rate. *Fertil Steril* 1981;35:409–412.

156. Wikland M, Hamberger L, Enk L, Nilsson L. Sonographic techniques in human in-vitro fertilization programmes. *Hum Reprod* 1988;3:65–68.

157. Salat-Baroux J, Tibi C, Alvarez S, Gomez A, Antoine JM, Cornet D. Ultrasonographic prediction of ovarian hyperstimulation (OHS) after IVF. In: Mashiach S, Ben-Rafael Z, Laufer N, Schenker JG, eds. *Advances in assisted reproductive technologies.* New York: Plenum Press; 1990:559–565.

158. Blankstein J, Shalev J, Saadon T, et al. Ovarian hyperstimulation syndrome: Prediction by number and size of preovulatory ovarian follicles. *Fertil Steril* 1987;47:597–602.

159. Fleischer AC, Kepple DM, Vasquez J. Conventional and color Doppler transvaginal sonography in gynecologic infertility. *Radiol Clin North Am* 1992;30:693–702.

160. Parsons J, Booker M, Goswamy RK, et al. Oocyte retrieval for in-vitro fertilization by ultrasonically guided needle aspiration via the urethra. *Lancet* 1985;1:1076–1077.

161. Steer CV, Campbell S, Tan SL, et al. Transvaginal color Doppler: A new technique for use after in vitro fertilization to identify optimum uterine conditions before embryo transfer. *Fertil Steril* 1992;57:372–376.

162. Baber RJ, McSweeney MB, Gill RW, et al. Transvaginal pulsed Doppler ultrasound assessment of blood flow to the corpus luteum in IVF patients following embryo transfer. *Br J Obstet Gynaecol* 1988;95:1226–1230.

163. Battaglia C, Larocca E, Lanzani A, Valentini M, Genazzani AR. Doppler ultrasound studies of the uterine arteries in spontaneous and IVF stimulated ovarian cycles. *Gynecol Endocrinol* 1990;4:245–250.

164. Kurjak A, Zalud I. Ectopic Pregnancy. In: Kurjak A, ed. *Transvaginal color Doppler: A comprehensive guide to transvaginal color Doppler sonography in obstetrics and gynecology.* New Jersey: Parthenon; 1991:83–92.

165. Kurjak A, Zalud I, Schulman H. Ectopic pregnancy: Transvaginal color Doppler of trophoblastic flow in questionable adnexa. *J Ultrasound Med* 1991;10:685–689.

166. Tekay A, Jouppila P. Color Doppler flow as an indicator of trophoblastic activity in tubal pregnancies detected by transvaginal ultrasound. *Obstet Gynecol* 1991;80:995–999.

167. Atri M, Bret PM, Tulandi T. Spontaneous resolution of ectopic pregnancy: Initial appearance and evolution at transvaginal ultrasound. *Radiology* 1993;186:83–86.

168. Rottem S, Thaler I, Timor-Tritsch IE. Classification of tubal gestations by transvaginal sonography. *Ultrasound Obstet Gynecol* 1991;1:197–201.

Doppler Ultrasound in Obstetrics and Gynecology,
edited by Joshua A. Copel and Kathryn L. Reed.
Raven Press, Ltd., New York © 1995.

CHAPTER 8

Color Applications and Limitations in Obstetrics

Alfred Z. Abuhamad and Joshua A. Copel

SCIENCE AND TECHNOLOGY

The latest advance in the field of diagnostic ultrasonography is color flow mapping (CFM). The technology of CFM is an extension of the Doppler effect, which is based on the change in frequency of sound with motion. In continuous and pulsed Doppler analysis, this frequency shift (Doppler effect) is displayed in a graphic form as a time-dependent plot of the frequency spectrum of the returning signal. Limitations of spectral Doppler include the time delay required to obtain a spectrum and the small sampling site.

CFM is a modified pulsed Doppler technique displaying the spatial characteristics of the direction and velocity of blood flow superimposed on the real-time gray scale ultrasound image. It employs new technology analyzing phase differences of the transmitted sound waves (1), thus deriving information regarding flow direction, velocity, and disturbance. A color convertor assigns colors based on the direction and variance of detected frequency shifts. Conventionally, flow toward the transducer is coded as red whereas flow away from the transducer is coded as blue. The velocity is directly proportional to the brightness of each color, which is displayed in different gradations. CFM therefore allows one to study three aspects of flow: direction, velocity, and turbulence in a panoramic, real-time display.

The quality of CFM is determined by the system's sensitivity to blood flow and the operator's understanding of color controls. Color controls include the color Doppler box size, color Doppler velocity scale, color Doppler velocity filter, and total color gain.

Adding color Doppler to gray scale imaging causes slowing of the frame rate. This is due to the added time needed to analyze the frequency shifts between pulse–echo cycles. If a large color box is selected for analysis, the image will be updated even less frequently. The clinical need for a high frame rate is greatest in the evaluation of the fetal heart, where abnormal flow patterns may be present only during a brief portion of the cardiac cycle. By using a narrow color box, reducing the image depth, and increasing the velocity scale, the frame rate can be increased to a desired level. The choice of the velocity scale is dependent on the blood flow velocity in the targeted vessel. With the exception of the fetal heart and great vessels, CFM of the fetus can be achieved by using low-velocity scales. The color Doppler velocity filter is used to reduce artifact produced by the movement of tissues around vessels. This motion artifact is usually produced at low-velocity scales. Finally, the amount of power necessary to generate the Doppler image is higher than that used for conventional gray scale imaging. This is mainly due to the fact that blood components do not reflect ultrasound energy in the same way that larger structures do. Although modern technology has allowed manufacturers to produce quality color imaging with low ultrasound power, the power may be increased if difficulty is encountered. Sonologists should be aware of the power limits and how each machine's output may be increased or decreased (2).

CLINICAL APPLICATIONS

The Fetal Heart

CFM has rapidly become incorporated into the standard ultrasound evaluation of congenital heart disease

A. Z. Abuhamad: Division of Maternal-Fetal Medicine, Eastern Virginia Medical School, 825 Fairfax Avenue, Norfolk, VA 23507-1912.

J. A. Copel: Department of Obstetrics and Gynecology, Yale University School of Medicine, 333 Cedar Street, New Haven, CT 06510.

in the pediatric population. In such studies, color flow information is generally applied to provide added physiologic information to the structural knowledge provided by the gray scale image. As fetal echocardiography has become an accepted and widely available technique for the diagnosis of fetal cardiac abnormalities (3–7), CFM has assumed an important role in similar applications.

Normal flow patterns can easily be seen in structurally normal hearts. These include flow into the right atrium from the inferior and superior vena cava, across the foramen ovale from right to left, into the ventricles across the atrioventricular (AV) valves (Fig. 1), and across the semilunar valves into the great vessels.

High-velocity, turbulent regurgitant flow can be demonstrated in cases of AV valve incompetence and some atrioventricular septal defects. In fetuses with obstructed flow, e.g., due to aortic or pulmonic valve atresia, the normal intracardiac and shunt flow patterns are disturbed. In pulmonic obstruction, there may be diminished ventricular filling across the tricuspid valve and/or tricuspid regurgitation (Fig. 2). With aortic obstruction similar patterns may be seen at the level of the mitral valve, and left-to-right (i.e., reversed) flow may be found across the foramen ovale. In addition, if the degree of stenosis is critical, there may not be normal forward flow across the semilunar valves, and filling of the great arteries may be abnormal (i.e., the ductus arteriosus may provide retrograde flow to the aortic arch). These patterns can be evaluated with pulsed Doppler, but CFM speeds the process and provides corroborating data. It may further be useful in directing a pulsed Doppler study, by defining areas of particular interest where abnormal patterns are present, or in identifying the location of abnormally small vessels.

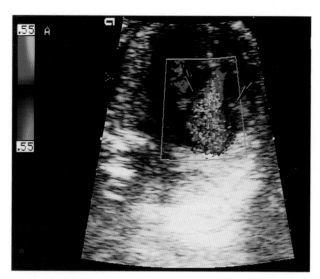

FIG. 2. Tricuspid regurgitation in the fetus with volume overload (recipient in twin-to-twin transfusion syndrome). Note the turbulence in the regurgitant jet. Arrows point to the leaflets of the tricuspid valve.

In some patients with ventricular septal defects, color can be helpful. The fetal ventricles normally function at the same systolic pressures (6). Thus, small muscular ventricular septal defects do not have the typical "jet" of flow across them that can be identified postnatally (7). There are exceptions to this rule, but these are found in the rare example of ventricular outflow obstruction with a restrictive ventricular septal defect (Fig. 3). In fetuses with a large inflow ventricular septal defect (atrioventricular septal defect, or atrioventricular canal defect) flow across the common atrioventricular valve can be seen to divide as it reaches the top of the interventricular septum (Fig. 4). Of course, any large ventricular septal defect will demonstrate color filling as blood occupies the space of

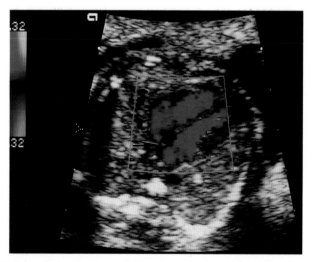

FIG. 1. Four-chamber view of the heart during diastole showing flow across the AV valves and the foramen ovale. The arrow points to the flow across the foramen ovale from the right atrium to the left atrium.

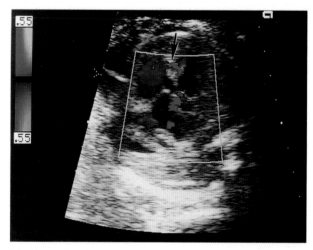

FIG. 3. Ventricular septal defect in a fetus with ventricular outflow obstruction. Arrow is pointing to the defect in the muscular part of the septum.

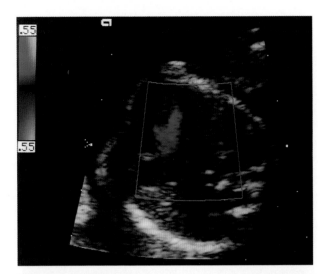

FIG. 4. Endocardial cushion defect in a fetus with Down syndrome during diastole. The flow across the common atrioventricular valve is dividing as it reaches the top of the interventricular septum.

the defect. Isolated, tiny muscular ventricular septal defects will not be identified with color flow mapping in the fetus, but are rarely hemodynamically significant.

The addition of CFM to clinical ultrasound equipment results in significant cost. In order to examine the value of color in the diagnosis of fetal heart disease, Copel et al. undertook a review of all fetal cardiac lesions diagnosed in an 18-month period (8). The contribution of CFM to the correct and complete diagnosis was graded as essential, helpful, or not helpful. Of 45 anomalies, color flow mapping was essential to the correct diagnosis in 13 (29%), helpful but not essential in 21 (47%), and not helpful in 11 (24%). The greatest impact of CFM was in the evaluation of distorted or obstructed great vessel anatomy, whereas intracardiac lesions were often more easily evaluated without CFM.

One further functional application of pulsed Doppler in the fetal heart is the evaluation of ductal patency when indomethacin is administered for control of preterm labor. Some authors have suggested that there is a high incidence of ductal constriction with maternal indomethacin treatment in the third trimester, which may occur rapidly after initiation of treatment and reverse when the medication is withdrawn (9,10). On occasion, the acute afterload increase may be severe enough to induce secondary tricuspid regurgitation. Detection is based on increased systolic and diastolic flow velocities in the ductus, which is easily identified at an optimal angle for evaluation with color guidance.

The addition of CFM to two-dimensional fetal echocardiography has not yet been shown conclusively to improve the already high sensitivity of ultrasound in the detection of fetal cardiac abnormalities. The information gained is nevertheless important in two ways. The

potential for enhanced accuracy of anatomic diagnosis allows for better counseling of the parents regarding the overall prognosis and potential surgical approaches. Truly informed consent for neonatal cardiac surgery may be impossible considering the stresses imposed on the parents, often without prior indication that anything was abnormal about the pregnancy. Any enhancement to the accuracy of prenatal diagnosis permits fuller exploration of all relevant issues with the parents. By far the most important benefit of color flow mapping lies in its ability to improve our understanding of fetal cardiovascular physiology. The overlay of cardiac flow information on the anatomic black-and-white image improves understanding of how the abnormal fetal circulatory system functions and may improve our ability to alter the management of the fetus through the transition to the neonatal circulation.

Umbilical Cord/Placental Circulation

Flow in the umbilical cord is clearly evident by CFM. Flow in the two umbilical arteries can be seen toward the placenta and in the umbilical vein back to the fetus (Fig. 5). CFM may also be helpful in localizing the site of placental cord insertion. This information is clinically useful when the cord insertion is being sought for fetal blood sampling or fetal transfusion. This is especially helpful during the second trimester, particularly with a posterior placenta.

CFM is also helpful in diagnosing abnormal cord insertion such as velamentous or vasa previa. Due to the high fetal mortality associated with vasa previa, its prenatal diagnosis is highly desirable (11). By using CFM,

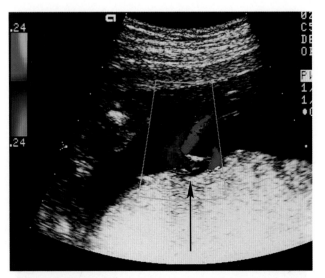

FIG. 5. Placental cord insertion. Note that the arteries are colored blue, reflecting flow to the posterior placenta, and the vein is colored red, reflecting flow to the fetus. Arrow is pointing to the cord insertion in the placenta.

the prenatal diagnosis of two cases of vasa previa have been reported (12). Patients at risk for vasa previa, such as those with placenta previa, velamentous insertion of the cord, multiple gestation, and succenturiate lobes of the placenta, should have a careful evaluation of the umbilical cord insertion into the placenta with possible CFM evaluation of the lower segment to rule out a vasa previa. Vaginal color Doppler sonography can be especially helpful in establishing the presence or absence of vessels overlying the cervical os. Recently, we were able to diagnose a vasa previa in a pregnant patient presenting with a succenturiate lobe of the placenta (Fig. 6).

The evaluation of the umbilical arteries around the fetal bladder using CFM is helpful in the occasionally difficult diagnosis of a single umbilical artery. CFM enables the examiner to identify the intraabdominal portion of the umbilical arteries, where congenital absence of one artery would be clearly visible as the vessels run past the bladder (Fig. 7). Another application that we have employed is looking for cord entanglement in monoamniotic twins using CFM. The presence of a large color-mapped area in the amniotic fluid that moves with movement of both twins can be indicative of cord entanglement (Fig. 8).

Although the insertion of the umbilical cord into the fetal abdomen is easily recognized using gray scale imaging, the presence of abdominal wall defects makes this task more difficult. The use of CFM may be helpful in differentiating gastroschisis from omphalocele. The visualization of a separate and distinct cord insertion into the abdominal wall in the presence of an abdominal wall defect virtually excludes omphalocele.

The advent of CFM has allowed the possibility of imaging blood flow in very small vessels. The combination

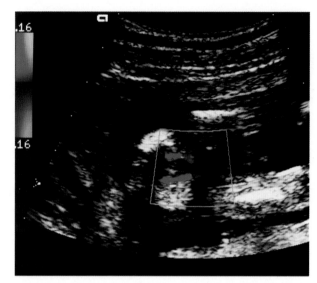

FIG. 7. Color flow mapping of a fetal pelvis in a transverse view, showing the umbilical arteries as they course along the bladder.

of pulsed and color flow Doppler can be used for the evaluation of vessels beyond the resolution of conventional gray scale ultrasound. An area of great promise, where such technical advances can be used, is the intraplacental fetal circulation. Abnormal development of the intraplacental fetal arterioles may be at the basis of some gestational diseases (e.g., preeclampsia). Using CFM, small fetal vessels within the placenta can be visualized and evaluated by flow velocity waveform analysis. To provide maximal sensitivity to flow detection, the placenta should be scanned perpendicular to the chorionic plate in order to align the ultrasound beam parallel to the fetal

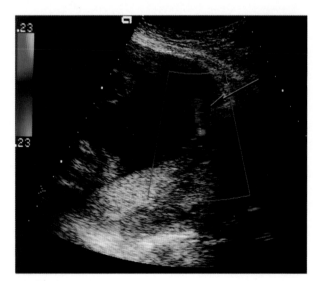

FIG. 6. Color flow mapping of the lower segment in a fetus with vasa previa. The arrow is pointing to the umbilical artery in the lower segment.

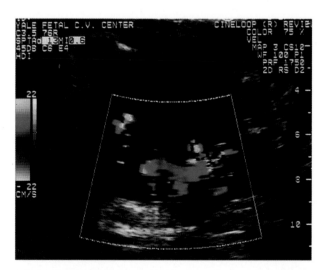

FIG. 8. Cord entanglement in monoamniotic twins detected by color flow mapping. The presence of a large color area in the amniotic fluid that moves with movement of both twins is very suspicious of cord entanglement.

vessels in main stem villi. The color setting should use the lowest frame rate and the smallest color area with the highest color gain. Documenting a flow rate synchronous with the fetal heart rate is essential, as maternal vessels are in close proximity (Fig. 9). Using the above techniques, Rotmensch et al. (13) evaluated the fetal intraplacental arteries in 138 uncomplicated and 22 growth-retarded pregnancies between 26 and 41 weeks of gestation. Failure to detect intraplacental color Doppler flow signals was associated with growth retardation and fetal distress. Flow velocity waveforms of detectable villous arteries were usually normal in growth-retarded fetuses, even in the presence of extremely abnormal umbilical artery Doppler indices. When such arteries were detected, fetal distress was not encountered.

Extracardiac Fetal Circulation

Blood flow within the fetal vessels can be detected using CFM. This allows for evaluation of the fetal cardiovascular system in great detail. CFM increases the overall efficiency of spectral Doppler evaluation, in a study evaluating whether the combined use of CFM and conventional pulsed Doppler improved the accuracy of blood velocity waveform analysis in the fetal circulation, Arduini et al. (14) studied 50 pregnant patients at 18–20 or 26–28 weeks. Recordings were performed at the level of the uterine arteries, umbilical arteries, descending aorta, and internal carotid artery. In all the vessels investigated, CFM allowed the authors to obtain a higher number of reliable recordings, to shorten the observation time, and to reduce the intra- and interobserver coefficients of variation.

Visualization of the intracerebral circulation is greatly

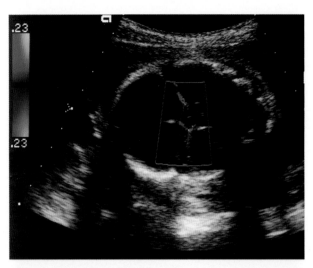

FIG. 10. Color flow mapping of the middle cerebral arteries. Note that the middle cerebral artery is running almost parallel to the ultrasound beam.

enhanced by CFM. The fetal middle cerebral artery (MCA) received detailed attention in the literature because of its accessibility to color imaging, as it runs parallel to the ultrasound beam when the fetal head is presenting in a transverse plane (Fig. 10). Mari and Deter (15) evaluated MCA flow velocity waveforms in 16 normal fetuses in a longitudinal study and 128 normal fetuses in a cross-sectional study. Their data indicated that the pulsatility index (PI) of the MCA in the normal human fetus has a parabolic pattern during pregnancy, with peak around 25–26 weeks of gestation, and does not change significantly after delivery. Furthermore, the authors speculate that the lower vascular impedance in the MCA during early and late gestation is caused by increased metabolic requirements in the fetal brain during periods of major cellular multiplication. Another clinical use of the MCA is in the management of the small-for-gestational-age (SGA) fetus. In some SGA fetuses, PI of the MCA is significantly below the normal range, suggesting a brain sparing effect. When the PI is abnormal, SGA fetuses had a greater incidence of adverse perinatal outcome.

CFM is helpful in localizing the renal arteries as they arise from the aorta (Fig. 11). The fetal renal artery PI decreases with advancing gestation (16). This decrease in PI with advancing gestation is a reflection of a decrease in renal vascular resistance and an increase in renal perfusion that also results in an increased fetal urine output. The renal artery flow velocity waveform in the fetus may play a role in the management of pregnancies complicated by oligohydramnios. In a study addressing the role of fetal renal artery flow velocity waveforms in pregnancies complicated by oligohydramnios, the presence of abnormal PI was associated with the worst fetal outcome (16).

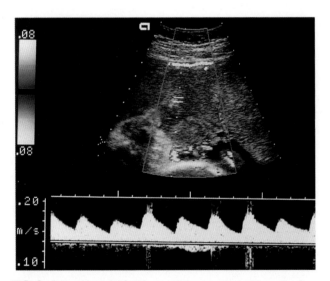

FIG. 9. Intraplacental fetal vessel demonstrated by color flow mapping. The combination of pulsed and color flow Doppler allows evaluation of this vasculature.

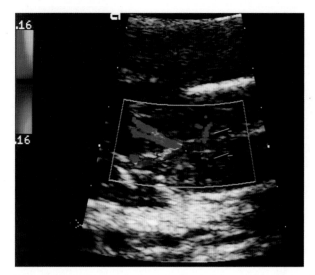

FIG. 11. Color flow mapping of a fetal abdomen in a coronal view showing the aorta, renal arteries (*arrows*), and common iliac arteries.

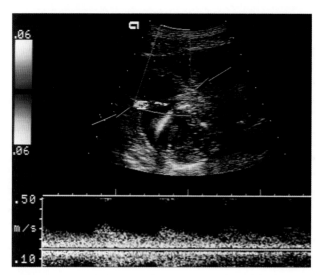

FIG. 13. An intrauterine reflective membrane (*arrows*) with color and pulsed Doppler. Note that flow along the membrane is synchronous with maternal pulse. This represents an intrauterine adhesion or uterine synechea.

Other fetal vessels evaluated with color and pulsed Doppler include internal carotid (17,18), inferior vena cava (19), ductus venosus (20), femoral artery (21), and superior mesenteric arteries (22).

Other Applications

As in fetal echocardiography, CFM plays an important role in prenatal sonography. It adds another dimension to the ultrasound examination by allowing the sonographer to determine the presence or absence of flow at specific sites. For instance, CFM was very helpful in establishing the diagnosis of a liver hemangioma in a fetus at 18 weeks of gestation presenting with a cystic mass in the left upper abdomen (23). The anatomic location of this

mass in the anterior abdomen together with the flow patterns noted on color Doppler sonography enabled us to diagnose a hepatic hemangioma (Fig. 12). Abuhamad et al. used CFM in the evaluation of pregnancies with intrauterine reflective membranes (24). Membranes of exclusively fetal origin (i.e., amniotic bands and apposing membranes of multiple pregnancies) should not have maternal blood flow signals. In contrast, reflective membranes with a central core of maternal tissue, e.g., uterine synechiae or a uterine septum, may have maternal blood flow, which can be identified by CFM (Fig. 13).

CONCLUSIONS

By combining functional and structural evaluation through ultrasound, color Doppler flow mapping represents the latest advance in diagnostic imaging. Current applications in the field of fetal echocardiography are similar to those already pioneered in pediatric and adult cardiology. Applications unique to obstetrics have already emerged, and the use of this new technology is very helpful in prenatal diagnosis. Although currently limited by an inability to obtain reproducible quantitative information, significant qualitative details can be acquired to allow a better understanding of the fetal behavior in physiologic and pathologic conditions.

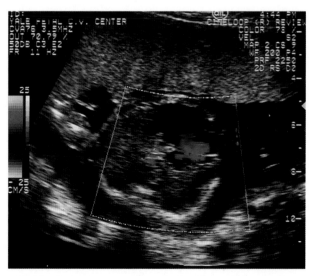

FIG. 12. Color flow mapping of a fetal hepatic hemangioma.

REFERENCES

1. Kasai C, Namekawa K, Koyano A, et al. Real-time two-dimensional blood flow imaging using an autocorrelation technique. *IEEE Trans Sonics Ultrasound SU* 1985;32:458.
2. AIUM/NEMA Safety Standard for Diagnostic Ultrasound Equipment. AIUM/NEMA Standards Publication UL1-1981. Bethesda,

MD: American Institute of Ultrasound in Medicine, or Washington, DC: National Electrical Manufacturer's Association. *J Ultrasound Med* 1983;2:S1.

3. Kleinman CS, Donnerstein RL, DeVore GR, et al. Fetal echocardiography for evaluation of in utero congestive heart failure: A technique for the study of non-immune fetal hydrops. *N Engl J Med* 1982;306:568–575.

4. DeVore GR. The prenatal diagnosis of congenital heart disease: A practical approach for the fetal sonographer. *J Clin Ultrasound* 1985;13:229–245.

5. Copel JA, Kleinman CS. The impact of fetal echocardiography on perinatal outcome. *Ultrasound Med Biol* 1986;12:327–335.

6. Rudolph A. *Congenital diseases of the heart.* Chicago: Yearbook, 1974.

7. Ortiz E, Robinson PJ, Deanfield JE, et al. Localization of ventricular septal defects by simultaneous display of superimposed color Doppler and cross-sectional echocardiographic images. *Br Heart J* 1985;54:53.

8. Copel JA, Morotti R, Hobbins JC, et al. The antenatal diagnosis of congenital heart disease using fetal echocardiography: Is color flow mapping necessary? *Obstet Gynecol* 1991;78:1–8.

9. Huhta JC, Moise KJ, Fisher DJ, et al. Detection and quantitation of constriction of the fetal ductus arteriosus by Doppler echocardiography. *Circulation* 1987;75:406–412.

10. Moise KJ, Huhta JC, Sharif DS, et al. Indomethacin in the treatment of premature labor: Effects on the fetal ductus arteriosus. *N Engl J Med* 1988;319:327–331.

11. Pent D. Vasa previa. *Am J Obstet Gynecol* 1979;134:151.

12. Harding JA, Lewis DF, Major CA, et al. Color flow Doppler: A useful instrument in the diagnosis of vasa previa. *Am J Obstet Gynecol* 1990;163:1566–1568.

13. Rotmensch S, Liberati M, Luo JS, Gollin Y, Hobbins JC, Copel JA. Villous artery flow velocity waveforms and color Doppler flow patterns in placentas of growth retarded fetuses. *Am J Obstet Gynecol;* in press.

14. Arduini D, Rizzo G, Boccolini MR, et al. Functional assessment of uteroplacental and fetal circulations by means of color Doppler ultrasonography. *J Ultrasound Med* 1990;9:249–253.

15. Mari G, Deter RL. Middle cerebral artery flow velocity waveforms in normal and small-for-gestational age fetuses. *Am J Obstet Gynecol* 1992;166:1262–1270.

16. Mari G, Kirshon B, Abuhamad A. Fetal renal artery flow velocity waveforms in normal pregnancies and pregnancies complicated by polyhydramnios and oligohydramnios. *Obstet Gynecol* 1993;81:560–564.

17. Wladimiroff JW, Tonge HM, Stewart PA. Doppler ultrasound assessment of cerebral blood flow in the human fetus. *Br J Obstet Gynaecol* 1986;93:471–475.

18. Van Den Wijingaard JAGW, Groenenberg IAL, Wladimiroff JW, Hop WCI. Cerebral Doppler ultrasound of the human fetus. *Br J Obstet Gynaecol* 1989;96:845–849.

19. Rizzo G, Arduini D, Romanini C. Inferior vena cava flow velocity waveforms in appropriate and small-for-gestational-age fetuses. *Am J Obstet Gynecol* 1992;166:1271–1280.

20. Kiserud T, Eik-Nes SH, Harm-Gerd KB, Hellevik LR. Ultrasonographic velocimety of the fetal ductus venosus. *Lancet* 1991;338:1412–1414.

21. Mari G. Arterial blood flow waveforms of the pelvis and lower extremities in normal and IUGR fetuses. *Am J Obstet Gynecol* 1991;165:143–151.

22. Cartier MS, Emerson DS, Felker RE, et al. Color and pulsed Doppler of the fetal superior mesenteric artery. *J Ultrasound Med* 1992;11:S93.

23. Abuhamad AZ, Lewis D, Inati MN, Johnson DR, Copel JA. The use of color flow Doppler in the diagnosis of fetal hepatic hemangioma. *J Ultrasound Med* 1993;4:223–226.

24. Abuhamad AZ, Romero R, Shaffer WK, Hobbins JC. The value of Doppler flow analysis in the prenatal diagnosis of amniotic sheets. *J Ultrasound Med* 1992;11:623–624.

Doppler Ultrasound in Obstetrics and Gynecology,
edited by Joshua A. Copel and Kathryn L. Reed.
Raven Press, Ltd., New York © 1995.

CHAPTER 9

Experimental Models Used to Investigate the Diagnostic Potential of Doppler Ultrasound in the Umbilical Circulation

R. J. Morrow, A. A. Hill, and S. L. Adamson

There is strong evidence that important information about fetal health is contained in the shape of the blood velocity waveform in the umbilical artery. In normal pregnancy near term, the decrease in blood velocity during diastole is modest, and end-diastolic velocity is about 50% of the systolic value. However, many growth-restricted fetuses and some fetuses with congenital anomalies exhibit dramatic decreases in blood velocity during diastole, so that absent or reversed blood velocity is observed (1–3). Abnormal blood velocity waveforms in the umbilical artery have proven helpful in identifying those fetuses with intrauterine growth restriction who are at high risk of a poor perinatal outcome (4) before conventional heart rate tests become abnormal (5). The diagnostic potential of this technique is limited if the pathophysiologic basis for these waveform changes is not fully understood.

This problem has been addressed using a number of experimental models to investigate the pathophysiologic causes of abnormal umbilical arterial velocity waveforms. Many studies have been performed on the most commonly used experimental animal model in perinatal medicine, the acutely or chronically instrumented fetal sheep. These studies have evaluated the effects of various pathophysiologic changes imposed on the fetus (e.g., hypoxia, hyperviscosity, vasoconstriction, or vasodilation) on the umbilical arterial velocity waveform. This approach has provided important information on which

factors can, and which cannot, directly result in abnormal velocity waveforms. This work will be outlined in the first section of this chapter. Other studies have taken a more basic, hemodynamic approach to the problem. They have sought to understand the pulsatile pressure–flow relations in the umbilical circulation in order to elucidate the underlying cardiovascular changes that result in abnormal velocity waveforms. To accomplish this goal, some investigators have used the instrumented fetal sheep as their model, and these studies will be outlined in the second part of this chapter. Others have used *in vitro* or computer models to address this issue and these studies will be outlined in the third part of this chapter.

In this chapter, we will use several indices that have been derived to quantify the degree of "pulsatility" of the umbilical arterial velocity waveform. These are the pulsatility index [$(S - D)$/mean], S/D, D/S, and the Pourcelot ratio [$(S - D)$/S] where S refers to the maximum velocity in systole, D refers to the minimum in diastole, and mean refers to the mean blood velocity averaged over the cardiac cycle. All these indices adequately quantify the degree of pulsatility of the waveform although S/D has the disadvantage that it becomes highly nonlinear when D is small (6). In some cases, these indices have been applied to flow rather than velocity waveforms. Although velocity and flow waveforms are not identical in theory (6), pulsatility indices derived from simultaneous measurements of the two waveforms proved to be similar under a wide variety of conditions (6,7). Thus, factors that control flow waveform shape will be discussed because these factors would have similar effects on velocity waveform shape.

R. J. Morrow, A. A. Hill, and S. L. Adamson: Samuel Lunenfeld Research Institute, Mount Sinai Hospital, 600 University Avenue, Toronto, Ontario, M5G 1X5, Canada.

PATHOPHYSIOLOGIC STUDIES

In clinical studies it is not possible to make many of the physiologic measurements that are fundamental to understanding the cause of abnormal velocity waveforms. Animal models enable the continuous measurement of such variables as fetal blood pressure and blood gases as well as placental blood flow and vascular resistance. The fetal sheep has been extensively used for this experimental model. Isolated physiologic changes may be made to assess how each may contribute to changes in the waveform.

Effects of Hypoxia and Acidosis

Clinical studies have shown that abnormal waveforms are correlated with fetal hypoxia (8) and it has therefore been suggested that abnormal umbilical waveforms are the consequence of redistribution of blood flow to maintain perfusion of vital organs. Fetal hypoxia has been induced by occluding the maternal internal iliac arteries (9), by embolizing the uteroplacental circulation (10), or by altering the maternal inspired oxygen concentration (11–13). Hypoxia induced by any of these methods does not cause any change in the umbilical velocity waveform (Fig. 1). In fact, even profound fetal acidosis does not

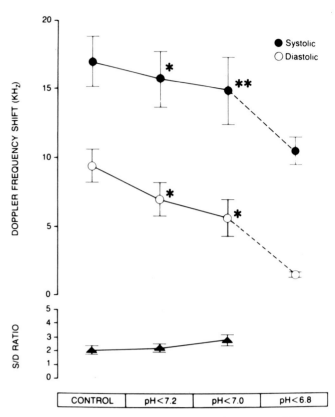

FIG. 2. Systolic and diastolic Doppler frequency shift and S/D ratio are shown for control and progressive acidemia. Only four of seven fetuses survived to pH ≤ 6.8 so data points are joined by dashed lines (these data were not subjected to statistical analysis). *p ≤ 0.025 compared with control. **p = 0.002 compared with control. From Morrow et al. (12).

cause changes in the waveform unless the fetus becomes hypotensive (12) (Fig. 2).

Occlusion of the Placental Microvasculature

Clinical studies have demonstrated a decrease in the number of small arteries and arterioles in the tertiary stem villus of the placenta when the umbilical waveform is abnormal (2,14). When plastic microspheres have been used to occlude the placental arterioles in fetal sheep (6,15–17), a progressive change in the waveform shape can be demonstrated (Fig. 3). These changes in waveform shape are correlated with increased downstream vascular resistance (6,16). However, when umbilicoplacental resistance is elevated by other techniques, such as the infusion of the vasoconstrictor angiotensin, indices of pulsatility are not well correlated with resistance (6,18). In the case of angiotensin II, a large increase in resistance and decrease in umbilical blood flow can occur with no significant change in the umbilical arterial blood flow pulsatility (6,19). This apparent paradox is explained by the fact that angiotensin primarily elevates

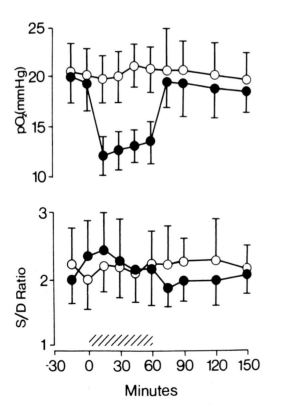

FIG. 1. Mean (±SEM) fetal arterial pO₂ and the umbilical S/D ratio during control experiments (open circles) and hypoxemia (closed circles). From Morrow et al. (13).

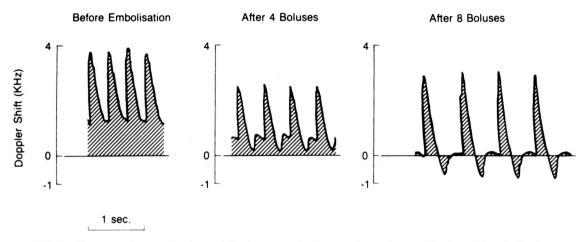

FIG. 3. Changes observed in the umbilical artery velocity waveform shape with placental embolization. From Morrow et al. (16).

umbilical artery resistance whereas embolization affects more peripheral vessels in the placental microcirculation (6). This observation is of importance since it has been assumed in clinical studies that infusion of vasoactive substances does not affect placental blood flow if the umbilical waveform shape does not change (20). Clearly, this assumption is not necessarily valid.

Hyperviscosity

Growth-restricted human fetuses tend to be polycythemic and thus have blood that is more viscous than normally grown fetuses. An association between abnormal umbilical waveforms and increased viscosity has previously been noted (21). Isovolemic exchange transfusion with concentrated donor erythrocytes in the fetal sheep to increase the hematocrit to 30–45% caused the placental vascular resistance to almost double. Despite this very large increase in placental resistance, the umbilical waveform shape remained unchanged (12).

Hypertension

Some clinical studies have suggested that the umbilical waveform shape may be modified by changes in maternal blood pressure (22). Infusion of angiotensin into the maternal circulation of the sheep causes a large increase in maternal blood pressure without affecting the umbilical Doppler waveform (12), suggesting that other factors may be involved.

These pathophysiologic studies have demonstrated some of the influences on umbilical waveform shape that are of clinical importance. Of fundamental importance to the understanding of waveform changes is their relationship to placental vascular resistance. Pulsatility indi-

ces are commonly interpreted to indicate the resistance of the circulatory bed supplied by the artery under examination (23). Indeed, one of these indices (the Pourcelot ratio) is sometimes referred to as the resistance index, and some investigators have used umbilical arterial velocity waveforms to draw conclusions relating to the effect of a drug treatment on umbilicoplacental vascular resistance (20). However, several studies have shown that in the umbilical circulation of the fetal sheep, the relationship between blood flow pulsatility and vascular resistance can be extremely poor depending on the method used to alter resistance (6,18,19). These results highlight the necessity to understand the functional link between waveform shape and vascular resistance. Basic hemodynamic studies of the fetal circulation have been performed to achieve this level of understanding.

HEMODYNAMIC STUDIES

Umbilicoplacental Hemodynamics

Pulsatile pressure–flow relationships in the umbilicoplacental circulation of chronically catheterized fetal sheep were determined by simultaneously monitoring pressure and flow at the input to the umbilical circulation using high-fidelity transducers (24). In addition, pressures in a small, cotyledonary artery and vein were measured at the placental end of the umbilical cord. These measurements enabled the propagation of the pressure pulse along the umbilical artery to be measured. They also enabled the contribution of the umbilical arteries, placental microcirculation, and the umbilical veins (including liver and ductus venous) to the overall umbilicoplacental vascular resistance to be determined. These studies revealed several unique features of the umbilical circulation that emphasize how hazardous it is to extrapolate conclusions based on other vascular beds to this highly specialized vascular bed.

Unlike other large-supply arteries, the umbilical arteries in sheep contribute significantly to the total vascular resistance of the umbilicoplacental circulation (30% of the total resistance resides in the large arteries) (24). This can be explained by the extreme length of the umbilical arteries ($\approx$45 cm; over twice the length of the fetal aorta) and by the low vascular resistance of the placental microcirculation. Another special feature is that the umbilical arteries and veins have thick muscular walls and are capable of complete closure when maximally stimulated (e.g., at birth), so that they are capable of providing significant regulatory control of blood flow. For example, angiotensin II infusion, which constricts the umbilical arteries while having minimal effects on the remainder of the umbilicoplacental circulation, can result in a marked decrease in umbilical blood flow (6,24). Norepinephrine, on the other hand, preferentially increases umbilical venous vascular resistance (25,26). Another consequence of the thick muscular wall and the length of the umbilical artery is that the pressure pulse wave is markedly attenuated by viscous damping as it propagates along the vessel (24).

Umbilicoplacental Vascular Input Impedance

In addition to these special features, hemodynamic studies have shown that the relationship between pulsatile pressure and pulsatile flow in the umbilicoplacental circulation is highly unusual. This information is derived from simultaneous, high-fidelity recordings of pressure and flow waveforms measured at the entrance to the umbilical circulation (24). The pressure and flow waveforms were then used to calculate the vascular input impedance of the umbilicoplacental vascular bed.

Analyzing pulsatile properties of an arterial bed introduces complex physical concepts (e.g., impedance, wave reflection, and interference) that are not encountered when only mean flow and mean pressure are considered. Resistance expresses the opposition to mean flow imposed by a vascular bed. It is equal to the ratio of the mean driving pressure to the resultant mean flow. Vascular input impedance is similar, except that it expresses the opposition to pulsatile flow and is equal to the ratio of the pulsatile pressure to the resulting pulsatile flow. Whereas resistance depends only on blood viscosity, and vessel diameter and length, impedance depends on these factors as well as on blood inertia, arterial distensibility (or compliance), wave propagation velocity, and wave reflection effects (23). Unlike resistance, impedance is not a single value. Instead it takes on different values at the heart rate frequency ("fundamental") and for frequencies that are multiples of the heart rate ("harmonics"); all these frequency components are contained

within the measured flow and pressure waveforms. In order to calculate impedance, it is necessary to break down the complete pulsatile waveforms into their component frequencies using Fourier analysis (23). At each frequency, impedance consists of a modulus that is a ratio of the amplitude of sinusoidal pressure to the amplitude of sinusoidal flow, and a phase that quantifies the degree to which the flow and pressure waves are out of synchrony. At zero frequency, the impedance modulus has the same meaning as the vascular resistance.

An example of an impedance spectrum obtained from the umbilical circulation under resting conditions in fetal sheep near term is shown in Fig. 4. The impedance modulus was only slightly below resistance to steady flow for frequencies up to 15 Hz, and the impedance phase was positive (flow led pressure) at the fundamental (or heart rate) frequency. Both of these characteristics are highly unusual when compared to impedance spectra obtained from all vascular beds studied to date in postnatal animals including the organ of gas exchange, the low-resistance pulmonary circulation (23). These obser-

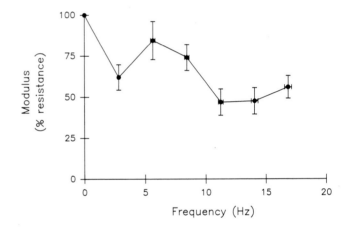

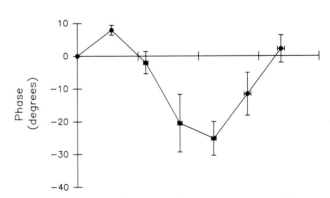

FIG. 4. Graphs showing umbilical impedance modulus (*top*) and phase (*bottom*) vs. frequency under control conditions. Impedance modulus is presented as a percentage of mean resistance to steady flow (0.077 ± 0.007 mm Hg ml⁻¹ min⁻¹). Data are averaged over seven fetuses. From Adamson et al. (24). Copyright 1992 American Heart Association.

vations again indicate the unique hemodynamic properties of the umbilicoplacental circulation.

Relationship Between Flow Pulsatility and Hemodynamics

One of the primary objectives of our detailed hemodynamic studies on the umbilical circulation was to determine the factors responsible for the shape of the umbilical arterial flow (or velocity) waveform. One problem with impedance analysis is that although it rigorously describes the relationship between pulsatile pressure and pulsatile flow, it results in a spectrum of values of modulus and phase rather than one value, so that it is difficult to relate it directly to waveform shape. However, we have shown that just one value of impedance, the impedance modulus at the heart rate frequency (or fundamental), closely describes the relationship between the measured pulse pressure divided by the measured pulse flow (19). Thus, this single value of impedance (the "fundamental impedance") describes the relationship between pulse pressure and pulse flow in a manner analogous to the way resistance describes the relationship between mean pressure and mean flow. This approximation was found to apply under a wide range of hemodynamic conditions (19), and it dramatically simplifies the interpretation of the effect of impedance on velocity waveform shape.

The functional link between the flow pulsatility index and various hemodynamic factors, including vascular resistance, were examined in experiments performed on catheterized fetal sheep near term (19). A specific goal was to explain why there is an excellent correlation between the flow pulsatility index when resistance is increased by embolization but not when it is increased by angiotensin II infusion (6). A wide range of hemodynamic conditions were tested in this study (including vasodilators, vasoconstrictors, and embolization) so that the factors identified would be as generally applicable as possible. Results indicated that there are three factors, in addition to vascular resistance, that are important determinants of the flow waveform in the umbilical artery. These are the arterial pulse pressure, the arterial mean pressure, and the fundamental impedance (i.e., impedance modulus at the heart rate frequency). They are related to the flow pulsatility index (flow PI) by the following equation:

$$\text{Flow PI} \approx \frac{\text{pulse pressure}}{\text{mean pressure}} \times \frac{\text{resistance}}{\text{impedance}}$$

The first term in this equation, the ratio of pulse pressure to mean pressure, depends on the characteristics of the heart and the circulatory system as a whole. It represents the input that drives flow in the umbilical circulation. With the interventions tested (vasodilator, vasoconstrictors, embolization), the ratio of pulse to mean pressure

did not change significantly (19). Thus, the primary determinant of the flow pulsatility index was the ratio of vascular resistance to fundamental impedance. Both these factors depend exclusively on the rheologic properties of blood and the properties of all vessels downstream of the recording site. Embolization increased resistance without changing impedance and, therefore, a close relationship between resistance and flow pulsatility index was observed. In contrast, angiotensin II increased both resistance and impedance approximately the same amount, so that no change in flow pulsatility occurred (19).

Heart Rate and Flow Pulsatility

There is an inversely proportional relationship between the pulsatility index in the umbilical artery and the fetal heart rate (27–30). The hemodynamic factors responsible for this relationship have been investigated in experiments using the anesthetized, acutely instrumented fetal sheep as the model (7). This model minimized spontaneous variations in heart rate by eliminating spontaneous fetal body movements and changes in sleep state, both of which are associated with changes in fetal heart rate (31). Changes in fetal heart rate were induced by either pacing the heart with electrodes implanted on the left atrium or by stimulating, on the cardiac side, the severed end of one vagus nerve. The umbilical arterial flow pulsatility index was a function of heart rate (slope = -0.007 (beat/min)$^{-1}$), and this relationship was similar to that observed previously during spontaneous changes in heart rate in human fetuses (27–30).

An intuitive argument has been proposed to explain this relationship as follows: A decrease in the interval between heart beats results in a higher end-diastolic velocity because there is less time for velocity to decrease between heart beats (32). Thus, as heart rate increases the difference between systole and diastole (i.e., the numerator of the pulsatility index) decreases, resulting in a decrease in the flow pulsatility index. However, experimentally, systolic flow decreased and diastolic flow was unchanged as heart rate increased (7) (Figs. 5 and 6). Changes in heart rate caused little change in umbilicoplacental vascular resistance or impedance. Instead, the ratio of pulse pressure to mean pressure was altered. Thus, the primary mechanism mediating the effect of heart rate on the umbilical arterial flow waveform is the change in driving pressure, which in turn is secondary to changes occurring upstream of the umbilicoplacental vascular bed.

These examples illustrate the valuable insights into the factors determining the shape of the umbilical arterial flow (or velocity) waveform which can be gained by examining the hemodynamic characteristics of the umbilicoplacental vascular bed in an animal model.

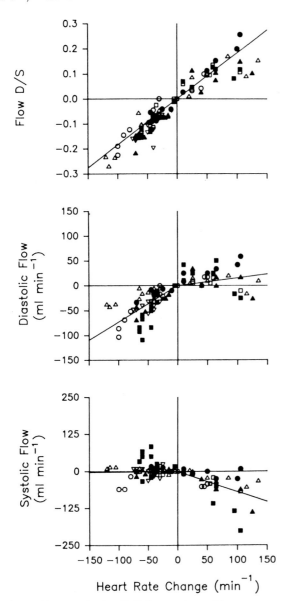

FIG. 5. Changes in the *D/S* flow ratio and its components with changing heart rate (*n* = 7). Values from different animals are depicted by different symbols. Lines depict the slope for each relationship. Where there was no significant difference between the slopes for acceleration and deceleration, a single overall slope is shown. From Morrow et al. (7). Copyright 1993, with permission from Pergamon Press Ltd.

IN VITRO AND COMPUTER MODELS

In animal models, it is very difficult to examine changes in the umbilical arterial velocity waveform that are caused by changing one variable in isolation. For example, factors that change peripheral vascular resistance often change arterial blood pressure and may change fetal heart rate as well (18). Also, it would be useful to predict, from a theoretical standpoint, which variables are most likely to influence velocity waveform shape so that subsequent *in vivo* studies can be based on theoretically

sound hypotheses. To this end, a number of *in vitro* and computer models of the umbilical circulation have been studied.

In Vitro Models

In vitro models, consisting of a pulsatile pump, a tube representing the insonated artery, and a peripheral resistance (tube or tubes in parallel whose resistance can be altered with clamps), have been studied (33–35). Studies using these simple models showed that when other fac-

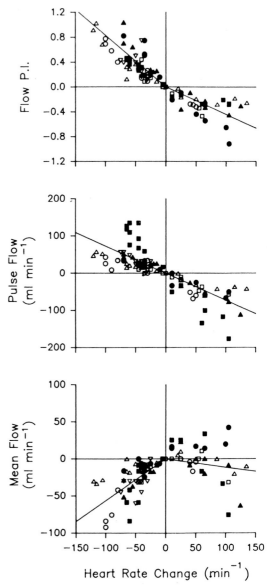

FIG. 6. Changes in the pulsatility index and its components with changing heart rate. Values from different animals are depicted by different symbols (*n* = 7). Lines depict the slope for each relationship. Where there was no significant difference between the slopes for acceleration and deceleration, a single overall slope is shown. From Morrow et al. (7). Copyright 1993, with permission from Pergamon Press Ltd.

tors are held constant, increases in peripheral resistance result in linear increases in the pulsatility index recorded in the supply artery (33,34), and that a decrease in pump rate (i.e., heart rate) results in an increase in the pulsatility index (35). Thus, results show similar trends to those observed in animal studies *in vivo*. The limitation of these models is that simple tubes and pumps do not accurately simulate the cardiovascular system, so that it is difficult to assess the degree to which results apply to the *in vivo* situation.

Computer Models

Computer models can be very simple (36,37) or they can incorporate more detailed representation of the physical characteristics of the umbilical vasculature and the input pressure waveform (38,39). They have the advantage over *in vitro* models that values for variables can be readily set and altered without requiring the substitution of materials with the necessary physical characteristics.

Windkessel Models

Several "windkessel"-type computer models of the human umbilical circulation have been developed. In this type of simulation, the artery or arterial system of interest is considered as a lumped elastic vessel, and peripheral vascular beds are represented by lumped resistive/compliant elements at the outlet of the elastic vessel. Pulsatile blood flow from the heart arrives at the entrance to the arterial vessel, which expands as blood pressure increases. During diastole, the vessel rebounds, pushing blood out through the peripheral resistive/compliant elements. The compliance of the windkessel transforms pulsatile flow from the heart into steady flow in the veins. The windkessel can be implemented as an electrical circuit analog, in which arteries are represented by lumped resistances and capacitances, and electrical voltage and electrical current are analogous to blood pressure and flow rate, respectively (see Fig. 7).

In the windkessel model of Thompson and Stevens (36), the resistance and compliance of the umbilical artery and the placental vascular bed were estimated from typical umbilical arterial dimensions, elastic properties of adult vascular beds, umbilical blood flow rates measured by Doppler ultrasound, and estimated fetal arterial blood pressures. Analytical expressions were derived for the pulsatility index of flow in the umbilical artery in terms of blood pressure, vascular resistance and compliance, and frequency when the blood pressure waveform was assumed to be a sine wave. The model was used to predict the effect of obliteration or radius reduction of vessels in the placental vascular bed on the flow pulsatility index in the umbilical artery. Pulsatility of flow in the

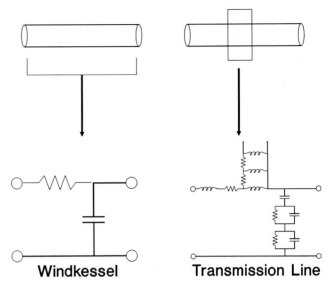

FIG. 7. Windkessel and transmission line models. The Windkessel represents an entire artery by a lumped resistance and capacitance. The transmission line model represents each small segment of artery by the electrical elements shown.

umbilical artery was found to be proportional to the ratio of placental vascular resistance to umbilical arterial vascular resistance over a wide range of hemodynamic conditions. Also, placenta vascular resistance was more sensitive to reductions in the radius of terminal blood vessels in the placenta than to obliteration of terminal vessels. For example, a 20% radius reduction in all terminal branches increased placental vascular resistance by the same amount as obliteration of 60% of the terminal vessels.

Guiot et al. (37) also investigated a windkessel-type model of the human umbilical artery and placentovascular bed. This model was similar to the model of Thompson and Stevens (36), with the exception that the placentovascular bed was simulated during development from approximately 8 weeks of gestation to term by the addition of successive generations of dichotomous branching vessels to the placental vascular tree in the model. The number of generations of branching in the placental bed was increased from 0 to 15 over this age range based on studies of placental morphology in the literature. The model was used to predict umbilical blood flow rate, mean umbilical blood velocity, total placental bed vascular resistance, and the pulsatility index of flow in the umbilical artery. The pulsatility index of flow for a sinusoidal input pressure waveform progressively increased or stayed nearly constant with increasing gestational age, which was contrary to the progressive decrease in pulsatility index with gestational age that had been observed *in vivo* using Doppler ultrasound (1). Guiot et al. (37) found that the predictions of their model were highly sensitive to the relative size of blood vessels in successive generations in the model placental vascular tree, but the results of their model confirmed the conclusion of Thompson and Stevens (36) that flow pulsatility index was dependent on both the hemodynamic characteristics of the umbilical vascular system and the blood pressure waveform.

The windkessel model's main advantage is its simplicity, but such a simple model cannot account for pulse wave propagation and reflection effects. For example, in the umbilical artery the arterial pressure pulse propagates down the length of the artery and is partially reflected back when it reaches the placental microcirculation. The time required for the pulse to travel down the artery and for the reflected pulse to return to the entrance of the vessel is a significant fraction (>30%) of the cardiac cycle. In addition, the input impedance of the sheep umbilical circulation, which is equal to the ratio of pusatile pressure to pusatile flow at the entrance of the common umbilical artery, shows characteristics indicative of significant wave reflection effects (24). The windkessel cannot account for these wave propagation effects, which may play a key role in determining the characteristics of arterial blood velocity waveforms. For this reason, some investigators have developed models of the umbilical circulation that incorporate wave propagation and reflection phenomena.

One-Dimensional Nonlinear Models

For example, Todros et al. (39) extended the work of Guiot et al. (37) by carrying out simulations using a one-dimensional nonlinear model of the umbilicoplacental circulation. In this type of model, both wave propagation effects and nonlinear effects arising from the fluid mechanics of blood flow are accounted for. The umbilical circulation was simulated as a single tube, whose cross-sectional area increased from the cross-section of the umbilical artery to the summed cross-section of the placental blood vessels, and then decreased back to the cross-section of the umbilical vein. When the blood pressure waveform was assumed to be a sine wave and the mean fetal arterial blood pressure was assumed to increase throughout pregnancy, then the model predicted a progressive decrease in flow pulsatility index with gestation. This prediction is in agreement with *in vivo* Doppler measurements (1). In addition, the effects of arrested placental vessel development and placental vessel obliteration on the pulsatility of flow in the umbilical artery were investigated. Arrested development of the placental vascular tree halted the decrease in flow pulsatility index if the mean arterial pressure also stopped increasing. Severe (>70%) occlusions of placental vessels produced large values of pulsatility index (>1.5) near term. However, the results of the model [like the results of Guiot et al. (37)] were highly sensitive to the relative cross-sectional areas of successive generations of vascular branches in the placental bed. The value of this area ratio

is not precisely known. If it was decreased from the assumed value of 1.3 to less than 1.2, then the flow pulsatility index increased throughout pregnancy and umbilical flow decreased near term. Both of these predictions contradict *in vivo* observations (1,40).

Like Todros et al., Vieyres et al. (38) used a one-dimensional nonlinear model, with a physiologic pressure waveform as input to the model. They investigated the effect of measurement location on the Pourcelot ratio of the Doppler velocity waveform at a number of points from the fetal end to the placental end of the umbilical artery. The Pourcelot ratio decreased by 15% (from 0.52 to 0.44) along the length of the umbilical artery from proximal to distal ends. This prediction is in qualitative agreement with the authors' *in vivo* measurements, which showed a decrease in the Pourcelot ratio of 30% along the length of the umbilical cord.

Transmission Line Models

We recently developed a transmission line model of the sheep umbilical circulation in our laboratory. In this type of model, each small length of an artery is simulated by a block of electrical elements that are similar to those used to model electrical transmission lines (see Fig. 7). Similar models of other circulations have been developed (41,42) and used to simulate the adult human arterial system (43–50). Our model of the sheep umbilical circulation incorporates wave propagation phenomena and has the advantage over previous models of the umbilical circulation that it is based on direct hemodynamic measurements taken under both baseline conditions and after experimental interventions in the sheep fetus (24). Input to the model was a physiologic pressure waveform at the proximal end of the umbilical artery rather than a simple sinusoidal waveform, so that complete blood flow waveform shape could be generated in the model rather than only simple indices of the flow waveform. The model was used to predict pressure and flow waveforms in the umbilical artery and input impedance of the umbilicoplacental circulation; these predictions were compared with direct experimental measurements of the same quantities. This model was successful in reproducing many of the measured changes in the pressure waveform recorded at the placental end of the umbilical artery, as well as changes in the flow waveform and the input impedance measured at the entrance of the artery, which were observed after embolization of the placenta with microspheres or after infusion of the vasoconstrictor angiotensin II into the fetal circulation.

In conclusion, it must be noted that hemodynamic models of the umbilical circulation are only as good as the data on which they are based. Hence, current models of the human umbilical circulation are limited by the lack of direct measurements of pressure, flow, and arterial and placental properties in this circulation. Up until the present time, hemodynamic models of the umbilical circulation have concentrated on examining the effect of changing arterial properties or vascular resistance on Doppler indices like the pulsatility index or the Pourcelot ratio. As discussed above, several computer models have predicted an increase in Doppler pulsatility indices when the distal placental vascular resistance is raised, confirming the results of experimental studies. In addition, models have demonstrated that pulsatility index is dependent on pressure pulsatility even if placental resistance is constant. This finding contradicts the widely held view that the Doppler pulsatility index is a simple measure of placentovascular resistance but it is in agreement with results from recent hemodynamic studies (19). Computer model studies have also pointed out the significant site dependence of Doppler measurements of blood flow pulsatility in the umbilical artery.

In the future, computer models like the one developed in our laboratory may allow more fundamental and detailed studies of umbilical hemodynamics under various normal and abnormal conditions using physiologic pressure and flow waveforms. Such studies have the potential not only to expand current understanding of the umbilical circulation but to improve clinical interpretation of Doppler ultrasound measurements of umbilical blood flow.

CONCLUSIONS

Animal, *in vitro*, and computer models enable us to study the mechanisms that cause changes in velocity waveform shape in the umbilical artery and to determine many of the physiologic variables that are inaccessible in the human circulation. Models are always limited by the fact that they do not exactly reproduce the human circulation and cannot tell us exactly which mechanisms are responsible for changes in the clinical situation. However, clinical interpretation of waveforms should be interpreted in the context of the considerable amount of physiologic data that are now available. This information should be used to design and interpret clinical studies of Doppler ultrasound so that this method can be more appropriately used in patient management.

REFERENCES

1. Erskine RLA, Ritchie JWK. Umbilical artery blood flow characteristics in normal and growth retarded fetuses. *Br J Obstet Gynaecol* 1985;92:605–610.
2. McCowan LM, Mullen BM, Ritchie K. Umbilical artery flow velocity waveforms and the placental vascular bed. *Am J Obstet Gynecol* 1987;157:900–902.
3. Trudinger BJ, Cook CM. Umbilical and uterine artery flow waveforms in pregnancy associated with major fetal abnormality. *Br J Obstet Gynaecol* 1985;92:666–670.
4. Al-Ghazali W, Chapman MG, Allan LD. Doppler assessment of the cardiac and uteroplacental circulations in normal and complicated pregnancies. *Br J Obstet Gynaecol* 1988;95:575–580.
5. Arabin B, Siebert M, Jimenez E, Saling E. Obstetrical characteristics of loss of end-diastolic velocities in the fetal aorta and/or umbilical artery using Doppler ultrasound. *Gynecol Obstet Invest* 1988;25:173–180.
6. Adamson SL, Morrow RJ, Langille BL, Bull SB, Ritchie JWK. Site-dependent effects of increases in placental vascular resistance on the umbilical arterial velocity waveform in fetal sheep. *Ultrasound Med Biol* 1990;16:19–27.
7. Morrow RJ, Bull SB, Adamson SL. Experimentally induced changes in heart rate alter umbilicoplacental hemodynamics in fetal sheep. *Ultrasound Med Biol* 1993;19:309–318.
8. Soothill PW, Bilardo CM, Nicolaides KH, Campbell S. Relation of fetal hypoxia in growth retardation to mean blood velocity in the fetal aorta. *Lancet* 1986;2:1118–1119.
9. Muijsers GJJM, Hasaart THM, Ruissen CJ, van Huisseling H, Peeters LLH, de Haan J. The response of the umbilical and femoral artery pulsatility indices in fetal sheep to progressively reduced uteroplacental blood flow. *J Dev Physiol* 1990;13:215–221.
10. Muijsers GJJM, Hasaart THM, van Huisseling H, de Haan J. The response of the umbilical artery pulsatility index in fetal sheep to acute and prolonged hypoxaemia and acidaemia induced by embolization of the uterine microcirculation. *J Dev Physiol* 1990;13:231–236.
11. van Huisseling H, Hasaart THM, Muijsers GJJM, de Haan J. Umbilical artery pulsatility index and placental vascular resistance during acute hypoxemia in fetal lambs. *Gynecol Obstet Invest* 1990;31:61–66.
12. Morrow RJ, Adamson SL, Bull SB, Ritchie JWK. Hypoxic acidemia, hyperviscosity, and maternal hypertension do not affect the umbilical arterial velocity waveform in fetal sheep. *Am J Obstet Gynecol* 1990;163:1313–1320.
13. Morrow RJ, Adamson SL, Bull SB, Ritchie JWK. Acute hypoxemia does not affect the umbilical artery flow velocity waveform in fetal sheep. *Obstet Gynecol* 1990;75:590–593.
14. Giles WB, Trudinger BJ, Baird PJ. Fetal umbilical artery flow velocity waveforms and placental resistance: pathological correlation. *Br J Obstet Gynaecol* 1985;92:31–38.
15. Trudinger BJ, Stevens D, Connelly A, et al. Umbilical artery flow velocity waveforms and placental resistance: the effects of embolization of the umbilical circulation. *Am J Obstet Gynecol* 1987;157:1443–1448.
16. Morrow RJ, Adamson SL, Bull SB, Ritchie JWK. Effect of placental embolization on the umbilical arterial velocity waveform in fetal sheep. *Am J Obstet Gynecol* 1989;161:1055–1060.
17. Copel JA, Schlafer D, Wentworth R, et al. Does the umbilical artery systolic/diastolic ratio reflect flow or acidosis? An umbilical artery Doppler study of fetal sheep. *Am J Obstet Gynecol* 1990;163:751–756.
18. Irion GL, Clark KE. Relationship between the ovine fetal umbilical artery blood flow waveform and umbilical vascular resistance. *Am J Obstet Gynecol* 1990;163:222–229.
19. Adamson SL, Langille BL. Factors determining aortic and umbilical blood flow pulsatility in fetal sheep. *Ultrasound Med Biol* 1992;18:255–266.
20. Erkkola RU, Pirhonen JP. Vascular resistance and the umbilical arterial velocity waveforms. *Am J Obstet Gynecol* 1992;166:910–916.
21. Giles WB, Trudinger BJ. Umbilical cord whole blood viscosity and the umbilical artery flow velocity waveforms: A correlation. *Br J Obstet Gynaecol* 1986;93:466–470.
22. Rochelson BL, Schulman H, Fleischer A. The clinical significance of Doppler umbilical artery velocimetry in the small-for-gestational-age fetus. *Am J Obstet Gynecol* 1987;156:1223–1226.
23. Nichols WW, O'Rourke MF. *McDonald's blood flow in arteries.* London: Edward Arnold; 1990:206, 270, 283, 381.
24. Adamson SL, Whiteley KJ, Langille BL. Pulsatile pressure-flow relations and pulse-wave propagation in the umbilical circulation of fetal sheep. *Circ Res* 1992;70:761–772.
25. Adamson SL, Morrow RJ, Bull SB, Langille BL. Vasomotor responses of the umbilical circulation in fetal sheep. *Am J Physiol* 1989;256:R1056–R1062.
26. Paulick RP, Meyers RL, Rudolph CD, Rudolph AM. Umbilical and hepatic venous responses to circulating vasoconstrictive hormones in fetal lamb. *Am J Physiol* 1991;260:H1205–H1213.
27. Mires G, Dempster J, Patel NB, Crawford JW. The effect of fetal

heart rate on umbilical artery flow velocity waveforms. *Br J Obstet Gynaecol* 1987;4:665–669.

28. Mulders LGM, Muijsers GJJM, Jongsma HW, Nijhuis JG, Hein PR. The umbilical artery blood flow velocity waveform in relation to fetal breathing movements, fetal heart rate and fetal behavioural states in normal pregnancy at 37 to 39 weeks. *Early Hum Dev* 1986;14:283–293.

29. Van Den Wijngaard JAGW, Eyck JV, Wladimiroff JW. The relationship between fetal heart rate and Doppler blood flow velocity waveforms. *Ultrasound Med Biol* 1988;14:593–597.

30. Yarlagadda P, Willoughby L, Maulik D. Effect of fetal heart rate on umbilical arterial Doppler indices. *J Ultrasound Med* 1989;8:215–218.

31. Visser GHA. Fetal behaviour and the cardiovascular system. *J Dev Physiol* 1984;6:215–224.

32. Hoskins PR, Johnstone FD, Chambers SE, Haddad NG, White G, McDicken WN. Heartrate variation of umbilical artery Doppler waveforms. *Ultrasound Med Biol* 1989;15:101–105.

33. Spencer JAD, Giussani DA, Moore PJ, Hanson MA. In vitro validation of Doppler indices using blood and water. *J Ultrasound Med* 1991;10:305–308.

34. Legarth J, Thorup E. Characteristics of Doppler blood-velocity waveforms in a cardiovascular in-vitro model. I. The model and the influence of pulse rate. *Scand J Clin Lab Invest* 1989;49:451–457.

35. Legarth J, Thorup E. Characteristics of Doppler blood-velocity waveforms in a cardiovascular in-vitro model. II. The influence of peripheral resistance, perfusion pressure and blood flow. *Scand J Clin Lab Invest* 1989;49:459–464.

36. Thompson RS, Stevens RJ. Mathematical model for interpretation of Doppler velocity waveform indices. *Med Biol Eng Comput* 1989;27:269–276.

37. Guiot C, Pianta PG, Todros T. Modelling the feto-placental circulation. 1. A distributed network predicting umbilical haemodynamics throughout pregnancy. *Ultrasound Med Biol* 1992;18:535–544.

38. Vieyres P, Durand A, Patat F, et al. Influence of the measurement location on the resistance index in the umbilical arteries: A hemodynamic approach. *J Ultrasound Med* 1991;10:671–675.

39. Todros T, Guiot C, Pianta PG. Modelling the feto-placental circulation. 2. A continuous approach to explain normal and abnormal flow velocity waveforms in the umbilical arteries. *Ultrasound Med Biol* 1992;18:545–551.

40. Erskine RLA, Ritchie JWK. Quantitative measurement of fetal blood flow using Doppler ultrasound. *Br J Obstet Gynaecol* 1985;92:600–604.

41. Chao JC, Hwang NHC. A review of the bases for the hydraulic transmission line equations as applied to circulatory systems. *J Biomechanics* 1972;5:129–134.

42. Cox RH. Comparison of linearized wave propagation models for arterial blood flow analysis. *J Biomechan* 1969;2:251–265.

43. Burattini R, Campbell KB. Modified asymmetric t-tube model to infer arterial wave reflection at the aortic root. *IEEE Trans Biomed Eng* 1992;36:805–814.

44. Einav S, Aharoni S, Manoach M. Exponentially tapered transmission line model of the arterial system. *IEEE Trans Biomed Eng* 1988;35:333–339.

45. Jager GN, Westerhof N, Noordergraaf A. Oscillatory flow impedance in electrical analog of arterial system. *Circ Res* 1965;16:121–133.

46. Krus P, Karlsson M, Engvall J. Modelling and simulation of the human arterial tree, using transmission line elements with viscoelastic walls. *Adv Bioeng* 1991;20:115–118.

47. Liu Z, Shen F, Yin FCP. Impedance of arterial system simulated by viscoelastic t-tubes terminated in windkessels. *Am J Physiol* 1989;256:H1087–H1099.

48. Mo LYL, Bascom PAJ, Ritchie K, McCowan LM. A transmission line modelling approach to the interpretation of uterine Doppler waveforms. *Ultrasound Med Biol* 1988;14:365–376.

49. Snyder MF, Rideout VC. Computer modeling of the human systemic arterial tree. *J Biomechan* 1968;1:341–353.

50. Westerhof N, Bosman F, de Vries CJ, Noordergraaf A. Analog studies of the human systemic arterial tree. *J Biomechan* 1969;2:121–143.

Doppler Ultrasound in Obstetrics and Gynecology,
edited by Joshua A. Copel and Kathryn L. Reed.
Raven Press, Ltd., New York © 1995.

CHAPTER 10

First-Trimester Fetal and Uterine Doppler

Giuseppe Rizzo, Domenico Arduini, and Carlo Romanini

In the past few years dynamic studies of fetal and maternal blood flow by Doppler ultrasound have added valuable information to the understanding of the pathophysiology underlying several diseases affecting pregnancy. The information gained from these studies has evidenced how the placenta plays a major role in the normal development of pregnancy and how placental dysfunction is generally caused by factors interfering with the normal growth of the uteroplacental and/or fetoplacental circulations. These abnormalities lead to a deficient supply of oxygen and nutrients to the fetus and to several complications of pregnancy.

Placental angiogenesis starts early in gestation and is considered completed by the end of the second trimester of pregnancy (1). In the past Doppler studies were limited to the late second and third trimester of pregnancy due to limitations of the conventional transabdominal approach in visualizing maternal vessels deep in the pelvis as well as small fetal vessels. More recently, the combined use of transvaginal ultrasound and color and pulsed Doppler techniques has allowed study of the uterine, placental, and fetal circulations as early as the first trimester of pregnancy. In the transvaginal approach, probes with a high carrier frequency are used because of the closer proximity to the region scanned. This results in a high image resolution allowing visualization of maternal and fetal vascular structures and thus enabling us to obtain early Doppler recordings of blood flow velocities.

This possibility has raised interesting and important questions on the normal hemodynamic evolution at the level of uterine and fetal vessels in physiologic pregnancies and opened future clinical applications in pathologic pregnancies.

G. Rizzo, and C. Romanini: Department of Obstetrics and Gynecology Università di Roma "Tor Vergata," Italy.
D. Arduini: Department of Obstetrics and Gynecology, Università di Ancona, Ancona, Italy.

In this chapter we will review the data on uterine and fetal circulations in early gestation so far obtained using Doppler techniques.

UTERINE CIRCULATION

The blood supply of the uterus is mainly provided by the uterine arteries. Both uterine arteries follow a tortuous course along the lateral margins of the uterus and then branch in the arcuate arteries. The arcuate arteries extend into the myometrium and encircle the uterus, forming anastomoses with branches of the same arteries from the contralateral side. The radial arteries arising from the arcuate arteries are directed towards the uterine cavity and terminate in the spiral arteries that feed the intervillous space.

In normal pregnancies the blood supply to the uterus remarkably increases from 50 ml/min in early pregnancy to approximately 500 ml/min at term (2). Systemic events occurring during pregnancy such as the expansion of maternal blood volume and the rise of cardiac output play a partial role in this increase of uterine blood flow but its main origin may be found in local factors decreasing uterine vascular resistance. In normal early pregnancy the trophoblastic cells invade the placental bed and migrate through the spiral arteries of the uterine circulation. The invading trophoblast destroys the elastic lamina and replaces the smooth muscle cells of the vascular wall of the spiral arteries (3). This transformation, completed by 20 weeks of gestation, leads to the formation of a low-resistance vascular system in which relatively large arteries pump blood directly to the placental intervillous space (4,5). Failure or impairment of trophoblastic invasion does not allow the fall of uterine vascular resistance and impairs the maternal–fetal exchange of nutrients and oxygen, thus leading to intrauterine growth retardation (IUGR) and/or maternal hypertension (6).

Transvaginal color Doppler ultrasonography allows visualization in early pregnancy of the main uterine arteries, arcuate arteries, radial arteries, and flows near the trophoblastic area believed to represent spiral arteries (7–9). The small dimensions of the uterine vessels and the difficulty of obtaining low angles of insonation have limited the analysis of blood flow velocity waveforms mainly to qualitative angle-independent indices considered directly related to vascular resistances, such as the S/D ratio (systolic velocity/diastolic velocity), resistance index [RI = (systolic velocity − diastolic velocity)/systolic velocity], or pulsatility index [PI = (systolic velocity − diastolic velocity)/mean velocity].

Velocity waveforms recorded from the various vascular districts of the uterine circulations showed significantly different morphology at similar gestational ages (Fig. 1). These differences are mainly related to the diastolic component, which is more prominent in distal vascular structures (i.e., spiral arteries) than in main branches of the uterine arteries. Possible explanations for these findings include either differences in vessel structure and distance from the heart, or the earlier trophoblastic invasion in distal vessels. As a consequence, the ratios of vascular resistances calculated from the spiral arteries are significantly lower than those from the arcuate and uterine arteries at similar gestational age (Fig. 2).

Furthermore there is a progressive decrease of Doppler indices of the different uterine districts with advancing gestation, and these changes are believed secondary to a fall of vascular resistances due to trophoblastic invasion (Fig. 2).

The possibility of studying the early physiologic development of the uterine circulation has turned attention to potential deviations from the norm that may be responsible for different complications of pregnancy such as early pregnancy failure, uteroplacental insufficiency, and trophoblastic disease.

Early Pregnancy Failure

It may be expected that major deviations from these patterns would probably lead to obstetric complications. Moreover, preliminary studies on pregnancies with early failure showed contradictory results. A study performed by the authors in 19 patients with early pregnancy failure (missed abortion, $N = 8$; anembryonic pregnancy, $N = 11$) showed that the S/D values calculated from spiral arteries always fell within the normal values (9). These findings are in agreement with the results of Stabile et al. who similarly found no significant modifications in the velocity waveforms obtained from the subplacental vessels of seven pregnancies with early failure (10). How-

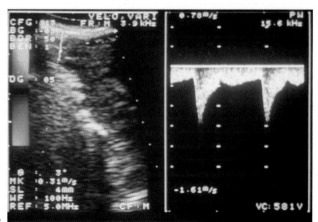

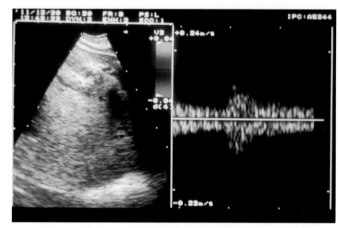

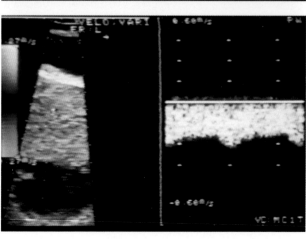

FIG. 1. Flow velocity waveforms from the main uterine artery (**A**), arcuate artery (**B**), and spiral arteries (**C**) at 9 weeks gestation.

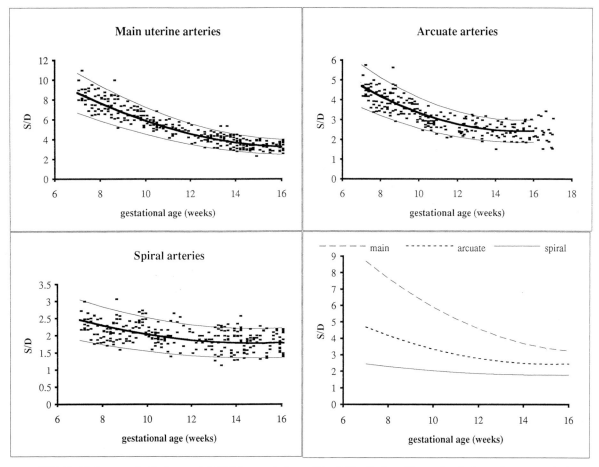

FIG. 2. Reference limits (mean ± 2 SD) for gestation of the *S/D* ratio from the main uterine artery, arcuate artery, and spiral artery. From Arduini et al. (9).

ever, Alfirevic and Kurjak reported the absence of trophoblastic flow in some patients with either anembryonic pregnancy or missed abortion (11). Of interest are the data of Jaffe and Warsof, who reported lower values of resistance to flow in anembryonic pregnancies when compared to missed abortions, suggesting a poorer vascularization in the latter group (12).

Although the number of cases studied is small and no serial recordings of pregnancies that eventually fail are available, it may be suggested that most of the cases of early pregnancy failure are not caused by failure of vascularization. However, in some cases a faulty vascularization may be the etiologic factor and may be evidenced by a nonvisualization of trophoblastic flow with color flow mapping, or by abnormal *S/D* ratios. Further studies will validate these concepts and will allow better definition of the pathophysiology of early pregnancy failure.

Early Prediction of Uteroplacental Insufficiency

Minor deviations of the vascularization process may lead to poor uterine perfusion and therefore to uteroplacental insufficiency. Early identification of these preg-

nancies is of great interest as it may allow prophylactic treatments (i.e., low-dose aspirin) theoretically able to reduce the frequency or delay the onset of related complications such as hypertension, preeclampsia, and IUGR. Doppler studies performed during the first trimester in those later developing hypertension and/or growth retardation showed that resistances to flow may be within normal ranges in the first trimester and deteriorate later, thus limiting the possibility of early screening (9). Moreover, Harrington et al. found evidence of abnormalities in uterine blood flow velocity waveforms in the late first trimester in pregnancies developing early onset preeclampsia and growth retardation (13). These results suggest that a normal Doppler velocity waveform does not exclude the later development of flow and pregnancy abnormalities. On the other hand, the finding of an abnormal flow pattern already in early gestation may well predict severe complications of pregnancy and thus justify pharmacologic treatments.

Trophoblastic Disease

Conventional real-time ultrasonography (in conjunction with serum β-hCG levels) is the established method for the diagnosis of abnormal trophoblastic proliferation. However, the possibility of using color and pulsed Doppler has been tested.

By invading the myometrium trophoblastic tissue erodes the muscular wall of the uterine arteries. This leads to a low impedance to flow resulting in increased uterine perfusion. The use of color Doppler allows evaluation of low resistances to flow and of hypervascularization within the uterus (14). These findings may be clinically useful to define the degree of trophoblastic invasion in terms of vessel penetration. Furthermore after curettage of the uterine cavity they may define the persistence of trophoblastic tissue. Finally, the success or failure of chemotherapy can be evaluated by serial recordings (15).

In summary, Doppler ultrasonography may not replace established methods of diagnosis of trophoblastic diseases but can provide additional information that may be useful to consider in the management of these pregnancies.

FETAL CIRCULATION

Fetal circulation in early gestation has been studied in different vascular beds among which are the umbilical circulation, peripheral arterial vessels, the heart, and the great veins. The different flow patterns found have provided important information allowing a better understanding of normal fetal physiology.

The normal development of flow patterns is different in the various areas investigated.

Umbilical Artery

At 6 completed menstrual weeks the villous vasculature is connected with the primitive fetal heart and the umbilical circulation starts (16). From this gestational age onward there is a progressive opening of small muscular arteries as demonstrated by the increased proportion of villi occupied by capillaries in morphometric studies (17).

The umbilical circulation may be studied by Doppler ultrasonography from 7 weeks of gestation (18,19) (Fig. 3). End-diastolic velocities are usually absent until 12 weeks of gestation. From this gestational age onward diastolic flow becomes progressively present in most of the cases while it is consistently present in all pregnancies after 15 weeks. The appearance of end-diastolic velocities induces an evident drop of Doppler indices such as pulsatility index (PI) (18). This latter finding has induced some authors to speculate on an abrupt passage from a high-resistance to a low-resistance placenta (20). Moreover, when the percentage of absent end-diastolic flow over the total cardiac cycle is calculated, a gradual fall of this index is evidenced from 7 to 16 weeks of gestation (19), a finding more in agreement with the existence of progressive changes in placental hemodynamics rather than abrupt modifications.

The increased number of small vessels and their progressive merging with the umbilical circulation play a key role in the gradual fall of impedance to flow evidenced by Doppler ultrasonography. Moreover, other factors such as changes in the pressure gradient of the intervillous space or modifications in fetal blood viscosity (i.e., reduction of nucleated red cells) may not be excluded (21).

Fetal Peripheral Arterial Vessels

Blood flow velocity waveforms in early gestation can be obtained from the descending aorta and intracerebral vessels. The descending aorta is directly connected with the umbilical circulation and its waveform profile may be greatly influenced by placental resistance.

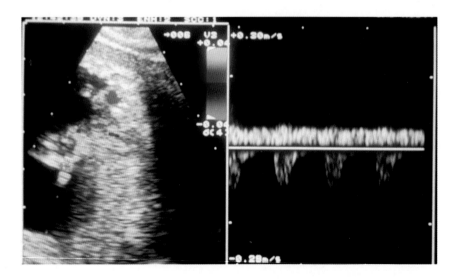

FIG. 3. Blood flow velocity waveforms in umbilical artery at 10 weeks gestation. Note the absence of end-diastolic flow.

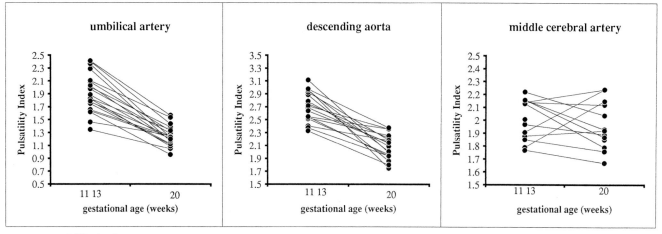

FIG. 4. Serial changes of pulsatility index from umbilical artery (**left**), descending aorta (**middle**), and middle cerebral artery (**right**) between 11–13 and 20 weeks gestation. From Rizzo et al. (23).

Similarly to the umbilical artery, the end-diastolic velocity is frequently absent in the aorta at 11–14 weeks of gestation and progressively appears with advancing gestation (22,23). Serial recordings from the umbilical artery and descending aorta have demonstrated a similar trend of PI values with advancing gestation (23,24) (Fig. 4).

Intracerebral blood flow velocity waveforms may be recorded as early as 11 weeks gestation (23,24). At this gestational age it is difficult to define which intracerebral vessel is insonated but the middle cerebral artery is probably the vessel most frequently insonated (Fig. 5). Of interest is the presence of end-diastolic velocities in blood flow velocity waveforms from this vessel in contrast to their absence in aorta and umbilical artery. Furthermore PI values remain constant during the first half of pregnancy (23,24) (Fig. 4). These findings suggest lower vascular resistances at the cerebral level than in the placenta or in splanchnic organs in early gestation that may explain or be a consequence of the ratio between head and body size at this time of gestation.

Cardiac Flows

Reliable recordings of velocity waveforms from atrioventricular valves, outflow tracts, and ductus arteriosus can already be obtained at 11 weeks of gestation (Fig. 6) (23,25).

At the level of the atrioventricular valves flow velocity waveforms are characterized by a low ratio between early (E) and active (A) ventricular filling. Serial recordings have shown a rapid increase of E/A ratios from both the mitral and tricuspid valves in early gestation (Fig. 7). The E/A ratio is a widely accepted index of ventricular diastolic function and it is influenced by several factors including preload, ventricular compliance, and afterload. The noninvasive nature of Doppler examination, without the possibility of obtaining simultaneous measurements of flow and pressure, does not allow a differentiation between these factors, but it may be suggested that all may contribute to induce these changes. The reduction of blood viscosity secondary to the decrease of nucleated red cells or an absolute increase of volume may

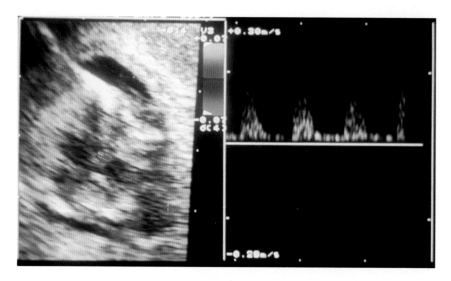

FIG. 5. Blood flow velocity waveforms from fetal cerebral vessel, presumably middle cerebral artery at 11 weeks of gestation. Note the presence of end-diastolic flow.

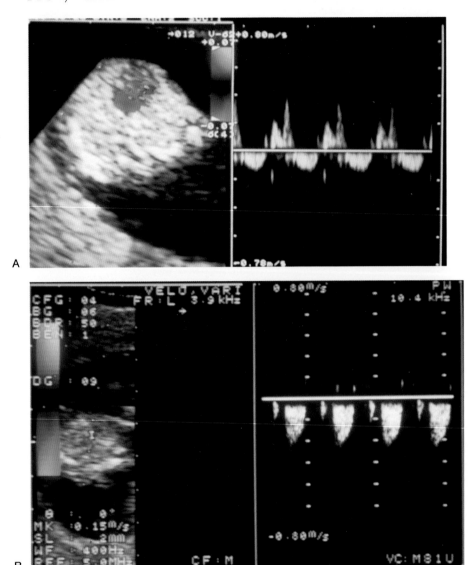

FIG. 6. Blood flow velocity waveforms from mitral valve (**A**) and pulmonary artery at 12 weeks of gestation (**B**).

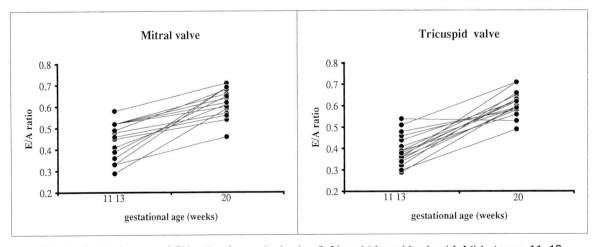

FIG. 7. Serial changes of *E/A* ratios from mitral valve (**left**) and tricuspid valve (**right**) between 11–13 and 20 weeks gestation. From Rizzo et al. (23).

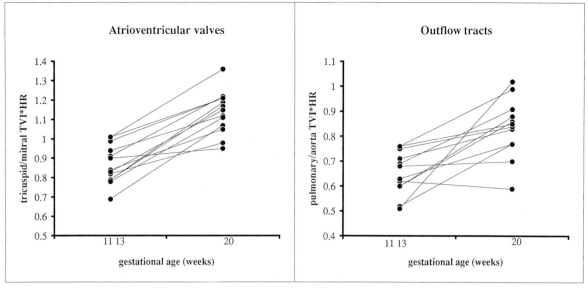

FIG. 8. Serial changes of right-to-left ratio of TVI*HR from atrioventricular valve (**left**) and outflow tract (**right**) between 11–13 and 20 weeks gestation. From Rizzo et al. (23).

explain an increased preload with advancing gestation and therefore the increase in E/A ratios values. On the other hand, an improvement of cardiac compliance may similarly explain the Doppler findings and is consistent with experimental studies showing a reduction of fetal heart stiffness with advancing gestation. Finally, the decrease of placental resistances may induce a decrease of cardiac afterload inducing an increase of E/A ratios.

Peak velocities in the outflow tracts similarly increase with advancing gestation (23). This may be due either to an increased myocardial contractility with advancing gestation or to an increased blood flow, or to a reduction of cardiac afterload. Again, differentiation between these factors is impossible in the human fetus.

Absolute cardiac output is given by the product of time velocity integral (TVI), heart rate (HR), and valve

area. This latter measurement is unreliable in early gestation due to the small dimensions of cardiac valves that are near the limits of ultrasound resolution. Moreover, the product TVI × HR is highly related to the cardiac output and may be used as an indirect measure of cardiac output. Serial recordings of TVI × HR showed a progressive increase with advancing gestation at the level of all four valves, suggesting an increase of fetal cardiac output in early gestation (23).

It is of interest that there is an increase also of the ratios between the right to left products of TVI × HR measured at the level of both great vessels and atrioventricular valves, suggesting a preferential streaming of blood to the right heart with advancing gestation (Fig. 8). Potential explanations for these findings include either an asymmetric growth of cardiac valves leading to nonsignificant

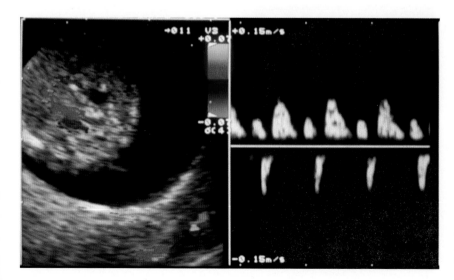

FIG. 9. Blood flow velocity waveforms from inferior vena cava at 13 weeks gestation. Note the high percentage of reverse flow during atrial contraction (*bottom*).

INFERIOR VENA CAVA

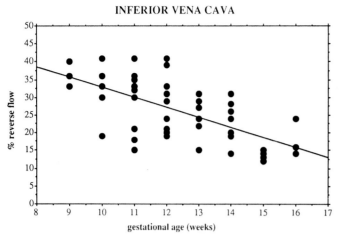

FIG. 10. Changes of % reverse flow in inferior vena cava from 11 to 16 weeks gestation. From Rizzo et al. (31).

changes of the distribution between right and left cardiac outputs or a shift in cardiac output in favor of the right ventricle (23). The former explanation seems unlikely on the basis of human studies showing a similar growth pattern between right and left cardiac valves (26). The latter hypothesis is also consistent with the selective modifications of cardiac afterload previously described. During fetal life the output of the left ventricle is directed through ascending aorta to upper body organs mainly represented by the brain, whereas the output of the right ventricle is directed through the patent ductus arteriosus to the lower body and placenta (27). The significant fall of Doppler-measured vascular resistances evidenced in umbilical artery and descending aorta not associated with similar changes in cerebral vascular resistances suggests a selective reduction of right ventricle afterload with respect to the left ventricle afterload, thus justifying the preferential blood streaming to the right heart.

Venous Blood Flow

Blood flow velocity waveforms were recorded in early gestation from the inferior vena cava, ductus venosus, and umbilical vein. Inferior vena cava flows exhibit a triphasic pattern characterized by a first forward peak during systole, a second forward flow concomitant with early diastole, and a third reverse flow with atrial contraction during late diastole (28) (Fig. 9). The percentage of reverse flow relative to total forward flow is the index more commonly used and it is believed to be related to pressure in the right atrium (29).

The percentage of reverse flow in the inferior vena cava significantly decreases with gestation, and this change may be secondary either to reduction in placental afterload or to an improvement of cardiac compliance (30,31) (Fig. 10). Both factors may contribute in reducing the pressure gradient in the right atrium and therefore the reverse flow during atrial contraction.

The ductus venosus has a pulsatile pattern with two forward components corresponding to systole and diastole (32). Of interest is the high velocity present in this vessel even in early gestation and the progressive increase that occurs with advancing gestation. This may be an expression of progressively increasing fetal volemia.

Umbilical vein flow patterns are usually continuous. The presence of a pulsatile pattern has been described in severely compromised fetuses as a result of cardiac decompensation (33). The suggested underlying pathophysiology of this phenomenon is impaired myocardial contractility resulting in increased pressure gradients leading to increased reversal of flow in the inferior vena cava that extends beyond the ductus venosus and the hepatic vein, causing regular end-diastolic pulsations in the umbilical vein (34). Recent studies in early gestation have demonstrated that these pulsations are physiologically present until 9 weeks of gestation (Fig. 11) and pro-

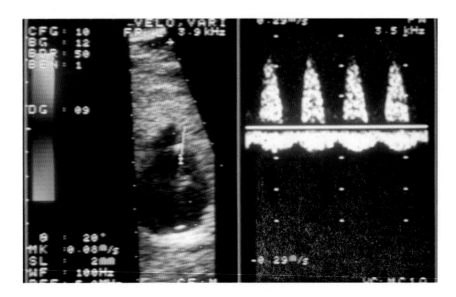

FIG. 11. Umbilical vein pulsations at 8 weeks gestation.

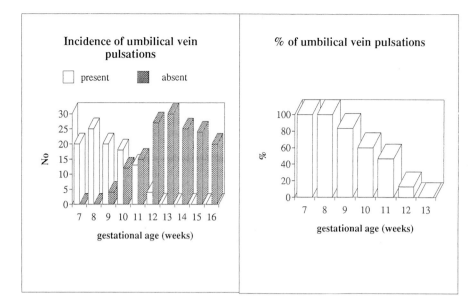

FIG. 12. Incidence of umbilical vein pulsations from 7 to 16 weeks gestation. Data are shown as absolute number (*left*) and percentage (*right*). From Rizzo et al. (31).

gressively disappear by 12 weeks of gestation (31) (Fig. 12). Their genesis is unclear but seems to be unrelated to Doppler-measured placental resistance or heart rate. The higher percentage of reverse flow in the umbilical artery in fetuses with pulsations compared with control fetuses without pulsations at corresponding gestational age suggests a mechanism similar to that described in pathologic fetuses (31). That is, the high reverse flow in the inferior vena cava may physiologically extend to the umbilical vein, causing pulsations in the first trimester of pregnancy.

CONCLUSIONS

The first part of pregnancy is characterized by profound hemodynamic changes both in uterine and fetal circulations. These changes are mainly secondary to the formation of the placenta, a vascular system characterized by low vascular resistance. The physiologic changes occurring in the different vascular districts and their relationships have been widely investigated by Doppler ultrasonography. It remains to be ascertained whether abnormalities in the physiologic development may be used to diagnose and predict pregnancy complications.

REFERENCES

1. Pijnenborg R, Dixon G, Robertson WB, Brosens I. Trophoblastic invasion of human decidua from 8 to 18 weeks of pregnancy. *Placenta* 1980;1:3–19.
2. Blechner JN, Stenger VG, Prystowsky C. Uterine blood flow in women at term. *Am J Obstet Gynecol* 1974;120:633–638.
3. Pijnenborg R, Bland JM, Robertson WB, Brosens I. Uteroplacental arterial changes related to interstitial trophoblast migration in early human pregnancy. *Placenta* 1983;4:397–414.
4. Robertson WB. Uteroplacental vasculature. *J Clin Pathol* 1976;29:9–17.
5. Hustin J, Schaaps JP, Lambotte R. Anatomical studies of utero-placental vascularization in the first trimester of pregnancy. *Trophoblast Res* 1988;3:49–60.
6. Khong TY, De Wolf F, Robertson WB, Brosens I. Inadequate maternal vascular response to placentation in pregnancies complicated by preeclampsia and small for gestational age infants. *Br J Obstet Gynaecol* 1986;93:1049–1059.
7. Jaffe R, Warsof SL. Transvaginal color Doppler imaging in the assessment of uteroplacental blood flow in the normal first-trimester pregnancy. *Am J Obstet Gynecol* 1991;164:781–785.
8. Jurkovic D, Jauniaux E, Kurjak A, Hustin J, Campbell S, Nicolaides KH. Transvaginal color Doppler assessment of uteroplacental circulation in early pregnancy. *Obstet Gynecol* 1991;77:365–369.
9. Arduini D, Rizzo G, Romanini C. Doppler ultrasonography in early pregnancy does not predict adverse pregnancy outcome. *Ultrasound Obstet Gynecol* 1991;1:180–185.
10. Stabile I, Grudzinskas J, Campbell S. Doppler ultrasonographic evaluation of abnormal pregnancies in the first trimester. *J Clin Ultrasound* 1990;18:497–501.
11. Alfirevic Z, Kurjak A. Transvaginal colour Doppler ultrasound in normal and abnormal early pregnancy. *J Perinat Med* 1990;18:173–180.
12. Jaffe R, Warsof SL. Color Doppler imaging in the assessment of uteroplacental blood flow in abnormal first trimester intrauterine pregnancies: an attempt to define etiologic mechanism. *J Ultrasound Med* 1992;11:41–44.
13. Harrington KF, Campbell S, Bewley S, Bower S. Doppler velocimetry studies of the uterine arteries in the early prediction of preeclampsia and intrauterine growth retardation. *Eur J Obstet Gynecol Reprod Med* 1991;42:S14–S20.
14. Aoki S, Hata T, Hata K, et al. Doppler color flow mapping of an invasive mole. *Gynecol Obstet Invest* 1989;27:52–54.
15. Long MG, Boulbtee JE, Begent RHJ, Hanson ME, Bagshawe KD. Preliminary Doppler studies of the uterine arteries and myometrium in trophoblastic tumors requiring chemotherapy. *Br J Obstet Gynaecol* 1990;97:686–689.
16. Benirschke K, Kauffmann P. *Pathology of the Human Placenta.* New York: Springer-Verlag; 1990.
17. Jauniaux E, Burton GJ, Moscoso GJ, Hustin J. Development of the early human placenta: a morphometric study. *Placenta* 1991;12:269–276.
18. Den Ouden M, Cohen-Overbeek TE, Wladimiroff JW. Uterine and fetal umbilical artery flow velocity waveforms in normal first trimester pregnancies. *Br J Obstet Gynaecol* 1990;97:716–719.
19. Arduini D, Rizzo G. Umbilical artery velocity waveforms in early pregnancy: a transvaginal color Doppler study. *J Clin Ultrasound* 1991;12:335–339.
20. Loquet Ph, Broughton Pipkin F, Symonds EM, Rubin PC. Blood

velocity waveforms and placental vascular formation (letter). *Lancet* 1988;2:1252.

21. Jauniaux E, Jurkovic D, Campbell S. In vivo investigation of the anatomy and the physiology of early human placental circulations. *Ultrasound Obstet Gynecol* 1991;1:435–445.

22. Wladimiroff JW, Huisman TWA, Stewart PA. Fetal and umbilical flow velocity waveforms between 10 and 16 weeks of gestation: A preliminary study. *Obstet Gynecol* 1991;78:812–814.

23. Rizzo G, Arduini D, Romanini C. Fetal cardiac and extra-cardiac circulation in early gestation. *J Mat-Fet Invest* 1991;1:73–78.

24. Wladimiroff JW, Huisman TWA, Stewart PA. Intracerebral, aortic and umbilical artery flow velocity waveforms in the late first trimester fetus. *Am J Obstet Gynecol* 1992;166:46–49.

25. Wladimiroff JW, Huisman TWA, Stewart PA. Cardiac Doppler flow velocity in the late first trimester fetus. *J Am Coll Cardiol* 1991;17:1357–1359.

26. Comstock CH, Riggs T, Lee W, Kirk J. Pulmonary to aorta diameter ratio in the normal and abnormal fetal heart. *Am J Obstet Gynecol* 1991;165:1038–1043.

27. Rudolph AM. Distribution and regulation of blood flow in the fetal and neonatal lamb. *Circ Res* 1985;57:811–821.

28. Reed KL, Appleton CP, Anderson CF, Shenker L, Sahn DJ. Doppler studies of vena cava flows in human fetuses: Insights into normal and abnormal cardiac physiology. *Circulation* 1990;81:498–505.

29. Rizzo G, Arduini D, Romanini C. Inferior vena cava flow velocity waveforms in appropriate and small for gestational age fetuses. *Am J Obstet Gynecol* 1992;166:1271–1280.

30. Wladimiroff JW, Huisman TWA, Stewart PA, Stijnen Th. Normal fetal Doppler inferior vena cava, transtricuspid and umbilical artery flow velocity waveforms between 11 and 16 weeks' gestation. *Am J Obstet Gynecol* 1992;166:46–49.

31. Rizzo G, Arduini D, Romanini C. Pulsations in umbilical vein: A physiological finding in early pregnancy. *Am J Obstet Gynecol* 1992;167:675–677.

32. Huisman THA, Stewart PA, Wladimiroff JW. Doppler assessment of normal early fetal circulation. *Ultrasound Obstet Gynecol* 1992;2:300–305.

33. Gudmundsson S, Huhta JC, Wood DC, Tulzer G, Cohen AW, Weiner S. Venous Doppler ultrasonography in the fetus with nonimmune hydrops. *Am J Obstet Gynecol* 1991;164:33–37.

34. Indick JH, Chen V, Reed KL. Association of umbilical venous with inferior vena cava blood flow velocities. *Obstet Gynecol* 1991;77:551–557.

Doppler Ultrasound in Obstetrics and Gynecology,
edited by Joshua A. Copel and Kathryn L. Reed.
Raven Press, Ltd., New York © 1995.

CHAPTER 11

Uteroplacental and Intraplacental Circulation

Siegfried Rotmensch, Marco Liberati, Joaquin Santolaya-Forgas,
and Joshua A. Copel

Uteroplacental insufficiency is a central concept in obstetric pathophysiology. Indeed, profound anatomic changes of the uterine vasculature during pregnancy are prerequisites for fetal growth and development, and lack thereof has been linked to intrauterine growth retardation (IUGR) and preeclampsia (1,2). When Doppler technology was first applied to the study of the uterine circulation (3), expectations were high that valuable information on screening, diagnosis, and management of affected pregnancies could be obtained. The first 10 years of experience, however, has been marked by an unfortunate lack of uniformity in technique and attention to confounding factors. Grossly contradictory studies on the utility of uterine artery Doppler in comparable populations have therefore appeared in the literature. The discrepancies are largely attributable to the limitations of continuous wave Doppler and gray scale sonography in the precise identification of sampled vessels in the highly vascular pelvis.

With the advent of color Doppler flow technology, localization of vessels in the uterine circulation has improved remarkably. We can anticipate, therefore, that more consistency of study results will become apparent over the next few years, provided that uniformity of the underlying pathophysiology in these fetal disorders exists. At present, however, the available body of knowledge consists largely of data obtained in the precolor Doppler era. We should bear this limitation in mind as we assess the current utility of uterine artery Doppler.

S. Rotmensch: Department of Obstetrics and Gynecology, Golda Meir Medical Center, Petach Tikuah, Israel.

M. Liberati and J. A. Copel: Department of Obstetrics and Gynecology, Yale University School of Medicine, New Haven, Connecticut 06511.

J. Santolaya-Forgas: Department of Obstetrics and Gynecology, University of Illinois at Chicago, Chicago, Illinois 60612.

FUNCTIONAL ANATOMY OF THE UTEROPLACENTAL CIRCULATION

Approximately 80% of the blood supply to the uterus is derived from the uterine arteries. Each of the main uterine arteries branches off the internal iliac arteries and reaches the uterus at the level of the internal cervical os. At this point, bifurcation into the cervical and corporal branches occurs, and the tortuous corporal branch ascends on the lateral border of the uterus, while remaining within the leaves of the broad ligament. At the uterine-tubal junction the uterine artery turns toward the ovary and terminates in a tubal and a mesoovarian branch, the latter anastomosing with the ovarian artery.

Throughout its course, the uterine artery gives rise to approximately eight arcuate arteries that run in parallel to encircle the surface of the uterus and form anastomoses with the contralateral vessel. These arcuate arteries supply the centripetal radial arteries, which penetrate the middle third of the myometrium and give rise to about 200 spiral arteries. The spiral arteries continue a convoluted course into the endometrium or decidua before breaking up into a network of capillaries from which blood is subsequently collected in endometrial veins.

As implantation proceeds, trophoblastic cells stream out from the tips of anchoring villi and penetrate into the lumina of the intradecidual portions of the spiral arteries. The musculoelastic architecture within the walls of maternal spiral arteries is replaced by a mixture of fibrinoid and fibrous tissue (4). This process, also called *physiologic change,* converts the spiral arteries to uteroplacental arteries, which are maximally dilated vascular channels of low resistance. It is considered a hallmark of normal placentation. These structurally altered spiral arteries are probably unable to respond to vasoactive stimuli (5), which further supports high-volume flow to the uteroplacental bed under varying physiologic condi-

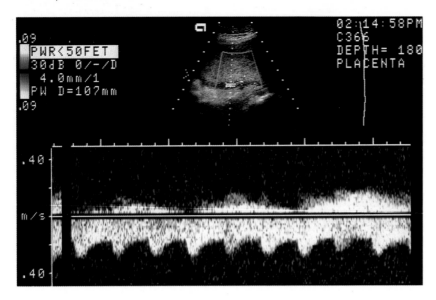

FIG. 1. Normal flow velocity waveform from a uteroplacental vessel in a term pregnancy. Abundant diastolic flow is observed.

tions. Therefore, a major characteristic of uterine blood flow after 20 weeks gestation is a progressively increasing, and rather extensive, diastolic flow.

Most of the trophoblastic invasion appears to occur in two waves, but the timing during gestation varies, and factors that control and limit the degree of invasion are incompletely understood. The initial wave of invasion is confined to spiral arteries within the decidua and occurs between 6 and 12 weeks gestation. Between 16 and 22 weeks gestation the endovascular trophoblast reaches the myometrial portion of the spiral artery in the second wave of vascular invasion. However, the invasion of the myometrial segments of the spiral arteries is not confined to the first two trimesters and seems to continue throughout pregnancy (6). Due to these and other anatomic changes within the uterus and its circulation, total uterine blood flow is estimated to increase from approximately 50 ml/min in early pregnancy to 500 ml/min at term (7).

While normal pregnancy is characterized by invasion of all spiral arteries in the placental bed, this process occurs in only a proportion of vessels in patients destined to develop preeclampsia and/or IUGR (8,9). Consequently, the high-resistance blood flow circuit in the placental bed is preserved, resulting in decreased uteroplacental perfusion. The failure to establish a low-resistance uterine circulation serves as the main pathophysiologic rationale for Doppler investigation of the uterine circulation.

GENERAL PRINCIPLES

As mentioned in previous chapters, considering the difficulty in determining the incident angle of sampled vessels, the tortuous anatomy, and the pulsatility of small vessels in the uterine circulation, Doppler shift in-

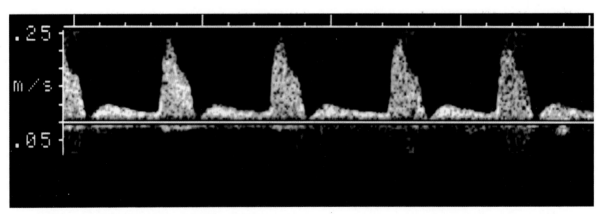

FIG. 2. Uteroplacental flow velocity waveform in a pregnancy with severe pregnancy-induced hypertension and IUGR. Diastolic notching is evident.

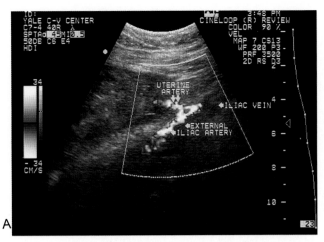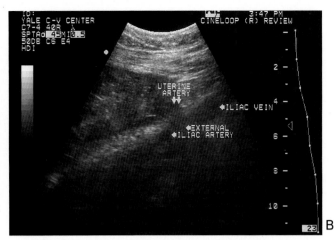

FIG. 3. A: Apparent "crossover" of the uterine and external iliac arteries, as seen with color Doppler flow equipment. **B:** Same image without color flow information illustrating difficulty in visualizing vessels without color.

formation is usually not translated into true flow velocities. Abnormally high Doppler indices, obtained from measurements on the "envelope" of Doppler flow velocity waveforms, correlate quite well with downstream impedance to flow (10) but do not allow for a quantitative assessment of volume flow.

Whether there is any practical difference between the various Doppler indices is uncertain. The *S/D* ratio and resistance index are probably less reliable than the pulsatility index in the presence of minimal diastolic flow. However, the uterine circulation typically has abundant diastolic flow (Fig. 1), in contrast to the fetal aorta and middle cerebral artery, for example. One advantage of using the resistance index is the normal distribution of obtained data, which makes the construction of nomograms and subsequent statistical analysis somewhat easier. The *S/D* ratio requires nonparametric statistics for data analysis. In the end, however, it is a matter of preference, as the differential use of the various Doppler indices in Europe, North America, and other areas demonstrates.

Direct visual impression of the flow velocity waveform is an important component of the uterine artery examination. Doppler indices do not convey potentially important information on systolic and diastolic notching (Fig. 2). Multiple studies have suggested that notching in the uterine artery flow velocity waveform correlates with increased Doppler index measurements (11,12). Furthermore, its presence improves the positive predictive value of the Doppler examination for preeclampsia, IUGR, and fetal distress in labor (11,12).

Continuous wave (CW) and pulse wave (PW) equipment have been extensively used for the examination of the uterine circulation. CW equipment is the least expensive, smallest, and most maneuverable device, which favors its use in screening programs. A major disadvantage of CW equipment, however, is that it does not per-

mit precise identification of the sampled vessel. Indeed, uteroplacental vessels are identified by their typical waveform, which makes it difficult to identify unusual flow dynamics in uterine vessels. It is impossible to determine whether a signal obtained by a CW device was derived from a uterine, arcuate, or spiral artery, and signals are best described as uteroplacental. PW equipment per se does not add substantially to a more precise localization of a desired vessel. The course of the uterine artery is tortuous, and the vessel is buried in the highly vascular and engorged tissues of the pregnant pelvis, which makes precise identification of most vessels by gray scale image alone virtually impossible.

Color Doppler equipment, however, adds a new dimension to uterine artery Doppler. With this technology, the uterine artery can usually be visualized throughout much of its course from the pelvic floor to the uterus (Fig. 3). This allows the precise identification of the sampling site. Furthermore, color flow mapping of small vessels in the uterine muscle or placental bed is feasible. It appears that color Doppler flow imaging improves the accuracy of Doppler measurements, as compared to PW ultrasound alone (13). Regardless of the Doppler equipment used, sampling should be optimized by auditory assessment of the Doppler shift signal, and adjustments in transducer position should be made until the crispest and loudest signal is achieved.

TECHNIQUE

Velocimetric studies of the uterine arteries can be performed by either the transabdominal or transvaginal route (14). First, a general obstetric scan should be performed. Placental location should be documented, as this has some bearing on the interpretation of Doppler indices of uterine arteries. Both CW and PW equipment can be used for the transabdominal examination. In the second and third trimesters of pregnancy, women should be examined in the semirecumbent position and care should be taken to avoid supine hypotension.

Transabdominal CW Doppler

The transducer should be placed 2–3 cm medial to the anterior superior iliac spine, directing the ultrasound beam to the lateral wall of the uterus and slightly downward toward the pelvis. An alternative technique is to locate the transducer immediately above and lateral to the pubis, directing the beam to the lateral wall of the uterus. The probe position should be altered with minute movements until the uteroplacental waveform is identified. CW signals can also be obtained from multiple predetermined locations in order to calculate an overall average Doppler index (15).

Transabdominal PW Doppler

PW Doppler can be used by itself or in conjunction with superimposed color Doppler flow mapping. If no color Doppler equipment is available, the search for the uterine artery is guided by the typical uteroplacental flow velocity waveform. In that sense, PW equipment in and of itself is not much help. Frequently, the outline of blood vessels presumed to be uterine can be seen adjacent to the uterus or within the myometrium. However, confirmation depends on the identification of the flow velocity waveform.

Color Doppler facilitates identification of the uterine artery substantially. When the transducer is positioned in the above-described fashion, an apparent "crossover" of the external iliac artery and the main uterine artery can be identified (Fig. 3). Even though this image is an artifact resulting from the diagonal scanning plane through the pelvis, it is extremely helpful in identifying the main uterine artery in a reproducible fashion.

Transvaginal PW Doppler

This technique utilizes the same PW system. The patient lies in a supine gynecologic position. The probe, covered by a lubricated condom, is introduced into the vaginal fornix and different segments of the main branch of the ascending uterine artery can easily be located along the side of the uterus. Transvaginal scanning is clearly the method of choice in the first trimester, when uterine blood flow is relatively small, compared to the second and third trimesters.

NORMAL UTERINE ARTERY DOPPLER FLOW VELOCITY WAVEFORMS

Flow velocity waveforms of the uteroplacental circulation undergo remarkable changes during the menstrual cycle and pregnancy. Absence of end-diastolic flow and early diastolic notching are frequently observed during the follicular phase of the menstrual cycle (16). Following ovulation, a decrease in the impedance to flow in the uterine artery is observed and is more pronounced in the uterine artery ipsilateral to the ovulating ovary (17).

During the first 10 weeks of pregnancy, Doppler index values remain high but quite stable, resembling the values of the secretory phase of the menstrual cycle. At the beginning of the second trimester, a sharp decrease in Doppler indices occurs. Concurrently, early diastolic notching disappears. Persistence of a diastolic notch can be a normal feature up to 26 weeks gestation.

Between 14 and 25 weeks gestation, significant differences exist between Doppler index values of arcuate and uterine arteries, and further differences exist in relation to the placental implantation site (15,18,19). After 24 weeks, the slope of decrease in uterine artery Doppler indices near the placenta is less prominent than those of the contralateral side. Little or no change is usually observed on either side after 26 weeks gestation (Fig. 4). However, data reference ranges in the published literature show considerable variation. Several studies did not

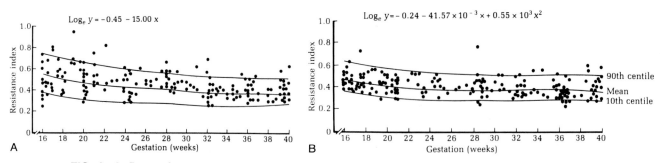

FIG. 4. A: Data reference range for the resistance index from the nonplacental side of the uterus. **B:** Reference range for the resistance index from the placental side of the uterus. From Pearce et al. (21).

demonstrate that Doppler index values continue to fall in the third trimester (16,20,21), whereas others show a continuing fall throughout the last two trimesters (22,23).

ABNORMAL UTEROPLACENTAL FLOW VELOCITY WAVEFORMS

Various parameters have been used in the literature as markers for abnormal uteroplacental flow dynamics detected by Doppler velocimetry. Since little or no change is seen in Doppler indices after 26 weeks, the use of a single cutoff value obtained from one uterine artery, corresponding to the 95th percentile, or 2 SD above the mean seems appropriate (24). Others have averaged values obtained from both uterine arteries and used the upper limit of the normal range. The presence of diastolic notching after 26 weeks also correlates with fetal compromise (11), and marked differences in Doppler indices between the placental and nonplacental sides are considered abnormal (16,25).

SCREENING WITH UTERINE ARTERY DOPPLER

The ability to identify mothers at risk for adverse pregnancy outcome is a major focus of obstetric research. Even though the efficacy of intervention strategies is still questionable, there is evidence to suggest that at least in the case of preeclampsia, low-dose aspirin may improve pregnancy outcome (26–28). On the other hand, it is certainly conceivable that overzealous testing and intervention could harm the mother and her fetus, particularly in the case of false-positive tests. Antenatal testing most definitely devours significant financial resources, and management policies have to be carefully evaluated for their cost–benefit ratio prior to implementation.

Decreased uteroplacental perfusion in pregnancies complicated by hypertension and IUGR has been demonstrated by a variety of techniques (29), including nitrous oxide diffusion studies, radioactive sodium tracing, and placental clearance of labeled dehydroepiandrosterone. The presumed pathophysiologic basis is increased resistance to blood flow. Since uterine artery Doppler indices seem to correlate with downstream resistance, it was hoped that this technique would detect the persistence of a high-resistance uteroplacental circulation secondary to abnormal placentation. At present, however, results are equivocal at best, and the role of the Doppler examination for screening is still evolving, particularly regarding the utilization of color Doppler equipment.

Analysis of the literature on uterine artery Doppler screening is hampered by a variety of methodologic and conceptual problems. It is of major importance that the target population for screening be clearly defined in the analysis of published data. Since the predictive power of a test correlates with the prevalence of the disease for which the test screens, marked differences can be expected when screening is done in normal gravidae, as opposed to women at high risk for pregnancy complications. Unfortunately, there is also no universal agreement on the definition of pregnancy outcome variables, which the Doppler examination is asked to predict. For example, widely discrepant definitions of "pregnancy-induced hypertension" have been used, and frequently proteinuric hypertensive patients were not stratified from the general group of hypertensive patients. As mentioned, the lack of agreement on the preferred sampling site within the uterine circulation certainly added to the variability of reported results. Conceptually, all Doppler screening studies assume that the disease process for which we test has a unidirectional natural history over the course of the gestation. However, it has been well established that vascular placental bed pathology can be focal and may not be universal (30). This implies that compensation for lack of "physiologic change" in the midtrimester is conceivable later in pregnancy, even though this possibility is speculative.

Campbell et al. (31) screened 149 presumably low-risk pregnancies at 16–18 weeks gestation for the subsequent occurrence of pregnancy-induced hypertension, IUGR, and birth asphyxia. Of the 50 women with resistance index (RI) values of 2 or more SD above the mean, 10 developed pregnancy-induced hypertension, another 10 developed isolated IUGR, and one fetus was asphyxiated at birth. An overall sensitivity and specificity of 68% and 69% were calculated, respectively, with corresponding positive and negative predictive values of 42% and 87%. Even though the results of this first screening study on the uterine circulation were rather encouraging, several authors have questioned the low-risk status of the study population, considering a complication rate of 25%. Similarly encouraging results were reported by Schulman et al. (32) who found a 78% positive predictive value for IUGR and hypertension in pregnancy, but no clear definition of the outcome variables was provided.

Harrington et al. (12) also demonstrated a significant correlation between uterine Doppler velocimetry studies and pregnancy-induced hypertension or IUGR. Interestingly, the 25% sensitivity of an abnormal RI (>95th percentile) with CW Doppler at 20 weeks was substantially improved to 76% by including color Doppler flow and considering diastolic notching in the 2437 screened patients. The high sensitivity at 20 weeks was retained at 24 and 26 weeks, with specificity improving from 86% to 97%.

In contrast to the above studies, Hanretty et al. (33) and Newnham et al. (34) did not find significant differences in uterine artery Doppler indices between normal pregnancies, and pregnancies complicated by hypertension or IUGR. Hanretty et al. performed 357 uterine Doppler examinations between 26 and 30 weeks gestation, and 395 examinations between 34 and 36 weeks. Two hundred and nine women were examined in both gestational age periods. The 95th percentile for S/D ratios was considered abnormal, which resulted in 6.5% and 2.8% abnormal Doppler indices in the two gestational age groups, respectively. Even though the birthweights of fetuses with abnormal Doppler indices in the umbilical artery were substantially lower, no other significant differences between the groups were found based on uterine Doppler indices. Contrary to other authors, however, Hanretty et al. chose the lowest Doppler index from the uterine circulation as representative for each patient. Furthermore, no stratification of hypertensive cases by severity was provided, and the definition of pregnancy-induced hypertension depended on whether the clinician arranged for further investigation or not. The statistical power of this study was also limited, based on the actual occurrence of pregnancy complications, despite the relatively large study populations.

Newnham et al. (34) reported on umbilical and subplacental Doppler velocimetry screening in 535 medium-risk pregnancies at 18, 24, 28, and 34 weeks gestation. The 24-week examination detected fetal hypoxia with a sensitivity of 24% and a specificity of 94%. However, examinations at other times did not correlate with hypoxia, nor did any examination correlate with pregnancy-induced hypertension or IUGR.

Since the discrepant results of the above studies could possibly be explained by varying insonation sites within the uterine circulation, Bewley et al. (15) constructed an averaged RI from four sites within the uterine circulation, consisting of the left and right uterine and arcuate arteries examined by CW Doppler. Data on 925 women between 16 and 24 weeks were available for statistical analysis. Main outcome measures included intrauterine fetal death, low birthweight, pregnancy-induced hypertension, and antepartum hemorrhage. An averaged RI above the 95th percentile had a positive predictive value of 67% for all pregnancy complications combined, but only 35% for IUGR and 17% for proteinuric hypertension. Even though this test identified a group of women at risk, the majority of women with disease were missed. However, the finding of abnormal flow velocity waveforms in a variety of pregnancy complications might suggest a common underlying pathophysiology, at least in a proportion of these cases.

Doppler screening of the uterine artery for adverse pregnancy outcome in low-risk populations with CW Doppler alone does not appear to be an efficient tool at the present time. Most studies, however, demonstrate an increased incidence of abnormal flow velocity waveforms in pregnancies destined for adverse pregnancy outcome. The contribution of color Doppler equipment to screening efficacy is still unclear, but the available data are encouraging.

HYPERTENSION IN PREGNANCY AND UTERINE ARTERY DOPPLER

Patients with chronic hypertension and documented pregnancy-induced hypertension with abnormal uteroplacental blood velocity waveforms have a significantly higher incidence of proteinuria, preterm delivery, cesarean sections, low 1-min Apgar scores, and lower birthweights, probably secondary to abnormal uteroplacental perfusion (3,22,25,31,35).

A classification scheme of hypertensive pregnancies based on uterine and umbilical artery Doppler velocimetry has been proposed (35). The implementation of this classification reveals that women with normal uteroplacental and umbilical artery Doppler indices delivered the heaviest babies and have the lowest incidence of cesarean sections and neonatal deaths; women with abnormal uteroplacental but normal umbilical Doppler indices delivered more frequently premature but adequate-for-gestational-age fetuses (24). Women with normal uteroplacental but abnormal umbilical flow velocity waveforms gave birth to more hypoxic and small-for-gestational-age newborns; and women with abnormal Doppler indices in both vessels had the worst prognosis due to early onset of pregnancy complications. Uteroplacental Doppler appears therefore to be valuable, both in our pathophysiologic understanding and in predicting clinical course. A randomized, controlled trial has demonstrated that knowledge of normal umbilical and uterine waveforms allows less interference in pregnancies, resulting in heavier babies (24). However, the precise role of uterine artery Doppler in the management of hypertensive pregnancies is still evolving.

PERIPARTUM UTEROPLACENTAL DOPPLER EVALUATION

Doppler indices of the uterine artery do not change during the latent and active phases of normal labor (36). During contractions, the end-diastolic component of the waveforms may disappear, but a diastolic notch does not recur. Interestingly, with Braxton–Hicks contractions only the resistance of the arcuate arteries in the nonplacental myometrium appears to change (37). These findings suggest that obliteration of the intervillous space during uterine contractions is responsible for the loss of end-diastolic velocities of the flow velocity waveform. Furthermore, they suggest that the diastolic notch depends on the presence of an elastic vessel in the placental bed. Studies performed during pregnancy and during the intrapartum period have not shown conclusive changes in the arcuate artery velocity signals with methyldopa or

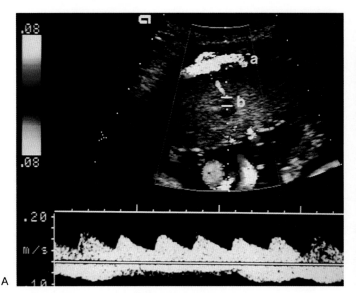 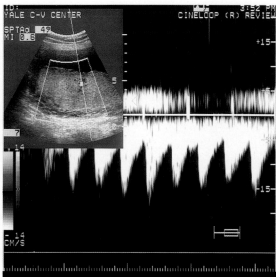

FIG. 5. A and B: Intraplacental color Doppler flow signals with superimposed pulse wave Doppler gate and spectral display of flow velocity waveforms.

β sympathomimetic administration, as well as epidural anesthesia (38,39,40). Following delivery, Doppler indices increase significantly during the first two postpartum days and the diastolic notch reappears. The indices continue to increase progressively until the end of the third month of the puerperal period (41) but continue to remain lower than in the nonpregnant state remote from a recent pregnancy.

DOPPLER VELOCIMETRY OF THE INTRAPLACENTAL CIRCULATION

Abnormal Doppler waveform indices of the umbilical artery have been demonstrated to be a measure of increased resistance in the umbilicoplacental circulation (42). The pathologic basis for this phenomenon appears to be a decrease in the number of tertiary villous arteries and arterioles (43). Decreased modal counts of muscular villous arteries in correlation with elevated umbilical artery Doppler waveform indices have indeed been observed in the setting of preeclampsia (43), IUGR (43–45), and fetal chromosome anomalies (46). It is presently unclear, however, whether the reduction in tertiary villous arteries is the result of primary failure of angiogenesis or of secondary vessel obliteration (47). The umbilical artery is the most extensively investigated fetal vessel in the assessment of fetal well-being by Doppler velocimetry. However, since the primary site of vascular pathology is further downstream in the tertiary villi of the placenta, alterations in umbilical artery Doppler waveforms merely reflect the distal vascular pathology and occur relatively late in the process. Thompson et al. calculated that 60% of the intraplacental fetal vasculature has to be occluded before significant changes in umbilical ar-

tery Doppler waveforms occur (48). This has been confirmed by placental embolization experiments in the sheep (10). It would be desirable, therefore, to examine the intraplacental villous vasculature by Doppler velocimetry directly, as opposed to examining the upstream umbilical artery. Until recently, intraplacental villous arteries have not been accessible to direct Doppler examination, since the small-vessel diameters (50–200 μm) are below the resolution of gray scale sonography. With the advent of color Doppler equipment, the detection of intraplacental blood flow and Doppler velocimetry has not become feasible (Fig. 5).

Rotmensch et al. (49) examined umbilical and intraplacental Doppler flow velocity waveforms in 211 cases, of which 192 were uncomplicated and 29 were affected by intrauterine growth retardation. Gestational

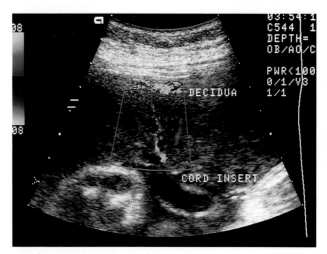

FIG. 6. Color Doppler flow signals from villous arteries in a normal placenta.

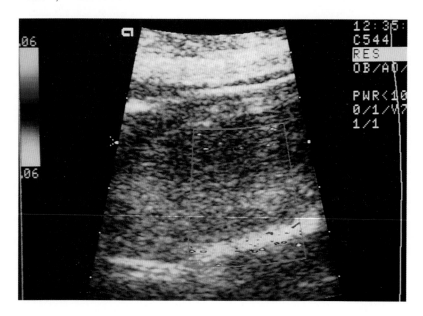

FIG. 7. Intraplacental color Doppler flow image in a pregnancy with severe IUGR. Only small-motion artifacts are noticeable at optimal system settings.

ages ranged between 26 and 41 weeks. The authors found that a minimum of two intraplacental fetal arteries could be detected by color Doppler flow in all 192 normal pregnancies (Fig. 6). In most cases 3 to 5 villous arteries were easily detectable. In 8 of 29 IUGR pregnancies (27.6%) no intraplacental fetal blood flow could be detected by color Doppler equipment (Fig. 7; $p < 0.0001$). Four of these 8 pregnancies were delivered by emergent cesarean sections for severe fetal distress prior to labor, as evident on antenatal fetal heart rate testing and biophysical profile scores of 0 and 2 out of 10. Umbilical vein blood gases confirmed fetal hypoxemia in all 4 cases (pO_2 range from 9 to 27 mm Hg) and all fetuses had low pH values (7.22–7.28), below the 5th percentile for gestational age in nonlaboring patients (50).

Doppler indices of the intraplacental arteries were found to be consistently lower than in the umbilical artery (Fig. 8), even though the difference narrowed with advancing gestational age. Interestingly, only 1 of 21 IUGR cases with detectable intraplacental color Doppler flow (4.8%) was associated with an abnormally high intraplacental artery Doppler index (Fig. 9), whereas 8 cases had abnormal umbilical artery Doppler indices. These findings suggest that failure to detect intraplacental color Doppler signals is associated with IUGR and fetal distress. However, flow velocity waveforms of detectable villous arteries are usually normal in IUGR, even in the presence of extremely abnormal umbilical artery Doppler indices.

Color Doppler investigation of the intraplacental circulation also revealed a variety of interesting incidental findings. Fetal breathing movements, for example, create flow velocity fluctuations in the umbilical vein, which are transmitted throughout the venous villous system, from the chorionic plate to the basal plate (Fig. 10). In the arterial compartment, reversed diastolic flow in the

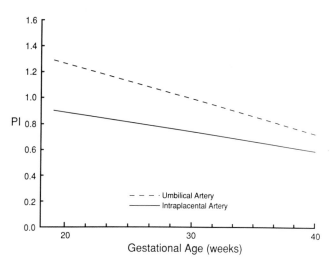

FIG. 8. Regression curves for mean umbilical artery and intraplacental artery pulsatility indices.

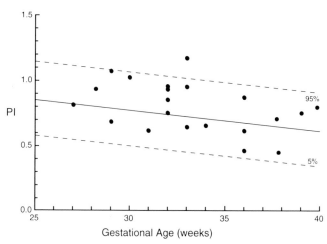

FIG. 9. Villous artery pulsatility indices (PI) of normal and IUGR pregnancies.

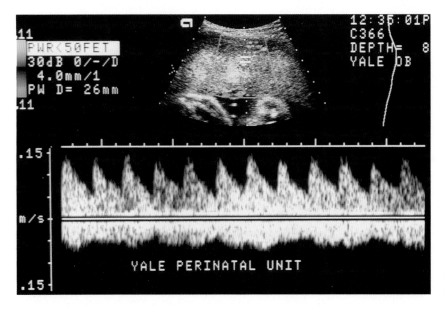

FIG. 10. Fetal breathing movements transmitted into venous system of placental villi.

umbilical artery was observed concurrently with normal diastolic forward flow in villous arteries. These findings appear to be contradictory but could suggest an uneven distribution of vascular occlusion among villous arteries in the placenta.

The studies by Hsieh et al. (51) and our own experience demonstrate that investigation of the intraplacental fetal circulation has become feasible with the advent of color Doppler flow technology. Whether the absence of intraplacental color Doppler flow patterns will prove to be useful as a predictor of fetal compromise in IUGR fetuses remains to be investigated prospectively.

CONCLUSIONS

The role of uterine artery Doppler velocimetry in the screening, diagnosis, and management of adverse pregnancy outcomes is still evolving and new information obtained by color Doppler equipment is needed. Currently available data do not justify large-scale screening of low-risk populations; however, a weak correlation between abnormal Doppler findings and adverse outcome appears to exist. Doppler signals of the maternal side of the placenta may become abnormal well before the fetus is metabolically compromised. On the other hand, one needs to be cognizant that not all adverse neonatal outcomes can be attributed to abnormal uteroplacental vascularization, and therefore Doppler velocimetry should not be expected to have perfect sensitivity to adverse outcomes due to the diversity in underlying pathophysiologies. The role of the intraplacental color Doppler examination is currently unclear. Based on our preliminary experience, abnormal color Doppler flow patterns probably occur late in the course of fetal compromise. It is unlikely, therefore, that the intraplacental examination can serve as a sensitive marker for antenatal assessment.

REFERENCES

1. Brosens I, Robertson WB, Dixon HG. The role of the spiral arteries in the pathogenesis of preeclampsia. *Obstet Gynecol Ann* 1972;1: 177–91.
2. Brosens I, Dixon HG, Robertson WB. Fetal growth retardation and the arteries of the placental bed. *Br J Obstet Gynecol* 1977;84: 656–663.
3. Campbell S, Griffin DR, Pearce JMF, Diaz-Recasens J, Cohen-Overbeek TE, Willson K. New Doppler technique for assessing uteroplacental blood flow. *Lancet* 1983;1:675–677.
4. Robertson WB, Brosens I, Dixon HG. Uteroplacental vascular pathology. *Eur J Obstet Gynecol Reprod Biol* 1975;5:47–65.
5. Rankin JHG. Interaction between the maternal and fetal placental blood flows. In: Rosenfeld CR, ed. *The uterine circulation.* Ithaca, NY: Perinatology Press; 1989;10:175–190.
6. Pijnenborg R, Bland JM, Robertson WB, Brosens I. Uteroplacental arterial changes related to interstitial trophoblast migration in early pregnancy. *Placenta* 1983;4:397–414.
7. Maini CL, Rosati P, Galli G, Bellati U, Bonetti MG, Moneta E. Non-invasive radioisotopic evaluation of placental blood flow. *Gynecol Obstet Invest* 1985;19:196–206.
8. Khong TY, Liddell HS, Robertson WB. Defective haemochorial placentation as a cause of miscarriage: a preliminary study. *Br J Obstet Gynecol* 1987;94:649–655.
9. Pijnenborg R, Anthony J, Davey DA, et al. Placental bed spiral arteries in the hypertensive disorders of pregnancy. *Br J Obstet Gynaecol* 1991;98:648–655.
10. Trudinger BJ, Stevens D, Connelly A, et al. Umbilical artery flow velocity waveforms and placental resistance: The effects of embolization of the umbilical circulation. *Am J Obstet Gynecol* 1987;157:1443–1448.
11. Thaler I, Weiner Z, Itskovitz J. Systolic or diastolic notch in uterine artery blood flow velocity waveforms in hypertensive pregnant patients: Relationship to outcome. *Obstet Gynecol* 1992;80:277–282.
12. Harrington KF, Campbell S, Bewley S, Bower S. Doppler velocimetry studies of the uterine artery in the early prediction of preeclampsia and intra-uterine growth retardation. *Eur J Obstet Gynecol Reprod Biol* 1991;42:S14–20.
13. Arduini D, Rizzo G, Boccolini MR, Romanini C, Mancuso S. Functional assessment of uteroplacental and fetal circulations by means of color Doppler ultrasonography. *J Ultrasound Med* 1990;9:249–253.
14. Rotmensch S, Copel JA, Hobbins JC. Introduction to Doppler velocimetry. *Obstet Gynecol Clin North Am* 1991;18:823–843.
15. Bewley S, Campbell S, Cooper D. Uteroplacental Doppler flow velocity waveforms in the second trimester. A complex circulation

[published erratum appears in *Br J Obstet Gynaecol* 1990 Mar;97(3):214]. *Br J Obstet Gynaecol* 1989;96:1040–1046.

16. Schulman H, Fleischer A, Farmakides G, Bracero L, Rochelson B, Grunfeld L. Development of uterine artery compliance in pregnancy as detected by Doppler ultrasound. *Am J Obstet Gynecol* 1986;155:1031–1036.

17. Santolaya-Forgas J. Physiology of the menstrual cycle by ultrasonography. *J Ultrasound Med* 1992;11:139–142.

18. Kurjack A, Zudenigo D, Funduk-Kurjack B, Shalan H, Predanic M, Sossic A. Transvaginal color Doppler in the assessment of the uteroplacental circulation in normal early pregnancy. *J Perinat Med* 1993;21:25–34.

19. Oosterhof H, Dijkstra K, Aarnoudse JG. Uteroplacental Doppler velocimetry during Braxton Hicks contractions. *Gynecol Obstet Invest* 1992;34:155–158.

20. McCowan LM, Ritchie K, Mo LY, Bascom PA, Sherret H. Uterine artery flow velocity waveforms in normal and growth-retarded pregnancies [published erratum appears in *Am J Obstet Gynecol* 1988 Aug;159(2):537]. *Am J Obstet Gynecol* 1988;158:499–504.

21. Pearce JM, Campbell S, Cohen-Overbeek T, Hackett G, Hernandez J, Royston JP. References ranges and sources of variation for indices of pulsed Doppler flow velocity waveforms from the uteroplacental and fetal circulation. *Br J Obstet Gynaecol* 1988;95:248–256.

22. Trudinger BJ, Giles WB, Cook CM. Uteroplacental blood flow velocity-time waveforms in normal and complicated pregnancy. *Br J Obstet Gynaecol* 1985;92:39–45.

23. Al-Ghazali W, Chapman MG, Allan LD. Doppler assessment of the cardiac and uteroplacental circulations in normal and complicated pregnancies. *Br J Obstet Gynaecol* 1988;95:575–580.

24. Pearce M. Doppler waveforms in normal pregnancy. In: Pearce M, ed. *Doppler ultrasound in perinatal medicine.* Oxford: Oxford University Press; 1992:82–94.

25. Fleischer A, Schulman H, Farmakides G, et al. Uterine artery Doppler velocimetry in pregnant women with hypertension. *Am J Obstet Gynecol* 1986;154:806–813.

26. Beaufils M, Uzan S, Donsimoni R, Colau JC. Prevention of pre-eclampsia by early antiplatelet therapy. *Lancet* 1988;1:840–842.

27. Wallenburg HCS, Rotmans N. Prevention of recurrent idiopathic fetal growth retardation by low-dose aspirin and dipyridamole. *Am J Obstet Gynecol* 1987;157:1230–1235.

28. Schiff E, Peleg E, Goldenberg M, et al. The use of aspirin to prevent pregnancy-induced hypertension and lower the ratio of thromboxane A2 to prostacyclin in relatively high risk pregnancies [see comments]. *N Engl J Med* 1989;321:351–356.

29. Chesley L. *Hypertensive disorders in pregnancy.* East Norwalk, CT: Appleton-Century-Crofts; 1978.

30. Khong TY, De-Wolf F, Robertson WB, Brosens I. Inadequate maternal vascular response to placentation in pregnancies complicated by pre-eclampsia and by small-for-gestational age infants. *Br J Obstet Gynaecol* 1986;93:1049–1059.

31. Campbell S, Pearce JM, Hackett G, Cohen-Overbeek T, Hernandez C. Qualitative assessment of uteroplacental blood flow: Early screening test for high-risk pregnancies. *Obstet Gynecol* 1986;68:649–653.

32. Schulman H, Winter D, Farmakides G, et al. Pregnancy surveillance with Doppler velocimetry of uterine and umbilical arteries. *Am J Obstet Gynecol* 1989;160:192–196.

33. Hanretty KP, Primrose MH, Neilson JP, Whittle MJ. Pregnancy screening by Doppler uteroplacental and umbilical artery waveforms [see comments]. *Br J Obstet Gynaecol* 1989;96:1163–1167.

34. Newnham JP, O'Dea MR, Reid KP, Diepeveen DA. Doppler flow velocity waveform analysis in high risk pregnancies: a randomized controlled trial. *Br J Obstet Gynaecol* 1991;98:956–963.

35. Ducey J, Schulman H, Farmakides G. A classification of hypertension in pregnancy based on Doppler velocimetry. *Am J Obstet Gynecol* 1987;157:680–685.

36. Meizner I, Levy A, Katz M. Assessment of uterine and umbilical artery velocimetry during latent and active phases of normal labor. *Isr J Med Sci* 1993;29:82–85.

37. Kofinas AD, Simon NV, Clay D, King K. Functional asymmetry of the human myometrium documented by color and pulsed-wave Doppler ultrasonographic evaluation of uterine arcuate arteries during Braxton Hicks contractions. *Am J Obstet Gynecol* 1993;168:184–188.

38. Montan S, Anandakumar C, Arulkumaran S, Ingemarsson I, Ratnam SS. Effects of methyldopa on uteroplacental and fetal hemodynamics in pregnancy-induced hypertension. *Am J Obstet Gynecol* 1993;168:152–156.

39. Alahuhta S, Rasanen J, Jouppila P, Jouppila R, Hollmen AI. Epidural sufentanil and bupivacaine for labor analgesia and Doppler velocimetry of the umbilical and uterine arteries. *Anesthesiology* 1993;78:231–236.

40. Schulman H. Uteroplacental flow velocity. In: Chervenak FA, Isaaacson GC, Campbell S, eds. *Ultrasound in obstetrics and gynecology.* 1st Ed. Boston: Little, Brown; 1993:569–577.

41. Tekay A, Jouppila P. A longitudinal Doppler ultrasonographic assessment of the alterations in peripheral vascular resistance of uterine arteries and ultrasonographic findings of the involuting uterus during the puerperium. *Am J Obstet Gynecol* 1993;168:190–198.

42. Trudinger BJ, Giles WB, Cook CM, Bombardieri J, Collins L. Fetal umbilical artery flow velocity waveforms and placental resistance: Clinical significance. *Br J Obstet Gynaecol* 1985;92:23–30.

43. Giles WB, Trudinger BJ, Baird PJ. Fetal umbilical artery flow velocity waveforms and placental resistance: pathological correlation. *Br J Obstet Gynaecol* 1985;92:31–38.

44. Bracero LA, Beneck D, Kirshenbaum N, Peiffer M, Stalter P, Schulman H. Doppler velocimetry and placental disease. *Am J Obstet Gynecol* 1989;161:388–393.

45. Fok RY, Pavlova Z, Benirschke K, Paul RH, Platt LD. The correlation of arterial lesions with umbilical artery Doppler velocimetry in the placentas of small-for-dates pregnancies. *Obstet Gynecol* 1990;75:578–583.

46. Rochelson B, Kaplan C, Guzman E, Arato M, Hansen K, Trunca C. A quantitative analysis of placental vasculature in the third-trimester fetus with autosomal trisomy. *Obstet Gynecol* 1990;75:59–63.

47. Trudinger BJ, Giles WB. Clinical and pathologic correlations of umbilical and uterine artery waveforms. *Clin Obstet Gynecol* 1989;32:669–678.

48. Thompson RS, Trudinger BJ. Doppler waveform pulsatility index and resistance, pressure and flow in the umbilical placental circulation: An investigation using a mathematical model. *Ultrasound Med Biol* 1990;16:449–458.

49. Rotmensch S, Liberati M, Luo JS, Gollin Y, Hobbins JC, Copel JA. Villous artery flow velocity waveforms and color Doppler flow patterns in placentas of growth-retarded fetuses. *Am J Obstet Gynecol* 1993;168:292.

50. Weiner CP, Sipes SL, Wenstrom K. The effect of fetal age upon normal fetal laboratory values and venous pressure. *Obstet Gynecol* 1992;79:713–718.

51. Hsieh FJ, Kuo PL, Ko TM, Chang FM, Chen HY. Doppler velocimetry of intraplacental fetal arteries. *Obstet Gynecol* 1991;77:478–482.

Doppler Ultrasound in Obstetrics and Gynecology,
edited by Joshua A. Copel and Kathryn L. Reed.
Raven Press, Ltd., New York © 1995.

CHAPTER **12**

Peripheral Fetal Circulation

Giancarlo Mari and Joshua A. Copel

The combination of color Doppler for vessel identification and pulsed Doppler spectral wave acquisition gives us the ability to evaluate numerous organ-specific vessels throughout the fetus. While the catalogue of such vessels grows at a rapid pace, we will review two specific areas in this chapter: the fetal kidneys and the musculoskeletal system as represented by lower extremity flow.

PHYSIOLOGY

In the lamb, the fetal carcass receives 32–40% of the combined ventricular output; 16% is distributed to the lower carcass, and 15–23% to the upper carcass (1). It has been shown that during fetal hypoxemia in the lamb there is a redistribution of the blood flow from the periphery to the brain (2). Therefore, the peripheral circulation in skin and muscles, which receives a large percentage of fetal cardiac output, is the major site where vasomotor responses effect redistribution of the fetal circulation.

The femoral artery provides flow to the muscles and skin of the lower extremities and may provide information regarding the vascular resistance of the lower extremities and may also contribute to our understanding of the fetal circulation in normal fetuses and fetuses with intrauterine growth retardation (IUGR).

ANATOMY BY COLOR DOPPLER OF PELVIC AND LOWER EXTREMITY CIRCULATION

The *aorta* descends on the bodies of the lumbar vertebrae, and in front of the fourth lumbar vertebra it divides into the two common iliac arteries (Fig. 1). The *common iliac arteries* run downward and laterally along the medial border of the psoas muscle. Each artery ends in front

of the sacroiliac joint by dividing into the external and internal iliac arteries (Figs. 1 and 2). The *external iliac artery* extends from the bifurcation of the common iliac artery to a point beneath the inguinal ligament, midway between the anterior superior iliac spine and the symphysis pubis. Entering the thigh below the inguinal ligament, the vessel then becomes the *femoral artery* (Figs. 2 and 3). The external iliac artery gives off few branches, the largest two being the *inferior epigastric* and the *deep iliac circumflex* (3). The femoral artery and the external iliac artery differ only in location (inside the pelvis, external iliac artery; outside the pelvis femoral artery).

The *internal iliac artery* in the fetus is positioned along the side of the bladder (Fig. 4). This artery is directed downward; then it becomes anterior to the bladder as it becomes the *umbilical artery* and runs superiorly on the inner aspect of the anterior wall of the abdomen to reach the umbilicus, converging toward the same vessel from the opposite side (Fig. 5). Having passed through the umbilical opening, the two arteries enter the umbilical cord and become coiled around the umbilical vein, to ramify ultimately in the placenta (3). Blood directed to the placenta passes through the internal iliac artery, whereas blood directed mainly to the lower extremities passes through the external iliac artery.

RECORDING TECHNIQUE OF THE FEMORAL ARTERY, INTERNAL ILIAC ARTERY, AND EXTERNAL ILIAC ARTERY

Doppler examination of the *femoral artery* can be performed with and without the use of color Doppler (4). After imaging a longitudinal section of the thigh and pelvis in which the bladder is visualized (Figs. 2 and 3), the sample volume is positioned on the femoral artery at the upper third of the thigh and Doppler waveforms of the femoral artery and vein are displayed on either side of the baseline (Fig. 6). In Fig. 7, two different waveforms

G. Mari and J. A. Copel: Department of Obstetrics and Gynecology, Yale University School of Medicine, New Haven, Connecticut 06511.

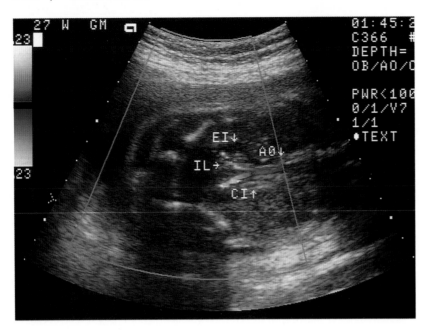

FIG. 1. Coronal section of fetal pelvis showing the relationship among the abdominal aorta (AO), the common iliac artery (CI), the internal iliac artery (IL), and the external iliac artery (EI).

are recorded simultaneously. This point corresponds to the bifurcation of the common iliac artery into internal and external iliac arteries. The waveforms with higher end diastole correspond to the *internal iliac artery* from which the *umbilical artery* takes its origin, whereas the waveforms with lower end-diastole correspond to the *external iliac artery*. In fact, from the point at which the two waveforms are imaged, the sample volume can be moved (a) toward the thigh, enabling the signal to be recorded at different levels along the external iliac artery (the waveforms of the external iliac artery are similar to those waveforms with lower end-diastolic flow obtained at the point of bifurcation of the common iliac artery) until it leaves the pelvis and becomes the common fem-

oral artery, or (b) toward the bladder enabling the signal to be recorded along the internal iliac artery (the waveforms of the internal iliac artery are similar to the waveforms with higher end-diastolic flow obtained at the point of bifurcation of the common iliac artery) until it leaves the fetal body and enters the umbilical cord.

Femoral and External Iliac Artery Flow Velocity Waveforms in Normal Fetuses

The pulsatility index of the fetal femoral artery increases linearly during gestation, which is consistent with the appearance of reverse flow in the diastolic component of the femoral artery waveform in the third trimester (Fig. 8) (4). We have been able to obtain fetal femoral artery flow velocity waveforms in 88% of attempts. Failure to obtain flow velocity waveforms may result from fetal body movements (especially before 30 weeks gestation) and fetal breathing.

The intraobserver error (coefficient of variation) for the pulsatility index of the femoral artery is 7.7% (5). The changes in femoral artery pulsatility index as a function of gestational age are presented in Table 1.

The reverse flow that appears in the fetal femoral artery velocity waveform in the third trimester could be due to an increase of the resistance in the lower extremities as has been shown by Rittenhouse et al. (6) in animals. The blood flow at the level of the common iliac encounters high resistance in the external iliac artery and therefore is primarily directed toward the placenta, which exhibits decreased vascular resistance with advancing gestation (7). Additionally, reverse flow at the level of the external iliac artery and femoral artery is a common pattern in newborn and adult.

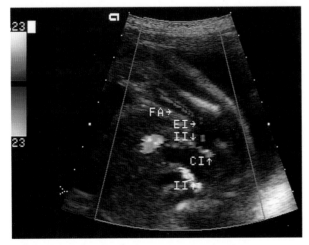

FIG. 2. Axial section of bladder and thigh showing the relationship among the common iliac artery (CI), the internal iliac artery (II), the external iliac artery (EI), the femoral artery (FA) (*in red*), and the femoral vein (*in blue*).

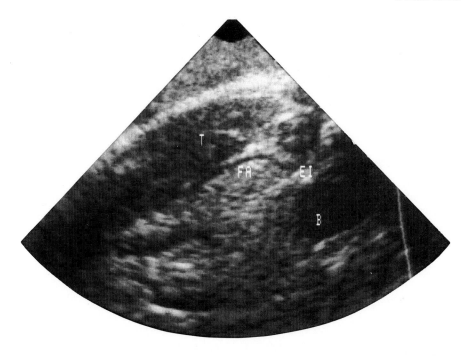

FIG. 3. Axial section of bladder (B) and thigh (T) without color Doppler showing the relationship between the fetal external iliac artery (EI) inside the pelvis, and femoral artery (FA) outside the pelvis. From Mari (4).

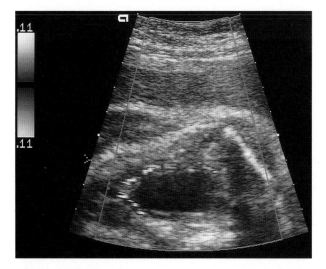

FIG. 4. Axial section of bladder showing the two internal iliac arteries.

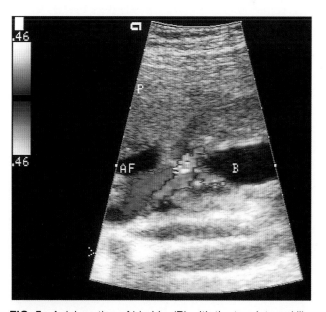

FIG. 5. Axial section of bladder (B) with the two internal iliac arteries that become umbilical arteries. AF, amniotic fluid.

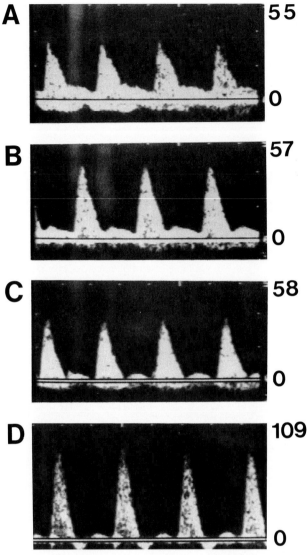

A 55 0

B 57 0

C 58 0

D 109 0

FIG. 6. Flow velocity waveforms from the fetal femoral artery at 18 (**A**), 24 (**B**), 30 (**C**), and 39 (**D**) weeks gestation with forward diastolic flow in A, presence of notch in B and C, and reverse flow in D. The values are in cm/sec. From Mari (4).

The reverse flow velocity waveforms obtained at the level of the external and femoral arteries explains why the pulsatility index of the fetal aorta does not change during gestation: the characteristics of flow velocity waveform in the fetal aorta in fact represent the summation of flow to the kidneys, other abdominal organs, the femoral arteries, and the placenta. The pulsatility index decreases in the umbilical artery (8) and renal artery (9) with advancing gestation. One would expect a decrease in the pulsatility index of the aorta; however, the pulsatility index of the fetal aorta does not change because the decrease of pulsatility index of the fetal renal artery and umbilical artery is balanced by the increased femoral artery pulsatility index.

A study by Stewart et al. (8) assessed the maximum velocity waveform in the external iliac artery. These authors stated that during normal pregnancy there is continuous forward flow throughout the cardiac cycle in the external iliac artery; this is associated with a decrease in the pulsatility index of this artery. The same authors demonstrated that in intrauterine growth retardation (IUGR) fetuses the pulsatility index of the external iliac artery increases, suggesting a redistribution of the blood flow from the lower extremities to the brain.

We found no difference between external iliac and femoral artery flow velocity waveforms (4). This discrepancy to Stewart's findings may be due to the fact that it is easy to visualize the internal iliac artery with color Doppler in virtually all cases; however, it is more difficult to visualize the external iliac artery and the femoral artery. There are two reasons for this. The first is anatomic: in the fetus, the internal iliac artery is twice as large as the external iliac artery (3). The second reason is the characteristic waveforms: the internal iliac and umbilical arteries display continuous diastolic flow, whereas the external iliac artery and the femoral artery have low/reverse diastolic flow indicating intermittent flow toward the thigh and leg.

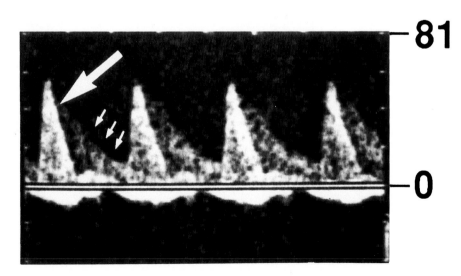

81 0

FIG. 7. Flow velocity waveforms obtained at the point of bifurcation of the common iliac artery in internal iliac artery and external iliac artery. The waveforms at higher diastole are those of the internal iliac artery (*large arrow*). The waveforms at lower diastole are those of the external iliac artery (*small arrows*). The values are in cm/sec. From Mari (5).

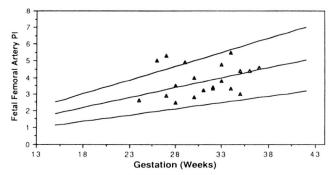

FIG. 8. Reference range (mean ± 2 SD) of femoral artery pulsatility index with gestation constructed from study of 12 normal fetuses followed longitudinally. The triangles represent the pulsatility index values of 20 IUGR fetuses. From Mari (4).

Femoral Artery Velocity Waveforms and Fetal Exercise

Lower extremity movements decrease the femoral artery pulsatility index (unpublished data) when the pulsatility index is obtained soon after the movement. This suggests that a vasodilation and an increase in blood flow to the lower extremities occurs during exercise. These results must be considered when the femoral artery pulsatility index is obtained. We suggest that the femoral artery be sampled when the fetus is at rest, when no activity has been observed to minimize this effect.

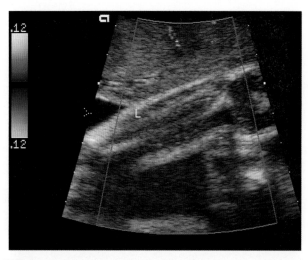

FIG. 9. Axial section of the fetal leg showing the tibial artery (*in blue*).

Internal Iliac and Umbilical Artery Flow Velocity Waveforms in Normal Pregnancies

In 30 normal fetuses the internal iliac artery pulsatility index was higher than that of the umbilical artery (4). The internal iliac artery reflects the waveforms of the umbilical artery; therefore it is not necessary to study the

TABLE 1. *Fetal femoral artery pulsatility index: Normal values*

Gestational age (wk)	Normal value		Predicted value	Normal value	
	−2 SD	−1 SD		+1 SD	+2 SD
15	1.1	1.4	1.8	2.1	2.5
16	1.2	1.5	1.9	2.3	2.6
17	1.2	1.6	2.0	2.4	2.8
18	1.3	1.7	2.1	2.5	3.0
19	1.4	1.8	2.2	2.7	3.1
20	1.5	1.9	2.4	2.8	3.3
21	1.5	2.0	2.5	3.0	3.5
22	1.6	2.1	2.6	3.1	3.6
23	1.7	2.2	2.7	3.3	3.8
24	1.8	2.3	2.9	3.4	4.0
25	1.8	2.4	3.0	3.6	4.1
26	1.9	2.5	3.1	3.7	4.3
27	2.0	2.6	3.2	3.8	4.5
28	2.1	2.7	3.3	4.0	4.6
29	2.1	2.8	3.5	4.1	4.8
30	2.2	2.9	3.6	4.3	5.0
31	2.3	3.0	3.7	4.4	5.1
32	2.4	3.1	3.8	4.6	5.3
33	2.4	3.2	3.9	4.7	5.5
34	2.5	3.3	4.1	4.8	5.6
35	2.6	3.4	4.2	5.0	5.8
36	2.7	3.5	4.3	5.1	6.0
37	2.7	3.6	4.4	5.3	6.1
38	2.8	3.7	4.5	5.4	6.3
39	2.9	3.8	4.7	5.6	6.5
40	3.0	3.9	4.8	5.7	6.6
41	3.0	4.0	4.9	5.9	6.8
42	3.1	4.1	5.0	6.0	7.0

Pulsatility index = 0.121 (gestational age) ($R^2 = 81 \pm 9$). 1 SD = 0.023.

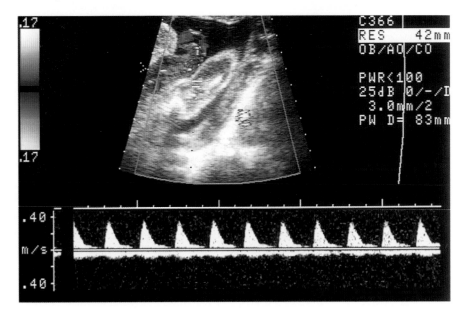

FIG. 10. Flow velocity waveforms of the tibial artery.

internal iliac artery if the umbilical artery is studied because the difference between these two arteries is only anatomic: inside the pelvis internal iliac artery, outside the pelvis umbilical artery. However, it is our opinion that internal iliac artery reverse diastolic flow precedes umbilical artery reverse flow in IUGR fetuses.

Femoral and External Iliac Artery Flow Velocity Waveforms in IUGR Fetuses

It has been reported that hypoxemia in the fetal lamb is associated with abnormal femoral artery flow velocity waveforms without appreciable effect on umbilical artery velocity waveforms (10).

In a study on 20 IUGR fetuses, Mari found that the femoral artery pulsatility index was higher than 2 SD above the mean for gestational age in 10% of the IUGR fetuses (Fig. 8) (4). The umbilical artery pulsatility index was abnormal in 50% of IUGR fetuses (i.e., presence of absent/reverse diastolic flow velocity waveform); four of the IUGR fetuses died, and four others developed fetal distress and/or were admitted to the neonatal intensive care unit.

These results suggest that the study of the femoral artery/external iliac artery of the human fetus does not appear to be as good an indicator of adverse fetal outcome as the umbilical artery velocity waveforms. In addition, we do not think that flow velocity waveforms of the arteries of the legs such as tibial artery (Figs. 9 and 10) will add any new information to our knowledge, especially

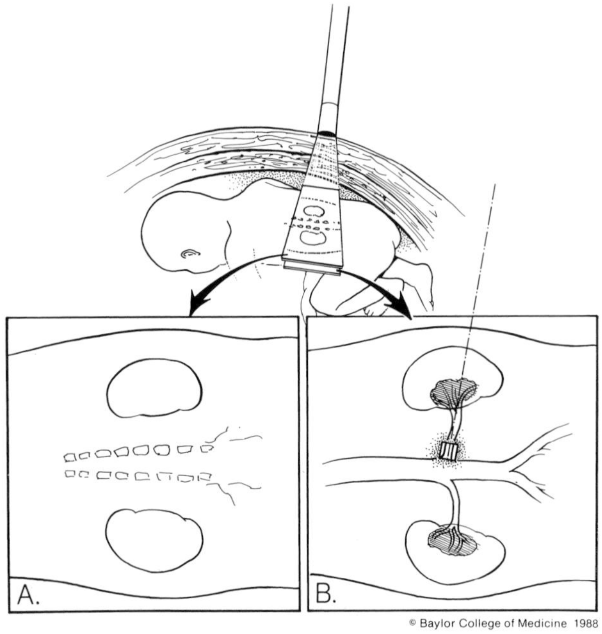

© Baylor College of Medicine 1988

FIG. 11. Drawing showing plane used in Doppler ultrasonographic studies of the renal artery.

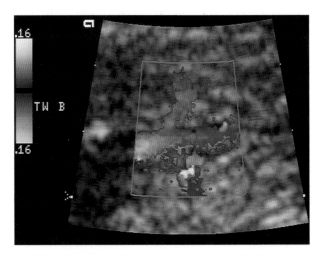

FIG. 12. Coronal section of the fetal aorta with the origin of the two renal arteries.

considering the increased difficulty of requiring appropriate signals from these small vessels.

Renal Artery

Recording Technique

Doppler examination of the renal artery can be performed with and without the use of color Doppler (11). After imaging a sagittal section of the fetal body, the ultrasound beam is directed lateral to the spine, obtaining a coronal section of the fetal body (Fig. 11). By moving the transducer anteriorly, a coronal section of the descending aorta and kidneys is imaged (Fig. 12). The sample volume is placed on the renal artery near the aorta and Doppler waveforms of the renal artery and vein are displayed on either side of the baseline (Fig. 13).

The intraobserver error (coefficient of variation) for the pulsatility index of the renal artery is 6.7% (11).

Renal Artery Flow Velocity Waveforms in Normal Fetuses

In normal fetuses, the pulsatility index of the renal artery decreases with advancing gestation (Fig. 14) (9, 11, 15). This suggests an increase in blood flow to the kidneys with advancing gestation. In adults, the reverse flow observed at level of the iliac arteries is necessary to maintain the blood flow to the kidneys. In the fetus, the high vascular resistance observed at level of the lower extremities in the third trimester does not explain the decreased renal vascular resistance with advancing gestation because the increased lower extremity vascular resistance is associated with a decreased umbilical artery vascular resistance. Placental resistance and lower extremity resistance may both influence the renal blood flow. However, prostaglandins produced by the fetal kidney may also play an important role in this regulation (12). In fact, in the human fetus prostaglandin inhibitors decrease the urine output (13) without altering the renal vascular re-

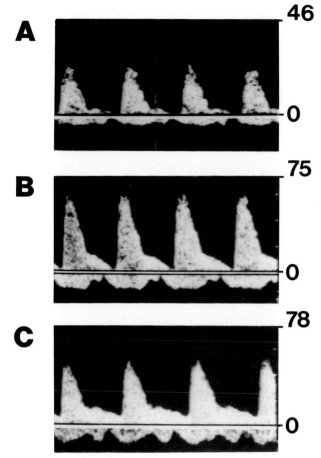

FIG. 13. Flow velocity waveforms of the renal artery at 20 weeks (**A**), 30 weeks (**B**), and at term of gestation (**C**). The values are in cm/sec.

sistance (14). The decreased renal vascular resistance with advancing gestation explains the decrease of the renal artery pulsatility index with advancing gestation.

Renal Artery Velocity Waveforms in IUGR Fetuses

Vyas et al. (15) reported that the renal artery pulsatility index is higher than normal in IUGR fetuses. The same

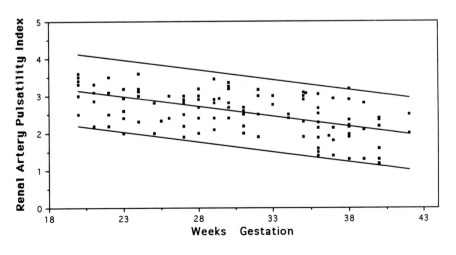

FIG. 14. Normal range of renal artery pulsatility index as a function of gestational age constructed from study of 121 normal fetuses. Mean ± 2 SE. From Mari et al. (11).

authors found a significant direct correlation between blood oxygen deficit and increased renal artery pulsatility index.

In our experience the renal artery pulsatility index is normal in many IUGR fetuses with brain-sparing effect documented by a lower pulsatility index at level of the fetal middle cerebral artery. A higher renal artery pulsatility index has been found in small-for-gestational-age fetuses with oligohydramnios who later died (11). It is our opinion that the renal blood flow decreases when the hypoxemia is prolonged. This concept is corroborated by animal data in which the blood flow to the kidneys becomes abnormal only with prolonged hypoxemia (16). The worst fetal outcome would be anticipated in those IUGR fetuses with abnormal renal artery pulsatility index and oligohydramnios (11).

Renal Artery Velocity Waveforms and Amniotic Fluid Volume

As human pregnancy progresses beyond the twentieth week, the fetus seems to become the primary source of both amniotic fluid production and elimination through the processes of urination and swallowing, thereby controlling the volume. It has been suggested that the renal perfusion may play an important role in the polyhydramnios-oligohydramnios observed in twin-to-twin transfusion syndrome (11). In fact, oligohydramnios could be a consequence of decreased renal perfusion and decreased urine output, whereas polyhydramnios may be a consequence of the increased renal perfusion and increased urine output.

Arduini and Rizzo (17) suggested that the etiology of amniotic fluid reduction differs between growth-retarded fetuses and postterm pregnancies. In the former group, the reduction of amniotic fluid volume appears to be related to Doppler-detectable changes in renal vascular resistance, whereas in the latter group there appear to be other changes such as an increased capability of tubular reabsorption.

We have found that in polyhydramnios the renal artery pulsatility index was in the normal range in all of the fetuses. These results suggest that the fetal renal perfusion is not the only factor that can influence the amniotic fluid volume. Other factors such as tubular reabsorption

may play an important role in fetuses with abnormal amniotic fluid volume.

REFERENCES

1. Rudolph AM, Heymann MA. Circulatory changes during growth in the fetal lamb. *Circ Res* 1970;26:289–299.
2. Cohn HE, Sacks EJ, Heymann MA, Rudolph AM. Cardiovascular responses to hypoxemia and acidemia in fetal lambs. *Am J Obstet Gynecol* 1974;120:817–824.
3. Gray H. The arteries. In: Clemente CD, ed. *Anatomy of the human body*. Philadelphia: Lea & Febiger; 1985:648–787.
4. Mari G. Arterial blood flow velocity waveforms of the pelvis and lower extremities in normal and growth-retarded fetuses. *Am J Obstet Gynecol* 1991;165:143–151.
5. Mari G, Moise JK, Deter RL, Kirshon B, Stefos T, Carpenter RJ. Flow velocity waveforms of the vascular system in the anemic fetus before and after intravascular transfusion for severe red blood cell alloimmunization. *Am J Obstet Gynecol* 1990;162:1060–1064.
6. Rittenhouse EA, Maixner W, Burr JW, Barnes RW. Directional arterial flow velocity: A sensitive index of changes in peripheral vascular resistance. *Surgery* 1976;79:350–335.
7. Trudinger BJ, Giles WB, Cook CM, Bombardieri J, Collins L. Fetal umbilical artery flow velocity waveforms and placental resistance: Clinical significance. *Br J Obstet Gynaecol* 1985;92:23–30.
8. Stewart PA, Wladimiroff JW, Stijnen T. Blood flow velocity waveforms from the fetal external iliac artery as a measure of lower extremity vascular resistance. *Br J Obstet Gynaecol* 1990;97:425–430.
9. Mari G, Moise JK, Kirshon B, Deter RL, Carpenter RJ. Doppler assessment of the renal blood flow in the normal human fetus (Abstract 293). In: *Proceedings of the 9th annual meeting of the Society of Perinatal Obstetricians*. New Orleans; 1989.
10. Muijsers GJJM, Hasaart THM, Ruissen GJ, van Huisseling H, Peeters LLH, de Haan J. The effect of hypoxemia on umbilical and femoral artery blood flow velocity waveforms in fetal sheep (Abstract 139). In: *Proceedings of the 36th annual meeting of the Society for Gynecologic Investigation*. San Diego; 1989.
11. Mari G, Kirshon B, Abuhamad A. Fetal renal artery flow velocity waveforms in normal pregnancies and pregnancies complicated by polyhydramnios and oligohydramnios. *Obstet Gynecol* 1993;81:560–564.
12. Millard RW, Baig H, Vatner SF. Prostaglandin control of the renal circulation in response to hypoxemia in the fetal lamb in utero. *Circ Res* 1979;45:172–179.
13. Kirshon B, Moise JK, Mari G, Willis R. Long term indomethacin decreases fetal urine output and results in oligohydramnios. *Am J Perinatal* 1991;8:86–88.
14. Mari G, Moise JK, Deter RL, Kirshon B, Carpenter RJ. Doppler assessment of the renal blood flow velocity waveforms during indomethacin therapy for preterm labor and polyhydramnios. *Obstet Gynecol* 1990;75:199–201.
15. Vyas S, Nicolaides KH, Campbell S. Renal flow-velocity waveforms in normal and hypoxemic fetuses. *Am J Obstet Gynecol* 1989;161:168–172.
16. Bocking AD, Gagnon R, White SE, Homan J, Milne KM, Richardson BS. Circulatory response to prolonged hypoxemia in fetal sheep. *Am J Obstet Gynecol* 1988;159:1418–1424.
17. Arduini D, Rizzo G. Fetal renal artery velocity waveforms and amniotic fluid volume in growth-retarded and post-term fetuses. *Obstet Gynecol* 1991;77:370–373.

Doppler Ultrasound in Obstetrics and Gynecology,
edited by Joshua A. Copel and Kathryn L. Reed.
Raven Press, Ltd., New York © 1995.

CHAPTER 13

Red Cell Alloimmunization

Kenneth J. Moise, Jr.

Since its advent, ultrasound has played an ever-increasing role in the management of the alloimmunized pregnancy. Today real-time ultrasound is used primarily to assist in needle guidance for such invasive procedures as amniocentesis, percutaneous umbilical blood sampling, and intrauterine transfusion. However, two-dimensional ultrasound has not proven useful in predicting the degree of fetal anemia unless overt hydrops is present (1,2). Doppler ultrasound has been beneficial in understanding the physiologic changes that occur in the fetus secondary to anemia. In addition, it has been instructive in the assessment of the cardiovascular alterations after intrauterine transfusion. Like two-dimensional ultrasound, Doppler has been disappointing in the prediction of fetal anemia.

FETAL ADAPTATION TO ANEMIA

Based on data in the animal model, it has long been suspected that the anemic human fetus compensates for its decreased oxygen-carrying capacity by increasing its cardiac output (3). However, it was not until the investigation of Kirkinen and Jouppila (4) in 1983 that this theory was substantiated. Using pulsed Doppler to measure umbilical venous velocity and two-dimensional ultrasound to measure the diameter of the umbilical vein, fetal umbilical venous flow (UVBF) was measured in 18 pregnancies complicated by Rhesus (Rh) alloimmunization. In seven of eight fetuses noted to be severely anemic at birth, the UVBF was found to be greater than the 97.5th percentile of the normal value for the corresponding gestational age. As real-time imaging techniques improved, direct measurements of the fetal cardiac output at the level of the atrioventricular valves became possible. Copel and coworkers (5) measured the biven-

tricular output in 11 severely anemic fetuses from Rh-alloimmunized pregnancies. These values were compared to a group of 35 normal fetuses matched for gestational age that were undergoing fetal echocardiography secondary to a history of a previous sibling with congenital heart disease. Combined ventricular output in the anemic fetuses was significantly higher than in their matched counterparts (879 ± 86 ml/kg/min vs. 644 ± 35.5 ml/kg/min). Since the heart rates were similar between the two groups, the authors concluded that the increased cardiac output in the anemic fetus was secondary to an elevated stroke volume. Rizzo et al. (6) compared right and left ventricular outputs in 12 anemic fetuses to reference ranges for gestational age determined from 187 normal controls. The mean hematocrit value at cordocentesis in the anemic fetuses was 30.5% (range: 24.9–39.4%). In the anemic fetuses, both right and left ventricular outputs were elevated 35% and 46% above norms, respectively. The authors then compared the ratio of right and left ventricular output to nonanemic fetuses. Right-sided ventricular dominance previously reported in the normal human fetus was maintained in the anemic fetus (7).

Movement of blood across the atrioventricular (AV) valves is represented by a Doppler waveform consisting of two blood velocity peaks—an E wave and an A wave. The early E wave represents the passive filling of the ventricle from the atrium during early diastole whereas the A wave represents the passage of blood related to the atrial contraction. In the nonanemic fetus, the A wave predominates making the calculation of the *E/A* ratio equal to less than 1 (7). In the anemic fetus, both Meijboom et al. (unpublished, abstract #17, Society of Perinatal Obstetricians, 1986) and Rizzo and coworkers (6) noted the *E/A* ratio to be increased over norms at both the mitral and tricuspid valves. The exact etiology of this finding has yet to be explained. Changes in the characteristics of the Doppler waveform of the AV valves depend on

K. J. Moise: Division of Maternal-Fetal Medicine, Baylor College of Medicine, One Baylor Plaza, Houston, Texas 77030.

complex interactions with such hemodynamic variables as preload, afterload, ventricular compliance, isovolumetric relaxation of the ventricle, heart rate, and end-systolic ventricular volume (8). Using a mathematical model, Thomas and coworkers (8) demonstrated that an increase in atrial pressure (preload) at the time of AV valve opening was associated with an increase in both the peak systolic velocity of the E wave and a higher ventricular stroke volume. As mentioned earlier, stroke volume appears to be increased in the anemic fetus (5). Therefore, the likely explanation for the increased E/A ratio of the AV valves of the fetus with anemia is an elevation in the preload that is presented to the ventricles.

FETAL ADAPTATION TO INTRAUTERINE TRANSFUSION

Although the intraperitoneal transfusion (IPT) for the treatment of severe fetal anemia secondary to Rh alloimmunization was first reported in 1963, investigations into the fetal adaptive response to such therapy were not undertaken until more than 20 years later (9). Two teams of investigators reported an acute increase in umbilical venous flow immediately after IPT (4,10). This elevation was noted to resolve over the 7 days following the transfusion. The authors speculated that these changes could be related to acute alterations in intraperitoneal pressure with resolution as the blood was absorbed from the peritoneal cavity.

In the mid-1980s, the advent of the intravascular transfusion (IVT) opened new frontiers for the study of fetal physiology (11,12). Unlike the IPT where donor red cells are absorbed slowly over several days, the IVT involves the acute correction of fetal anemia with an associated rapid expansion of the fetoplacental volume. One

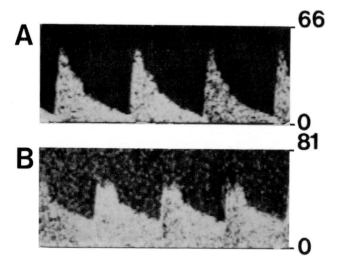

FIG. 1. Doppler velocity waveforms of the fetal middle cerebral artery before (**A**) and within 2 hr after intravascular transfusion (**B**). From Mari et al. (14).

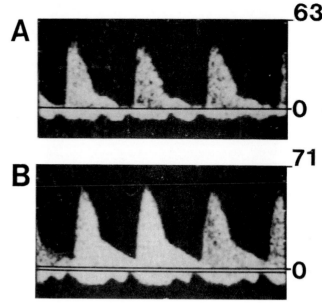

FIG. 2. Doppler velocity waveforms of the fetal renal artery before (**A**) and within 2 hr after intravascular transfusion (**B**). From Mari et al. (15).

would expect that such changes would call for major cardiovascular adaptation by the fetus. Indeed, this has been noted to be the case.

Weiner and Anderson (13) measured the systolic/diastolic (S/D) ratio of the umbilical artery before and immediately following 19 intravascular transfusions for fetal hemolytic disease. A significant decline in the S/D ratio was noted to occur after the procedure. A significant correlation was noted between this change in the S/D ratio and the increase in fetal hematocrit secondary to the intrauterine transfusion. No correlation could be demonstrated between the volume of transfused blood and the alteration in the S/D ratio. Our group was the first to report the effects of IVT on the pulsatility index (PI) of various fetal regional circulations (14). The PI of the fetal middle cerebral, anterior cerebral, internal carotid, and umbilical artery was studied in 13 fetuses just before, within the first 2 hr following and the day after IVT. A significant decrease in the PI of all vessels studied was noted immediately following IVT with a return to baseline values by the next day after the procedure (Fig. 1). In a subsequent investigation in nine fetuses, a similar acute reduction of the PI of the fetal renal artery was detected after IVT (15). Again the PI was noted to return to pretransfusion levels within 24 hr after completion of the procedure (Fig. 2). In a third study at our institution, pulsed Doppler assessment of the PI of multiple fetal vessels was undertaken in 16 anemic fetuses at the time of IVT (16). Flow velocity waveforms were obtained from the fetal middle cerebral artery, anterior cerebral artery, internal carotid artery, thoracic aorta, abdominal aorta, renal artery, femoral artery, and umbilical artery prior to IVT and the day following the procedure. The PI values in the various vessels were not significantly different 24 hr after IVT as compared to baseline values. The findings of the four aforementioned studies are indicative of a fall in vascular impedance after IVT as a fetal compensatory mechanism for the abrupt changes in volume and viscosity.

We have studied fetal cardiac output just prior to IVT and immediately following the procedure (17). The relative change in right- and left-sided cardiac output was assessed by pulsed Doppler measurement of the time velocity integral and heart rate at the level of the pulmonary and aortic valves. Right-sided output was reduced by 22% and left-sided by 19%. No alteration in heart rate was noted after IVT leading us to deduce that stroke volume was transiently depressed. Our findings were confirmed by a subsequent investigation by Rizzo et al. (6) in which AV valve areas were measured with real-time ultrasound and blood velocities were assessed by pulsed Doppler. In this study, the nadir of the decreased cardiac output occurred at 15–45 min after the intrauterine transfusion with resolution to near baseline values by 2 hr. Again, no change in the fetal heart rate was found after the intrauterine transfusion indicating that cardiac stroke volume was reduced. In another study, Copel et al. (5) noted no change in fetal cardiac output by 12 hr after IVT when compared to baseline values. The summation of the findings of these three studies would indicate that fetal cardiac output is transiently decreased after IVT with a recovery to baseline levels by the day following the correction of the anemia.

In addition to an acute decrease in cardiac output after IVT, Rizzo et al. (6) also noted a transient rise in the E/A ratio of both the mitral and tricuspid valves. Thomas et al. (8) found that an increase in either atrial pressure or end-systolic ventricular volume will generate an elevation in the peak velocity of the E wave of the Doppler spectrum of the AV valves. We have proposed that relative hyperviscosity secondary to the acute correction of anemia during an IVT produces an increase in cardiac afterload (17). A secondary increase in the end-systolic volume of the ventricles would be expected. With each cardiac cycle, the stroke volume will be reduced leading to an overall decrease in cardiac output. An elevation in atrial pressure will be produced and may account for the acute rise in umbilical venous pressure found by several investigators after the direct IVT of donor red blood cells (17–19). Vasodilation of regional vascular beds occurs in response to such an acute increase in afterload. Atrial naturietic hormone and vasodilatory prostanoids have been noted to increase acutely after IVT and probably account for this generalized vasodilation (20–22). Resolution of these acute changes begins by 2 hr after an IVT and is completed within the first 24 hr postprocedure.

PREDICTION OF FETAL HEMATOCRIT

Probably the greatest amount of Doppler investigation has been in the area of prediction of fetal hematocrit. Vessels studied have included the umbilical vein, fetal descending thoracic aorta, fetal common carotid artery, and fetal middle cerebral artery.

Kirkinen and Jouppila (4) were the first to report a correlation between blood velocities in the fetus and the fetal hematocrit. Umbilical venous blood flows (UVBFs) were measured in 18 fetuses within 4 days of delivery. A negative correlation ($r = -0.65$) was noted between the umbilical venous blood flow per kilogram of birthweight and the cord hemoglobin at delivery. The authors proposed that their technique represented a noninvasive method of monitoring the anemic fetus. In a later series, Warren et al. (10) followed 51 Rh-alloimmunized pregnancies with weekly fetal UVBF determinations. Based on amniotic fluid bilirubin analysis, intraperitoneal transfusions were necessary in 14 of the pregnancies. In the 51 patients, 35% developed UVBFs above the 90th percentile for gestational age, 55% had no abnormal flows, and 10% had one or more low flows (less than 10th percentile). Eleven of the 18 patients with high flows were noted to develop ultrasound evidence of fetal hydrops within a week. The authors arbitrarily defined a significant change in UVBF between weekly assessments as an increase of 20% or more. In four of five cases that required intrauterine transfusions based on rising amniotic fluid bilirubin evaluation, flow rates increased by more than 20%. Further work by the authors revealed that serial umbilical venous flows could be used to decide when to perform a subsequent intrauterine transfusion.

Rightmire and coworkers (23) were the next to attempt to use Doppler to predict the severity of fetal anemia. The mean velocity in the fetal descending aorta, inferior vena cava, and intraabdominal portion of the umbilical vein was measured in 21 fetuses found to be anemic secondary to red cell alloimmunization. In addition, the PI of the umbilical artery was also evaluated. Measurements were performed with duplex Doppler equipment capable of calculating the intensity-weighted mean of the Doppler shift frequency. Both the mean blood velocity in the aorta ($r = 0.67$) and the PI of the umbilical artery ($r = 0.78$) were found to correlate inversely with the fetal hematocrit determined at the time of fetoscopy. Velocity measurements in the fetal inferior vena cava and umbilical vein did not correlate with the degree of fetal anemia. The authors proposed the following equation for the prediction of the fetal hematocrit:

$$-1.07 \times \text{aortic blood velocity}$$
$$+ 895.72 \times \text{PI of the umbilical artery}$$
$$- 708.72 \times (\text{PI})^2 - 219.91; \quad (r = 0.82)$$

The mean error in the predicted hematocrit value was $3.8 \pm 3.0\%$. The authors subsequently studied the usefulness of their technique in a prospective investigation (24). A normal curve for fetal aortic velocity in relation to gestational age was established from 218 pregnancies. Mean velocities were then measured in fetuses of 68 pregnancies complicated by red cell alloimmunization at the time of hematocrit determination by cordocentesis. A positive correlation was noted between the fetal hemoglobin deficit from the mean for gestational age and the deviation in aortic velocity from the mean value for gestational age ($r = 0.46$). However, when fetuses were divided into those with and without hydrops, the correlation no longer proved valid. In fact, hydropic fetuses were noted to have decreasing mean aortic velocities as the hematocrit was noted to decline. If one defines fetal anemia as a hematocrit value of less than 2 SD from the mean for a particular gestational age, then only 9% of anemic fetuses would be detected by an increased mean abdominal aortic velocity (>2 SD from the mean value for gestational age). It would therefore appear that fetal aortic mean velocity is not likely to be useful in the prediction of fetal anemia in erythroblastosis fetalis.

Following the lead of the British investigators, Copel and coworkers (25) studied the descending aorta and umbilical artery in anemic fetuses. These authors measured the peak aortic velocity as compared to the intensity-weighted mean aortic velocity used by their British counterparts. Sixteen fetuses were studied prior to the first intravascular transfusion. Multiple regression yielded the following two equations for the prediction of fetal hematocrit in the nonhydropic fetus:

$$7.778 - (0.088 \times \text{peak velocity in descending aorta})$$
$$+ (0.968 \times \text{gestational age [weeks]})$$
$$- (10.911 \text{ if hydrops present}); \qquad r = 0.88$$

and

$$45.312 - (56.261 \times \text{umbilical artery PI})$$
$$- (0.128 \times \text{peak velocity in the descending aorta})$$
$$+ (1.042 \times \text{gestational age in weeks}); \qquad r = 0.82$$

The authors critically examined their formula to assess whether it could predict those fetuses with a hematocrit above or below 25%. Formula 1 correctly achieved this prediction in 14 of 16 fetuses (sensitivity = 90%, specificity = 69%). Using the second formula, 12 of the 16 fetuses with this hematocrit were correctly predicted (sensitivity 100%, specificity 20%). Further analysis of the second formula prior to subsequent transfusions revealed that it was a very poor predictor of the actual hematocrit as determined by cordocentesis. Copel and coworkers (25) concluded that their Doppler technique held promise as a tool for predicting the need for the first intrauterine transfusion. In a subsequent prospective

evaluation, this group of investigators studied 13 fetuses prior to first intravascular transfusion (26). Predicted fetal hematocrit using the second formula from the previous investigation failed to correlate with the actual fetal hematocrit; $r = 0.29$. Formula 1 was found to be somewhat more predictive of the actual fetal hematocrit with an r value of 0.71. Further analysis of the components of this equation revealed that the presence of fetal hydrops was the major factor contributing to the ability to forecast the fetal hematocrit. Since hydrops fetalis has been associated with severe fetal anemia (27), the authors concluded that their previously described formulas utilizing Doppler indices were unable to assist in accurately predicting the severity of fetal anemia.

Finally, various researchers have studied the fetal cerebral circulation in an effort to predict the degree of fetal anemia. Bilardo and coworkers (28) measured the time-averaged mean velocity in the common carotid artery in 12 fetuses prior to cordocentesis. A negative correlation ($r = -0.64$) was found between the carotid velocity and the hemoglobin concentration of the fetus expressed as the number of standard deviations from the normal mean value for gestational age. Another British group (29) measured the middle cerebral artery intensity-weighted mean velocity in 24 nonhydropic fetuses prior to cordocentesis. A negative correlation ($R = -0.72$) was noted between middle cerebral artery (MCA) mean velocities and hemoglobin corrected for gestational age. This represents one of the best correlations reported to date between a blood velocity and the fetal hematocrit. However, on closer inspection of the data, the usefulness of the technique must be questioned. Only 12 of the 24 fetuses studied were correctly predicted to be anemic by this technique. Mari and coworkers (unpublished, abstract #313, Society for Gynecologic Investigation, 1990) evaluated the maximal systolic velocity of the fetal MCA as a predictor of fetal anemia. In the 18 fetuses studied, the hematocrit ranged between 10% and 30%. Twelve of the fetuses exhibited MCA peak velocities above the 95% tolerance limit for the appropriate gestational age. A linear correlation was noted between the fetal hematocrit and the MCA velocity ($r = -0.57$); however, the equation estimated the true fetal hematocrit with an error of up to 50%. The authors concluded that peak MCA was not sensitive for predicting the actual fetal hematocrit in pregnancies complicated by red cell alloimmunization.

Therefore, attempts to date at predicting the fetal hematocrit from Doppler velocities in the various regions of the fetal circulation have not been promising. Published investigations share a common error of being retrospective. The availability of percutaneous umbilical blood sampling has led investigators to search for a noninvasive tool that is accurate in forecasting the actual fetal hematocrit. The onset of fetal anemia secondary to maternal red cell alloimmunization is variable and probably is dependent on multiple factors including the

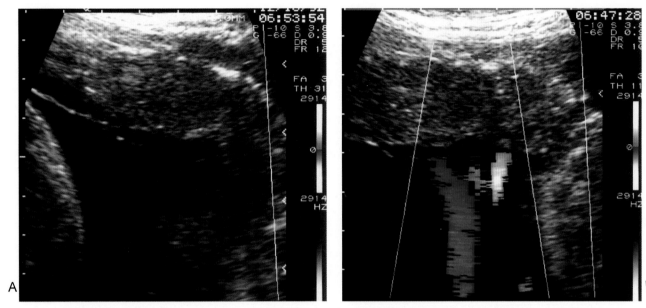

FIG. 3. Amniotic fluid pocket as visualized by real-time ultrasound (**A**) and after addition of color flow Doppler (**B**). The umbilical vein at its placental insertion site can be easily discerned as a blue vessel.

amount of maternal antibody present, the transplacental passage of the antibody, the affinity of the antibody for the fetal red cell antigen, and the ability of the fetal erythropoietic system to respond to the anemia. It is therefore not surprising that a variable fetal cardiovascular response to anemia has been observed. Perhaps future investigations should be modeled after the study of Warren et al. (10) and assess fetal blood velocities in a prospective, serial fashion to detect changes from baseline observations.

DOPPLER DURING INTRAUTERINE TRANSFUSION

What, then, is the role of Doppler in the management of the anemic fetus? Both color and pulsed Doppler are useful tools during intravascular transfusion. In situations in which the umbilical cord or its placental insertion is difficult to visualize, color Doppler can be used to distinguish between amniotic fluid and the umbilical vessels (see Fig. 3). In addition, fetal cardiac pulsations can be used to monitor the fetal heart rate response to IVT. If fetal bradycardia is noted, the infusion of packed red blood cells can be slowed or discontinued. Pulsed Doppler can also be used to assess the fetal heart rate at the site of needle puncture of the umbilical vessel and negates the need for moving the transducer to visualize the fetal heart during crucial moments of the fetal transfusion (30).

REFERENCES

1. Frigoletto FD, Greene MF, Benacerraf BR, Barss VA, Saltzman DH. Ultrasonographic fetal surveillance in the management of the isoimmunized pregnancy. *N Engl J Med* 1986;315:430–432.
2. Nicolaides KH, Fontanarosa M, Gabbe SG, Rodeck CH. Failure of ultrasonographic parameters to predict the severity of fetal anemia in rhesus isoimmunization. *Am J Obstet Gynecol* 1988;158: 920–926.
3. Fan F-C, Chen RY, Schuessler GB, Chien S. Effects of hematocrit variations on regional hemodynamics and oxygen transport in the dog. *Am J Physiol* 1980;238:H545–552.
4. Kirkinen P, Jouppila P. Umbilical vein blood flow in rhesus-isoimmunization. *Br J Obstet Gynaecol* 1983;90:640–643.
5. Copel JA, Grannum PA, Green JJ, et al. Fetal cardiac output in the isoimmunized pregnancy: A pulsed Doppler-echocardiographic study of patients undergoing intravascular intrauterine transfusion. *Am J Obstet Gynecol* 1989;161:361–365.
6. Rizzo G, Nicolaides KH, Arduini D, Campbell S. Effects of intravascular fetal blood transfusion on fetal intracardiac Doppler velocity waveforms. *Am J Obstet Gynecol* 1990;163:1231–1238.
7. Reed KL, Sahn DJ, Scagnelli S, Anderson CF, Shenker L. Doppler echocardiographic studies of diastolic function in the human fetal heart: Changes during gestation. *J Am Coll Cardiol* 1986;8:391–395.
8. Thomas JD, Choong CP, Flachskampf FA, Weyman AE. Analysis of the early transmitral Doppler velocity curve: Effect of primary physiologic changes and compensatory preload adjustments. *J Am Coll Cardiol* 1990;16:644–655.
9. Liley AW. Intrauterine transfusion of foetus in haemolytic disease. *Br Med J* 1963;2:1107–1109.
10. Warren PS, Gill RW, Fisher CC. Doppler flow studies in rhesus isoimmunization. *Semin Perinatol* 1987;11:375–378.
11. Grannum PA, Copel JA, Plaxe SC, Scioscia AL, Hobbins JC. In utero exchange transfusion by direct intravascular injection in severe erythroblastosis fetalis. *N Engl J Med* 1986;314:1431–1434.
12. Berkowitz RL, Chitkara U, Goldberg JD, Wilkins I, Chervenak FA, Lynch L. Intrauterine intravascular transfusions for severe red blood cell isoimmunization: Ultrasound-guided percutaneous approach. *Am J Obstet Gynecol* 1986;155:574–581.
13. Weiner CP, Anderson TL. The acute effect of cordocentesis with or without fetal curarization and of intravascular transfusion upon umbilical artery waveform indices. *Obstet Gynecol* 1989;73:219–224.
14. Mari G, Moise KJ, Deter RL, Carpenter RJ. Flow velocity waveforms of the umbilical and cerebral arteries before and after intravascular transfusion. *Obstet Gynecol* 1990;75:584–589.
15. Mari G, Moise KJ, Deter RL, Carpenter RJ. Doppler assessment of renal blood flow velocity waveforms in the anemic fetus before

and after intravascular transfusion for severe red cell alloimmunization. *J Clin Ultrasound* 1991;19:15–19.

16. Mari G, Moise KJ, Deter RL, Kirshon B, Stefos T, Carpenter RJ. Flow velocity waveforms of the vascular system in the anemic fetus before and after intravascular transfusion for severe red blood cell alloimmunization. *Am J Obstet Gynecol* 1990;162:1060–1064.

17. Moise KJ, Mari G, Fisher DJ, Huhta JC, Cano LE, Carpenter RJ. Acute fetal hemodynamic alterations after intrauterine transfusion for treatment of severe red blood cell alloimmunization. *Am J Obstet Gynecol* 1990;163:776–784.

18. Nicolini U, Talbert DG, Fisk NM, Rodeck CH. Pathophysiology of pressure changes during intrauterine transfusion. *Am J Obstet Gynecol* 1989;160:1139–1145.

19. Weiner CP, Pelzer GA, Heilskov J, Wenstrom K, Williamson RA. The effect of intravascular transfusion on umbilical venous pressure in anemic fetuses with and without hydrops. *Am J Obstet Gynecol* 1989;161:1498–1501.

20. Robillard JE, Weiner C. Atrial natriuretic factor in the human fetus: Effect of volume expansion. *J Pediatr* 1988;113:552–555.

21. Kingdom JC, Ryan G, Whittle MJ, et al. Atrial natriuretic peptide: A vasodilator of the fetoplacental circulation? *Am J Obstet Gynecol* 1991;165:791–800.

22. Weiner CP, Robillard JE. Effect of acute intravascular volume expansion on human fetal prostaglandin concentrations. *Am J Obstet Gynecol* 1989;161:1494–1497.

23. Rightmire DA, Nicolaides KH, Rodeck CH, Campbell S. Fetal blood velocities in Rh isoimmunization: Relationship to gestational age and to fetal hematocrit. *Obstet Gynecol* 1986;68:233–236.

24. Nicolaides KH, Bilardo CM, Campbell S. Prediction of fetal anemia by measurement of the mean blood velocity in the fetal aorta. *Am J Obstet Gynecol* 1990;162:209–212.

25. Copel JA, Grannum PA, Belanger K, Green JJ, Hobbins JC. Pulsed Doppler flow-velocity waveforms before and after intrauterine intravascular transfusion for severe erythroblastosis fetalis. *Am J Obstet Gynecol* 1988;158:768–774.

26. Copel JA, Grannum PA, Green JJ, Belanger K, Hobbins JC. Pulsed Doppler flow-velocity waveforms in the prediction of fetal hematocrit of the severely isoimmunized pregnancy. *Am J Obstet Gynecol* 1989;161:341–344.

27. Nicolaides KH, Thilaganathan B, Rodeck CH, Mibashan RS. Erythroblastosis and reticulocytosis in anemic fetuses. *Am J Obstet Gynecol* 1988;159:1063–1065.

28. Bilardo CM, Nicolaides KH, Campbell S. Doppler studies in red cell isoimmunization. *Clin Obstet Gynecol* 1989;32:719–727.

29. Vyas S, Nicolaides KH, Campbell S. Doppler examination of the middle cerebral artery in anemic fetuses. *Am J Obstet Gynecol* 1990;162:1066–1068.

30. Rotmensch S, Liberati M, Luo J-S, Hobbins JC. Monitoring of intravascular fetal transfusions with Doppler velocimetry. *Am J Obstet Gynecol* 1992;167:1314–1316.

Doppler Ultrasound in Obstetrics and Gynecology,
edited by Joshua A. Copel and Kathryn L. Reed.
Raven Press, Ltd., New York © 1995.

CHAPTER 14

Multiple Pregnancy

Jorge E. Tolosa and Abraham Ludomirski

The availability of diagnostic ultrasound has improved the accuracy of prenatal diagnosis of multiple pregnancy (1–3). Early confirmation of a multiple pregnancy is very important for the obstetrician and the patient, given the known increased risk for low birthweight, the result of intrauterine growth retardation and premature delivery, as well as a higher incidence of malpresentation, placental abruption, congenital anomalies, and pregnancy-induced hypertension. The combination of such risk factors explains the higher perinatal mortality associated with multiple pregnancies—6.3% for twins, 16.4% for triplets (4,5), significantly higher than that expected for singletons (6)—even after adjusting for weight as determined in a recent study by Buekens and Wilcox (7) using birth and death certificate information and comparing weight-specific perinatal mortality rates of twins and singletons. It is encouraging, though, that mortality rates have decreased (8), presumably as a result of a combination and added effects of factors such as early diagnosis of a multiple pregnancy, identification of significant growth discordance with ultrasound, intense fetal surveillance with tools like electronic fetal monitoring (9), and improved neonatal care. Whether or not screening with Doppler ultrasound (10) contributes to this trend toward improvement is the concept that we will now discuss.

FETAL GROWTH

Twins follow a pattern of growth similar to that of singletons, up to 29–30 weeks (11,12); although there is continued growth beyond that point, it occurs at a slower rate than that of the singleton fetus (13). Possible explanations include a restrictive effect of "crowding," a deterioration of placental function, or the effect of the differ-

ent genetic potential of each twin. Twins are either monozygotic (MZ), whereby they originate from a single ovum and in consequence have identical genetic material except for very rare exceptions and share the same genetic potential; or dizygotic (DZ), whereby two separate ova share some of the same genetic material, as is seen in siblings. When significant discordance in growth between fetuses occurs, which has been defined as 15% (14) or the more accepted figure of 20% (15,16), an association with increased perinatal morbidity and mortality is found (17,18). We use the following formula to determine the difference in estimated fetal weight (EFW) (19):

$$\frac{\text{EFW large twin} - \text{EFW smaller twin}}{\text{EFW large twin}} \times 100$$

Identification of a multiple pregnancy complicated by significant discordance increases the likelihood of morbidity or mortality. A weight discordance can suggest one fetus complicated by intrauterine growth retardation (IUGR), or one fetus with a chromosomal anomaly accompanied by a normal cotwin, or both fetuses normal in spite of the discordance, as the result of differences in genetic potential. It is also possible for both twins to be growth-retarded and hence not show a significant discordance (20). There is an association between the small-for-gestational-age singleton fetus with abnormal umbilical artery velocimetry and poor outcome, such as a higher incidence of abnormal fetal heart rate tracings, oligohydramnios, pregnancy-induced hypertension, and admission to the neonatal intensive care unit (21,22). In addition to these complications, there is an association between IUGR and poor academic achievement later in life (23). It has been shown that there are no differences in the normal ranges for the velocimetric parameters of the umbilical artery between normal twins and singleton fetuses (11,15,24,25). The above observations from the singleton fetus have also been made in the IUGR twin (25); this explains why the concept of trying to identify

J. E. Tolosa and A. Ludomirski: Department of Obstetrics and Gynecology, Pennsylvania Hospital, 800 Spruce Street, Philadelphia, PA 19107.

significant growth discordance through the utilization of Doppler ultrasound has been a main concern of several investigators.

Farmakides et al. (26) studied 43 twin pregnancies with continuous wave Doppler of the umbilical artery and subtracted the value for the systolic/diastolic ratio (S/D) of one twin from the other. Use of a cutoff of >0.4 in the difference of the S/D ratio predicted a difference of at least 349 gms, with a sensitivity of 73% and a specificity of 82%; the positive predictive value was 68%. This early report was not able to use technical advances such as a pulsed Doppler duplex system instead of a continuous wave system that would allow each fetus to be identified in a more precise way. It must be stressed that very important work in this field has been done with the use of continuous wave Doppler, which is still being used (10,27,28). In this study it was also noted that if both twins were IUGR, the proposed guideline did not apply.

Gerson et al. (15) studied 56 multiple pregnancies and found elevated S/D ratios in 9 of 11 sets of discordant twins; in 6 of those, abnormal S/D ratios were detected prior to the identification of significant discordant growth. The sensitivity of the test was 81.8%, its specificity 97.9%; the positive predictive value of an abnormal Doppler was 90% and the negative predictive value was 95.6%. Opposite findings have been reported (4). Hastie et al. (28) studied 89 consecutive twin pregnancies; his results showed a sensitivity for the prediction of a small-for-gestational-age (SGA) fetus of 29%, with a positive predictive value of 34%. An important observation within this study was the association between absent end diastolic velocities and increased risk for SGA or intrauterine death.

Saldana et al. (29) used the parameters set by Farmakides et al. (26) to test the accuracy of a difference in S/D ratio of >0.4 in identifying a discordance in birth weight of at least 350 gms; the predictive value was only 42%.

Gaziano et al. (30) combined 94 pairs of twins and 7 sets of triplets. Seventeen fetuses showed abnormal S/D ratios in the study group, of which seven were SGA while five were appropriate for gestational age but products of pregnancies complicated by twin-to-twin transfusion syndrome (TTTS), and another one had multiple congenital anomalies. An association was found between abnormal S/D ratios and earlier delivery (3–4 weeks) than those fetuses with normal S/D ratios.

Nimrod et al. (31) utilized Doppler ultrasound of the descending aorta in addition to the umbilical artery in 30 twin pregnancies. Only by combining many variables, including biparietal diameter, peak end-diastolic velocity, volume flow (an unsatisfactory parameter with high inherent variability), and aortic and umbilical peak systolic/end-diastolic velocities, was the sensitivity high, i.e., 82% for detection of an unsatisfactory outcome,

which was defined as premature delivery before 32 weeks, weight difference at birth of 500 g or more, birthweight below the 10th percentile, or admission to the neonatal intensive care unit.

The utilization of other peripheral vessels for the study of fetal well-being or to identify fetuses at risk has been of interest in singletons more than in multiple pregnancies (32,33).

Mari et al. (34) studied the flow velocity waveforms in the renal arteries of 121 normal fetuses, 10 with oligohydramnios, 10 with polyhydramnios, and 8 sets of diamniotic twins with discordance in amniotic fluid. Interobserver variability for the Doppler examination of the renal arteries was established at 6.7% at the level of the hilium and 12% inside the renal parenchyma, which would make this measurement a useful parameter given its reproducibility. The Pulsatility Index (PI) of the renal artery in twins with polyhydramnios was significantly lower than that in twins with oligohydramnios. Seven fetuses with oligohydramnios were also SGA and three deaths occurred in this group, of which four had an abnormal renal artery PI.

Degani et al. (35) studied the fetal internal carotid artery with Doppler ultrasound in 17 sets of twins. He concluded that the study of the PI of the internal carotid artery provides evidence of a brain-sparing effect in the growth-retarded fetus. Using a cutoff level of a PI < 1.2 the sensitivity of the test to identify an SGA fetus was 83%, with a specificity of 95%, a positive predictive value of 91%, and a negative predictive value of 91%.

Divon et al. (14) analyzed the effectiveness of Doppler ultrasound in combination with ultrasound biometry to predict discordance in 58 third-trimester twin pregnancies; the combination of a difference of at least 15% in the S/D ratio and a difference in the EFW of at least 15% had the best positive predictive value (73%) and a negative predictive value of 90%.

Giles has been one of the most active investigators in the area of Doppler ultrasound and multiple pregnancy (10,11,24,25,36–38). Using a historic cohort study design, 272 twin pregnancies were studied. After the first 100 cases the information of umbilical artery Doppler values was used for clinical management. A significant difference in perinatal mortality was detected, dropping from 42.1 per 1000 initially to 8.9 per 1000 in the latter phase of the study. The difference was suggested to be a result of recognition of the potentially compromised fetus through the use of Doppler ultrasound (10). Giles also studied umbilical Doppler ultrasound in 20 sets of triplets (37). He suggests that this is one situation when the utilization of pulsed Doppler is not enough to identify correctly the fetus being examined, but that the use of continuous wave Doppler with simultaneous matching of the fetal heartbeat to real-time ultrasound permits the operator to make a distinction. He recently showed a significant association between abnormal *S/D* ratios and a reduction in placental tertiary stem villi vessels, when studying 41 twin pregnancies (38).

Recent publications in this area tend to favor the utilization of Doppler ultrasound as a tool to identify those fetuses that are at higher risk for increased morbidity or mortality. Jensen (39) studied the correlation between an abnormal umbilical artery resistance index (RI) and the presence of late fetal heart decelerations in 50 pairs of twins. An RI greater than or equal to 80% above the normal value was associated with late decelerations in seven of nine fetuses. An association between a high RI and low birthweight was also identified.

Shah et al. (40) compared the *S/D* ratio of the umbilical artery in 63 pairs of concordant and 17 discordant twins with those of 277 appropriate-for-gestational-age fetuses. The *S/D* ratio for the smaller of the discordant twins increased throughout gestation. Using an *S/D* ratio above the 95% as abnormal, the characteristics of the test for discordancy were the following: sensitivity 75%, specificity 83.3%, and positive predictive value 75%.

Chang et al. (41) conducted a literature review to identify which ultrasonic parameter was better at identifying the SGA fetus. A comparison of two-dimensional and Doppler ultrasound highlights enormous difficulties given differences in operator experience, equipment, and methodology used to determine specific ultrasound parameters. Nevertheless two important results emerged: an abdominal circumference (AC) and the EFW below the 10th percentile were the most accurate identifiers of SGA; and abnormal Doppler velocimetry was significantly associated with risk, but less so than AC and EFW.

The AC had a common odds ratio (OR), (a statistic that provides a measure of risk) of 18.4 with 95% confidence intervals (CI) 9.8 to 34.3; the EFW showed even better characteristics, with a common OR of 39.1 (95% CI 28.9 to 52.8). Although the common ORs of the Doppler studies analyzed were lower than those of the AC and EFW < 10%, they were still within the boundaries of a positive finding. An umbilical artery *S/D* ratio > 3 showed a common OR of 6.9 (95% CI 4.8 to 10.0); similar results were obtained when the definition of abnormality used was that of an *S/D* ratio above the 95th percentile for gestational age, with a common OR of 5.8 (95% CI 4.8 to 7.0). When an evaluation of the uteroplacental circulation was considered, an RI > 0.5 showed a common OR of 2.3 (95% CI 1.2 to 4.3). This information is very interesting in the sense that it suggests that if both parameters are combined (i.e., the biometric evaluation of the AC and EFW with umbilical artery Doppler studies), those fetuses at higher risk to be SGA will be identified.

Beattie et al. (42) looked at the predictive value of biometry, the umbilical artery *S/D* ratio, and the biophys-ical profile together to predict perinatal mortality, morbidity, and discordant or retarded growth through a retrospective analysis of 134 twin pairs. Discordant *S/D* ratios following the definitions of Farmakides et al. (26) and Saldana et al. (29) were not associated with discordant birthweight, but there was an association between an abnormal *S/D* ratio in one or both twins with neonatal depression, perinatal mortality, neonatal intensive care unit admission, and the need for mechanical ventilation. Again, an association between absent end-diastolic velocity and increased morbidity was found. IUGR has also been associated with absent end-diastolic velocities in the umbilical cord in work done by Tyrell et al. (43). Nicolaides et al. (44) were able to correlate this abnormal umbilical artery waveform with fetal hypoxia through fetal blood sampling. Bell et al. (45) demonstrated how umbilical artery Doppler can be used to monitor pregnancies at high risk or those that show other abnormal results indicative of fetal compromise. He evaluated 40 fetuses (all singleton pregnancies) with absent end-diastolic velocities at our institution. In 11 (27%), antenatal improvement occurred and a significant correlation with more advanced gestational age, higher birthweight, and a clinically significant difference in neonatal death was observed in comparison to those fetuses in which there was no improvement in the umbilical artery waveform, under the same treatment, i.e., hospitalization, bed rest, and intense fetal monitoring. There is no reason to expect that a similar pattern might not be present in the twin pregnancy in which there is IUGR and absent end-diastolic velocity, although to our knowledge work in this particular area has not been done.

ACARDIAC ANOMALY

A rare complication of monozygotic twin gestations is that of an acardiac anomaly, thought to occur in 1/35,000 pregnancies (46) and associated with a very high mortality rate of around 50% (47). Two possible explanations for the development of this anomaly have been postulated. One suggests that acardia is a primary anomaly resulting from an unknown etiology, while the second suggests that as a result of the passage of nonoxygenated blood to the fetus through vascular connections in the placenta, this "recipient" twin suffers the effects of lack of oxygen at a critical time in the development of the heart; this would be a very severe expression of the twin-to-twin transfusion syndrome (TTTS) very early in the pregnancy. The circulatory pattern, known as twin reversed arterial perfusion sequence (TRAP), involves reversal of normal blood flow to the abnormal twin. Sherer et al. (48) described abnormal umbilical Doppler velocities in one patient with this complication at 29 weeks gestation. Donnenfeld et al. (49) reported his experience with the diagnosis and management of four cases of acardiac anomaly. Doppler ultrasound confirmed the diagnosis in three cases in which the normal fetus was viable, documenting retrograde arterial perfusion of the acardiac twin, with normal S/D ratios in the umbilical cords of both twins. He proposed for future studies the utilization of fetal echocardiography, specifically that of Doppler flow studies of the tricuspid valve, to identify signs of congestive heart failure in the normal twin, given that this is a known complication for the normal fetus.

TWIN-TO-TWIN TRANSFUSION SYNDROME

A complication almost unique to monozygotic-monochorionic twins is that of the TTTS. Monozygotic twins occur in approximately 4/1000 pregnancies, and of those two-thirds are monochorionic. Vascular anastomoses between the circulations of the fetuses that can be superficial, deep, or both have been thought to be responsible for this serious complication. It has been shown that the most frequent type of anastomoses are artery-to-artery and artery-to-vein (50), the latter being the most significant type. It has been hypothesized that a hemodynamically unbalanced arteriovenous shunt develops. For reasons that are not clear, only rarely does this condition develop in spite of the very frequent finding of vascular communications between fetuses (51). Blickstein (52) recently published a thorough review of this topic.

In a pathologic condition in which there is an alteration of blood flow between fetuses, as the TTTS is thought to be, Doppler velocimetry would appear to be an appropriate tool to diagnose and monitor the progression of the disease. Several authors have approached this problem and the results have been conflicting, perhaps because the definition of the TTTS has varied between authors and also because the number of cases analyzed tends to be small, given the rarity of the condition. Weiner (53) described the antenatal diagnosis of TTTS. Neilson (4) also emphasized the need for a strict definition of the TTTS.

Farmakides et al. (26) reported finding a difference in Doppler signals between twins when using continuous wave Doppler of the umbilical cord, with high and low resistance values in two cases of TTTS.

Erskine et al. (54) reported discordant Doppler signals in the umbilical cord in a patient with a pregnancy complicated by TTTS. After the death of the small twin, who showed absent end-diastolic velocities, no change in the Doppler signal of the surviving twin occurred, but no confirmation of the diagnosis was made by hematologic or pathologic exam.

Neilson et al. (55) looked at the significance of vascular anastomoses in monochorionic placentas in the absence of TTTS. He compared a group of monozygotic twins with monochorionic placentas with those having dichorionic placentas. Of 63 monozygotic pregnancies, 48 were monochorionic and 15 were dichorionic. Doppler ultrasound studies were available in 22 monochorionic and 10 dichorionic pairs. No difference in S/D ratios was found when those cases showing absent end-diastolic velocities were excluded.

Pretorius et al. (56) studied eight twin pairs suspected of having TTTS by ultrasonographic criteria. Variable Doppler findings were observed; a specific pattern of change was not detected.

Giles et al. (36) analyzed a group of 11 twin pairs diagnosed with TTTS. Using continuous wave Doppler of the umbilical cord he found no difference in the S/D ratios of the twins. The mean gestational age of the group was 34 weeks, so we have to consider that if indeed these were all cases of TTTS, they were not those more severely affected. Postnatal diagnosis was used based on placental and hematologic differences.

Gaziano et al. (30) used newborn information, analyzing the placenta and obtaining hematologic information on the twins, to conclude that the more frequently found pattern of Doppler velocimetry of the umbilical cord was for the small fetus (or donor) to present with elevated values (seen in 7 of 11 donor twins), but that varying Doppler findings in both the donor and the recipient twin could be expected.

In light of these discrepancies in findings among authors, D'Alton and Mercer (57) questioned the use of Doppler ultrasound in TTTS.

Yamada et al. (58) studied 31 pairs of twins, of which 6 were diagnosed as TTTS based on neonatal data with histologic exam of the placenta and hematologic differences in the twins. He found that the individual value of the PI for each fetus was not able to discriminate between the presence of TTTS or its absence, but when intertwin differences were analyzed, a statistically significant difference was detected when there was a discordance of 0.5 or greater in the PI of the umbilical cords; the characteristics of the test for this purpose showed a sensitivity of 75%, a specificity of 96%, and a positive predictive value of 86%. This difference in umbilical artery PI is clearly changed in the presence of hydrops, probably as a result of heart failure of the hydropic fetus.

Ludomirski et al. (59) reported an elevation of the S/D ratio in the donor twin that was significantly associated with nonsurvival, when studying 15 twin pairs and making the antenatal diagnosis of TTTS with cordocentesis and detailed ultrasonography.

The information available about Doppler ultrasonography in the diagnosis of TTTS appears to be conflicting, since the definitions used have not been consistent, but there is enough ultrasonographic data and experience to conclude that a twin pregnancy complicated by significant discordance in EFW (20% or more), with a clear discordance in the amount of amniotic fluid in each sac (i.e., one fetus showing polyhydramnios and the other oligohydramnios), monochorionicity, and fetuses with the same gender, has a significant probability of being complicated by TTTS. Other etiologies that could be responsible for such a clinical picture are placental insufficiency of one twin, intrauterine infection, or a chromosomal abnormality. Weiner (53) discussed this spectrum of the disease. The most common pattern followed by this condition involves a donor fetus who demonstrates IUGR and anemia, and a recipient fetus that suffers the consequences of volume overload and possibly the transfusion of other biological substances like hormones or proteins (52,60,61). As the condition worsens the large fetus develops hydrops fetalis and dies. The perinatal management of this serious complication of pregnancy is very controversial and certainly frustrating for the perinatologist, given the very high perinatal mortality associated with the disease, reported to be higher than 50% (58). Several therapies have been attempted, including laser occlusion of placental vessels (62), feticide of one twin (63), and therapeutic amniocentesis (64–66). None of those therapies appear to be highly effective, except for serial amniocentesis in occasional cases, as has been our experience.

Since none of the therapies available are definitely useful and all are invasive in nature, a different approach to improving mortality and morbidity by changing the perinatal management with the utilization of fetal echocardiography was recently reported by Tolosa et al. (67). The rationale for this work has been that in light of the lack of an effective therapy, the timing of delivery is especially important in preventing the development of hydrops in the large fetus, since hydrops fetalis and prematurity are almost invariably associated with perinatal death. Other authors have also suggested the potential use of echocardiography in the evaluation of the TTTS or the fetus with IUGR.

Achiron et al. (68) reported the echocardiographic evaluation of a patient with suspected twin-to-twin transfusion; he estimated the ventricular output by pulsed Doppler ultrasound on both twins and found that the hydropic fetus had an increased cardiac output with evidence of tricuspid and mitral regurgitation as well as cardiomegaly. Although in this case report the diagnosis of TTTS was not conclusive, since the fetuses were concordant in size, had concordant hemoglobin concentrations at birth, and the hydropic twin recovered spontaneously (indeed, a rare development in TTTS), the author suggests that hydrops might have been the result of volume overload. Naeye (69) conducted postmortem studies on 11 pairs of twins with a diagnosis of TTTS and found cardiovascular abnormalities in all cases. Myocardial enlargement with hyperplasia of the myocardial fiber was a common finding, as was thickening of pulmonary and systemic arteries, suggesting increased peripheral resistance. He postulated that the findings of

myocardial hyperplasia were possibly the result of systemic and pulmonary arterial hypertension.

Reed et al. (70) studied the deceleration time in the tricuspid and mitral valves in normal and IUGR fetuses from pulsed Doppler velocity waveforms and associated this information with ventricular function. In fetuses with IUGR and absent end-diastolic velocities, tricuspid and mitral valve deceleration times were longer than normal. The author explained this findings as a result of prolongation of ventricular relaxation, secondary to an increased afterload, due to an elevated placental resistance. Reed et al. (71) also studied the Doppler signals of the inferior vena cava (IVC) in 15 normal and 15 IUGR fetuses, and documented an increased reversal in flow during atrial contraction as well as an increased S/D ratio of the IVC forward time velocity integrals (TVI).

Gudmundsson et al. (72) reported his results on venous Doppler ultrasound by studying 18 fetuses with nonimmune hydrops fetalis. Of these, 6 were recipient twins in pregnancies complicated by TTTS. A clear pattern of umbilical vein pulsations was observed in 14 (Fig. 1). These pulsations are explained as a result of abnormal reversal of flow starting in the central veins and extending into the umbilical vein, the product of an abnormal wave of blood generated after atrial systole (Fig. 2). The shortening fraction of the right ventricle was calculated from an M-mode measurement as follows: diastolic dimension − systolic dimension ÷ diastolic dimension. Decreased ventricular shortening was documented in

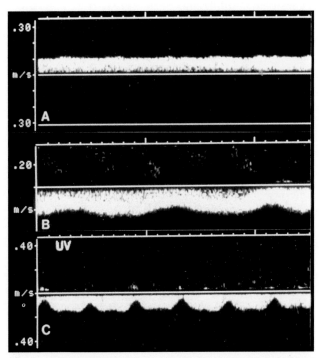

FIG. 1. Blood velocity in fetal umbilical vein. **A:** Normal blood velocity pattern. **B:** Blood velocity influenced by fetal breathing. **C:** Venous pulsations in nonimmune hydrops. From Gudmundsson et al. (72).

those with umbilical vein pulsations, suggesting congestive heart failure.

Rizzo et al. (73,74) reported similar findings in fetuses with IUGR; 79 SGA fetuses were studied and of those 20 had absent end-diastolic velocities; his results suggested that the degree of cardiac dysfunction necessary to alter the IVC Doppler signal might be associated with the temporal duration of the hemodynamic abnormality and not necessarily to the degree of change in peripheral vascular resistance only.

Tulzer et al. (75) also explored the association of Doppler echocardiography and perinatal mortality in fetuses with hydrops fetalis; of 24 fetuses with nonimmune hydrops fetalis, 7 were hydropic fetuses of TTTS pairs. The percentage of retrograde flow in the IVC: 10.7 in the survivors and 49 in the nonsurvivors ($p < 0.001$), the IVC E/V wave velocity ratio: 0.63 in the survivors and 0.04 in the nonsurvivors ($p < 0.001$) and the presence of umbilical vein pulsations: 4 of 11 of the survivors and 12 of 13 of the nonsurvivors ($p < 0.001$) were all associated with an increased perinatal mortality.

Tolosa et al. (67) reported the results of venous Doppler studies in 11 pairs of discordant twins, defined as >20% different in EFW (10/11), with evidence of polyhydramnios in the large twin and oligohydramnios in the small twin (9/11) and with monochorionic diamniotic placentation (10/11); the average gestational age was 28 weeks with a range of 25–34 weeks. Using serial two-dimensional ultrasound, M-mode and Doppler echocardiography, measurements of the ratio of the area of the heart relative to the area of the thorax (C/T), thickness of the left ventricular free wall (LVW), Doppler ultrasound of the IVC and the umbilical vein were obtained.

Using color and continuous wave Doppler a tricuspid regurgitation (TR) signal was sought and the peak velocity was converted to a peak ventricular pressure (VP), using the modified Bernoulli equation (76). Patterns observed in the large twin included heart enlargement: C/T area ratio > 0.33 in 54%, myocardial hypertrophy: LVW > 2 SD (77) in all cases, increased reversed flow in the IVC in 73%, umbilical vein pulsations in 36%, and elevated VP (55–88 mm Hg) in 45%. Neonatal hypertension was present in all the large twins during the first 24 hr after birth and was always associated with myocardial hypertrophy. Hydrops fetalis was present in the first two fetuses studied. Since we incorporated these echocardiographic parameters into the antenatal monitoring plan for the management of twins complicated with TTTS, of nine sets of twins followed, none of the large twins have developed hydrops fetalis at the time of delivery.

In summary, then, Doppler ultrasound in twins needs a more rigorous analysis with appropriately designed studies, but it appears from the current evidence as presented by Neilson (78) that Doppler ultrasonography can contribute to a decrease in perinatal mortality in the IUGR fetus. Serial two-dimensional ultrasonography for the detection of IUGR in twins is indicated, and in the circumstance of discordance in growth between the twins being clinically significant or both twins falling below their expected growth curves, Doppler ultrasonography of the umbilical cord can help in identifying those fetuses who are at even higher risk for increased perinatal morbidity and mortality. In the management of the TTTS, Doppler echocardiography and Doppler ultrasound of the venous circulation of the fetus appears to be a useful tool to improve the perinatal management of this serious complication of pregnancy.

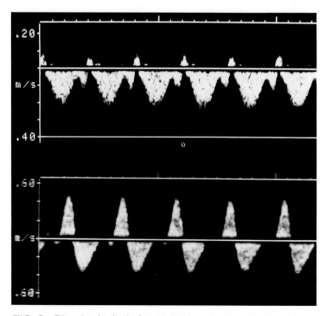

FIG. 2. Blood velocity in fetal inferior vena cava. **Top:** Normal blood velocity. **Bottom:** Reversal of venous flow in nonimmune hydrops. From Gudmundsson et al. (72).

REFERENCES

1. Chervenak FA, Youcha S, Johnson RE, Berkowitz RL, Hobbins JC. Antenatal diagnosis and perinatal outcome in a series of 385 consecutive twin pregnancies. *J Reprod Med* 1984;29:727–730.
2. Eik-nes SH, Okland O, Aure JC. Ultrasound screening in pregnancy: A randomized controlled trial. *Lancet* 1984;1:1347.
3. Bakketeig LS, Jacobsen G, Brodtkorb CJ, et al. Randomized controlled trial of ultrasound screening in pregnancy. *Lancet* 1984;2:207–210.
4. Neilson JP. Prenatal diagnosis in multiple pregnancies. *Curr Opin Obstet Gynecol* 1992;4(2):280–285.
5. Botting BH, McDonald-Davies I, McFarlane AJ. Recent trends in the incidence of multiple births and associated mortality. *Arch Dis Child* 1987;62:941–950.
6. Kiely J. The epidemiology of perinatal mortality in multiple births. *Bull NY Acad Med* 1990;66:618–637.
7. Buekens P, Wilcox A. Why do small twins have a lower mortality rate than small singletons? *Am J Obstet Gynecol* 1993;168:937–941.
8. Alvarez M, Berkowitz RL. Multifetal gestation. *Clin Obstet Gynecol* 1990;33:79–87.
9. Devoe LD, Azer H. Simultaneous nonstress fetal heart rate testing in twin pregnancy. *Obstet Gynecol* 1981;58:450–455.
10. Giles WB, Trudinger BJ, Cook CM, Connelly A. Umbilical artery flow velocity waveforms and twin pregnancy outcome. *Obstet Gynecol* 1988;72:894–897.

11. Giles WG. Doppler assessment in multiple pregnancy. *Semin Perinatol* 1987;11(4):369–374.
12. McKeown YT, Record RG. Observations on foetal growth in multiple pregnancy in man. *J Endocrinol* 1952;8:386–401.
13. Neilson JP. Detection of the small-for-dates twin fetus by ultrasound. *Br J Obstet Gynaecol* 1981;88:27–32.
14. Divon MY, Girz BA, Sklar A, Guidehi DA, Langer O. Discordant twins: A prospective study of the diagnostic value of real-time ultrasonography combined with umbilical artery velocimetry. *Am J Obstet Gynecol* 1989;161:757–760.
15. Gerson AG, Wallace DA, Bridgens NK, Ashmead GC, Weiner S, Bolognese RJ. Duplex Doppler ultrasound in the evaluation of growth in twin pregnancies. *Obstet Gynecol* 1987;70:419–423.
16. Socol M, Tamura R, Sabbagha R, Chen T, Vaisrub N. Diminished biparietal diameter and abdominal circumference growth in twins. *Obstet Gynecol* 1984;64:235–238.
17. Crane J, Tomich P, Kopta M. Ultrasonic growth patterns in normal and discordant twins. *Obstet Gynecol* 1980;55:678–683.
18. Erkkola R, Ala-Mello S, Piiroinen O, Kero P, Sillanpa M. Growth discordancy in twin pregnancies: A risk factor not detected by measurements of biparietal diameter. *Obstet Gynecol* 1985;66:203–206.
19. Storlazzi E, Vintzileos AM, Campbell WA, Nochimson DJ, Weinbaum PJ. Ultrasonic diagnosis of discordant fetal growth in twin gestations. *Obstet Gynecol* 1987;69:363–367.
20. Divon MY, Hsu HW. Maternal and fetal blood flow velocity waveforms in intrauterine growth retardation. *Clin Obstet Gynecol* 1992;35:156–171.
21. Rochelson BL, Schulman H, Fleisher A, et al. The clinical significance of Doppler umbilical artery velocimetry in the small for gestational age fetus. *Am J Obstet Gynecol* 1987;156:1223–1226.
22. Berkowitz GS, Mehalek KE, Chitkara U, et al. Doppler umbilical velocimetry in the prediction of adverse outcome in pregnancies at risk for intrauterine growth retardation. *Obstet Gynecol* 1988;71:742–746.
23. Low JA, Handley-Derry MH, Burke SO, et al. Association of intrauterine fetal growth retardation and learning deficits at age 9 to 11 years. *Am J Obstet Gynecol* 1992;167:1499–1505.
24. Giles WB, Trudinger BJ, Cook CM. Umbilical waveforms in twin pregnancy. *Acta Genet Med Gemellol* 1985;34:233–237.
25. Giles WB, Trudinger BJ, Cook CM. Fetal umbilical artery flow velocity-time waveforms in twin pregnancies. *Br J Obstet Gynecol* 1985;92:490–496.
26. Farmakides G, Schulman H, Saldana LR, Bracero LA, Fleischer A, Rochelson B. Surveillance of twin pregnancy with umbilical artery velocimetry. *Am J Obstet Gynecol* 1985;153:789–792.
27. Snijders RJM, Sherrod C, Gosden CM, Nicolaides KH. Fetal growth retardation: Associated malformations and chromosomal abnormalities. *Am J Obstet Gynecol* 1993;168:547–555.
28. Hastie SJ, Danskin F, Neilson JP, Whittle MJ. Prediction of the small for gestational age twin fetus by Doppler umbilical artery waveforms analysis. *Obstet Gynecol* 1989;74:730–733.
29. Saldana LR, Eads MC, Schaefer TR. Umbilical blood waveforms in fetal surveillance of twins. *Am J Obstet Gynecol* 1987;157:712–715.
30. Gaziano EP, Knox E, Bendel RP, Calvin S, Brandt D. Is pulsed Doppler velocimetry useful in the management of multiple gestation pregnancies? *Am J Obstet Gynecol* 1991;164:1426–1433.
31. Nimrod C, Davies D, Harder J, et al. Doppler ultrasound prediction of fetal outcome in twin pregnancies. *Am J Obstet Gynecol* 1987;156:402–406.
32. Wladimiroff JW, Tonge HM, Stewart PA. Doppler assessment of cerebral blood flow in human fetus. *Br J Obstet Gynaecol* 1986;93:471–475.
33. Wladimiroff JW, Van Den Wijngaard JAGW, Degani S, Noordam NJ, Van Eyck J. Cerebral and umbilical arterial blood flow velocity waveforms in normal and growth retarded pregnancies; A comparative study. *Obstet Gynecol* 1987;69:705–709.
34. Mari G, Kirshon B, Abuhamad A. Fetal renal artery flow velocity waveforms in normal pregnancies and pregnancies complicated by polyhydramnios and oligohydramnios. *Obstet Gynecol* 1993;81:560–564.
35. Degani S, Paltiely J, Lewinsky R, Shapiro I, Sharf M. Fetal internal carotid artery flow velocity time waveforms in twin pregnancies. *J Perinat Med* 1988;16:405–409.
36. Giles WB, Trudinger BJ, Cook CM, Connelly AJ. Doppler umbilical artery studies in the twin-twin transfusion syndrome. *Obstet Gynecol* 1990;76:1097–1099.
37. Giles WB, Trudinger BJ, Cook CM, Connelly AJ. Umbilical artery waveforms in triplet pregnancy. *Obstet Gynecol* 1990;75:813–816.
38. Giles W, Trudinger B, Cook C, Connelly A. Placental microvascular changes in twin pregnancies with abnormal umbilical artery waveforms. *Obstet Gynecol* 1993;81:556–559.
39. Jensen OH. Doppler velocimetry in twin pregnancy. *Eur J Obstet Gynecol Reprod Biol* 1992;45(1):9–12.
40. Shah YG, Gragg LA, Moodley S, Williams GW. Doppler velocimetry in concordant and discordant twin gestations. *Obstet Gynecol* 1992;80:272–276.
41. Chang TC, Robson SC, Boys RJ, Spencer JAD. Prediction of the small for gestational age infant: Which ultrasonic measurement is best? *Obstet Gynecol* 1992;80:1030–1038.
42. Beattie RB, McDowell MJ, Ritchie JWK. Optimizing fetal surveillance in twin pregnancy. *J Mat-Fet Invest* 1993;3:53–57.
43. Tyrell S, Obaid AH, Lilford RJ. Umbilical artery Doppler velocimetry as a predictor of fetal hypoxia and acidosis at birth. *Obstet Gynecol* 1989;74:332–337.
44. Nicolaides KH, Bilardo CM, Soothill PW, Campbell S. Absence of end diastolic frequencies in umbilical artery: A sign of fetal hypoxia and acidosis. *Br Med J* 1988;297:1026–1027.
45. Bell JG, Ludomirski A, Bottalico J, Weiner S. The effect of improvement of umbilical artery absent end-diastolic velocity on perinatal outcome. *Am J Obstet Gynecol* 1992;167:1015–1020.
46. Severn CB, Holyoke EA. Human acardiac anomalies. *Am J Obstet Gynecol* 1973;116:358–365.
47. Moore TR, Gale S, Benirschke K. Perinatal outcome of forty-nine pregnancies complicated by acardiac twinning. *Am J Obstet Gynecol* 1990;163:907–912.
48. Sherer DM, Armstrong S, Shah YG, Metlay LA, Woods JR. Prenatal sonographic diagnosis, Doppler velocimetric umbilical cord studies, and subsequent management of an acardiac twin pregnancy. *Obstet Gynecol* 1989;74:472–475.
49. Donnenfeld AE, Van De Woestijne J, Craparo F, Smith CS, Ludomirski A, Weiner S. The normal fetus of an acardiac twin pregnancy: Perinatal management based on echocardiographic and sonographic evaluation. *Prenat Diagn* 1991;11(4):235–244.
50. Benirschke K, Driscoll SG. *The pathology of the human placenta.* Berlin: Springer-Verlag; 1967.
51. Robertson EG, Neer KJ. Placental injection studies in twin gestation. *Am J Obstet Gynecol* 1983;147:170–173.
52. Blickstein I. The twin-twin transfusion syndrome. *Obstet Gynecol* 1990;76:714–722.
53. Weiner CB. Challenge of twin-twin transfusion syndrome. *Contemp Ob Gyn* 1992;83–104.
54. Erskine RLA, Ritchie JWK, Murnaghan GA. Antenatal diagnosis of placental anastomosis in a twin pregnancy using Doppler ultrasound. *Br J Obstet Gynaecol* 1986;93:955–959.
55. Neilson JP, Danskin F, Hastie SJ. Monozygotic twin pregnancy: Diagnostic and Doppler ultrasound studies. *Br J Obstet Gynaecol* 1989;96:1413–1418.
56. Pretorius DH, Manchester D, Barkin S, Parker S, Nelson TR. Doppler ultrasound of twin transfusion syndrome. *J Ultrasound Med* 1988;7:117–124.
57. D'Alton ME, Mercer BM. Antepartum management of twin gestation: Ultrasound. *Clin Obstet Gynecol* 1990;33(1):42–51.
58. Yamada A, Kasugai M, Ohno Y, Ishizuka T, Mizutani S, Tomoda Y. Antenatal diagnosis of twin-twin transfusion syndrome by Doppler ultrasound. *Obstet Gynecol* 1991;78:1058–1061.
59. Ludomirski A, Weiner S, Craparo F, Bhutani V. Twin to twin transfusion syndrome: Role of Doppler flow and fetal hyperviscosity in predicting outcome. *Am J Obstet Gynecol* 1991;1645:243.
60. Nageotte MP, Hurwitz SR, Kaupke CJ, Vaziri ND, Panchian MR. Atriopeptin in the twin transfusion syndrome. *Obstet Gynecol* 1989;73:867–870.
61. Ervin MG. Perinatal fluid and electrolyte regulation: Role of arginine vasopressin. *Semin Perinatol* 1988;12:134–142.
62. DeLia JE, Cruikshank DP, Keye WF. Fetoscopic neodymium: Yag laser occlusion of placental vessels in severe twin-twin transfusion syndrome. *Obstet Gynecol* 1990;75:1040–1053.
63. Wittmann BK, Farquharson DF, Thomas WDS, Baldwin VJ, Wadsworth LD. The role of feticide in the management of severe

twin transfusion syndrome. *Am J Obstet Gynecol* 1986;155:1423–1426.

64. Elliott JP, Urig MA, Clewell WH. Aggressive therapeutic amniocentesis for treatment of twin–twin transfusion syndrome. *Obstet Gynecol* 1991;77:537.

65. Feingold M, Cetrulo CL, Newton ER, Weiss J, Shakr C, Shmoys S. Serial amniocentesis in the treatment of twin-to-twin transfusion complicated with acute polyhydramnios. *Acta Genet Med Gemellol* 1986;35:107–113.

66. Saunders NJ, Sniders RJ, Nicolaides KH. Therapeutic amniocentesis in twin–twin transfusion syndrome appearing in the second trimester of pregnancy. *Am J Obstet Gynecol* 1992;166:820–824.

67. Tolosa JE, Zoppini C, Ludomirski A, Bhutani V, Weil SR, Huhta JC. Fetal hypertension and cardiac hypertrophy in the discordant twin syndrome. *Am J Obstet Gynecol* 1993;168:292.

68. Achiron R, Rabinovitz R, Aboulafia Y, Diamant Y, Glaser Y. Intrauterine assessment of high-output cardiac failure with spontaneous remission of hydrops fetalis in twin–twin transfusion syndrome: Use of two-dimensional echocardiography, Doppler ultrasound, and color flow mapping. *J Clin Ultrasound* 1992;20:271–277.

69. Naeye RL. Human intrauterine parabiotic syndrome and its complications. *N Engl J Med* 1963;268:804–809.

70. Reed KL, Appleton CP, Sahn DJ, Anderson CF. Human fetal tricuspid and mitral deceleration time: Changes with normal pregnancy and intrauterine growth retardation. *Am J Obstet Gynecol* 1989;161:1532–1535.

71. Reed KL, Appleton CP, Anderson CF, Shenker L, Sahn DJ. Doppler studies of vena cava flows in human fetuses insights into normal and abnormal cardiac physiology. *Circulation* 1990;81:498–505.

72. Gudmundsson S, Huhta JC, Wood DC, Tulzer G, Cohen AW, Weiner S. Venous Doppler ultrasonography in the fetus with nonimmune hydrops. *Am J Obstet Gynecol* 1991;164:33–37.

73. Rizzo G, Arduini D, Romanini C. Doppler echocardiographic assessment of fetal cardiac function. *Ultrasound Obstet Gynecol* 1992;2:434–445.

74. Rizzo G, Arduini D, Romanini C. Inferior vena cava flow velocity waveforms in appropriate and small-for-gestational-age fetuses. *Am J Obstet Gynecol* 1992;166:1271–1280.

75. Tulzer G, Gudmundsson S, Wood DC, Cohen AW, Weiner S, Huhta JC. Doppler in fetal hydrops fetalis; submitted.

76. Goldberg SJ. Doppler echocardiography. In: Moss AJ, Adams FH, Emmanouilides GC. Riemenscneider TA, eds. *Heart diseases in infants, children and adolescents.* Baltimore: Williams & Wilkins; 1989:81–93.

77. Allan LD. *Manual of fetal echocardiography.* London: MTP Press Ltd; 1986.

78. Neilson JP. Doppler ultrasound study of umbilical artery waveforms in high risk pregnancies. In: Chalmers I, ed. *Oxford database of perinatal trials.* Version 1.3, Disk Issue 8, Autumn 1992, Record 3889.

Doppler Ultrasound in Obstetrics and Gynecology,
edited by Joshua A. Copel and Kathryn L. Reed.
Raven Press, Ltd., New York © 1995.

CHAPTER 15

Hypertension

Elizabeth P. Schneider and Harold Schulman

Hypertensive disease occurs in 5–15% of all pregnancies and continues to cause significant fetal and maternal morbidity and mortality. During pregnancy, hypertension encompasses a range of disorders including essential hypertension, acute pregnancy-induced hypertension, preeclampsia, and eclampsia. Although the exact etiology of hypertension in pregnancy is unknown, several theories have been suggested including abnormal trophoblast invasion, coagulation abnormalities, vascular endothelial damage, cardiovascular maladaptation, abnormal immunologic reaction, genetic predisposition, and dietary influences (1).

Classification of the hypertensive disorders has been problematic due to inconsistent clinical presentations and confusing terminology. The management of the disease has been somewhat arbitrary based on severity as defined by clinical and laboratory criteria. Separation of maternal and fetal risks in women with hypertension have not been clearly enunciated.

The development of the uteroplacental and umbilical circulation is essential for the achievement of a normal pregnancy. Compromised uteroplacental or fetal circulation has been shown to play an important role in hypertensive disorders of pregnancy. Doppler technology provides a noninvasive tool to assess maternal and fetal hemodynamics.

By differentiating normal vs. abnormal flow in the uteroplacental and umbilical circulation we can follow changes in a human pregnancy in a dynamic fashion. Doppler velocimetry studies complement years of basic studies in animals and demonstrate the effects of an incomplete evolution of placental vessels. Important information about the uterine and umbilical circulation in

pregnancies complicated by hypertension can be provided by Doppler studies.

The objective of this chapter is to review the current understanding of the measures of maternal and fetal blood flow velocity used in the clinical assessment of women with hypertension disorders of pregnancy. This information may further clarify the pathophysiologic changes and help in classification and management of these pregnancies based on the presence or absence of vasculopathy.

UTEROPLACENTAL CIRCULATION

The blood supply to the uterus comes from the uterine arteries. Peripheral branches give rise to the arcuate arteries, which give off multiple branches of penetrating vessels called the radial arteries. As the radials approach the cavity they become the spiral arteries, the direct feeders of the endometrium (Fig. 1).

Dramatic histologic changes happen in the spiral arteries after conception. The first change is the disappearance of the internal elastic lamina. Remaining is a thin layer of basement membrane between the endothelium and smooth muscle in the media of the vessels. This is true whether vessels are basal branches supplying the decidua or spiral arteries directly communicating with the emerging intervillous space (2). Next the trophoblast penetrates the expanded spiral arteries, and the media is replaced by a matrix containing cytotrophoblasts, cellular debris, and fibrin fibers. Brosens believes that these changes are limited to the decidua in the first trimester and extend into the myometrial part in the early second trimester. Of interest is that trophoblast cells also replace the endothelial cells of the distal artery entering the intervillous space (3). Ramsey has shown the evolution of the arterial supply to the primate uterus using serial sections of plastic casts of the vessels (4). Since Doppler waveforms primarily reflect resistance, it is instructive to

E. P. Schneider: Department of Obstetrics and Gynecology, North Shore University Hospital, Manhasset, New York 11030.

H. Schulman: Department of Obstetrics and Gynecology, Winthrop University Hospital, Vero Beach, Florida 32963.

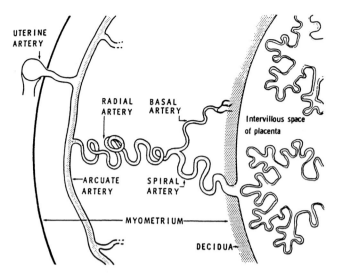

FIG. 1. Anatomy of the arcuate, radial, and spiral arteries in pregnancy. From Schulman et al. (2).

compare Ramsey's work with this physical parameter. In the fifteenth week (of a 23-week gestation) there are clinically definable intervillous spaces, but there is still considerable coiling of the spiral arteries. Coiling of the vessel probably contributes to resistance to flow. By the nineteenth week, the coiling is gone and the vessel is uniformly dilated. Ramsey stated that in the first two-thirds of pregnancy "continued growth and progressive narrowing of the endometrium by pressure of the conceptus produce increased coiling with back and forth looping of the arteries. . . . In the last trimester of pregnancy, as the uterine wall stretches, the coils of the arteries become extended and their course becomes circumferential and undulating" (Fig. 2). Reynolds believed that these latter changes happen because the shape of the uterus changes from spheroidal to cylindrical as it grows (5). Barcroft and Barron described the vascular changes in the sheep and stated that the real pattern of the maternal vessels changes little except for increasing distention during the first three-fifths of pregnancy (6). In the last two-fifths of pregnancy, however, the bed of maternal placenta was

described as "increasing steadily" and being "most spectacular" (5).

These studies suggest that at a point between two-thirds and three-fifths of the way through pregnancy, there is a definite pattern of vessel development that serves to diminish the resistance to flow. Important and still unclear is the relative contribution of the trophoblast as compared to those changes in resistance produced by the enlargement of the uterus.

DOPPLER AND THE NORMAL UTEROPLACENTAL CIRCULATION

When Doppler instruments are used to evaluate the pelvic vasculature, a variety of patterns can be detected. Pulsed Doppler can be used to identify specific vessels in the nonpregnant state. But as pregnancy advances, the lower segment of the uterus is embraced by a web-like curtain of arteries and veins, particularly after midgestation. The patterns of the waveforms are specific; thus the use of direct imaging offers little advantage.

Accurate measures of blood flow, although the ideal, have been abandoned in clinical studies of human pregnancies due to methodologic problems. Maternal and fetal blood flow velocity indices avoid the major sources of error. These indices are independent of the angle of insonation and do not require a measurement of vessel diameter. There is a close correlation in normal pregnancies between the three indices (S/D, RI, PI) used in most clinical studies. However, in pregnancies with abnormal flow (AEDV), errors increase due to the inability to express mathematically the absence of diastolic flow.

Doppler signals of maternal and fetal waveforms are distinct and can be obtained by either pulsed wave or continuous wave with similar results. No significant differences have been reported when looking at inter- and intraobserver variation. The waveform analysis yields information relating to the condition of the proximal circulation and the impedance of the distal vascular bed.

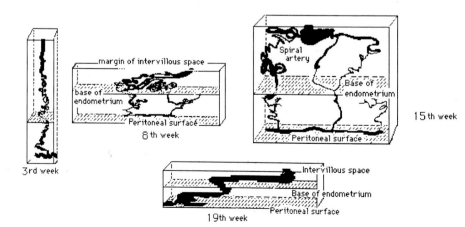

FIG. 2. Evolution of the uteroplacental circulation in the primate. Modified from Ramsey (4).

The evolution of the uterine arteries was studied through the menstrual cycle and pregnancy (2). Pregnancy does not produce significant changes in the main uterine branches until there is a well-developed intervillous circulation. Approximately 4 weeks after implantation, well-defined low-resistance vessels are seen at the site of the future placenta. Decreases in resistance can be seen in feeding radial arteries as the pregnancy progresses (7,8).

Dramatic changes occur in the second trimester. The uterus begins to grow rapidly, uncoiling the main uterine and spiral arteries. The trophoblast invades the myometrial portion of the spiral vessels and dissolves the smooth muscle and collagen in the vessel wall, thereby allowing maximum flow into the intervillous space. The placentation process continues until the 24th–26th week of pregnancy after which there is only a small decrease in values in the main uterine branch, reflecting the sum of all the radial and spiral vessels (8,9).

The uterine artery, a more complex waveform, changes from a high-resistance vessel with one or more diastolic notches to a low-resistance vessel with no dia-

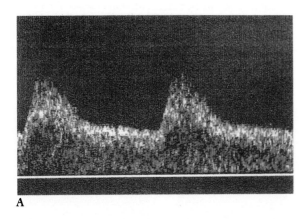

A

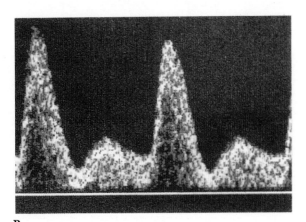

B

FIG. 3. Uterine artery flow velocity waveforms. **A:** Normal pregnancy. **B:** High-impedance pattern with a well-defined diastolic notch and reduced end-diastolic velocity. From Chervenak et al. (41).

stolic notches (Fig. 3). The changes in end-diastolic velocity may be primarily regulated by intervillous space flow. After delivery, the uterine artery returns to its prepregnant level in 4–6 weeks.

The diastolic notch is an important characteristic of vessels having resistance. These notches are seen in peripheral vessels and are a manifestation of forward and reverse waves caused by the reflections at distal branches and blockage points. Disappearance of the notch will happen first in the uterine artery, which is directly under the placenta. If the notch has not been lost by 24–26 weeks, most women will develop a hypertensive complication of pregnancy. During normal labor, when there is a maximum uterine contraction, the end-diastolic part of the waveform disappears but the diastolic notch does not recur (10). These findings suggest that there are two main sites of resistance to velocity flow. Since the intervillous space is obliterated during a uterine contraction, Fleisher and colleagues suggested that this was the site controlling the end-diastolic part of the waveform. The diastolic notch represents the elasticity of the vessel, which is generally lost in the second trimester. Simple changes of pressure do not make it reappear, perhaps because the elastic tissue and smooth muscle have been replaced by fibrin.

ABNORMAL UTEROPLACENTAL CIRCULATION

Robertson and associates developed a hypothesis regarding the normal and abnormal development of the uteroplacental circulation in pregnancy (11). It is their belief that under normal and abnormal circumstances, the trophoblast invades the spiral artery only as far as the decidua in the first trimester and it then advances into the myometrial part of the vessel in the early part of the second trimester. They postulated that a failure of trophoblastic invasion to the myometrial level is associated with maternal hypertension and intrauterine growth retardation (IUGR). Also, they suggested that acute atherosis of the vessels occurs primarily in women with albuminuric pregnancy hypertension. Sheppard and Bonnar disagreed with the conclusions of Robertson and associates by expressing the opinion that the changes between the decidua and myometrial part of the vessels were more random. Also, they argued that the similar changes could be seen in pregnancies with normal outcomes (12). In a later study using placental bed biopsy specimens, both groups collaborated and offered another possibility, that of the approximately 100 spiral arteries, only some were "converted to uteroplacental arteries," whereas in preeclampsia–eclampsia and in IUGR a significant proportion escape or resist involvement with endovascular trophoblast migration (13). Doppler velocimetry data would tend to support this latter hypothesis.

Impaired uterine artery flow velocity can be identified

by a persistent abnormal index, a persistent notch, and a significant difference between the indices in the two vessels (14). Adverse outcomes associated with an abnormal uterine artery flow velocity include preeclampsia, and fetal growth retardation and its sequelae. If the fetus has normal umbilical flow, the growth delay will be mild, and the risk of fetal distress slightly above normal. The most common indication for intervention is maternal, not fetal. The most significant abnormality of the waveform in terms of abnormal outcome is the diastolic notch. Presumably the persistence of the notch is a manifestation of unaltered vascular tone or spasm, and is analogous to the vascular response seen in the angiotensin infusion test. In other words, the normal adaptation of pregnancy has not occurred. Since the majority of abnormal uterine artery waveforms are associated with unilateral implantation of the placenta, it can be hypothesized that normal pregnancy changes require both uterine arteries to be involved in the development of the placenta. It reminds us of the situation in the kidney, where one-sided flow reduction is also associated with hypertension.

CLINICAL UTEROPLACENTAL VELOCIMETRY

There are numerous reports describing the use of uteroplacental flow velocity wave forms in the predic-

tion, diagnosis, and management of hypertensive disorders of pregnancy. Campbell and coworkers can be credited with the first clinical application of Doppler ultrasound to the study of uteroplacental blood flow (15). They used a pulsed Doppler duplex approach, described the waveform from subplacental vessels only, and used a calculation called the "frequency index profile." Measurements were carried out in women in the second and third trimester. They suggested that an abnormal waveform was characterized by a higher systole, a lower end diastole, and the presence of a diastolic notch. When there were abnormal waveforms, there was a higher occurrence of maternal proteinuria, early delivery, and low birthweight.

Trudinger and associates using a continuous wave Doppler system also examined the subplacental vessels (16,17) and described the waveform as the diastolic flow velocity as a percentage of systole. In 9 of 12 women with severe hypertensive disease of pregnancy, there was reduced uterine artery diastolic velocity. In a later study they looked at both the uterine and umbilical circulations, and commented that when there was severe maternal hypertension there were abnormal uterine and umbilical artery waveforms. Noted also was a decrease in the small muscular arteries without a decrease in tertiary stem villi (18).

After defining a normal value for the combined left–right uterine artery waveforms, Fleischer and associates

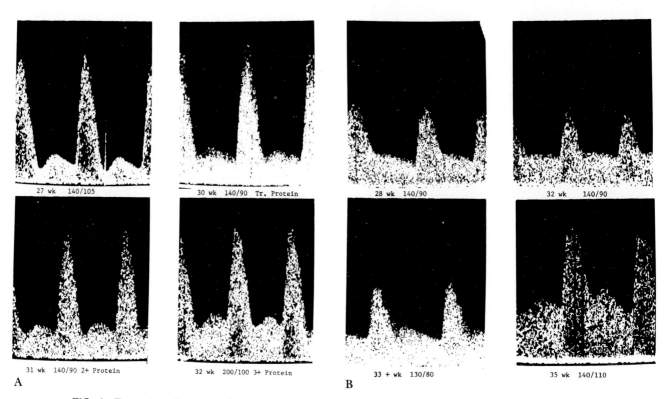

FIG. 4. Examples of the waveform evolution in women with chronic hypertension. **A:** The early pattern of pregnancy persisted and the preeclampsia became obvious at 31 weeks. **B:** In this woman, a mature waveform was achieved, but an acute vasospastic or degenerative process appeared at 33 weeks. From Chervenak et al. (41).

analyzed 71 pregnant women with various diagnosis of hypertension (19). They designated an *S/D* ratio of higher than 2.6 from 26 weeks onward as abnormal. When the ratio exceeded this level, there was usually a notch in the waveform, and the pregnancies were complicated by maternal preeclampsia, stillbirths, premature birth, and IUGR (20). The abnormal waveform preceded the onset of disease, showing that in most circumstances the uterine artery never finished its evolution to a mature placental vessel. However, in an occasional case a normal waveform reverted to an abnormal contour (Fig. 4).

Abnormality of the uterine artery flow velocity waveforms has been reported to precede maternal hypertension, (21,22), but not all authors support the observation that the degree of abnormality is related to the severity of the hypertension. Hanretty et al. using a matched cohort study compared 32 patients with untreated pregnancy-induced hypertension with 32 patients with normal blood pressure and did not demonstrate an association between uteroplacental blood flow velocity and hypertensive disorders (23). Trudinger also reported that many women with severe hypertension had normal uteroplacental artery flow velocity waveforms. Conflicting data may in part be due to results from different techniques, different location in relation to placental vessels, and laterality of the placenta (24).

Schulman et al., in 1987, evaluated the left and right uterine arteries independently (14). An abnormal difference between the two was associated with earlier gestational age at delivery, lower fetal weight, and higher incidence of pregnancy-induced hypertension, proteinuria, and IUGR when compared to normals. This difference was shown to have had an adverse impact on the pregnancy, even when the combined ratio was normal.

Kofinas et al. (25) found that in both normal and hypertensive pregnancies the flow indices of the uterine artery on the same side as the placenta was significantly lower than the contralateral artery *S/D* ratio. A centrally located placenta demonstrated similar indices on both sides. Later the relationship between pregnancy outcome and vascular resistance in both uterine arteries was evaluated (26). In patients with unilateral placentas, the placental uterine artery was found to be a better predictor of poor pregnancy outcome than the nonplacental uterine artery, or the mean of the two arteries.

MATERNAL RENAL CIRCULATION

There has been some speculation that preeclampsia is associated with elevations in maternal renal vascular resistance. In order to determine whether renal artery blood flow indices can accurately identify pregnancies complicated by or destined to develop hypertensive disease, Levine et al. compared the blood flow characteristics in the maternal renal artery as a function of gesta-tional age in normotensive, chronic hypertensive, and preeclamptic women (27). Using a pulsed Doppler scanner, evaluation of the maternal renal artery was performed in normotensive nonpregnant, normotensive pregnant, pregnant chronic hypertensive, and preeclamptic women. Maternal renal artery Doppler waveforms are not significantly altered by either pregnancy or hypertensive complications in pregnancy.

UMBILICAL CIRCULATION

The basic foundation of the placenta is laid down by the twelfth week of gestation. The remainder of gestation is characterized by increased size and proliferation of small muscular arteries resulting in lowered resistance and increased blood flow.

NORMAL UMBILICAL CIRCULATION

The decrease in umbilical placental resistance with advancing gestational age has been attributed to growth of the placenta with the development of new vascular channels. The development of the small arteries and arterioles of the tertiary villi are responsible for the major drop in arterial pressure across the umbilical placental vascular bed. The umbilical vessels are not innervated and are relatively refractory to catecholamines, and dependent on reduced resistance of the placental bed relative to other fetal vascular sites to facilitate normal growth. Umbilical flow velocity indices are lower at the placental than the fetal end of the cord. Indices prior to 20 weeks gestation are of limited value because of low or absent end-diastolic velocity. Although variation has been reported, there is a decrease in mean values of all indices during the latter half of pregnancy (28).

ABNORMAL UMBILICAL CIRCULATION

Abnormal flow may represent failure of angiogenesis resulting in increased resistance. Flow abnormalities can be mild to severe, with either absent diastolic component or reversal of diastolic flow seen in the umbilical circulation. Abnormal umbilical artery flow patterns with reduced diastolic flow is associated with the presence of maternal hypertension and IUGR. This change in flow indicates an increase in the resistance in the umbilical placental vascular bed. Giles and others have looked at the changes in these vessels as they related to umbilical Doppler flow (18). Small arterial vessel number was significantly less in the abnormal umbilical Doppler group as compared to the normal and control group, which did not differ. The umbilical artery Doppler studies identified a lesion of vascular sclerosis in the fetal placenta. Blood flow pattern may indicate placental pathology responsible for the maternal and fetal sequelae of hypertensive disorders of pregnancy.

CLINICAL UMBILICAL VELOCIMETRY AND HYPERTENSION

Severe pregnancy hypertension is associated with elevated umbilical Doppler velocimetry indices. These observations demonstrate the relationship between the placental vascular lesions and maternal disease. In most cases the abnormal umbilical artery waveform precedes the clinical manifestation of maternal disease. But investigators have realized that a comprehensive analysis of pregnancy-associated hypertension requires evaluation of both the uterine and the umbilical circulations (20).

Ducey et al. (20) classified both uterine and umbilical Doppler flow studies with their associated maternal and newborn events (Table 1). These findings have been substantiated by others (29,30). This type of analysis is instructive because it suggests that this hypothetical grouping may have a clinical reality. Most often there is maternal hypertension with normal blood flow velocity (49–78%). Most of these women received a clinical diagnosis of chronic hypertension; 35% were thought to have a more serious disorder, such as pregnancy-induced hypertension or preeclampsia. However, the clinical result is usually a normal delivery and normal newborn. A knowledge of velocimetry in this group of women should therefore encourage the clinician to complete medical management and not interrupt the pregnancy because of a belief that there is maternal or fetal danger. Proteinuria can be seen despite normal velocimetric findings.

The next most common group are those women having abnormal blood flow velocity in the uterine and umbilical arteries (23%). The severity of the clinical outcomes that this group has suggests early onset disease in which there is a failure of maturation of both the umbilical and uterine circulations. As mentioned earlier, this would be early in the second trimester for the uterine arteries. Since the basic skeleton of the umbilical-cotyledonary vascular tree is also established by the early part of the second trimester, the arrest in maturation may also begin there for the fetal side or the placental blood flow.

When either uterine or umbilical velocimetry demonstrates abnormal findings, adverse events are to a certain extent dependent on which side of the placenta is abnormal. Patients with abnormal results on uterine artery velocimetry only comprised the least common group of patients encountered (9%). This is counter to the general belief that the uterine ischemia present in pregnancy-induced hypertension originates on the maternal side. The presence of a normal umbilical circulation offers considerable protection, as the fetus is not severely growth-retarded and there is no increase in fetal distress during labor. Proteinuria is present in 75–80%, and thrombocytopenia seems more common when either

TABLE 1. *Velocimetry and hypertension and pregnancy*

	Normal flow velocity in uterine artery		Abnormal flow velocity in uterine artery	
	NL UMB (66)	ABNL UMB (27)	NL UMB (12)	ABNL UMB (31)
Maternal data				
Age (yr)	29 ± 7	27 ± 6	24 ± 7	27 ± 6
Nulliparas (%)	57	52	80	63
MAP (2nd trimester) (mm Hg)	97 ± 12	95 ± 13	105 ± 21	96 ± 21
Abnormal platelets (%)	0	26[a]	13	0
Uric acid (mg/dl)	5.6 ± 1.1	6.5 ± 2.2	6.0 ± 1.4	6.5 ± 1.5[a]
Proteinuria (%)	24	71[b]	75[b]	86[c]
Uterine artery S/D ratio	2 ± 0.3	2.1 ± 0.3	3.4 ± 9.0[c]	4.1 ± 1.5[c]
Fetal neonatal data				
Birth weight (g)	3261 ± 522	2098 ± 811[c]	2464 ± 722[c]	1627 ± 697[c]
Gestational age (wk)	39 ± 2	35.7 ± 3.2[c]	36.3 ± 3.0[b]	33.3 ± 2.7[c]
Del (<37 wk) (%)	11	61[c]	67[c]	84[c]
SGA (%)	2	29[b]	17	51[c]
C/S fetal distress (%)	8	39[b]	8	62[c]
NICU (%)	12	68[c]	50[a]	89[c]
Umbilical artery S/D ratio	2.4 ± 0.3	4.2 ± 1.1[c]	2.5 ± 0.3	4.6 ± 1.1[c]
Clinical diagnoses (%)				
Chronic hypertension (43)	65[c]	23	5	7
PIH (34)	59[c]	15	6	21
Preeclampsia (51)	20	24	16	41

MAP = mean arterial pressure; NL UMB = normal flow velocity in umbilical artery; ABNL UMB = abnormal flow velocity in umbilical artery; S/D = systolic-diastolic; SGA = small for gestational age; C/S = cesarean section; NICU = neonatal intensive care unit; PIH = pregnancy-induced hypertension.
[a] $p < 0.05$.
[b] $p < 0.01$.
[c] $p < 0.001$.
From Chervenak et al. (41).

circulation is compromised, but rarely with normal flow. The etiology of these vasculopathies may be acute or chronic, i.e., a failure of development, acute vasospasm, or a degenerative process.

The most intriguing group of patients comprised those with abnormal flow in the umbilical artery only. A detailed study by Guzman and associates clarified this entity (31). It was concluded that the majority of pregnant women with vasculopathy have involvement or initiation of the process from the fetal side of the placental circulation. Bracero and colleagues examined the muscular artery–placental pathology issue in relationship to uterine and umbilical velocimetry (32). Recall that Giles and associates showed that when there is abnormal blood flow velocity in the umbilical artery, there are a reduced number of small muscular arteries in the tertiary villi. They also showed that this count was stable throughout the third trimester (18). Bracero *et al.* confirmed these observations. The fact that the number is low from the late part of the second trimester through the third trimester implies developmental failure, not degeneration. When the muscular artery count was compared to normal or abnormal findings on uterine velocimetry, it was reduced in both circumstances. Therefore reduced uterine flow velocimetry may contribute in some way to abnormal umbilical vascular development, but it may also be an independent event.

It became apparent, as more cases accumulated, that most patients with abnormal flow velocity in the uterine artery had significant differences between the left and right vessels. This is caused by unilateral placental implantation in which one uterine artery supplies most of the intervillous circulation. Presumably the other vessel is not invaded by trophoblast or it does not establish effective anastomoses. This may explain why many of these fetuses have normal growth for most of the pregnancy, as the placenta received normal flow from one artery.

DOPPLER AS A SCREENING TEST FOR HYPERTENSION

Uterine artery flow velocity can be applied as a screening tool for women at risk of developing hypertension. Campbell's group examined the potential of using uteroplacental flow velocity waveforms for screening on 127 high-risk women at 16–18 weeks gestation (21). A statistical difference was found for a grouping of adverse perinatal events, but there was a 40% false-positive rate. Arduini et al. evaluated the uteroplacental velocimetry in 64 high-risk patients at 18–20 weeks gestation (33). The 22 patients who subsequently developed hypertension showed a higher resistance index than those in the normotensive group. The sensitivity of this measurement was 64%, specificity was 84%, and positive predictive value was 70%. The authors suggested that this screening test can be useful in identifying those patients who will remain normotensive. The weak predictive value of these studies may be a result of screening too early in gestation and that the adverse outcome parameters were too diffuse. Endpoints for outcome should be limited to pregnancy-induced hypertensive syndromes and growth retardation.

Fleischer, as previously mentioned, had a positive predictive value of 93% when the *S/D* ratio exceeded 2.6 and there was notching in the uterine artery waveform (19).

Screening on 255 women in a general obstetric population found nine positive results. Seven of these were true positive for hypertensive syndromes, but the most significant disease was seen when there was a coexisting abnormal flow velocity in the umbilical artery (34).

In 1991, Harrington reported on two midpregnancy screening studies assessing the use of Doppler velocimetry studies in predicting subsequent development of pregnancy-induced hypertension and IUGR (35). There was a significant association between abnormal flow (RI higher than the 95th percentile) and subsequent development of hypertension and IUGR in 925 patients. There was no significant association with nonproteinuric hypertension. To improve the sensitivity, color flow imaging and use of the diastolic notch as well as elevated RI was introduced. In 2437 patients, studied at 20 weeks gestation, 16% had abnormal waveforms; 5.4% persisting at 24 weeks and 4.6% persisting at 26 weeks gestation. Therefore the high sensitivity (76%) at 20 weeks was maintained at 24 and 26 weeks, while the specificity improved from 86% to 97%. These screening studies may play an important role in targeting populations at risk and requiring treatment or therapeutic intervention.

FLOW FOR THOUGHT

Velocimetry has provided some insight into the pathophysiology of hypertensive disorders of pregnancy. Since vasculopathy appears on both sides of the placenta independently, it suggests that the responsible substance or lack of it may originate in the placenta. Vasculopathy appears because of unilateral placental implantation or arrested development of the umbilical circulation. Although trophoblastic invasion into the myometrial spiral arteries probably plays a role, the data are probably made inconclusive by the dominance of the umbilical circulation in growth retardation and maternal hypertension. Both pregnancy-induced hypertension and preeclampsia can occur without vasculopathy, but this usually happens near term when the vessels are so widely dilated that the pathogenic agent may not effect enough reduction in flow for it to be detected by velocimetry.

An interesting concept is that preeclampsia is associated with a deficient generation of prostacyclin. When seven women were given intravenous infusions of prostacyclin, no changes in flow velocity were noted in maternal and fetal vessels (36). It may be that the prostacyclin deficiency is merely a manifestation of a smaller vascular tree and not a true metabolic derangement.

USE OF ASPIRIN

Prevention of hypertension or at least modification of the disease sequelae is an important clinical goal. This requires the ability to both identify an at-risk group and have safe effective therapy available. As greater understanding of the pathogenesis and pathologic lesions associated with hypertension in pregnancy was gained, interest developed in the prospect of manipulating the prostaglandin/thromboxane system in an effort to alter placental thromboxane production and possibly reverse the associated placental vascular lesions.

The early recognition by Doppler studies of the placental vascular lesions that precede fetal compromise has identified patients at risk of developing severe hypertensive disorders of pregnancies. This has allowed studies of a targeted population suitable for potential treatment and prophylaxis of hypertension and IUGR with aspirin.

Trudinger et al. carried out a randomized, placebo-controlled, double-blind trial to evaluate the fetal benefits of low-dose aspirin (150 mg/day) in patients identified by elevated S/D ratio in the third trimester. Aspirin therapy was associated with a significant increase in birthweight (526 g), head circumference, and placental weight (136 g). Aspirin therapy did not result in a different outcome if the initial S/D ratio was higher than the 99.95th percentile. Trudinger stated that if "treatment is to be adopted clinically . . . early recognition of the abnormality is most important" (37).

McParland et al. screened 1226 nulliparous women in early pregnancy by means of Doppler uteroplacental waveforms and identified 12% as being high risk for pregnancy-induced hypertension. After exclusions, 100 women were randomly allocated to either aspirin (75 mg) or placebo for the remainder of the pregnancy. Although the frequency of pregnancy-induced hypertension (13% vs. 25%) did not achieve significance, there were significant decreases in the frequency of proteinuric hypertension (2% vs. 19%) and hypertension occurring before 37 weeks (0% vs. 17%). Fewer aspirin-treated women had low-birthweight babies, although the difference was not statistically significant. Only one perinatal death occurred in the aspirin group due to a cord accident during labor, whereas the placebo group had three perinatal deaths, all due to severe hypertensive disease (38).

Uzan et al. reported on a randomized, placebo-controlled, double-blind trial of low-dose aspirin, aspirin and dipyridamole, and placebo in preventing fetal growth retardation (39). Three hundred twenty-three women at 15–18 weeks were selected on the basis of previous pregnancy history and begun on therapy for the remainder of the pregnancy. Mean birthweight was significantly higher in the treated groups compared to the placebo group (2751 g vs. 2526 g; $p < 0.02$). The frequency of fetal growth retardation in the placebo group was twice that in the treated group (26% vs. 13%; $p < 0.02$). The frequencies of stillbirth and abruptio placentae were higher in the placebo than in the treated group. No significant differences were found comparing aspirin to aspirin/dipyridamole, and there were no significant maternal or neonatal side effects in the treated patients (39). In 1991, Imperiale et al. performed a meta-analysis of the six published controlled trials to estimate the magnitude of protection of aspirin from pregnancy-induced hypertension and its risks and adverse effects. According to their analysis, low-dose aspirin reduced the risks of pregnancy-induced hypertension and severe low birthweight with no observed risk of maternal or neonatal adverse effects (40).

IUGR is a frequent complication in pregnancies associated with hypertension Doppler velocimetry of the uteroplacental circulation in early pregnancy. To identify these women allows preventive therapy such as low-dose aspirin to be assessed in well-planned studies where study entry is based on a pathophysiologic finding and thereby determine the role of aspirin and other antiprostaglandins in the prevention of hypertension during pregnancy.

CONCLUSION

Hypertension in pregnancy continues to cause significant fetal and maternal morbidity and mortality. The clinical definition and classification of the hypertensive disorders of pregnancy have been cumbersome and most diagnoses have been determined in retrospect offering no value for clinical management. Not all pregnant patients with hypertension develop similar sequelae and this leads to uncertainty concerning the best methods of managing this medical complication of pregnancy. Study of the uteroplacental circulation in patients with hypertension helps discriminate between mild and severe forms of the disease and should form the basis of a classification. Doppler velocimetry, although it has generated considerable controversy, has potential clinical usefulness in obstetric care not only as a screening test but to elucidate the vascular abnormalities in women with hypertensive disease during pregnancy. Many studies have suggested that Doppler velocimetry can play a significant role in defining the pathophysiology of hypertensive disease in pregnancy. Doppler velocimetry can also aid in the classification of the different hypertensive disorders found in pregnancy. Testing may distinguish pregnancies at serious risk that warrant urgent delivery from those not at risk that may be followed with medical management.

REFERENCES

1. Sibai Baha M, Anderson GD. *Normal and problem pregnancies.* New York: Churchill Livingstone; 1991.
2. Schulman H, et al. Development of uterine artery compliance in pregnancy as detected by Doppler ultrasound. *Am J Obstet Gynecol* 1986;155:1031.
3. Brosens IA. Morphological changes in the utero-placental bed in pregnancy hypertension. *Clin Obstet Gynecol* 1977;4:573.
4. Ramsey EM. The story of the spiral arteries. *J Reprod Med* 1981;26:393.
5. Reynolds SRM. *Physiology of the uterus.* 2nd Ed. New York: Hafner; 1965. p. 329.
6. Barcroft J. *Researches on prenatal life.* Oxford: Blackwell Scientific; 1946. Chap. 5.
7. Hustin J, Schaaps JP. Echocardiographic and anatomic studies of the maternotrophoblastic border during the first trimester of pregnancy. *Am J Obstet Gynecol* 1987;157:162.
8. Juaniaux E, et al. Investigation of placental circulations by color Doppler. *Am J Obstet Gynecol* 1991;64:486.
9 Thaler I, et al. Changes in uterine blood flow during human pregnancy. *Am J Obstet Gynecol* 1990;162:121.
10. Fleischer A, et al. Uterine and umbilical velocimetry during normal labor. *Am J Obstet Gynecol* 1987;157:40.
11. Robertson WB, et al. The making of the placental bed. *Eur J Obstet Gynecol Reprod Biol* 1984;18:255.
12. Sheppard BL, Bonnar J. An ultrastructural study of uteroplacental spiral arteries in hypertensive and normotensive pregnancy and fetal growth retardation. *Br J Obstet Gynaecol* 1981;88:695.
13. Robertson WB, et al. The placental bed biopsy: Review from three European centers. *Am J Obstet Gynecol* 1986;155:401.
14. Schulman H, et al. Uterine Doppler velocimetry. The significance of divergent S/D ratios. *Am J Obstet Gynecol* 1987;157:1539.
15. Campbell S, et al. New Doppler technique for assessing uteroplacental blood flow. *Lancet* 1983;1:675.
16. Trudinger BJ, Giles WB, Cook C. Flow velocity waveforms in the maternal uteroplacental and fetal umbilical circulations. *Am J Obstet Gynecol* 1985;152:155.
17. Trudinger BJ, Giles WB, Cook CM. Uteroplacental blood flow velocity-time waveforms in normal and complicated pregnancy. *Br J Obstet Gynaecol* 1985;92:39.
18. Giles WB, Trudinger BJ, Baird PJ. Fetal umbilical artery flow velocity waveforms and placental resistance: Pathologic correlation. *Br J Obstet Gynaecol* 1985;92:39.
19. Fleischer A, et al. Uterine artery Doppler velocimetry in pregnant women with hypertension. *Am J Obstet Gynecol* 1986;154:806.
20. Ducey J, et al. A classification of hypertension in pregnancy based on Doppler velocimetry. *Am J Obstet Gynecol* 1987;157:680.
21. Campbell S, et al. Qualitative assessment of uteroplacental blood flow: Early screening test for high-risk pregnancies. *Obstet Gynecol* 1986;68:649.
22. Steel AA, et al. Maternal blood viscosity and uteroplacental blood flow velocity waveforms in normal and complicated pregnancies. *Br J Obstet Gynaecol* 1988;95:747.
23. Hanretty KP, et al. Doppler uteroplacental waveforms in pregnancy-induced hypertension: A re-appraisal. *Lancet* 1988;1:850.
24. Trudinger BJ, Cook CM. Doppler umbilical and uterine flow waveforms in severe pregnancy hypertension. *Br J Obstet Gynaecol* 1990;97:142.
25. Kofinas AD, et al. The effect of placental location on uterine artery flow velocity waveforms. *Am J Obstet Gynecol* 1988;159:1504.
26. Kofinas A, et al. Interrelationship and clinical significance of increased resistance in the uterine arteries in patients with hypertension or preeclampsia or both. *Am J Obstet Gynecol* 1992;166:601.
27. Levine AB, et al. Maternal renal artery Doppler velocimetry in normotensive pregnancies and pregnancies complicated by hypertensive disorders. *Obstet Gynecol* 1992;79:264.
28. Low JA. The current status of maternal and fetal blood flow velocimetry. *Am J Obstet Gynecol* 1991;164:1049.
29. Schneider EP, et al. Use of Doppler in the management of hypertension during pregnancy. Abstract Soc Perinat Obstet. *Am J Obstet Gynecol* 1992.
30. Kofinas AD, et al. Uterine and umbilical artery flow velocity waveform analysis in pregnancies complicated by chronic hypertension or preeclampsia. *South Med J* 1990;83:150.
31. Guzman E, et al. Maternal hypertension associated with the Doppler pattern of normal and abnormal umbilical artery velocimetry. *J Mat–Fet Invest* 1991;1:19.
32. Bracero L, et al. Doppler velocimetry and placental disease. *Am J Obstet Gynecol* 1989;161:388.
33. Arduini D, et al. Uteroplacental blood flow velocity waveforms as predictors of pregnancy-induced hypertension. *Eur J Obstet Gynecol Reprod Biol* 1987;26:335.
34. Schulman H, et al. Pregnancy surveillance with uterine-umbilical Doppler velocimetry. *Am J Obstet Gynecol* 1989;160:192.
35. Harrington KF, et al. Doppler velocimetry studies of the uterine artery in the early prediction of pre-eclampsia and intra-uterine growth retardation. *Eur J Obstet Gynecol Reprod Biol* 1991;42:S14.
36. Jouppila P, et al. Failure of exogenous prostacyclin to change placental and fetal blood flow in preeclampsia. *Am J Obstet Gynecol* 1985;151:661.
37. Trudinger BJ, et al. Low dose aspirin therapy improves fetal weight in umbilical placental insufficiency. *Am J Obstet Gynecol* 1988;159:681.
38. McParland P, et al. Doppler ultrasound and aspirin in recognition and prevention of pregnancy-induced hypertension. *Lancet* 1990;335:1552.
39. Uzan S, et al. Prevention of fetal growth retardation with low dose aspirin: Findings of the EPREDA trial. *Lancet* 1991;337:1427.
40. Imperiale TF, Stollenwerk Petrulis A. A meta-analysis of low dose aspirin for the prevention of pregnancy-induced hypertensive disease. *JAMA* 1991;226:260.
41. Chervenak et al. *Textbook of ultrasound in obstetrics and gynecology.* Boston: Little, Brown; 1992.

Doppler Ultrasound in Obstetrics and Gynecology,
edited by Joshua A. Copel and Kathryn L. Reed.
Raven Press, Ltd., New York © 1995.

CHAPTER 16

Diabetes Mellitus

Rosemary E. Reiss, Mark B. Landon, and Steven G. Gabbe

Antepartum surveillance and interventions in pregnancies complicated by maternal diabetes mellitus have intensified over the past decades, resulting in improved perinatal outcome. In the United States, the standard of care for pregnant insulin-requiring diabetic women includes meticulous blood glucose monitoring, twice weekly nonstress testing (NST), frequent ultrasounds, and sometimes early delivery. In patients compliant with this stringent regimen perinatal mortality rates have declined, with much of the remaining excess mortality due to congenital malformations. However, stillbirth rates remain high in less carefully followed patients. A population-based study found the fetal death rate ninefold higher in diabetic pregnancies than in nondiabetic controls (1).

Intrauterine death late in pregnancy has contributed to a significant portion of perinatal mortality in pregnancies complicated by diabetes mellitus. Fetal demise has been observed to occur unexpectedly within a week of a normal NST more often in diabetic women than in other high-risk pregnancies (2,3). In diabetic gravidas, uteroplacental insufficiency may be difficult to detect by ultrasound assessment of fetal growth since fetal weight gain can be excessive due to abnormal fuel metabolism even when uteroplacental circulation is compromised. Finally, the incidence of preeclampsia, a major contributor to fetal and maternal mortality, is high in diabetes, and its diagnosis may be obscured by diabetic vasculopathy or nephropathy. These problems prompt interest in seeking alternate modalities to assess fetal well-being. Since Doppler ultrasound is specifically directed at assessment of the uteroplacental circulation, it has potential to improve our evaluation of these pregnancies. This chapter will examine the available data regarding the performance of Doppler ultrasound in this context and suggest areas where more investigation is warranted.

PATHOPHYSIOLOGY OF INTRAUTERINE DEATH IN DIABETES MELLITUS

Although the exact mechanisms of intrauterine death among infants of diabetic mothers are still uncertain, we know that maternal diabetes predisposes the fetus to hypoxia and acidosis in several ways. Maternal arterial oxygen saturation and tension are lower than in pregnant controls, perhaps due to abnormal interaction between glycosylated hemoglobin and 2,3-diphosphoglyceric acid (4). Reduced uterine blood flow is believed to be a cause of fetal growth retardation in patients with diabetic vasculopathy. Even in the absence of vasculopathy, Nylund et al., using a radioactive tracer technique, found reduced uterine blood flow and suggested a correlation with hyperglycemia (5). Placental abnormalities may also impair oxygen diffusion.

Metabolic derangements caused by abnormal carbohydrate metabolism also increase fetal vulnerability to hypoxia. Unexpected fetal deaths rarely occur when maternal glucose levels have been kept in tight control. Poor control of maternal blood glucose leads to hyperglycemia and hyperinsulinemia in the fetus. Fetal pancreatic islet cell hyperplasia, which develops in the first half of pregnancy in response to maternal hyperglycemia, renders the fetus prone to hyperinsulinemia even if good maternal glucose regulation is achieved later. In a study of fetal lambs, insulin infusion led to an increase in oxygen consumption and a decrease in arterial oxygen content (6). Animal models have also shown that hyperglycemia results in increased fetal glycolysis and accumulation of lactate (7–9). When accompanied by minimal degrees of hypoxemia, this combination can result in fetal death (10). β-Hydroxybutyrate infusion into the uterine arteries can produce fetal hypoxia and lactic acidosis in sheep (11).

R. E. Reiss, M. B. Landon, and S. G. Gabbe: Department of Obstetrics and Gynecology, Ohio State University, Columbus, OH 43210-1228.

In human diabetic pregnancies, fetal blood sampling by cordocentesis has suggested that acidemia is often present and is only sometimes accompanied by hypoxia (12,13). In a study of diabetic pregnancies complicated by nephropathy, Salvesen et al. found low pH and pO_2 in umbilical venous blood samples obtained at cordocentesis in all six fetuses examined (14). Evidence for chronic hypoxia of the fetus of a diabetic mother is also provided by Naeye's finding of increased extramedullary hematopoiesis on autopsy of stillborn infants of diabetic mothers (15). Polycythemia and increased erythropoietin are common in diabetic progeny both in cordocentesis samples (13) and in the immediate neonatal period (16). Salvesen et al. suggested that the increased platelet aggregation and the hyperviscosity caused by polycythemia seen in these infants may account for their predilection to intravascular thrombosis (13). Thrombotic events may also occur *in utero* and may be another reason for the excess perinatal mortality observed among infants of diabetics (17,18).

WHY DOPPLER MIGHT BE A GOOD TOOL

In nondiabetic pregnancies, not surprisingly, ultrasound biometry has proved more sensitive and more accurate than Doppler ultrasound in the detection of small-for-gestational-age (SGA) infants since biometry directly examines fetal size. However, Doppler aids in discriminating the small infants who are constitutionally small but well from those suffering from *in utero* nutritional deprivation (19). In addition, some fetuses with weights above the 10th percentile for gestational age are hypoxic and may have uteroplacental dysfunction (20). It is reasonable to suppose that fetuses of diabetic mothers may often fall into this category. As discussed above, hyperglycemia and hyperinsulinemia can paradoxically lead to both hypoxia and macrosomia in these fetuses. Ultrasound biometry could thus document apparently "normal" fetal weight in a poorly controlled diabetic pregnancy where fetal islet cell hyperplasia and vascular insufficiency coexist. Such macrosomic fetuses are especially prone to acidosis. Normal nonstress testing of such a fetus does not ensure continuing fetal well-being if the metabolic condition of the mother is unstable. The question is whether Doppler techniques, which assess placental or uterine vascular resistance or redistribution of blood flow, will identify these fetuses when other modalities fail.

Vascular resistance can be affected by either physiologic or structural changes in vessels. In the nondiabetic pregnancy, elevated umbilical artery (UA) resistance indices have been shown to identify a specific structural placental lesion: a paucity of small muscular arteries in tertiary villi (21,22). Most investigators believe that this finding represents gradual obliteration of these small vessels. Small fetuses with abnormal umbilical artery velocimetry show this deficiency, while small fetuses with normal UA indices have muscular artery counts similar to their normally grown counterparts. Fetuses with increased umbilical artery resistance have lower arterial pO_2 and higher lactate levels than fetuses with normal velocimetry (23), and are more likely to be stillborn or exhibit fetal distress in labor (24). In the uterine circulation, elevated Doppler resistance indices reflect abnormal trophoblastic invasion of spiral arteries and a predilection to preeclampsia and growth retardation (25).

In addition to detecting these fixed placental lesions, Doppler might be expected to detect more transient changes in resistance in the uterine or umbilical circulations. Transient decreases in uterine blood flow, e.g., with uterine contractions, do alter both uterine and umbilical artery waveforms. Though mild hypoxemia does not have a significant effect, tissue hypoxia severe enough to produce metabolic acidosis increases placental resistance (26). However, the induction of hypoxia and acidosis over periods of approximately 120 min in fetal sheep did not significantly increase the systolic/diastolic ratio (S/D) in the umbilical artery until fetal pH was <6.8 and myocardial contractility was impaired (27). These investigators did not simultaneously examine waveforms in other fetal vessels to determine whether Doppler might be able to detect redistribution of blood flow induced by the hypoxia and acidosis.

PLACENTAL CHANGES IN DIABETIC PREGNANCY

Placental anatomy and histology is very variable in diabetes mellitus and is not closely correlated to severity of disease (28,29) or tightness of control (30–32). Unlike maternal vessels exposed to many years of altered glucose metabolism, placental vessels do not show the changes characteristic of diabetic angiopathy (28). There are no placental lesions pathognomonic for diabetes. Nor is there unanimity among investigators regarding interpretation of the findings.

Placentas of diabetic gravidas are usually large with an increased ratio of placental weight to fetal weight (6), except in settings of maternal vascular disease when the placental size may be decreased (33). The large placenta of the diabetic has increased surface area for nutrient exchange (32). However, combinations of villous immaturity, with increased distance between fetal capillaries and the intervillous space, premature senescence due to hypoxic damage and repair, and abnormalities of levels and function of enzymes of carbohydrate and lipid metabolism, may impair placental transfer functions (31,33,34). The most commonly described finding in placentas from diabetic pregnancies is villous immaturity. Though abnormal maturation is seen focally in many placentas from diabetic pregnancies without adverse sequelae, extensive areas of immature villi may predispose to uteroplacental insufficiency as manifested by late decelerations and stillbirth (31). Salafia has suggested that the large inefficient placenta of the diabetic is a liability because it competes with the fetus for fuel (34).

Placental vascularity is variable (28,35). Bjork and Persson used angiography to show abnormal distribution and caliber of placental stem arteries in diabetes (30). This may be a reflection of villous immaturity (36) or of the obliterative-end arteritis to which the diabetic is also prone (28). These abnormalities might lead to alterations in blood flow detectable with Doppler. Stoz et al. (32) found the number of vessels in terminal villi in the placentas of diabetics to be significantly reduced, a finding that has been correlated with elevated umbilical artery S/D in IUGR (21,22). Other abnormalities in diabetic placentas that might be reflected in altered resistance to umbilical artery flow include increased capillary tortuosity (33), and increased frequency of infarction and intervillous thrombosis. Infarction is more commonly observed in the presence of maternal diabetic vasculopathy. There is controversy as to whether the intervillous space is increased or decreased in diabetes (28,30).

Just as little consensus exists regarding the effects of diabetes on uterine vascular histology. Some studies have found abnormalities in the spiral arteries (33,35,37), while others have not (38). Looking at the placental bed histologically and with immunofluorescence, Kitzmiller et al. found fibrinoid necrosis and atherosis in decidual arteries in a third of the 30 normotensive diabetic patients they examined, changes originally described as pathognomonic for preeclampsia (37). One would expect placental bed abnormalities to be common in light of the finding of Nylund et al. that there is reduced uteroplacental blood flow in patients of all White diabetic classes (5).

DOPPLER FINDINGS

Umbilical and Uterine Artery Waveforms in Uncomplicated Diabetic Pregnancies

Several large studies have now confirmed that ranges for UA waveform indices are no different in a diabetic population without pregnancy complications than in normal controls (39–42). Umbilical artery resistance indices show a normal decline with advancing gestational age. No association has been found between duration of diabetes and Doppler indices (43).

Only a few investigators have examined uterine artery waveforms in diabetic pregnancies (14,44–46). The limited data available suggest that it is appropriate to use uterine artery reference ranges derived from the nondia-

betic population. Johnstone and Steel studied pregnancies in 113 insulin-dependent diabetics without hypertension and compared them to nondiabetic controls (45). Averaging measurements from right and left uterine arteries, they found the third-trimester mean value for the uterine artery resistance index (RI) to be 0.4 ± 0.06 for both groups.

Doppler and Glycemic Control

In the earliest study examining Doppler velocimetry in diabetic pregnancies, Bracero et al. suggested that there was a correlation between UA S/D and glycemic control (47). Forty-three patients with White's class A–D diabetes were serially examined with continuous wave Doppler from 30 to 40 weeks gestation. Simple regression analysis found a positive correlation between mean third-trimester S/D ratios and serum glucose measurements averaged over the last 2 weeks of pregnancy ($r = 0.52$, $p < 0.001$). Using a cutoff of 3.0 as their upper limit of normal for UA S/D, they found elevated mean UA S/D in 5 of 9 patients with mean glucose measurements above 120 mg/dl. Only 2 of 34 patients with more tightly controlled diabetes had $S/D > 3.0$. However, in this study assessment of glycemic control was based only on small numbers of random blood glucoses.

Other investigators have not confirmed an association between glycemic control and UA resistance. Landon et al. (42), studying 35 insulin-dependent diabetic women, found that mean third-trimester S/D ratios correlated neither with mean third-trimester blood glucose nor with glycosylated hemoglobin at 32–34 weeks gestation in 35 insulin-dependent diabetics. Dicker and colleagues studied 108 pregnancies in insulin-dependent diabetic patients with varying degrees of control (39). Twenty-three patients had a mean third-trimester S/D above 3.0. They found no correlation between mean third-trimester S/D and mean glucose or glycosylated hemoglobin. However, inspection of their scatterplots does show that the highest S/D ratios were found in patients with a hemoglobin $A_{1c} > 7.0$. Since 10 of the 23 patients with elevated S/D also had chronic vascular disease and 10 of the remaining 13 developed preeclampsia, it is probable that the elevated UA resistance in these patients was related to vascular disease and only indirectly to glycemic control.

Kofinas et al. (44) used continuous wave Doppler to examine the umbilical and uterine arteries in 31 gestational and 34 insulin-dependent diabetic patients. Abnormal UA S/D was not found significantly more often in patients with poor control, defined as a hemoglobin $A_{1c} > 8.5\%$. Mean UA S/D ratios were similar in patients with good and poor control. Simple regression analysis found only a weak positive correlation between hemoglobin A_{1c} and UA S/D ($r = 0.30$, $p < 0.02$). UA S/D was more strongly correlated with the presence of proteinuria or hypertension than with hemoglobin A_{1c}. Similarly, these investigators found no correlation between uterine artery S/D and glycemic control, though there was a significant correlation with preeclampsia (uterine artery $S/D = 3.5 \pm 2.2$ in preeclamptic patients, 2.4 ± 1.3 in normals, $p < 0.05$). Johnstone et al., in a study of 128 insulin-dependent diabetic women, showed no correlation between uterine artery RI, measured at 30 weeks and at 36 weeks, and glycosylated hemoglobin measured at 28–34 weeks (41).

In an especially careful study, Zimmerman et al. (43) used serial pulsed Doppler to measure RI in 53 insulin-requiring diabetic pregnancies, White's classes B to FR, from 17 weeks to term. At the time of each Doppler study short-term glycemic control was assessed with a 24-hr blood glucose profile consisting of the mean of six to eight blood glucose measurements. Long-term control was assessed with hemoglobin A_{1c}, with 6.5% as their upper limit of normal. There were no significant differences in RI at any gestational age between patients with 24-hr glucose profiles above and below their cutoff for tight control (6.3 mmol/L). Hemoglobin A_{1c} levels were stratified into three groups: <6.5%, 6.5–8.0%, and >8.0%. Only 11 of 153 hemoglobin A_{1c} measurements were above 8.0%. Though the highest RI values were measured in patients with hemoglobin $A_{1c} > 8.0\%$, there were again no statistically significant differences between the groups at any gestational age.

Though well-designed studies have demonstrated no correlation between long-term glucose regulation and chronic changes in placental resistance, they leave room to question whether acute or extreme changes in blood glucose can affect the placental vasculature in ways that might be detectable by Doppler. In a study of 16 insulin-dependent diabetics without vascular disease, Ishimatsu et al. found two patients with mean daily serum glucose > 300 mg/dl at the time of enrollment (40). Both patients had elevated UA resistance indices when pulsed Doppler studies were performed. A few weeks later when better control was achieved (mean glucose < 200 mg/dl), each patient's RI had declined into the normal range.

This clinical observation is intriguing in view of animal and *in vitro* studies of the effects of glucose on the placental vasculature. In a sheep model Crandell et al. induced maternal and fetal hyperglycemia by glucose infusion (9). When the glucose concentration in the ewe was elevated to two to three times normal range, fetal hypoxemia and mixed metabolic and respiratory acidemia developed, and umbilical blood flow was significantly decreased. To elucidate whether the reduction in blood flow was locally controlled or mediated by vasoactive substances released by the hypoxic fetus, the same investigators examined vascular resistance in isolated human placental cotyledons (48). Cotyledons perfused with 80 mg/dl and then 160 mg/dl glucose solutions

maintained constant placental vascular resistance. However, within 12 min of perfusion with 320 mg/dl glucose, vascular resistance more than doubled. Two cotyledons perfused with mannitol solutions of similar concentrations showed no increase in resistance, excluding the possibility that the changes were simply an osmotic effect. The authors proposed that high glucose levels caused a local decrease in prostacyclin production promoting vasoconstriction. Studies showing decreased prostacyclin production from placentas of women with gestational diabetes (49) and from human trophoblast cultures exposed to elevated glucose levels (50) support this theory.

Thus it is possible that severe hyperglycemia can produce transient, humorally mediated changes in placental blood flow that could be detected by simultaneous Doppler studies, even though average glycemic control does not correlate with UA resistance. Testing this hypothesis would require an animal model. Doppler interrogation of other fetal vessels to determine whether acute hyperglycemia causes flow redistribution would also be of interest.

Doppler as a Tool to Predict Fetal Compromise

Evidence that UA Doppler does not correlate with maternal glycemic control has been presented. Similarly, Doppler has poor ability to predict neonatal complications such as hypoglycemia and macrosomia (39,42,44). How does Doppler perform in diabetic pregnancies in predicting IUGR, fetal distress, or stillbirth, endpoints more directly related to uteroplacental insufficiency?

Doppler findings have been reported in four diabetic pregnancies culminating in fetal death (43,47,51). Two of 43 pregnancies described by Bracero et al. ended as third-trimester stillbirths; both had elevated UA S/D (47). One demise occurred at 40 weeks gestation in a setting of chronic hypertension and poor compliance. The last UA S/D at 37 weeks was 5.1; mean third-trimester S/D was 4.2. Birthweight was 4760 g and multiple congenital anomalies were present. The other fetal death occurred at 35 weeks in a class B diabetic with poor glycemic control. Third-trimester UA S/D was modestly elevated at 3.7. A nonstress test was equivocal a week before fetal death. The stillborn weighed 2250 g. Zimmerman et al. (43) found pathologic umbilical artery waveforms in only 1 of their 53 tightly controlled diabetics. That patient was found to have antiphospholipid antibody syndrome, and the pregnancy ended in fetal death at 22 weeks. However, Tyrrell reported an unexpected fetal demise in a diabetic pregnancy at 35 weeks with normal UA Doppler findings 3 days before (51).

Table 1 displays test properties for UA Doppler in predicting manifestations of uteroplacental insufficiency such as IUGR or fetal distress before labor in those stud-

TABLE 1. *Umbilical artery Doppler prediction of fetal/pregnancy compromise*

Study	n	Outcome variable	PPV[a]	NPV[b]	Sens[c]	Specificity
Bracero (22)	33	IUGR[d] or PET[e]	0.66	0.96	0.66	0.96
Dicker (38)	108	IUGR or PET	0.78	—	—	—
Landon (42)	35	IUGR or PET or AP FD[f]	0.88	1.00	1.00	0.96
Johnstone (41)	128	AP FD	0.33[g]	0.97	0.43	0.96

[a] Positive predictive value.
[b] Negative predictive value.
[c] Sensitivity.
[d] Intrauterine growth retardation.
[e] Preeclampsia.
[f] Antepartum fetal distress.
[g] If preeclampsia included as a predicted outcome, PPV = 0.44.

ies providing data sufficient for their calculation. The small number of patients in each study and the differences in populations and endpoints account for the variation in positive predictive value and sensitivity. Overall the accuracy appears comparable to that observed when umbilical artery Doppler is applied to other high-risk populations (52).

In the largest investigation screening diabetic pregnancies with Doppler velocimetry ($n = 128$), Johnstone et al. compared the accuracy of weekly UA Doppler to biophysical profile (BPP) testing in detection of fetal compromise (41). Nine patients had abnormal UA Doppler, defined as RI > 2 SD above the mean in 50% of that patient's studies, or any RI more than 4 SD above the mean. None of these newborns had birthweight below the 10th percentile. Three of the nine fetuses with abnormal Doppler had abnormal fetal heart rate tracings before labor. One fetus with absent end-diastolic flow for 6 weeks before delivery was delivered at 32 weeks because of maternal preeclampsia and myocardial infarction. Biophysical assessment including NST for this fetus was normal. Another fetus in this group had normal heart rate tracings but fetal distress in labor. Two pregnancies were complicated only by placenta previa and two were without any fetal or maternal complications.

Of seven patients delivered by emergency cesarean section for abnormal BPP, four had normal UA Doppler, including the only two patients in the series whose infants had Apgar scores below 7.0. Umbilical cord pH was obtained only for three newborns. One, with normal Doppler, had a pH of 7.28. The two who had abnormal UA RI had pH values of 7.22 and 7.15, respectively.

Since BPP, antepartum fetal heart rate testing, and Doppler velocimetry all have high false-positive rates, it is difficult to judge their accuracy by internal comparisons. Thus in one of the cases just described, one might claim that the absence of end-diastolic flow on UA Doppler correctly predicted fetal jeopardy before the development of maternal preeclampsia and myocardial infarction, a finding missed by fetal heart rate testing. Alternatively, the same case could be interpreted as a Doppler false positive in view of the normal heart rate tracing and Apgar scores. Similarly, a fetus with normal Doppler delivered at 36 weeks because of fetal tachycardia and poor BPP who had normal Apgar scores and cord pH may represent either an unnecessary intervention or a false-negative Doppler.

The confounding effects of delivery interventions can be avoided somewhat by comparing tests of fetal status with fetal pH assessed antepartum by cordocentesis. In a very interesting but small study, Salvesen et al. used serial color flow Doppler studies to examine both the uteroplacental and fetal circulations in six diabetic patients with preexisting nephropathy (14). Five patients were delivered before 33 weeks because of worsening hypertension. Two patients had abnormal fetal heart rate testing at the time of delivery. Two infants were SGA. Waveform indices from the umbilical and fetal circulations were normal in five of the six cases. The only case of Doppler abnormality was a growth-retarded fetus with abnormal fetal heart rate testing who had elevated umbilical artery pulsatility index (PI) and showed redistribution in the fetal circulation, with increased PI in the descending thoracic aorta and decreased middle cerebral artery PI. Cordocentesis performed on the day of delivery showed all fetuses to have an umbilical venous pH below the 5th percentile (range 7.23–7.37). Umbilical vein pO_2 was also below the 5th percentile in five of six fetuses (15.0–25.3 mm Hg). Hemoglobin and nucleated red blood cell counts were above the 50th percentile in all cases.

These findings document that some diabetic pregnancy fetuses can have apparently normal growth despite mild to moderate hypoxia and acidosis. To explain the absence of Doppler findings characteristic of uteroplacental insufficiency, the authors proposed that the fetal hypoxia and acidemia were metabolic in origin, or that the poor maternal renal function led to increased intervillous edema and impaired placental transport despite Doppler evidence of normal perfusion. The presence of normal Doppler flow despite mild to moderate fetal hypoxia suggests that Doppler will not prove more successful than fetal heart rate testing as a tool for the surveillance of fetal well-being in diabetic pregnancies.

Doppler as a Tool to Predict Pregnancy-Induced Hypertension

The diagnosis of preeclampsia is difficult in diabetics with vasculopathy, since proteinuria usually increases with advancing gestation even in the absence of preeclampsia. In nondiabetic patients with preeclampsia, increased resistance indices have been found in both the umbilical and the uteroplacental circulations (53–56). Abnormalities in the uterine artery waveforms, including persistence of a notch at the end of systole and elevated S/D or RI, have been reported at the end of the second trimester in 24–76% of patients destined to develop overt preeclampsia (57). Chronic hypertensives without superimposed preeclampsia usually have normal uterine artery waveforms. Doppler might therefore prove useful in differentiating diabetic patients with bona fide preeclampsia, for whom delivery might be indicated, from those with chronic hypertension and nephropathy who would benefit from medical management. Unfortunately, the difficulty in making a clear diagnosis of preeclampsia in diabetes also hampers the interpretation of studies looking at Doppler's predictive abilities, especially as some studies present data without distinguishing between patients with preeclampsia and those with nephropathy and chronic hypertension.

Most investigators have found higher mean UA resistance indices among diabetic patients with hypertension and proteinuria (39,42–44) (see Tables 1 and 2). In some cases elevated indices were present in the second trimester before clinical signs of maternal or fetal deterioration (39,42). In Landon's study, 5 of 10 patients with vascular disease (class F/R or chronic hypertension) had elevated UA S/D. The five whose S/D ratios were normal did not have fetal distress in labor and delivered appropriately grown infants. Of the five with abnormal UA resistance, one with a nonreactive NST and oligohydramnios devel-

oped fetal distress in labor and the other four had growth-retarded infants. Three of these patients had elevated S/D in the second trimester, before the onset of growth failure. Among their 25 patients without vascular disease, only 3 had abnormal S/D and 2 of these developed preeclampsia. Thus, in this study the positive predictive value of an elevated UA S/D was 89% using preeclampsia or growth retardation as endpoints.

Less information is available about uterine artery Doppler in predicting hypertensive complications in diabetic pregnancies. Of 33 patients studied by Bracero et al. (22), one had an elevated uterine artery S/D and developed preeclampsia. Kofinas et al. (44) found significant differences between uterine artery S/D in patients with and without preeclampsia (uterine artery S/D = 3.5 ± 2.2 in preeclamptics, 2.4 ± 1.3 in normals, $p < 0.05$). However, the six diabetic patients with nephropathy studied by Salvesen et al. had uterine artery resistance indices in the normal range despite worsening hypertension and proteinuria (14). In one patient who required dialysis for renal failure after delivery, uterine artery resistance rose steeply from 26 to 30 weeks instead of showing the normal decline. The authors concluded that in nephropathic diabetes, proteinuria and hypertension may worsen in pregnancy in the absence of the placental bed lesions characteristic of preeclampsia. However, they did not report histologic findings in these placentas, relying instead on normal uterine artery waveforms in drawing this conclusion.

It appears that in pregnant diabetics, as in nondiabetics, abnormal uterine or umbilical artery flow velocity waveforms may predict or accompany preeclampsia as well as uteroplacental insufficiency. Since patients with chronic hypertension or vasculopathy are more prone to preeclampsia and IUGR it is not surprising that this group had higher mean UA or uterine artery S/D in some studies. Further investigation is needed to deter-

TABLE 2. *Doppler indices in diabetics with hypertensive or vascular disorders*

Study (criteria)	Index	Hypertensives (n)	Normotensives (n)	p
Landon (42) (Cl F/R[a] or HTN[c])	UA S/D[b] 2nd TM[d]	4.34 ± 0.7 (10)	3.72 ± .42 (25)	<0.03
	UA S/D 3rd TM	3.2 ± 0.65 (10)	2.55 ± .32 (25)	<0.03
Dicker (39) (Cl F/R)	UA S/D 2nd TM	4.10 ± 0.70 (22)	3.8 ± .44 (86)	<0.05
	UA S/D 3rd TM	3.32 ± 0.61 (22)	2.58 ± .37 (86)	<0.05
Kofinas (44) (PET[e])	UA S/D	3.1 ± 0.9 (11)	2.4 ± 0.5 (54)	<0.002
	Ut A S/D[f]	3.5 ± 2.2 (11)	2.4 ± 1.3 (54)	<0.05
Zimmerman (43) (proteinuric HTN)	UA RI	0.635 ± 0.01 (7)	0.596 ± .06 (35)	NS

[a] White class F or R.
[b] Umbilical artery S/D ratio.
[c] Hypertension.
[d] Second trimester.
[e] Preeclampsia.
[f] Uterine artery S/D ratio.

mine whether Doppler might be a useful tool to identify patients at increased risk for preeclampsia or to distinguish preeclampsia from worsening diabetic nephropathy. More investigation of uterine artery waveforms in diabetic pregnancies is warranted to evaluate its utility in early prediction or diagnosis of preeclampsia.

CONCLUSION

Though abnormal umbilical artery Doppler can indicate classical uteroplacental insufficiency in diabetic pregnancies, sometimes in advance of antepartum fetal heart rate abnormalities (12,47), it reliably identifies neither fetuses jeopardized by acidemia of metabolic origin nor neonates at increased risk of hypoglycemia. Just as with nonstress testing, normal Doppler umbilical artery waveforms have been reported within a week of fetal demise. Severe hyperglycemia may cause transient vasoconstriction in the placental circulation, but this would be detectable only by Doppler studies performed at the time of hyperglycemia and might be missed with routine Doppler surveillance. Long-term poor glycemic control, while predisposing the fetus to hypoxia or intrauterine death, is not reflected in abnormal waveforms. This observation is not surprising since the placental and decidual abnormalities of diabetes are not consistently related to tightness of glucose regulation, nor are they always the lesions that Doppler has been shown to detect. Though several of the poorly controlled patients in the literature have had abnormal umbilical artery Doppler indices, these patients have often also had preeclampsia or IUGR. The discovery that Doppler flow can be normal in both the uteroplacental and umbilical circulations at the time of documented, albeit mild, fetal acidosis and hypoxemia is a useful contribution to our understanding of fetal demise in diabetic pregnancy, though one that diminishes the clinical promise of Doppler. Uterine artery Doppler does have promise to refine the diagnosis of preeclampsia, especially in the setting of diabetic nephropathy. More investigation of its accuracy is warranted, with Doppler findings compared to clinical presentation and histologic findings in the placental bed.

REFERENCES

1. Connell FA, Vadheim C, Emmanuel I. Diabetes in pregnancy: A population-based study of incidence, referral for care, and perinatal mortality. *Am J Obstet Gynecol* 1985;151:598–603.
2. Lavery JP. Nonstress fetal heart rate testing. *Clin Obstet Gynecol* 1982;25:689–705.
3. Miller JM, Horger EO. Antepartum heart rate testing in diabetic pregnancy. *J Reprod Med* 1985;30:515–518.
4. Madsen H, Ditzel J. Changes in red blood cell oxygen transport in diabetic pregnancy. *Am J Obstet Gynecol* 1982;143:421–424.
5. Nylund L, Lunell NO, Lewander R, Persson B, Sarby B. Uteroplacental blood flow in diabetic pregnancy: measurements with indium 113m and a computer-linked gamma camera. *Am J Obstet Gynecol* 1982;144:298–302.
6. Carson BS, Phillipps AF, Simmons MA, et al. Effect of sustained insulin infusion upon glucose uptake and oxygenation of the bovine fetus. *Pediatr Res.* 1980;14:147–152.
7. Phillips AF, Porte PJ, Stabiusky S, Rosenkrantz TS, Raye JR. Effects of chronic fetal hyperglycemia upon oxygen consumption in the ovine uterus and conceptus. *J Clin Invest* 1984;74:279–286.
8. Robillard JE, Sessions C, Kennedy RL, Smith FG. Metabolic effects of constant hypertonic glucose infusion in well oxygenated fetuses. *Am J Obstet Gynecol* 1978;130:199–203.
9. Crandell SS, Fisher DJ, Morris FH. Effects of ovine maternal hyperglycemia on fetal regional blood flows and metabolism. *Am J Physiol* 1985;249:E454–E460.
10. Shelley JH, Bassett JM, Milner RD. Control of carbohydrate metabolism in the fetus and newborn. *Br Med Bull* 1975;31:37–43.
11. Miodovnik M, Lavin JP, Harrington D, et al. Effect of maternal ketoacidemia on the pregnant ewe and the fetus. *Am J Obstet Gynecol* 1982;144:585–593.
12. Bradley RJ, Nicolaides KH, Brudenell JM, Campbell S. Early diagnosis of chronic fetal hypoxia in diabetic pregnancy. *Br Med J* 1988;296:94–95.
13. Salvesen DR, Brudenell MJ, Nicolaides KH. Fetal polycythemia and thrombocytopenia in pregnancies complicated by maternal diabetes mellitus. *Am J Obstet Gynecol* 1992;166:1287–1292.
14. Salvesen DR, Higueras MT, Brudenell JM, Drury PL, Nicolaides KH. Doppler velocimetry and fetal heart rate studies in nephropathic diabetics. *Am J Obstet Gynecol* 1992;167:1297–1303.
15. Naeye RL. Infants of diabetic mothers: A quantitative morphologic study. *Pediatrics* 1965;35:980–988.
16. Shannon K, Davis J, Kitzmiller JL, Fulcher SA, Koenig HM. Erythropoiesis in infants of diabetic mothers. *Pediatr Res* 1986;20:161–165.
17. Oppenheimer EH, Esterly JR. Thrombosis in the newborn; comparison between diabetic and nondiabetic mothers. *J Pediatr* 1965;67:549–556.
18. Van Allen MI, Jackson JC, Knopp RH, Cone R. In utero thrombosis and neonatal gangrene in an infant of a diabetic mother. *Am J Med Genet* 1989;33:323–327.
19. Burke G, Stuart B, Crowley P, Scanaill SN, Drumm J. Is intrauterine growth retardation with normal umbilical artery blood flow a benign condition? *Br Med J* 300:1044–1045.
20. Trudinger BJ, Giles WB, Cook CM, Bombardieri J, Collins L. Fetal umbilical artery flow velocity waveforms and placental resistance: Clinical significance. *Br J Obstet Gynaecol* 1985;92:23–30.
21. Giles WB, Trudinger BJ, Baird PJ. Fetal umbilical artery flow velocity waveforms and placental resistance: A pathological correlation. *Br J Obstet Gynaecol* 1985;92:31–38.
22. Bracero LA, Beneck D, Kirshenbaum N, Peiffer M, Stalter P, Schulman H. Doppler velocimetry and placental diseases. *Am J Obstet Gynecol* 1989;161:388–393.
23. Marconi AM, Cetin I, Ferrazzi E, Pardi G, Battaglia FC. Lactate metabolism in normal and growth retarded human fetuses. *Pediatr Res* 1990;28:652–656.
24. Pattison R, Dawes G, Jennings J, Redman C. Umbilical artery resistance index as a screening test for fetal well-being: Prospective revealed evaluation. *Obstet Gynecol* 1991;78:353–357.
25. Khong TY, Pearce JMF. Development and investigation of the placenta and its blood supply. In: Lavery JP, ed. *The human placenta*. Rockville, MD: Aspen; 1987:35–46.
26. Dawes GS. The umbilical circulation. *Am J Obstet Gynecol* 1962;84:1634–1648.
27. Morrow RJ, Adamson SL, Bull SB, Ritchie JWK. Hypoxic acidemia, hyperviscosity and maternal hypertension do not affect the umbilical artery velocity waveform in fetal sheep. *Am J Obstet Gynecol* 1990;163:1313–1320.
28. Fox H. The placenta in diabetes mellitus. In: Sutherland HW, Stowers JM, Pearson DWM, eds. *Carbohydrate metabolism in pregnancy and the newborn*. London: Springer-Verlag, 1989:109–117.
29. Stoz F, Schuhmann RA, Haas B. Morphohistometric investigations in placentas of gestational diabetes. *J Perinat Med* 1988;16:205–209.
30. Bjork O, Persson B. Placental changes in relation to the degree of metabolic control in diabetes mellitus. *Placenta* 1982;3:367–378.
31. Laurini RN, Visser GHA, Van Ballegooie E, Schoots CJF. Mor-

phological findings in placentae of insulin-dependent diabetic patients treated with continuous subcutaneous insulin infusion. *Placenta* 1987;8:153–165.

32. Stoz F, Schuhmann RA, Schultz R. Morphohistometric investigations of placentas of diabetic patients in correlation to metabolic adjustment of the disease. *J Perinat Med* 1988;16:211–216.

33. Driscoll SG. The pathology of pregnancy complicated by diabetes mellitus. *Med Clin North Am* 1965;49:1053–1067.

34. Salafia CM. The fetal, placental, and neonatal pathology associated with maternal diabetes mellitus. In: Reece EA, Coustan DR, eds. *Diabetes mellitus in pregnancy: principles and practice.* New York: Churchill Livingstone; 1988:143–181.

35. Labarrere CA, Faulk WP. Diabetic placentae: Studies of the battlefield after the war. *Diabetes/Metab Rev* 1991;7:253–263.

36. Singer DB. The placenta in pregnancies complicated by diabetes. *Persp Pediatr Pathol* 1984;8:199–212.

37. Kitzmiller JL, Watt N, Driscoll SG. Decidual arteriopathy in hypertension and diabetes in pregnancy: immunofluorescent studies. *Am J Obstet Gynecol* 1990;162:110–144.

38. Pinkerton JHM. The placental bed arterioles in diabetes. *Proc R Soc Med* 1963;56:1021–1022.

39. Dicker D, Goldman JA, Yeshaya A, Peleg D. Umbilical artery velocimetry in insulin-dependent diabetes mellitus pregnancies. *J Perinat Med* 1990;18:391–395.

40. Ishimatsu J, Yoshimura O, Manabe A, et al. Umbilical artery blood flow velocity waveforms in pregnancy complicated by diabetes mellitus. *Arch Gynecol Obstet* 1991;248:123–127.

41. Johnstone FD, Steel JM, Haddad NG, Hoskins PR, Greer IA, Chambers S. Doppler umbilical artery flow velocity waveforms in diabetic pregnancy. *Br J Obstet Gynecol* 1992;99:135–140.

42. Landon MB, Gabbe SG, Bruner JP, Ludmir J. Doppler umbilical artery velocimetry in pregnancy complicated by insulin-dependent diabetes mellitus. *Obstet Gynecol* 1989;73:961–965.

43. Zimmerman P, Kujansuu E, Tuimala R. Doppler velocimetry of the umbilical artery in pregnancies complicated by insulin-dependent diabetes mellitus. *Eur J Obstet Gynecol Reprod Biol* 1992;47:85–93.

44. Kofinas A, Penry M, Swain M, et al. Uteroplacental doppler flow velocity waveform analysis correlates poorly with glycemic control in diabetic pregnant women. *Am J Perinatol.* 1991;8:273–277.

45. Johnstone F, Steel JM. Use of doppler ultrasound in the management of diabetic pregnancy. In: Pearce JM, ed. *Doppler ultrasound in perinatal medicine.* Oxford: Oxford University Press; 1992:178–188.

46. Bracero LA, Jovanovic L, Rochelson B, Bauman W, Farmakides G. Significance of umbilical and uterine artery velocimetry in the well-controlled pregnant diabetic. *J Reprod Med* 1989;34:273–276.

47. Bracero LA, Schulman H, Fleischer A, Farmakides G, Rochelson R. Umbilical artery velocimetry in diabetes and pregnancy. *Obstet Gynecol.* 1986;68:654–658.

48. Roth JB, Thorp JA, Palmer SM, Brath PC, Walsh SW, Crandell SS. Response of placental vasculature to high glucose levels in the isolated human placental cotyledon. *Am J Obstet Gynecol.* 1990;163:1828–1830.

49. Walsh SW, Parisi VM. The role of prostanoids and thromboxane in the regulation of placental blood flow. In: Rosenfeld C, ed. *The uterine circulation.* Ithaca, NY: Perinatology Press; 1989:273–298.

50. Rakoczi I, Tihanyi K, Gero G, Czeh I, Rozsa I, Gati I. Release of prostacyclin from trophoblast in tissue culture: The effect of glucose concentration. *Acta Physiol Hung* 1988;71:545–549.

51. Tyrrell SN. Doppler studies in diabetic pregnancy. *Br Med J* 1988;296:428.

52. Ng A, Trudinger B. The application of umbilical artery studies to complicated pregnancies. In: Pearce JM, ed. *Doppler ultrasound in perinatal medicine.* Oxford: Oxford University Press; 1992:142–158.

53. Bewley S, Campbell S, Cooper D. Doppler investigation of uteroplacental blood flow resistance in the second trimester: A screening study for preeclampsia and intrauterine growth retardation. *Br J Obstet Gynaecol* 1991;88:871–879.

54. Ducey J, Schulman H, Farmakides G, et al. A classification of hypertension in pregnancy based on Doppler velocimetry. *Am J Obstet Gynecol.* 1987;157:680–685.

55. Steel SA, Pearce JM, McParland P, Chamberlain GVP. Early Doppler ultrasound screening in prediction of hypertensive disorders of pregnancy. *Lancet 1:* 1990;1548–1551.

56. Trudinger BJ, Cook CM. Doppler umbilical and uterine flow velocity waveforms in severe pregnancy hypertension. *Br J Obstet Gyneacol* 1990;97:142–148.

57. Bewley S, Bower S. The application of continuous wave screening to the uteroplacental circulation. In: Pearce JM, ed. *Doppler ultrasound in perinatal medicine.* Oxford: Oxford University Press; 1992:112–141.

Doppler Ultrasound in Obstetrics and Gynecology,
edited by Joshua A. Copel and Kathryn L. Reed.
Raven Press, Ltd., New York © 1995.

CHAPTER 17

Postterm Pregnancy

Carl Nimrod and Andree Gruslin-Giroux

---

*"To everything there is a season . . . . A time to be
born, and a time to die"*

Ecclesiastes 3:1–2

Considerable variability exists in the length of gestation in mammals. The determinants of the length of gestation in various species are unclear; however, a similar degree of maturation of the fetus is present across species by the time that delivery occurs. In the past it was not possible to identify the precise length of gestation in each pregnancy. However, since the advent of diagnostic ultrasound in pregnancy and *in vitro* fertilization, the opportunity to document accurately gestational age has come about. Early, accurate fetal biometric parameters have provided a precise estimation of the incidence of postterm pregnancies. To this end, the verification of gestational age is therefore critical to the interpretation of the results of any trial addressing the issue of postdates. In those trials in which this is lacking, significant limitations in the interpretation of results will result.

POSTTERM PREGNANCY

The phenomenon of postterm pregnancy is mainly applicable to primiparous pregnancies as an extremely small number of accurately dated multiparous patients maintain a pregnancy beyond 294 days. However, there is an increased risk of reoccurrence of postdatism if a previous pregnancy was prolonged (1). Earlier reports underscored a prevalence as high as 14%, but the accurate establishment of dates now reveals an occurrence that is more in the range of 3.5%.

In 1904, Ballantyne (2) described the features now known to be associated with postdatism. The neonatal characteristics include abundant scalp hair, absent la-

nugo, a relative absence of vernix with desiccation and absence of the normal red coloration of skin, and long fingernails. When the outcomes of these pregnancies were assessed, it became apparent that an increase in fetal loss occurred when gestation had advanced beyond 290 days in pregnancies with no identifiable risk (3). This loss rate is further increased as the length of gestation exceeds this point.

Exposure to increased fetal jeopardy in the intrapartum period and early neonatal life continues to be a concern particularly because of the increased presence of meconium in the amniotic fluid in postterm pregnancies. Despite preventative steps to avoid meconium aspiration syndrome, its increased occurrence in the postterm gestation with the attendant risk of hypoxia does generate some concern.

This background information forms the basis for the management approach commonly utilized in providing care for these patients. A consensus exists governing the decision path of patients with a favorable Bishop score. Induction of labor is effective, is well accepted by patients, and can be accomplished with minimal risk. For the small proportion of patients in which this intervention is not acceptable, awaiting the onset of spontaneous labor is appropriate while diligently maintaining an effective fetal welfare surveillance strategy. For the subgroup of patients in which labor induction is expected to fail this conservative approach is most appealing. This approach acknowledges the position of Gibberd (4) who stated that "we must accept that postmaturity carries an increased risk to the fetus but this is not necessarily a reason for forcing the fetus out of the frying pan of postmaturity into the fire of induction."

The satisfactory assessment of fetal health in the postdate population has been guided by two different schools of thought. Pierce et al. (5) recently brought into focus the issue of whether postmaturity is merely a reflection of intrauterine growth restriction occurring late in pregnancy secondary to uteroplacental insufficiency. Leveno

---

C. Nimrod and A. Gruslin-Giroux: Department of Obstetrics and Gynecology, Division of Perinatology, University of Ottawa, Ottawa General Hospital, Ottawa, Ontario, Canada.

et al. (6) argue that the findings can best be explained by compromised umbilical cord perfusion secondary to oligohydramnios. Arguments in support of the latter theory are plausible in light of the evidence of reduced Wharton's jelly around the cord in these older gestations.

This chapter will examine the application of Doppler technology in the elucidation of the various aspects of this problem to clarify the pathophysiology, management strategies, and relationship between the Doppler information and other parameters of fetal assessment.

EXTRACARDIAC DOPPLER

Several fetal vessels have been studied both by pulsed and continuous wave Doppler.

Descending Thoracic Aorta

Under normal situations, there is a deepening of the incisural notch between the deceleration phase of systole and diastole in late gestation. This is probably due to the diminishing vascular compliance of the proximal aorta.

Griffin et al. (7) in a cross-sectional study of 92 normal singleton pregnancies with verified dates by second-trimester ultrasound demonstrated a fall in the time-averaged maximum and mean velocities in the descending thoracic aorta (Fig. 1) and decreased flow per kilogram of fetal weight toward term.

Rightmire and Campbell (8) studied pulsed Doppler blood flow characteristics three times weekly in 35 pregnancies exceeding 42 weeks gestation and reported similar findings. The velocity in the fetal aorta correlated significantly with pregnancy duration beyond 280 days ($r = -0.41$, $p = 0.015$). Pregnancies with meconium in labor had a significantly lower mean velocity than those without (24.8 ± 1.26 vs. 28.8 ± 1.22 cm/sec, $p = 0.057$). Fetuses in this study with compromised outcomes displayed a trend toward lower mean aortic velocities, the development of which appeared to be a gradual process and was probably related to hypovolemia and hyperviscosity.

Battaglia and associates (9) published the most comprehensive evaluation of this problem to date. In 82 patients at 287 days gestation and beyond, they evaluated fetal health by a series of biochemical and biophysical parameters. Hematocrit was the most relevant biochemical marker and nonstress testing (NST), amniotic fluid assessment, and fetal and maternal vessel Doppler studies were also performed. The 58 normal patients had a time-averaged mean velocity of 28.78 ± 2.66 vs. 23.06 ± 2.01 in the abnormal group of 24 patients ($p < 0.01$). The data showed statistically significant differences in oligohydramnios, meconium-stained amniotic fluid, and the proportion of abnormal nonstress tests and cesarean section for fetal distress. No differences were seen in fetal weights and waveform indices for the fetal aorta or any other fetal (umbilical, middle cerebral, and renal) vessels or the uterine artery. The diagnostic and predictive value of this tool as evaluated by Battaglia is shown in Table 1.

In our own work, we previously demonstrated a similar decline in parameters of mean, peak, and end-diastolic velocities and volume flow at 40 weeks and beyond (10). In addition, in a prospective study of 243 gestations beyond 41 weeks, the subgroup of patients with elevated S/D ratios ($N = 40$) in the descending thoracic aorta had outcomes that were significantly different from those with normal S/D ratios. The frequency of neonatal hyperbilirubinemia requiring phototherapy was 6/40 vs. 12/203 ($p < 0.02$) in the patients with normal aortic S/D (11). This information is supportive of the hypothesis that hypovolemia and hemoconcentration are possible causes for the altered findings in fetal thoracic mean velocity.

Finally, in a cross-sectional study of 20 near-term fetal lambs (12), the observation previously described of decreased mean and peak thoracic velocities was also observed (Fig. 2).

These findings from several different laboratories both with human and animal data all clearly point to a decrease in aortic velocities in the normal postterm fetus.

Fetal Umbilical Artery Studies

The umbilical artery has received more attention than any other fetal vessel.

The consistent theme from this large group of studies is that when outcomes in this population are stratified on the basis of normal and compromised, the umbilical artery Doppler evaluation shows values that are often in the normal range (8,13–18). The indices may be statistically higher in the abnormal group [e.g., in the Rightmire and Campbell study (8) the Pourcelot index was 0.56 ± 0.027 vs. 0.49 ± 0.017, $p < 0.05$, and in Fischer's study (17) the S/D was 2.4 vs. 2.19, $p = 0.03$], but these differences were not clinically significant. However, it was Fischer's contention that the cutoff value for an abnormal S/D ratio in the postdate population be altered to 2.4

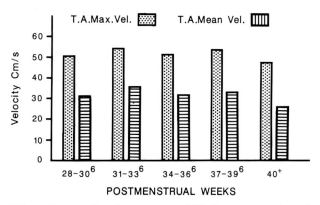

FIG. 1. Descending thoracic aorta (TA) time-averaged maximum and mean velocity as gestation advances.

TABLE 1. *Global evaluation of Doppler velocimetry of the fetal descending thoracic aorta as a diagnostic and predictive tool[a]*

Characteristic	Oligohydramnios	Meconium-stained amniotic fluid	Abnormal nonstress test	Cesarean delivery	Cesarean for fetal distress
Sensitivity	64	92	100	58	80
Specificity	86	97	84	50	78
Positive predictive value	67	92	54	58	33
Negative predictive value	84	97	100	83	96
Concordance	78	95	87	76	78
Prevalence	30	29	16	29	12

[a] Data are presented as percentages. A test is considered positive when the observed velocity is less than 24 cm/sec.
From ref. 9, with permission.

rather than 3.0 based on a receiver operating characteristic curve analysis. This would result in a sensitivity of 57.1% and a specificity of 77.8% for the umbilical artery Doppler identification of pregnancy compromise.

Devoe et al. (19) took a novel approach to the interpretation of umbilical artery Doppler data. They contended that serial evaluations were important and that given the normal trend toward a decrease in *S/D* ratios with advancing gestation a change in the direction of this trend may represent a reason for concern. It is evident from these data that the pattern of compromise in postdate gestation is clearly different from the placental insufficiency pattern seen in association with intrauterine growth restriction.

Overall, umbilical artery velocimetry seems to be of little or no benefit in the assessment of the otherwise uncomplicated postdate gestation.

Cerebral Blood Flow

Satoh et al. (20) established the characteristics of blood flow in the middle cerebral artery in the third trimester. The RI (Fig. 3) and PI both show a consistent and statistically significant decline to 42 weeks gestation. This vessel is the largest of the intracranial vessels and it supplies wide areas of the fetal brain including the parietal, temporal, and frontal lobes.

Few studies are available regarding the impact of mid-

dle cerebral artery velocimetry in the postterm population. In 47 well-dated pregnancies beyond 41 weeks gestation, Shyken and colleagues (21) observed that the Pourcelot index (RI) was statistically different in two groups of patients with normal and abnormal neonatal morbidity outcomes (0.74 ± 0.01 vs. 0.64 ± 0.03, $p < 0.005$). Neonatal morbidity was defined as having two of the following: umbilical artery pH < 7.2, low 1-min or 5-min Apgar score, or neonatal intensive care unit admission.

The changes that occur in the internal carotid artery have been documented by Wladimiroff et al. (22) and Brar et al. (16). The latter demonstrated an abnormally low cerebral *S/D* ratio in compromised postdate patients. Even though the incidence of abnormal umbilical artery blood flow indices in their study was low, the ratio of cerebral/umbilical resistance was significantly lower—1.1 ± 0.3 in the compromised group compared to 1.8 ± 0.3 in the normals $p < 0.05$.

This cerebral-to-placental resistance relationship holds some potential for the assessment of pregnancies with growth restriction. Its role in postdate pregnancies will require validation.

Because the fetal thoracic aorta blood flow pattern is a reflection of the sum of the flow in the lower limbs and carcass of the fetus and the placenta, expressing the middle cerebral artery flow in relation to the descending thoracic aorta was explored in our laboratory. Figure 4 shows a linear relationship in normal gestation in the

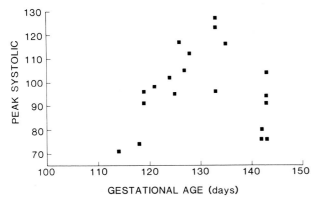

FIG. 2. Peak systolic velocities in the descending thoracic aorta in 20 near-term (143 days) fetal lambs.

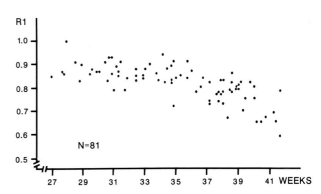

FIG. 3. Resistance index (RI) in the middle cerebral artery as gestation advances.

TABLE 2. *Characteristics of the postterm pregnancies studied according to the response in internal carotid artery to maternal oxygen administration[a]*

Characteristic	Oxygen responders (n = 9)	Oxygen nonresponders (n = 36)	Significance[b]
Meconium staining (no.)	66.6% (6)	25.0% (9)	0.05
Emergency cesarean section for fetal distress (no.)	77.7% (7)	11.1% (4)	0.001
1-min Apgar score < 7 (no.)	55.5% (5)	13.9% (5)	0.05
5-min Apgar score < 7 (no.)	33.4% (3)	2.7% (1)	0.05
Neonatal resuscitation (no.)	44.4% (4)	5.5% (2)	0.02
Newborns admitted to intensive care nursery (no.)	33.3% (3)	0% (0)	0.005

[a] Data are mean ± 1 SD. Ranges are in parentheses.
[b] Fisher's exact probability test.
From ref. 23, with permission.

term to postterm situation in cross-sectional studies. The utility of this in pregnancies at risk will require evaluation.

Further work utilizing the fetal internal carotid artery was advanced by the examination of the role of oxygen therapy in 45 postdate patients by Arduini and colleagues (23). The fetuses of nine patients responded to oxygen therapy by significantly altering their internal carotid PI (mean change 24.3 ± 2%). Table 2 demonstrates the substantially increased fetal morbidity of these when compared to nonresponders.

Maternal oxygen challenge of 60% oxygen appeared to be an effective discriminator of fetuses likely to have an adverse outcome when the fetal vascular response in the internal carotid artery is examined (Table 3).

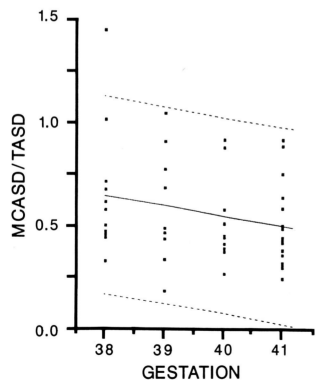

FIG. 4. Relationship between middle cerebral artery (MCASD) and descending thoracic aorta (TASD) *S/D* ratios in late-gestational-age fetuses.

Fetal Renal Artery

The assessment of Doppler flow in fetal renal vasculature and its relationship to amniotic fluid volume was examined by Arduini and Rizzo (24). Even though the fetal renal artery PI decreases up to 42 weeks gestation, no significant differences were noted in the PI among normal postterm patients with adequate amniotic fluid volume (AFV), and those with reduced AFV or oligohydramnios (Fig. 5).

Fetal Venous Circulation

The venous circulation of term and postterm fetuses were examined to characterize the Doppler pattern that exists in normal gestation. A fourth-degree polynomial fit (Fig. 6) best explained the changes in the hepatic vein waveform. A similar pattern was seen in the ductus venosus. There was no detectable change in the pattern of flow seen in the distal inferior vena cava in the normal postterm fetus.

Maternal Vasculature

The uterine (16) and arcuate (18) arteries have been assessed in separate studies to determine their utility in

TABLE 3. *Efficacy of the fetal response to maternal hyperoxygenation to predict fetal distress requiring emergency cesarean section (CS) and low 5-min Apgar score (<7)*

Characteristic	Emergency CS for fetal distress	5-min Apgar score < 7
Specificity	94.1	85.3
Sensitivity	63.6	75.0
Predictive value positive	77.8	33.3
Predictive value negative	88.9	97.2
Accuracy	86.6	84.4
Prevalence	24.4	8.9

From ref. 23, with permission.

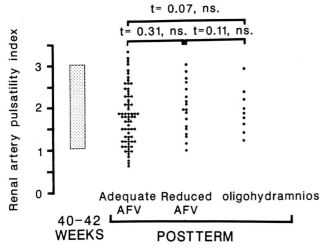

FIG. 5. Relationship between amniotic volume at term and postterm, and fetal renal artery pulsatility index.

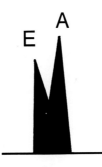

FIG. 7. Typical flow velocity waveform across tricuspid valve in early third-trimester fetus.

postdates gestation. No benefit could be demonstrated in the assessment of fetal well-being.

Intracardiac Flow

The assessment of flow across the tricuspid and mitral valves has been popularized by Reed et al. (25). If the sample volume is placed in the right ventricle just apical to the valve leaflets, a pattern as shown in Fig. 7 is ob-

tained. The passive filling phase *E* is smaller than the active filling phase *A* prior to term. As term is approached this relationship is altered and the *E/A* ratio approaches 1. In early neonatal life, the prenatal relationship of *E/A* is reversed with *E* becoming much greater than *A*.

From this limited number of studies several areas of consensus are now apparent. The vascular changes seen as gestation advances beyond 40 weeks reflect a path that was developing in the near-term gestation, and is dissimilar to that of the growth-restricted fetus. As a result umbilical artery velocimetry alone may not be beneficial. However, if serial studies demonstrate an upward trend in the *S/D* ratio this may be useful in assessing fetal health.

The changes seen in the descending thoracic aorta are consistent with the slow redistribution of blood away from the limbs and fetal gut and to the fetal brain. This suggests a chronic hypoxic situation giving rise to hemoconcentration (higher fetal bilirubin levels) and an increase in end-diastolic flow in all of the cerebral vessels studied. The intracardiac flow studies further document the maturation processes that are occurring in these fetuses.

Doppler velocimetry has been useful to document the normal physiologic changes in the normal term and postterm fetus. Limited information is available regarding the fetus with pathology.

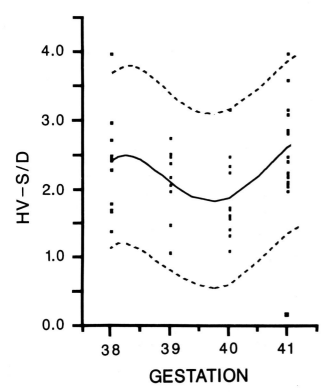

FIG. 6. Fetal hepatic vein Doppler studies in late gestation demonstrating a fourth degree polynomial fit.

REFERENCES

1. Bakketeig LS, Hoffman HJ, Hailey EE. The tendency to repeat gestational age and birth weight in successive births. *Am J Obstet Gynecol* 1979;135:1086–1103.
2. Ballantyne JW. The problems of the postmature infant. *J Obstet Gynecol Br Empire* 1902;2:521–544.
3. Crowley P. Post-term pregnancy: Induction or surveillance? In: Chalmers I, Enkim M, Keirse M, eds. *Effective care in pregnancy and childbirth.* Oxford: Oxford University Press; 1989;1:776–791.
4. Gibberd GF. The choice between death from postmaturity and death from induction of labor. *Lancet* 1958;1:64–66.
5. Pierce JM, McParland PJ. A comparison of Doppler flow velocity waveforms, amniotic fluid columns and the non stress test as a means of monitoring post dates pregnancies. *Obstet Gynecol* 1991;77:204–207.
6. Leveno K, Quick JG, Cunningham G. Prolonged pregnancy. *Am J Obstet Gynecol* 1984;150:465–473.
7. Griffin D, Cohen-Overbeek T, Campbell S. Fetal and uteroplacental blood flow. *Clin Obstet Gynecol* 1983;10:565–602.

8. Rightmire D, Campbell S. Fetal and maternal Doppler blood flow parameters in post-term pregnancies. *Obstet Gynecol* 1987;69:891.

9. Battaglia C, Larocca E, Lanzani A, et al. Doppler velocimetry in prolonged pregnancy. *Obstet Gynecol* 1991;77:213–216.

10. Cameron A, Nicholson S, Nimrod C, et al. Duplex ultrasonography of the fetal aorta, umbilical artery and placental arcuate artery throughout normal human pregnancy. *J Can Assoc Radiol* 1989;40:145–149.

11. Nimrod C, Yee J, Hopkins C, et al. The utility of pulsed Doppler studies in the evaluation of post-date pregnancies. *J Mat-Fet Invest* 1991;1:127.

12. Cameron A. The influence of heart rate and gestational age on Doppler flow parameters in the fetal lamb in clinical and experimental studies of the fetal and uteroplacental circulations using doppler ultrasound. MD thesis, University of Glasgow, 1990:109–114.

13. Stokes H, Roberts R, Newnham J. Doppler flow velocity waveform analysis in postdate pregnancies. *Aust NZ Obstet Gynecol* 1991;31:27–30.

14. Guidetti A, Divon M, Cavalieri RL, et al. Fetal umbilical artery flow velocimetry in postdate pregnancies. *Am J Obstet Gynecol* 1987;157:1521–1523.

15. Farmakides G, Schulman H, Ducey J, et al. Uterine and umbilical artery Doppler velocimetry in post term pregnancy. *J Reprod Med* 1988;33:259–261.

16. Brar H, Horenstein J, Medearis A, et al. Cerebral, umbilical and uterine resistance using Doppler velocimetry in post-term pregnancy. *J Ultrasound Med* 1989;8:187–191.

17. Fischer R, Kuhlman K, Depp R, et al. Doppler evaluation of umbilical and uterine-arcuate arteries in the postdates pregnancy. *Obstet Gynecol* 1991;78:363–368.

18. Forouzan I, Cohen A. Can umbilical and arcuate artery Doppler velocimetry predict fetal distress among prolonged pregnancies? *J Ultrasound Med* 1991;10:15–17.

19. Devoe L, Gardner P, Dear C, et al. The significance of increasing umbilical artery systolic-diastolic ratios in third trimester pregnancy. *Obstet Gynecol* 1992;80:684–687.

20. Satoh S, Koyanagi T, Hara K, et al. Developmental characteristics of blood flow in the middle cerebral artery in the human fetus in utero, assessed using linear array pulsed Doppler method. *Early Hum Dev* 1988;17:195–203.

21. Shyken J, Lieberman S, Kivikoski A, et al. Low middle cerebral artery (MCA) resistance index of Pourcelot (RI) predicts neonatal morbidity in post-term pregnancies. *Am J Obstet Gynecol* 1992;166:334.

22. Wladimiroff JW, Tonge HM, Stewart PA. Doppler ultrasound assessment of cerebral blood flow in the human fetus. *Br J Obstet Gynecol* 1986;93:471–475.

23. Arduini D, Rizzo G, Romanini C, et al. Doppler assessment of fetal blood flow velocity waveforms during acute maternal oxygen administration as a predictor of fetal outcome in post-term pregnancy. *Am J Perinatol* 1990;7:258–262.

24. Arduini D, Rizzo G. Fetal renal artery velocity waveforms and amniotic fluid volume in growth retarded and post-term pregnancies. *Obstet Gynecol* 1991;77:370–373.

25. Reed K, Meijboom EJ, Sahn DJ, et al. Cardiac Doppler flow velocities in human fetuses. *Circulation* 1986;73:41–46.

Doppler Ultrasound in Obstetrics and Gynecology,
edited by Joshua A. Copel and Kathryn L. Reed.
Raven Press, Ltd., New York © 1995.

CHAPTER 18

Intrauterine Growth Retardation

Diagnosis

Raphael N. Pollack and Michael Y. Divon

The association between intrauterine growth retardation (IUGR) and increased perinatal morbidity and mortality has received considerable attention in recent years (1). The accurate and timely identification of the growth-retarded fetus is an important goal that may optimize pregnancy outcome.

There are several methods available to the obstetrician that assist in the identification of the growth-retarded fetus. Historically, these methods have involved measurement of uterine size using the symphyseal fundal height and clinical estimation of fetal weight. These methods may be inaccurate, particularly in the presence of maternal obesity, uterine leiomyomata, and polyhydramnios. The advent of real-time ultrasound has allowed for sonographic estimation of fetal weight using a variety of computer-generated formulas (2–4). In the setting of accurate pregnancy dating, the sonographic estimation of fetal weight may prove to be of great value in the identification of the growth-retarded fetus (5).

Doppler analysis of the uteroplacental and fetal circulations is a technique that may be particularly well suited to the identification of the growth-retarded fetus. IUGR is a condition that may result from a broad variety of pathophysiologic mechanisms. Placental insufficiency is one such condition. Creasy et al. (6) demonstrated that when the placental circulation of fetal lambs was embolized using microspheres, a 30% decrease in birthweight occurred. Microsphere embolization is thought to decrease the placental surface area available for nutrient and gas exchange, and may be associated with an increase in impedance to blood flow. During the progress of a normal pregnancy an increase in placental size and blood flow has been demonstrated. Deficient placental growth and function may clearly result in the development of IUGR. These placental abnormalities may be detected using Doppler velocimetry. This, in fact, is the theoretical basis on which the use of Doppler velocimetry to diagnose IUGR has been proposed. In this chapter the current status of Doppler velocimetry in the diagnosis of IUGR is reviewed.

UMBILICAL ARTERY VELOCIMETRY

Umbilical artery velocimetry has been the subject of extensive investigation over the past decade. The umbilical cord may be easily interrogated using either continuous wave or pulsed wave Doppler velocimetry techniques. The flow velocity waveforms (FVWs) generated are assessed as to the extent of downstream impedance to flow presented by the placenta. The impedance may be characterized by a number of empiric indices including the systolic/diastolic (S/D) ratio, the resistance index (RI), and the pulsatility index (PI). Measurement of these indices is associated with an error of 10–20% (7). Recording of the umbilical arterial FVW is commonly obtained from a free loop of umbilical cord. Although some differences in measurements may be noted depending on whether the fetal, placental, or central areas of the umbilical cord are interrogated, these differences are minor and usually do not have a significant impact on clinical decision making (8). A characteristic umbilical flow velocity waveform has a rapid upstroke during

R. N. Pollack: Department of Obstetrics and Gynecology, The Sir Mortimer B. Davis Jewish General Hospital, McGill University, Montreal, Canada.

M. Y. Divon: Department of Obstetrics and Gynecology, Jack D. Weiler Hospital, Albert Einstein College of Medicine, Montefiore Medical Center, Yeshiva University, Bronx, NY.

systole and gradually declines during diastole, while maintaining continuous forward flow. Since blood flow during diastole is largely passive and relates in large measure to the number of tertiary stem villi available to absorb the circulating volume, a decrease in peripheral impedance results in an increase in end-diastolic flow velocity. Conversely, increased peripheral impedance, as may be seen in cases of placental insufficiency is likely to result in abnormalities such as decreased, absent, or reversed end-diastolic flow. As gestational age advances and placental growth continues, a significant increase in the number of small arterial channels and tertiary stem villi occurs. This results in a placental vascular tree that is expanding with advancing gestational age and whose impedance to flow is decreasing. Since decreasing impedance to flow increases the passive diastolic component of the waveform, we note that end-diastolic velocities characteristically increase with advancing gestational age. Thus, the indices used to describe the FVW, such as S/D, decrease with advancing gestational age (9).

Giles et al. (10) studied the relationship between the placental vasculature and umbilical artery FVWs. Placental vascular resistance was quantitated by counting the number of small muscular arteries in the tertiary stem villi. The number of these vessels was significantly decreased in the placentas of fetuses who had abnormal umbilical artery FVWs (one to two arteries per high-power field) when compared to placentas of fetuses with normal umbilical artery FVWs (seven to eight arteries per high-power field). The authors suggested that abnormal umbilical artery FVWs serve to identify a specific placental microvascular lesion characterized by obliteration of the small muscular arteries in the tertiary stem villi. This placental lesion of vascular sclerosis with partial or complete obliteration of the small muscular arteries of the tertiary stem villi was recently identified by other investigators (11,12) and could theoretically result in increased placental impedance to flow resulting in increased fetal cardiac afterload. Trudinger et al. (13) also reported that microsphere embolization of the umbilical circulation in the fetal lamb is associated with increased impedance to blood flow in the umbilical artery, which may be detected by the presence of abnormally elevated S/D ratios. These data provide the scientific basis that has led to the use of umbilical artery Doppler velocimetry in the detection of IUGR.

A number of investigators have examined the relationship between IUGR and abnormal umbilical artery FVWs (Table 1). Unfortunately, the multiple studies in the literature that address the utility of Doppler velocimetry to detect IUGR are difficult to compare due to different definitions of IUGR, inconsistent protocols for the measurement of umbilical artery velocimetry, different definitions of abnormal Doppler results, and, lastly, varied study populations. The fact that IUGR may have many different etiologies also complicates the comparison of studies attempting to delineate the role of Doppler velocimetry in detecting IUGR.

Fleischer et al. (9) studied a series of 189 high-risk pregnancies with umbilical artery velocimetry and showed that as the S/D ratio increased, the birthweight percentile decreased. The sensitivity and specificity of an S/D ratio of >3 in identifying the IUGR fetus was 78% and 85%, respectively. Based on these data, an S/D ratio of >3 was proposed as being abnormal beyond 30 weeks gestation.

Similarly, Trudinger et al. (14) studied 179 high-risk pregnancies and noted that 64% of IUGR fetuses had an S/D ratio greater than the 95th percentile for gestational age. Trudinger's group recently updated its experience and reported on 2178 high-risk pregnancies in which Doppler studies of the umbilical arteries were performed (22). The incidence of IUGR in this population (defined as a birthweight of less than the 10th percentile) was 27%. Half of all growth-retarded fetuses studied had an S/D ratio greater than the 95th percentile for gestational age. In this group of patients the odds ratio (OR) of a fetus with an elevated S/D ratio having IUGR was 5.9 (95% confidence interval = 4.7–7.3). They also observed that preterm infants with abnormal S/D ratios spent twice as long in the neonatal intensive care unit as preterm infants who had normal S/D ratios.

TABLE 1. *Identifying the IUGR fetus with umbilical artery velocimetry*

Reference	No. of pts	Definition of abnormal waveform	Sensitivity	Specificity	PPV	NPV
Trudinger (14)	172	S/D > 95th% for GA	64	77	55	83
Fleischer (9)	189	S/D > 3.0	78	85	49	95
Marsal (15)	142	PI > 2 SD above mean for GA	57	85	80	64
Arduini (16)	75	PI > 1 SD above mean	61	73	50	81
Al-Ghazali (17)	371	>95th%	72	87	82	79
Berkowitz (18)	168	S/D > 3.0	45	89	58	86
Gaziano (19)	256	S/D > 4.0	79	66	79	96
Divon (20)	127	S/D > 3.0	49	94	81	77
Schulman (21)	255	S/D > 3.0	65	91	43	96

IUGR, intrauterine growth retardation; PPV, positive predictive value; NPV, negative predictive value; GA, gestational age; S/D, systolic/diastolic ratio; PI, pulsatility index.
SD, standard deviation.

The utility of umbilical artery Doppler velocimetry in the screening of "low-risk" populations for IUGR has recently been studied by Beattie and Dornan (23). Two thousand ninety-seven pregnancies of confirmed gestational age were studied at 28, 34, and 38 weeks gestation. The sensitivity of Doppler velocimetry in detecting IUGR ranged from 31% to 40%. Bruinse et al. (24) recently performed a similar screening study on 405 unselected patients. They noted a sensitivity of 17% for an examination performed at 28 weeks gestation and a sensitivity of 22% for an examination performed at 34 weeks gestation.

The combined use of Doppler velocimetry and real-time ultrasound for the diagnosis of IUGR was studied by Divon et al. (20). The study population included 127 patients referred for the clinical suspicion of IUGR. Thirty-five percent of these patients delivered infants who were growth-retarded by birthweight criteria. These authors found that a sonographic estimated fetal weight below the 10th percentile for gestational age had the greatest sensitivity in detecting IUGR. The sensitivity of this measure was 87%. In contrast, an S/D ratio of >3 was associated with a sensitivity of only 49%. The positive predictive value of either of these two tests in predicting IUGR was similar and approximated 80%.

Various authors have explored the use of Doppler velocimetry in predicting the outcome in fetuses identified sonographically as being growth-retarded. Berkowitz et al. (25) noted that 50% of the fetuses identified as being growth-retarded had abnormal umbilical artery velocimetry. These fetuses were found to be at elevated risk for adverse perinatal outcome. Burke et al. (26) recently performed Doppler velocimetry on 179 fetuses identified sonographically as being growth-retarded. Abnormal umbilical artery velocimetry, defined as an S/D ratio above the 95th percentile, was associated with a marked increase in perinatal mortality (54.5/1000) relative to fetuses with a normal umbilical artery FVW, in whom no perinatal mortality was observed. These data suggest that Doppler velocimetry is a useful adjunct in the clinical management of the growth-retarded fetus. Management of such fetuses may be individualized on the basis of umbilical artery FVWs. Fetuses with abnormal FVWs should be subjected to more intensive fetal surveillance. These fetuses are more likely to require early delivery and are at increased risk of cesarean section for fetal distress. In contrast, the IUGR fetus with normal umbilical artery FVWs may be at a decreased risk for adverse perinatal outcome.

A recent report by Trudinger's group addressed the issue of serial assessment of umbilical artery FVWs over time (22). Seven hundred ninety-four patients were subjected to serial evaluations of FVWs. Of the 567 patients with normal FVWs, the incidence of IUGR was 17%. One hundred seventeen patients were noted to have abnormal FVWs on first examination but showed lower $S/$ D ratios on subsequent testing. In this group of patients the incidence of IUGR was 40%. One hundred ten patients were noted to have abnormal umbilical artery FVWs and on serial examination deterioration in FVWs was observed. In this subset of patients, the incidence of IUGR was highest (71%). Patients who showed progressive deterioration over time had the least favorable perinatal outcomes. The perinatal mortality in this group was 63.6/1000, a fivefold increase relative to the fetuses with normal umbilical artery FVWs. Similarly, these infants were more likely to require admission to the neonatal intensive care unit and were more likely to spend a longer time there.

Based on the studies reviewed, an integrated approach to umbilical artery velocimetry for the detection and management of the growth-retarded fetus may be proposed. At this time there appears to be no basis in the literature for universal screening with umbilical artery velocimetry to identify the growth-retarded fetus. Pregnancies at risk for IUGR are best identified by history, by clinical examination of symphyseal-fundal height, and by sonographic estimation of fetal weight. Fetuses identified sonographically as being growth-retarded should be followed with serial estimations of fetal weight and by serial measurements of umbilical artery velocimetry. Normal umbilical artery FVWs should be considered to be reassuring but may still be associated with adverse perinatal outcome. Fetuses with an abnormal umbilical artery FVW may be triaged based on the severity of FVW pattern and the evolution of the FVW pattern over time. Fetuses identified as having absent end-diastolic flow or reverse end-diastolic flow are at highest risk of adverse perinatal outcome. These fetuses should be subjected to a regime of intensive fetal surveillance on a daily basis using nonstress testing or biophysical profile assessment. Fetuses with abnormal umbilical artery FVWs who do not demonstrate an absence of end-diastolic flow or reverse end-diastolic flow should be followed carefully. A deterioration in FVWs over time should be viewed with concern and should prompt intensified fetal surveillance to detect any further deterioration to an absent or reverse end-diastolic flow pattern. A prospective controlled evaluation of the role of umbilical Doppler velocimetry in the management of IUGR has yet to be published.

It should be noted that Doppler velocimetry may be particularly useful in the diagnosis of IUGR in the patient with uncertain dates. Since the diagnosis of IUGR is dependent on gestational age, these patients constitute a diagnostic challenge. Doppler velocimetry provides a useful adjunct to sonographic estimation of fetal weight. Patients who are identified as having abnormal umbilical artery FVWs in the setting of uncertain dates must be considered to be at elevated risk for IUGR. Scorza et al. (27) recently provided nomograms for the interpretation of S/D ratios in pregnancies with uncertain dates.

The sensitivity of this technique approximated that obtained when sonographic estimation of fetal weight was compared with gestational age in accurately dated pregnancies.

FETAL CEREBRAL CIRCULATION

The development of duplex Doppler combining real-time two-dimensional imaging with a steered Doppler-sample volume has allowed the sonographer to direct the Doppler sample volume to specific sites and thereby select with great precision the vessels to be studied. The fetal cerebral circulation is a vascular bed that has attracted the interest of investigators because of its capacity for autoregulation. Campbell and Thomas (28) drew attention to the fact that fetuses that are growth-retarded may be classified broadly as belonging to one of two categories: the symmetrically growth-retarded in whom growth of the abdomen and head are proportionally decreased, or the asymmetrically growth-retarded in whom the growth of the abdomen is decreased while that of the head remains normal. The phenomenon of asymmetric growth retardation, in which the growth of the head continues unimpaired, has been referred to as "head sparing." The physiologic basis for this phenomenon may be related to an ability of the fetal cerebral circulation to assure preferred access to cardiac output. This finding is somewhat analogous to the mammalian "dive reflex" which preferentially redirects cardiac output to the brain during hypoxic stress. Vasodilation of the cerebral vasculature reduces the impedance of the cerebral vascular bed and assures the developing fetal brain a constant supply of oxygen and glucose (Fig. 1).

Flow velocity waveforms obtained from fetal internal carotid arteries have been studied by various investigators. van den Wijngaard et al. (29) recently defined nor-

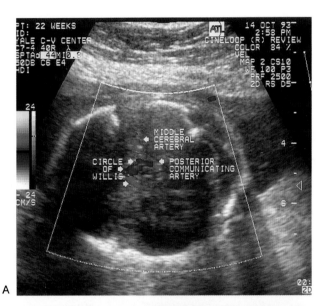

A

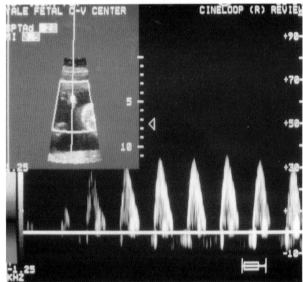

B

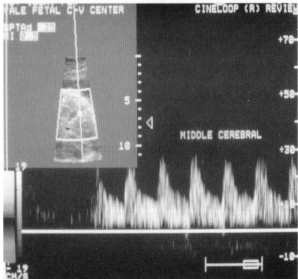

C

FIG. 1. A: Color Doppler image of central cerebral circulations of fetal head taken at 22 weeks gestation in a normal pregnancy. B: Pulsed Doppler waveform from umbilical artery of a severely growth-retarded 29-week fetus. Note absence of end-diastolic flow. C: Pulsed Doppler waveform from the middle cerebral artery of the same 29-week growth-retarded fetus. There is enhanced diastolic flow.

mal flow velocity parameters for a group of normally grown fetuses. Wladimiroff et al. (30) examined internal carotid artery FVWs in 35 growth-retarded fetuses and observed that 54% of these fetuses had abnormally low PIs, indicating that growth retardation may be associated with decreased impedance of the cerebral circulation to flow. These investigators also compared the umbilical artery FVWs with carotid artery FVWs in IUGR fetuses. They noted that abnormalities of the umbilical artery FVW were much more common than abnormalities of the internal carotid artery FVW. Abnormalities of the umbilical artery FVW were also found to correlate better with adverse perinatal outcome than abnormalities of the internal carotid artery flow.

Mari and Deter (31) studied the middle cerebral artery FVWs in 128 normally grown fetuses, and noted that in the normal pregnancy the PI of the middle cerebral artery FVW has a parabolic pattern over time, increasing to a maximum at 25–30 weeks gestation. They suggest that this increase in PI is correlated with the period of increased fetal cerebral cellular multiplication. Thirty-three growth-retarded fetuses were also studied and 27.3% of these fetuses had abnormally low middle cerebral artery PIs. This indicates the presence of decreased impedance of the cerebral circulation to blood flow. The growth-retarded fetuses with abnormalities of middle cerebral arterial FVWs were subsequently found to be at greater risk of adverse perinatal outcome. These authors have concluded that abnormalities of the fetal middle cerebral artery FVWs are useful in the prediction of adverse perinatal outcome, defined as admission to the neonatal intensive care unit for more than 12 hr. The sensitivity and positive predictive value of an abnormal middle cerebral artery PI in predicting adverse outcome were 60% and 67%, respectively. Hadjiev et al. (32) corroborated these findings and noted a decrease in impedance to flow in the middle cerebral artery associated with IUGR. They observed that the sensitivity and positive predictive value of an abnormal middle cerebral artery PI in predicting IUGR were 88% and 91%, respectively. It should be noted that decreased impedance to cerebral flow in the setting of IUGR has not been uniformly reported. Veille et al. (33) studied middle cerebral artery waveforms in 17 IUGR and 25 normally grown fetuses and were unable to demonstrate any difference in S/D ratios.

The increase in cerebral arterial end-diastolic flow that some investigators have observed in the setting of fetal growth retardation has been postulated to result from redistribution of cardiac output. This redistribution is a feature of asymmetric growth retardation and would not be expected to occur in fetuses with symmetric patterns of IUGR. Interestingly, Wladimiroff (34) and Hadjiev et al. (32) both noted that cerebral resistance to flow in fetuses with symmetric patterns of growth retardation was no different than in normally grown fetuses.

FETAL AORTA

Normal blood flow in the fetal descending aorta is highly pulsatile with a minimal end-diastolic component. The fetal descending aorta perfuses the abdominal viscera, the lower limbs, and the placental vascular bed. Redistribution of blood flow associated with fetal growth restriction has been demonstrated in the descending aorta FVWs. Tonge et al. (35) noted that the PI in normally grown fetuses was constant throughout the third trimester. In contrast, 42% of the 12 growth-retarded fetuses studied had decreased descending aorta end-diastolic flow. Similar results have been noted by other investigators (36). Diminished end-diastolic flow has also been shown to be associated with an increase in the incidence of adverse perinatal outcome. Soothill (37) showed that this may be mediated by fetal hypoxia, which is often observed in the fetus with diminished end-diastolic flow. Nicolaides et al. (38) observed that institution of chronic oxygen therapy to the mother resulted in improvements in fetal oxygenation that were associated with improved descending aorta end-diastolic flow patterns. Interestingly, the detection of abnormal descending aorta FVWs was associated with the appearance of abnormal fetal heart rate patterns in 30 growth-retarded fetuses studied by Arabin et al. (39). The FVW abnormalities in these growth-retarded fetuses preceded fetal heart rate tracing abnormalities by an average of 8 days.

A subset of patients at particularly high risk of adverse perinatal outcome has been identified by Joupilla and Kirkinen (40). They observed that 14% of the 608 high-risk pregnancies that they studied demonstrated absent end-diastolic flow in the descending aorta. The perinatal mortality rate in this population was 150/1000 and the cesarean section rate was 72%. The sensitivity and specificity for the detection of IUGR complicated by fetal distress were 85% and 81%, respectively.

FETAL RENAL ARTERY

Redistribution of blood flow in the setting of fetal growth restriction may also be associated with decreased fetal renal blood flow. This may ultimately result in oligohydramnios. Pulsed Doppler velocimetry was used to assess renal blood flow in 22 normally grown and 11 IUGR fetuses by Veille et al. (41). The renal artery PI was significantly elevated in the growth-retarded fetuses, a finding that is consistent with vascular redistribution away from the kidneys. Arduini and Rizzo (42) studied renal artery FVWs and amniotic fluid volume in 114 growth-retarded fetuses. The PI was significantly increased in the IUGR group, a finding that was accentuated when both IUGR and oligohydramnios were observed. Vyas et al. (43) corroborated these findings and demonstrated that abnormal renal artery PI is associated with fetal hypoxemia.

UTEROPLACENTAL CIRCULATION

Pregnancy is associated with a significant increase in uterine blood flow from 50 ml/min at conception to approximately 700 ml/min at term. This increase in blood flow is associated with a decrease in uteroplacental impedance that is brought about by dilation of the spiral arteries. Invasion of these arteries by trophoblast occurs early in the second trimester and is thought to mediate this vasodilation. This marked vasodilation of the spiral arteries allows for the development of a low-impedance vascular bed that is characterized by continuous forward flow throughout the cardiac cycle.

Schulman et al. (44,45) examined the characteristics of the uterine vascular bed with advancing gestation and noted that as gestation advances the end-diastolic component of uterine blood flow increases. These authors suggested that the failure to observe the characteristic third-trimester increase in end-diastolic flow may herald the ultimate appearance of IUGR.

Campbell's group also explored the utility of screening for pregnancy complications using Doppler ultrasound to assess the flow characteristics of the uterine arteries (46). The abnormal outcomes for which they screened included preeclampsia and IUGR. One hundred and twenty-six patients were studied during the second trimester and the sensitivity and specificity of an abnormal uterine artery FVW were 68% and 69%, respectively.

Bewley et al. (47) performed a screening study of 977 patients who had Doppler velocimetry performed on the uteroplacental vasculature during the second trimester. This study measured the average RI at four sites, which included both uterine and arcuate arteries. Thirteen percent of patients studied delivered growth-retarded infants, defined as a birthweight of less than the 10th percentile for gestational age. The sensitivity of an abnormal average RI in diagnosing IUGR was only 15% and the positive predictive value of this test was only 35%. On the other hand, patients having an abnormal average RI had a threefold increase in relative risk of having a growth-retarded infant. Based on these data the authors concluded that the introduction of Doppler velocimetry of the uteroplacental vasculature as a screening test for IUGR is not justified at this time.

Newnham et al. (48) compared the utility of Doppler velocimetry of the uterine artery with ultrasonographic biometry in the detection of IUGR. The sensitivity of uterine artery FVWs in detecting IUGR was 8.6%, whereas the sensitivity of an abdominal circumference of less than the 5th percentile in detecting IUGR was 47.2%. The odds ratio of a fetus with an abnormal uterine artery FVW being growth-retarded was 2.2 (95% confidence interval 0.5–6.1). In marked contrast, the odds ratio of a fetus with an abnormal abdominal circumference being growth-retarded was 13.6 (95% confidence interval 6.2–29.6). These data suggest that the efficacy of uterine artery Doppler velocimetry in the diagnosis of IUGR is very limited when compared to that of sonographic biometry.

Much of these data confirm an association between abnormalities of uteroplacental blood flow and the development of IUGR. This association is, however, weak and does not justify population screening with uteroplacental Doppler velocimetry in an attempt to identify the growth-retarded fetus. The role of uteroplacental Doppler velocimetry has yet to be well defined. Further research may clarify the role of uteroplacental Doppler velocimetry in patients who are at elevated risk of IUGR.

SUMMARY

The development of Doppler velocimetry has afforded the perinatologist a valuable tool by which insights into fetal growth retardation may be obtained in a noninvasive manner. The multiple etiologies that contribute to abnormalities of fetal growth, the varied study populations, as well as the methodologic differences employed by different investigators have led to discrepancies between individual studies. Nonetheless, there remains little doubt that abnormal Doppler velocimetry is significantly associated with IUGR. At this time the role of Doppler velocimetry in the diagnosis of IUGR is not fully defined. As a result, the introduction of Doppler velocimetry of the umbilical artery or uteroplacental vasculature as a screen for IUGR in populations at low risk for this disorder cannot be endorsed. The addition of Doppler velocimetry to the diagnostic armamentarium may, however, contribute to improved perinatal outcome. The optimal choice of the vessels to be studied has yet to be defined. This technique may prove to be particularly useful in defining the sonographically identified IUGR fetuses at highest risk for adverse perinatal outcome. These fetuses may then be subjected to either increased surveillance or early delivery in order to optimize perinatal outcome. In contrast, this technique may also serve to define the fetus that, despite being growth-retarded, is *not* at elevated risk for morbidity or mortality. This should serve to minimize interventions and iatrogenic complications in this group of patients. Further research aimed at delineating strategies for the diagnosis and management of the growth-retarded fetus is urgently needed to guide the intelligent integration of Doppler velocimetry into clinical perinatal practice.

REFERENCES

1. Williams RL, Creasy RK, Cunningham GC, Hawes WE, Norris MA, Tashiro MS. Fetal growth and perinatal viability in California. *Obstet Gynecol* 1982;59:624–632.
2. Warsof SL, Gohari P, Berkowitz RL, et al. The estimation of fetal weight by computer assisted analysis. *Am J Obstet Gynecol* 1977;128:881–892.

3. Shepard MJ, Richard VA, Berkowitz RL, et al. An evaluation of two equations for predicting fetal weight by ultrasound. *Am J Obstet Gynecol* 1982;142:47–54.

4. Hadlock FP, Harriet RB, Carpenter RJ, et al. Sonographic estimation of fetal weight. *Radiology* 1984;150:535–540.

5. Warsof SL, Cooper DJ, Little D, et al. Routine ultrasound screening for the antenatal detection of intrauterine growth retardation. *Obstet Gynecol* 1987;67:33–39.

6. Creasy RK, Barrett CT, de Sweet M. Experimental intrauterine growth retardation in the sheep. *Am J Obstet Gynecol* 1972;112:566–573.

7. Thompson RS, Trudinger BJ, Cook CM. Doppler ultrasound waveform indices. AB ratio, pulsatility index, and Pourcelot ratio. *Br J Obstet Gynecol* 1988;95:581–588.

8. Trudinger BJ. Doppler ultrasonography and fetal wellbeing. In: Reece EA, Hobbins JC, Mahoney M, Petrie RH, eds. *Medicine of the fetus and mother.* Philadelphia: JB Lippincott Co.; 1992.

9. Fleischer A, Schulman H, Farmakides G, Bracero L, Blattner P, Randolph G. Umbilical artery waveforms and intrauterine growth retardation. *Am J Obstet Gynecol* 1985;151:502–505.

10. Giles WB, Trudinger BJ, Baird PJ. Fetal umbilical artery flow velocity waveforms and placental resistance: Pathological correlation. *Br J Obstet Gynecol* 1985;92:31–38.

11. McCowan LM, Mullen MB, Ritchie K, et al. Umbilical artery flow velocity waveforms and the placental vascular bed. *Am J Obstet Gynecol* 1987;157:900–902.

12. Fox RY, Pavlova Z, Benirschke K, et al. The correlation of arterial lesions with umbilical artery Doppler velocimetry in the placentas of small for dates pregnancies. *Obstet Gynecol* 1990;75:578–583.

13. Trudinger BJ, Stevens D, Connelly A, et al. Umbilical artery flow velocity waveforms and placental resistance: The effect of embolization of the umbilical circulation. *Am J Obstet Gynecol* 1987;157:1443–1448.

14. Trudinger BJ, Giles WB, Cook C. Flow velocity waveforms in the maternal uteroplacental and fetal umbilical placental circulations. *Am J Obstet Gynecol* 1985;152:155–163.

15. Marsal K. Ultrasound assessment of the fetal circulation as a diagnostic test: A review. In: Lipshitz J, Maloney J, Nimrod C, Carson G, eds. *Perinatal development of the heart and lung.* Ithaca, NY: Perinatology Press; 1987.

16. Arduini D, Rizzo G, Romanini C, Mancuso S. Fetal blood flow velocity waveforms as a predictor of growth retardation. *Obstet Gynecol* 1987;70:7–10.

17. Al-Ghazali W, Chapman MG, Allan LD. Doppler assessment of the cardiac and uteroplacental circulation in the normal and complicated pregnancies. *Br J Obstet Gynecol* 1988;95:575–580.

18. Berkowitz GS, Chitkara U, Rosenberg J, et al. Sonographic estimation of fetal weight and Doppler analysis of umbilical artery velocimetry in the prediction of intrauterine growth retardation: A prospective study. *Am J Obstet Gynecol* 1988;158:1149–1153.

19. Gaziano E, Knoz GE, Wager GP, Bendel RP, Boyce DJ, Olson J. The predictability of small-for-gestational age infant by real-time ultrasound-derived measurements combined with pulsed Doppler Umbilical artery velocimetry. *Am J Obstet Gynecol* 1988;158:1431–1439.

20. Divon MY, Guidetti DA, Braverman JJ, Oberlander E, Langer O, Merkatz IR. Intrauterine growth retardation: A prospective study of the diagnostic value of real-time sonography combined with umbilical artery flow velocimetry. *Obstet Gynecol* 1988;72:611–614.

21. Schulman H, Winter D, Farmakides G, et al. Pregnancy surveillance with uterine umbilical Doppler velocimetry. *Am J Obstet Gynecol* 1989;160:192–196.

22. Trudinger BJ, Cook CM, Giles WB, et al. Fetal umbilical artery velocity waveforms and subsequent neonatal outcome. *Br J Obstet Gynecol* 1991;98:378–384.

23. Beattie RB, Dornan JC. Antenatal screening for intrauterine growth retardation with umbilical artery Doppler ultrasonography. *Br Med J* 1989;298:631–635.

24. Bruinse HW, Sijmons EA, Reuwer PJHM. Clinical value of screening for fetal growth retardation by Doppler ultrasound. *J Ultrasound Med* 1989;8:207–209.

25. Berkowitz GS, Mehalek KE, Chitkara U, Rosenberg J, Cogswell C, Berkowitz RL. Doppler umbilical velocimetry in the prediction of adverse outcomes in pregnancies at risk for intrauterine growth retardation. *Obstet Gynecol* 1988;71:742–746.

26. Burke G, Stuart B, Crowley P, Scanaill SN, Drumm J. Is intrauterine growth retardation with normal umbilical artery blood flow a benign condition? *Br Med J* 1990;300:1044–1045.

27. Scorza WE, Nardi T, Vintzileos AM, Fleming AM, Rodis JF, Campbell WA. The relationship between umbilical artery Doppler velocimetry and fetal biometry. *Am J Obstet Gynecol* 1991;165:1013–1019.

28. Campbell S, Thoms A. Ultrasound measurement of the fetal head to abdominal circumference ratio in the assessment of growth retardation. *Br J Obstet Gynecol* 1977;84:165–174.

29. van den Wijngaard JAGW, Groenenberg IAL, Wladimiroff JW, Hop WCJ. Cerebral Doppler ultrasound of the human fetus. *Br J Obstet Gynecol* 1989;96:845–849.

30. Wladimiroff JW, Noordam MJ, van den Wijngaard JAGW, Hop JCW. Fetal internal carotid and umbilical blood flow velocity waveforms as a measure of fetal well-being in intrauterine growth retardation. *Pediatr Res* 1988;24:609–612.

31. Mari G, Deter R. Middle cerebral artery flow velocity waveforms in normal and small-for-gestational-age fetuses. *Am J Obstet Gynecol* 1992;166:1262–1270.

32. Hadjiev C, Ishikawa M, Sasaki K, Sengoku K, Shimizu T. Pulsatility indexes of the middle cerebral, umbilical, internal iliac, and femoral arteries as predictors of intrauterine growth retardation. *J Mat–Fet Invest* 1992;1:271.

33. Veille JC, Cohen I. Middle cerebral artery blood flow in normal and growth retarded fetuses. *Am J Obstet Gynecol* 1990;162:391.

34. Wladimiroff JW. Fetal cerebral blood flow. *Clin Obstet Gynecol* 1989;32:710–718.

35. Tonge HM, Wladimiroff JW, Noordam MJ, van Kooten C. Blood flow velocity waveforms in the descending fetal aorta: Comparison between normal and growth retarded pregnancies. *Obstet Gynecol* 1986;67:851–855.

36. Laurin J, Lingman C, Marsal K, Persson P. Fetal blood flow in pregnancies complicated by intrauterine growth retardation. *Obstet Gynecol* 1987;69:895–902.

37. Soothill PW, Bilardo CM, Nicolaides KH, Campbell S. Relation of fetal hypoxia in growth retardation to mean blood velocity in the fetal aorta. *Lancet* 1986;2:1118–1120.

38. Nicolaides KH, Campbell S, Bradley RD, et al. Maternal oxygen therapy for intrauterine growth retardation. *Lancet* 1987;1:942–945.

39. Arabin B, Siebert M, Jimenez E, Saling E. Obstetrical characteristics of a loss of end-diastolic velocities in the fetal aorta and/or umbilical artery using Doppler ultrasound. *Gynecol Obstet Invest* 1988;25:173–180.

40. Joupilla P, Kirkinen P. Non-invasive assessment of fetal aortic blood flow in normal and abnormal pregnancies. *Clin Obstet Gynecol* 1989;32:703–709.

41. Veille JC, Kanaan C. Duplex Doppler ultrasonographic evaluation of the fetal renal artery in normal and abnormal fetuses. *Am J Obstet Gynecol* 1989;161:1502–1507.

42. Arduini D, Rizzo G. Fetal renal artery velocity waveforms and amniotic fluid volume in growth retarded and post term fetuses. *Obstet Gynecol* 1991;77:370–373.

43. Vyas S, Nicolaides KH, Campbell S. Renal artery flow-velocity waveforms in normal and hypoxemic fetuses. *Am J Obstet Gynecol* 1989;161:168–172.

44. Schulman H, Fleischer A, Farmakides G, et al. Development of uterine artery compliance in pregnancy as detected by Doppler ultrasound. *Am J Obstet Gynecol* 1986;155:1031–1036.

45. Schulman H. Doppler ultrasound. In: Eden RD, Boehm RH, eds, *Assessment and care of the fetus.* Norwalk, CT: Appleton and Lange; 1990.

46. Campbell S, Pearce JM, Hackett G, Cohen-Overbeek T, Hernandez C. Qualitative assessment of uteroplacental blood flow: Early screening test for high-risk pregnancies. *Obstet Gynecol* 1986;68:649–653.

47. Bewley S, Cooper D, Campbell S. Doppler investigation of uteroplacental blood flow resistance in the second trimester: A screening study for pre-eclampsia and intrauterine growth retardation. *Br J Obstet Gynecol* 1991;98:871–879.

48. Newnham JP, Patterson LL, James IR, Diepeveen DA, Reid SE. An evaluation of Doppler flow velocity waveform analysis as a screening test in pregnancy. *Am J Obstet Gynecol* 1990;162:403–410.

Doppler Ultrasound in Obstetrics and Gynecology,
edited by Joshua A. Copel and Kathryn L. Reed.
Raven Press, Ltd., New York © 1995.

CHAPTER 19

Intrauterine Growth Retardation

Management

Brian J. Trudinger

The umbilical cord is the lifeline of the fetus, connecting with its placenta for supply of oxygen and nutrients. In it the two umbilical arteries spiral down to the placenta carrying some 40% of the combined ventricular stroke volume. The term *placental insufficiency* has been developed to cover the circumstance when fetal compromise occurs, usually in late pregnancy as a result of inadequate oxygen and nutrient supply. The fetal consequences include death in utero, growth failure, and perinatal asphyxia. Early neonatal complications and long-term developmental deficit may follow as well. Yet the pathologic basis for this situation has not been well defined. The insufficiency implied by this situation could be reduced blood flow through either the maternal uteroplacental or fetal umbilical-placental circulations, or disturbed exchange between the maternal and fetal circulations. Whichever of these vascular inadequacies is primary is debated and may vary from case to case. It is strongly likely that blood flow on the fetal and maternal sides of placental exchange is in balance. Doppler ultrasound provides a means to study blood flow in the umbilical (and uterine) arteries. It was a very logical step to examine the relationships between umbilical blood flow and fetal compromise and to explore the value of such Doppler studies as a clinical test in placental insufficiency.

Although it is possible to measure both volume blood flow in the umbilical vein and the flow velocity waveform (FVW) of the umbilical artery, it is the FVWs that have entered into clinical practice. Well-understood er-

rors in measurement of volume blood flow have limited its clinical utility, although future development may alter this.

UMBILICAL DOPPLER STUDIES AND FETAL IUGR

The Fundamental Observation

The umbilical artery FVW of normal pregnancy has a characteristic "low-resistance" pattern with high forward flow velocities in both systolic and diastolic phases of the cardiac cycle (Fig. 1). Growth of the placenta (and its villus vascular tree) is associated with a decreasing resistance. The umbilical artery FVW reflects this in that the diastolic flow velocities increase relative to the systolic peak with advancing gestation (Fig. 2). In the presence of fetal compromise the umbilical FVWs reveal a pattern of decreased diastolic velocities (Fig. 3) (1). This is quantified by a high index of resistance.

The Meaning of an Abnormal Umbilical Artery Doppler FVW

The Doppler umbilical artery waveform provides a guide to the presence of a placental pathology important in terms of the equation

$$\text{Placental lesion} \rightarrow \text{fetal effect}$$

Such umbilical studies are not a direct fetal test and should not in themselves be used as a measure of fetal condition, but rather an indication of the need for detailed assessment of fetal welfare.

The meaning of an abnormal umbilical FVW has been

B. J. Trudinger: Department of Obstetrics and Gynaecology, The University of Sydney at Westmead Hospital, Westmead NSW 2145, Australia.

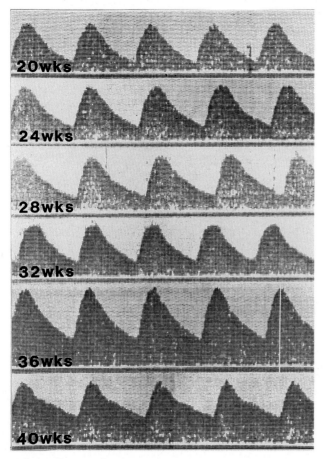

FIG. 1. The umbilical artery flow velocity waveform recorded from one normal fetus at varying gestational ages during pregnancy.

assessed in terms of placental pathology. Experimental and modeling approaches have also been undertaken to understand the change.

PATHOLOGIC CORRELATIONS OF ABNORMAL UMBILICAL ARTERY FVWs

Throughout pregnancy the overall increase in placental size and associated increase in number of villi results in a continuing expansion of the umbilical-placental vascular tree and so a decreasing vascular resistance. Since the major drop in arterial pressure across the umbilical-placental vascular bed occurs in the small arteries and arterioles of the tertiary villi, these are the resistance vessels (2).

Giles et al. (3) carried out a study to correlate the umbilical artery FVW pattern with these "resistance" vessels in the umbilical-placental vascular tree. Differences in these vessels were found in normal and complicated pregnancy. The modal tertiary villus small arterial vessel count was significantly less in the group with the abnormal umbilical artery FVW (1–2 arteries/high-power field) compared with the normal (7–8 arteries/field). This placental lesion of vascular sclerosis with obliteration of the small muscular arteries of the tertiary stem villi could be expected to cause an increase in flow resistance in the umbilical circulation. Obliterative changes in the walls of these vessels have also been described (4). This lesion in the fetal placenta can best be described as umbilical-placental insufficiency. The failure to recognize this lesion in the past may be due to the fact that patients were classified by maternal disease or fetal effect rather than the disturbance in arterial flow pattern produced by the vascular pathology.

EXPERIMENTAL MODELS

Experimental models have been created in which the meaning of the waveform indices can be explained by manipulating a variety of governing parameters influencing blood flow. Physical and animal models have been used.

Animal studies have been carried out in fetal lambs. Vessel obliteration in the fetal placental circulation produced by microsphere embolization resulted in a change in the FVW to a high resistance pattern with low diastolic flow velocities (5). A feature of these studies was the very large number of microspheres that were required to produce this effect suggesting immense placental vascular reserve. Others have repeated this work with larger microspheres and bigger doses (6).

Physical modeling of the placental vasculature using a lumped electrical circuit equivalent with detailed attention to the branching of the umbilical arteries in the villus tree has been reported (7). The great strength of this approach is that the effects of various parameters on the FVWs can be examined individually. Demonstrations that the model predicted realistic volume flow rates for input parameters in the physiologic range established the validity of this approach.

A pulsatile input pressure waveform was applied. The FVW resulting from this was predicted. Placental vascular pathology was created by assuming obliteration of an increasing fraction of the small arterial branches of the model. It was demonstrated that obliteration of an increasing fraction of vessels caused an increase in pulsatility index. For a model with vessel branch numbers similar to a 28-week placenta there was initially little change in the pulsatility index. Above 50% obliteration of the vascular bed the pulsatility index rose above the normal range and thereafter climbed steeply (Fig. 4). Doppler umbilical flow waveforms are regarded as early predictors of vascular disease and potential fetal compromise (relative to other fetal tests). Yet the results of such modeling studies demonstrate that extensive disease must be present even in mild cases because of the large reserve of the placenta. In these modeling studies it was demon-

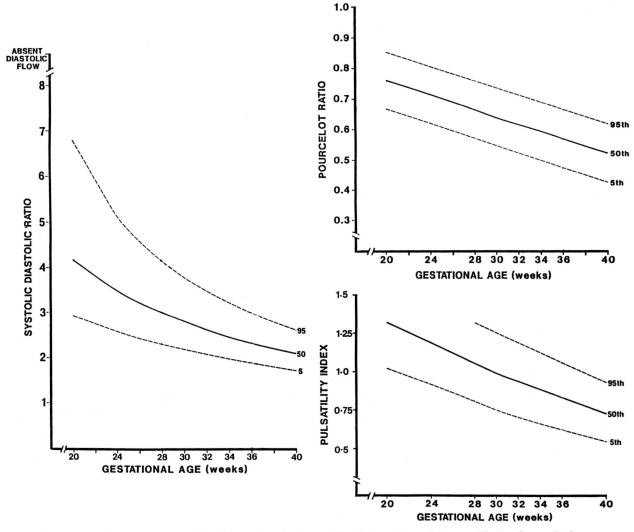

FIG. 2. The normal range for the various indices of ''resistance'' used to quantify the flow velocity waveform pattern of the umbilical artery during pregnancy. Derived from data reported by Thompson et al. (40).

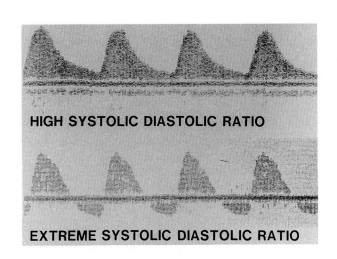

FIG. 3. Examples of two abnormal umbilical artery flow velocity waveforms recorded at 32–34 weeks. In the lower panel the example shows diastolic flow velocities that are reversed in direction.

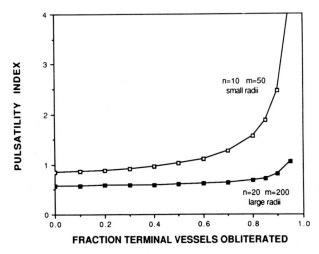

FIG. 4. The increase in pulsatility index of the umbilical artery with progressive vessel obliteration in the placenta. The figures **n** and **m** refer to the number of first-order and second-order branches of the umbilical artery in the villus tree of the placenta and were chosen to correspond approximately to late second- and late third-trimester placentae. From Thompson and Trudinger (7).

strated that increasing the size of the placenta (increasing the number of vascular channels), as might occur with growth and advancing gestational age, altered this relationship. In larger placentas it was necessary to obliterate a greater fraction of vessels before the pulsatility index increased beyond the normal range. The concept of the pulsatility index (or systolic/diastolic ratio, S/D) as a reflection of the number of small arterial channels in the umbilical-placental circulation is based on these studies. If the placenta is growing the number of channels will increase and the pulsatility index decrease. In the presence of an obliterative vascular process the pulsatility index increases.

Another prediction from such modeling relates to the altered capacitance of the umbilical-placental vascular bed in association with arterial vessel obliteration. It is increased, i.e., compliance is reduced. A consequence of this is the transmission of arterial pulses into the venous system so that they appear on the venous flow waveform. This theoretical prediction has been observed clinically (8). The pulsatility of the FVW can be shown to be related to the pulsatility of the input pressure waveform.

PATHOGENESIS OF (DOPPLER) UMBILICAL-PLACENTAL INSUFFICIENCY

Vessel obliteration of the microcirculation is a feature of umbilical placental insufficiency. This is associated with fetal platelet consumption. Platelet counts in fetuses at the time of cesarean delivery were lower in the group in whom the umbilical artery S/D ratio was high (9). This finding was independent of maternal platelet levels and whether or not pregnancy hypertension was present. Further work has demonstrated that the reduced platelet count is indeed due to platelet consumption. Using a glycocalicin measurement of platelet life span (10), it was clearly demonstrated that consumption was present in increased amounts even in fetuses with only mildly elevated S/D ratios. The cause of vessel spasm and obliteration and platelet consumption in the umbilical placental circulation remains speculative. It is attractive to implicate the vasoactive prostanoids. In preeclampsia, the study of thromboxane and prostacyclin generation rates by pieces of placenta demonstrates a shift to thromboxane excess (11). Reduced prostacyclin production by umbilical artery rings has been demonstrated in association with fetal growth retardation (12). *In vivo* studies in fetal lambs have demonstrated that thromboxane promotes vessel constriction and a high S/D ratio in the umbilical artery flow waveform (13), matching *in vitro* observations in perfused placentas (14). It is therefore quite possible that the release of locally acting vasoactive prostanoids occurs in umbilical-placental insufficiency. It remains to be determined as to what triggers this step.

CLINICAL ASSOCIATIONS: FETAL CONDITION AND UMBILICAL ARTERY FVWs

Many publications have looked at the clinical correlates of an abnormal umbilical Doppler study (15–19). Small size at birth is the most consistent finding. The author has reviewed the experience of his unit (20) over a 6-year period. A high S/D ratio was associated with small size at birth and reduced centile birthweight. Morbidity as measured by the requirement for neonatal intensive care, corrected for gestation, was increased. Perinatal mortality was strongly associated with an abnormal result. If instead of a single study the trend of results from serial studies was used, these associations became more clear-cut. At least three study results were required for this. A deteriorating trend was defined as one in which the S/D ratio was moving away from the normal range. In contrast, an improving trend was one in which the direction was toward normal, even if the study results themselves were abnormal. It was the deteriorating trend that was most strongly associated with adverse outcomes such as perinatal mortality and neonatal morbidity (20). These findings are not surprising if one thinks in terms of vessel obliteration. A deteriorating trend implies progressive obliteration whereas an improving trend, even if the results are abnormal, implies vascular expansion and placental growth. Serial studies would then appear to offer more information than a single study and may be used to determine the significance of a single abnormal result. It is the author's practice to carry out studies at weekly intervals in high-risk pregnancies.

Among small fetuses an abnormally high-resistance aortic Doppler study identified those at increased risk of necrotizing enterocolitis (21). It has been suggested that intrauterine growth retardation (IUGR) with normal umbilical studies is a benign condition (22).

Studies of fetal blood gas tensions have been related to the results of the umbilical Doppler FVW (23,24). This has been done in situations of small fetal size where fetal blood sampling was considered ethically indicated. The studies therefore carry a risk of ascertainment bias. Nonetheless it has been shown that the most severe disturbance of the umbilical artery FVW pattern is associated with the lowest fetal blood pH and oxygen tension. To answer the question of fetal condition and mild to moderate abnormality in the umbilical Doppler result, Wilcox and Trudinger (25) adopted a different approach. The red blood cell count and hemoglobin concentration were measured at birth. These were used as indices of erythropoietin production, and so fetal hypoxemia. It was shown that both mild (S/D more than the 95th percentile) and severe (S/D more than the 99.95th percentile) abnormality in the last umbilical FVW study was associated with similar but significantly increased levels relative to the normal study result group. The extent of the placental vascular lesion even when the indices were mildly increased has been commented on above. These results indicate that impaired oxygen transfer to the fetus occurs in this circumstance. This fetal effect precedes growth failure and adverse fetal outcome.

UMBILICAL ARTERY DOPPLER STUDIES AND OTHER FETAL WELFARE TESTS

Tests of fetal welfare exist to identify the potentially compromised fetus, sometimes termed the "at-risk" fetus, and to quantitate fetal condition. The recognition of imminent fetal demise (i.e., the fetus in a terminal state) may be too late to prevent damage or loss of potential. It has been stated above that the umbilical Doppler study recognizes a vascular pathology in the fetal placenta that may lead to a fetal effect. Evaluative studies against other fetal tests support this.

Antenatal nonstressed fetal heart rate (FHR) monitoring is widely used in fetal surveillance protocols for high-risk pregnancy. In the recognition of the small-for-gestational-age (SGA) fetus several comparative studies (26,27) have demonstrated a greater sensitivity (the proportion of abnormal outcomes identified by the test) for umbilical Doppler in comparison to nonstressed FHR monitoring. Since antenatal FHR monitoring is not a test to recognize the SGA fetus, this may not be the correct endpoint to examine. It is important to identify the small fetus before birth, but it is even more important to identify those fetuses at risk of further morbidity. In the author's study (26), the predictive value of an abnormal Doppler was similar to that of an abnormal FHR tracing in relation to such measures of prenatal asphyxia as operative delivery for fetal distress, low 5-min Apgar score, and admission to neonatal level 3 care. However, the Doppler study had a greater sensitivity. A high sensitivity for umbilical artery Doppler in predicting antenatal and intrapartum fetal distress has been noted in prospective evaluation (27). The association of an abnormal nonstressed FHR test with an abnormal Doppler study selects a group with a very high risk of morbidity. These observations suggest that the abnormal FHR monitoring occurs later in fetal compromise than the abnormal umbilical Doppler study. This interval has been variously estimated at 3 weeks (28) and 17 days.

The relationship between umbilical Doppler and ultrasonic estimation of fetal size has been examined. Sonographic biometry was a more sensitive technique for identifying the small fetus than the umbilical artery S/D ratio (29,30). Serial studies in complicated pregnancy suggest the umbilical Doppler study is abnormal at a significantly earlier gestation (31). It has been demonstrated that among a group of fetuses clinically suspected of being SGA, Doppler umbilical studies identified the fetus

at risk for adverse perinatal outcome in comparison to ultrasonic abdominal circumference, which better identified the small size only. A Swedish study of all small fetuses identified from a total obstetric population, screened for ultrasound weight estimation at 32 weeks, reported operative delivery for fetal distress more likely in the group also exhibiting an abnormal Doppler study. Good fetal outcome has been reported in the ultrasonically small fetus with a normal umbilical Doppler study (32). Serial umbilical Doppler studies in such cases should reveal the normal decrease in S/D ratio as the placenta grows.

Since fetal compromise is not confined to the SGA fetus, larger fetuses in which growth has stopped may also be identified by umbilical Doppler FVWs. In this situation the ultrasonic measurements are not small but serial ultrasound measurements may reveal failure of growth. Identification of growth failure requires at least a 2-week interval between studies. Doppler umbilical studies provide earlier identification. The genetically small fetus of low growth potential may not present with any abnormal measure of fetal welfare apart from the small size and reduced ultrasonic estimates of fetal weight. Serial ultrasonic measurement should demonstrate growth. Doppler studies may be normal. The biophysical profile has not been widely compared to umbilical Doppler studies. It has been suggested that first the umbilical artery Doppler, then the fetal abdominal circumference measurement, and finally the biophysical profile changes with deteriorating fetal condition (33).

The use of umbilical Doppler studies at or beyond term has not proven helpful. Poor discrimination of potential fetal compromise has been reported (34). On the basis of observations made using models of the placenta, it has been reported that the larger the placenta (and so, the number of arterial branches), the greater is the fraction of vessels which need to be obliterated before the Doppler index of resistance becomes abnormal (7). A large fraction of the vascular villus tree may be obliterated and significant hypoxia may be present with the index still within normal limits. It is also likely that the mature fetus is more susceptible to hypoxia than the immature fetus. This would explain the poor sensitivity of umbilical Doppler studies in this group. In this group of pregnancies the amniotic fluid index and nonstressed FHR monitoring are more appropriate tests.

EVALUATION CLINICAL UTILITY: RESULTS OF RANDOMIZED TRIALS

To date there have been four randomized controlled trials evaluating umbilical Doppler studies. It is important to understand that such trials are specific to their design and clinical setting. We conducted the first such trial to be performed (35). In this study clinicians had access to all other fetal welfare assessments with the availability of the umbilical Doppler studies randomized. Such Doppler studies were not associated with earlier delivery and intervention rates were similar in the groups with and without Doppler umbilical studies available. There was a significantly reduced incidence of fetal distress in labor and emergency cesarean section in the group in whom Doppler studies were available. This information was interpreted to provide reassurance that the availability of umbilical Doppler did not lead to unnecessary early intervention. It also provided evidence that Doppler studies were associated with better antenatal management in that the incidence of fetal distress in labor was reduced. A Dutch study (36) was performed with patients randomized at the onset of pregnancy. Again a high-risk patient group was examined. One group could have Doppler performed should an indication occur during the pregnancy and in the other group all other fetal welfare assessments were available except Doppler. There was a significant reduction in fetal death in the group with access to umbilical Doppler studies. In a third trial of high-risk pregnancy, patients referred to an ultrasound department for fetal biometry were randomized after the ultrasound results were known (37). The umbilical Doppler studies were either performed or not. All other fetal welfare data were available in both groups. In this trial there were no differences apparent in outcome between the two groups. These are interesting results suggesting that umbilical Doppler adds little to clinical management if the fetus is known to have a problem prior to performance of the Doppler study. This third trial contrasts with the first two in which the patients in the trial had been selected from a high-risk group but not on the basis of specific fetal welfare tests. Umbilical Doppler was compared to nonstressed FHR monitoring in a Swedish study as a method of surveillance of fetuses identified as small by third-trimester ultrasound biometry (38). The Doppler group had a lesser rate of emergency cesarean section for fetal distress, and neonates required less level 3 care. Taken together the results of these four trials support the clinical value of umbilical Doppler studies in determining which high-risk fetuses require further surveillance.

CLINICAL STRATEGIES USING UMBILICAL ARTERY DOPPLER IN THE MANAGEMENT OF THE IUGR FETUS

Potential for fetal compromise is recognized when a risk factor is identified in a pregnancy from either history or clinical examination. It is at this point that umbilical Doppler FVW study is of most use. Such studies identify the truly at-risk pregnancy in whom there is a placental vascular lesion present. This assumes that the placental pathology underlies the fetal threat. There are other circumstances in pregnancy that can put the fetus at risk. These include fetal anemia whether associated with isoimmunization or fetomaternal hemorrhage, acute placental abruption, and acutely reduced uterine perfusion. One cannot expect umbilical Doppler FVW studies to offer useful information here. The circumstance of fetal growth constraint usually implies a slowly progressive vascular restriction and it is this that is identified by umbilical Doppler studies.

Beyond this point along the pathway of deteriorating fetal condition the choice of fetal welfare tests to confirm compromise and define its extent is not standard. It would be unreasonable to expect one test to provide all this information. Currently ultrasound measurements are most widely used to confirm small fetal size. The biophysical profile or a combination of some of its components (particularly amniotic fluid volume and fetal movements) is used to assess fetal function, and so the safety of a policy of continuing with the pregnancy. This allows the fetus to develop further. Fetal heart rate monitoring alone is of very low sensitivity in the recognition of growth retardation. It does, however, identify the preterminal state. Currently, most obstetricians would wait for abnormality of the FHR tracing before delivery if this is necessary before 37 weeks. Unequivocal cessation of ultrasound growth would also constitute fetal grounds for intervention. Gestational age has an important influence on such management. Since the risk of elective delivery after 37 weeks is small, suspicion of fetal compromise from any abnormal fetal welfare study may precipitate delivery. Such an attitude is hard to criticize although it will result in higher intervention rates. In the postterm fetus the time course for demise appears much shorter than for premature fetuses. In these fetuses detection of any compromise should prompt delivery.

Low-dose aspirin has been used as a therapy for the placental vascular pathology identified by abnormally elevated index of a resistance of the umbilical Doppler waveform (39). The demonstrated placental vascular obliteration and fetal platelet consumption suggested the possibility of thromboxane release in the umbilical-placental circulation. This was the rationale behind the use of low-dose aspirin in such cases. Our study demonstrated that the group of pregnancies treated with low-dose aspirin yielded infants with a 25% greater birthweight than the placebo-treated group. Placental size was also greater, suggesting that placental growth and repair might be occurring. Low-dose aspirin might then provide a means of treatment for umbilical-placental insufficiency if the Doppler diagnosis is early and before marked fetal effect has occurred.

Cesarean delivery is liberally used for the compromised fetus because of the high risk of fetal distress in labor. Umbilical Doppler studies do identify fetuses at high risk of fetal distress in labor and hence worthy of consideration for elective cesarean delivery.

REFERENCES

1. Trudinger BJ, Giles WB, Cook CM, Bombardieri J, Collins L. Fetal umbilical artery flow velocity waveforms and placental resistance: Clinical significance. *Br J Obstet Gynaecol* 1985;92:23–30.
2. Dawes GS. The umbilical circulation. In: *Fetal and neonatal physiology.* Chicago: Year Book; 1968:66–78.
3. Giles WB, Trudinger BJ, Baird P. Fetal umbilical artery flow velocity waveforms and placental resistance: Pathological correlation. *Br J Obstet Gynaecol* 1985;92:31–38.
4. Fok RY, Pavlova Z, Bernischke K, Paul RH, Platt LD. The correlation of arterial lesions with umbilical artery Doppler velocimetry in the placenta of small for dates pregnancies. *Obstet Gynecol* 1990;75:578–583.
5. Trudinger BJ, Stevens D, Connelly A, et al. Umbilical artery flow velocity waveforms and placental resistance: The effects of embolization of the umbilical circulation. *Am J Obstet Gynecol* 1987;157:1443–1449.
6. Morrow RJ, Adamson SL, Bull SB, Ritchie JWK. Effect of placental embolization on the umbilical arterial velocity waveform in fetal sheep. *Am J Obstet Gynecol* 1989;161:1056–1060.
7. Thompson RS, Trudinger BJ. Doppler waveform pulsatility index and resistance, pressure and flow in the umbilical placental circulation: An investigation using a mathematical model. *Ultrasound Med Biol* 1990;16:449–458.
8. Reed KL, Anderson CF, Shenker L. Changes in intracardiac Doppler blood flow velocities in fetuses with absent umbilical artery diastolic flow. *Am J Obstet Gynecol* 1987;157:774–779.
9. Wilcox GR, Trudinger BJ, Cook CM, Wilcox WR, Connelly AJ. Reduced fetal platelet counts in pregnancies with abnormal Doppler umbilical flow waveforms. *Obstet Gynecol* 1989;75:639–643.
10. Wilcox GR, Berndt MC, Mehrabani PA, Exner T, Trudinger BJ. An improved method for measuring plasma glycocalicin in the investigation of causes of thrombocytopaenia. *Platelet* 1991;2:45–50.
11. Walsh SW. Preeclampsia: An imbalance in placental prostacyclin and thromboxane production. *Am J Obstet Gynecol* 1985;154:335–340.
12. Stuart MJ, Clark DA, Sunderji SG, et al. Decreased prostacyclin production: A characteristic of chronic placental insufficiency syndromes. *Lancet* 1981;1:1126–1128.
13. Trudinger BJ, Connelly AJ, Giles WB, Hales JR, Wilcox GR. The effects of prostacyclin and thromboxane analogue (U46619) on the fetal circulation and umbilical flow velocity waveforms. *J Devel Physiol* 1989;11:179–184.
14. Mak KKW, Gude NM, Walters WAW, Boura ALA. Effects of vasoactive autocoids on the human umbilical-fetal placental vasculature. *Br J Obstet Gynaecol* 1984;91:99–106.
15. Fleischer A, Schulman H, Farmakides G, et al. Umbilical velocity wave ratios in intrauterine growth retardation. *Am J Obstet Gynecol* 1985;151:502–506.
16. Reuwer PJHM, Bruinse HW, Stoutenbeek, et al. Doppler assessment of the feto-placental circulation in normal and growth retarded fetuses. *Eur J Obstet Gynecol Reprod Biol* 1984;18:199–205.
17. Erskine RLA, Ritchie JWK. Umbilical artery blood flow characteristics in normal growth retarded fetuses. *Br J Obstet Gynaecol* 1985;92:605–610.
18. Trudinger BJ, Giles WB, Cook CM. Flow velocity waveforms in the maternal uteroplacental and fetal umbilical placental circulation. *Am J Obstet Gynecol* 1985;152:155–163.
19. Gudmundsson S, Marsal K. Umbilical and uteroplacental blood flow velocity waveforms in pregnancies with fetal growth retardation. *Eur J Obstet Gynecol Reprod Biol* 1988;27:187–196.
20. Trudinger BJ, Cook CM, Giles WB, et al. Fetal umbilical artery velocity waveforms and subsequent neonatal outcome. *Br J Obstet Gynaecol* 1991;98:378–384.
21. Hackett GA, Campbell S, Gamsu H, Cohen-Overbeek T, Pearce JM. Doppler studies in the growth retarded fetus and prediction of neonatal necrotising enterocolitis, haemorrhage, and neonatal morbidity. *Br Med J* 1987;294:13–16.
22. Burke G, Stuart B, Crowley P, Scanuill SN, Drumin J. Is intrauterine growth retardation with normal umbilical artery blood flow a benign condition? *Br Med J* 1990;300:1044–1045.
23. Nicolaides KH, Bilardo CM, Soothill PW, Campbell S. Absence of end diastolic frequencies in umbilical artery: A sign of fetal hypoxia and acidosis. *Br Med J* 1988;297:1026–1027.
24. Nicolini U, Nicolaidis P, Fisk NM, Vaughan JI, et al. Limited role of fetal blood sampling in prediction of outcome in intrauterine growth retardation. *Lancet* 1990;336:768–772.
25. Wilcox GR, Trudinger BJ. Erythrocytes in fetuses with abnormal umbilical artery flow velocity waveforms. *Am J Obstet Gynecol* 1993;169:379–383.
26. Trudinger BJ, Cook CM, Jones L, Giles WB. A comparison of fetal heart rate monitoring and umbilical artery waveforms in the recognition of fetal compromise. *Br J Obstet Gynaecol* 1986;93:171–175.
27. Pattinson R, Dawes G, Jennings J, Redman C. Umbilical artery resistance index as a screening test for fetal well-being. I. Prospective revealed evaluation. *Obstet Gynecol* 1991;78:353–358.
28. Anyaegbunam A, Brustman L, Langer O. A longitudinal evaluation of the efficacy of umbilical Doppler velocimetry in the diagnosis of intrauterine growth retardation. *Int J Gynecol Obstet* 1991;34:121–125.
29. Divon MY, Girz BA, Lieblich R, Langer O. Clinical management of the fetus with markedly diminished umbilical artery end-diastolic flow. *Am J Obstet Gynecol* 1989;161:523–527.
30. Chambers SE, Hoskins PR, Haddad NG, Johnstone FD, McDicken WN, Muir BB. A comparison of fetal abdominal circumference measurements and Doppler ultrasound in the prediction of small-for-dates babies and fetal compromise. *Br J Obstet Gynaecol* 1989;96:803–808.
31. Berkowitz GS, Chitkara U, Rosenberg J, et al. Sonographic estimation of fetal weight and Doppler analysis of umbilical artery velocimetry in the prediction of intrauterine growth retardation: A prospective study. *Am J Obstet Gynecol* 1988;158:1149–1153.
32. Berkowitz GS, Mehalek KE, Chitkara U, et al. Doppler velocimetry in the prediction of adverse outcome in pregnancies at risk for intrauterine growth retardation. *Obstet Gynecol* 1988;71:742–746.
33. James DK, Parker MJ, Smoleniec JS. Comprehensive fetal assessment with three ultrasonographic characteristics. *Am J Obstet Gynecol* 1992;166:1486–1495.
34. Guidetti DA, Diven MY, Cavalieri RL, et al. Fetal umbilical artery flow velocimetry in postdate pregnancies. *Am J Obstet Gynecol* 1987;1157:1521–1523.
35. Trudinger BJ, Cook CM, Giles WB, Connelly A, Thompson RS. Umbilical artery flow velocity waveforms in high-risk pregnancy: Randomized controlled trial. *Lancet* 1987;1:188–190.
36. Omtzigt AWJ. Clinical value of umbilical Doppler velocimetry. PhD thesis, University of Utrecht, 1990.
37. Newnham JP, O'Dea M, Reid K, Diepeveen DA, James I. Doppler waveform analysis in high risk obstetric cases: A randomized controlled trial. *Br J Obstet Gynaecol* 1991;98:956–963.
38. Almstrom H, Axelsson O, Cnattingius S, et al. Comparison of umbilical artery velocimetry and cardiotocography for surveillance of small for gestation age fetuses. *Lancet* 1992;340:936–939.
39. Trudinger BJ, Cook C-M, Thompson RS, Giles WB, Connelly A. Low dose aspirin therapy improves fetal weight in umbilical placental insufficiency. *Am J Obstet Gyn* 1988;159:681–685.
40. Thompson RS, Trudinger BJ, Cook CM, Giles WB. *Br J Obstet Gyn* 1988;95:589–591.

Doppler Ultrasound in Obstetrics and Gynecology,
edited by Joshua A. Copel and Kathryn L. Reed.
Raven Press, Ltd., New York © 1995.

CHAPTER 20

Absent and Reversed Umbilical Artery End-Diastolic Velocity

Dan Farine, Edmond N. Kelly, Greg Ryan, Robert J. Morrow,
and J. W. Knox Ritchie

It was first suggested in 1977 that Doppler flow velocity assessment of the umbilical artery (UA) may have a role in fetal surveillance (1). The most ominous waveform patterns occur when there is absence (AEDV) (Fig. 1) or reversal (REDV) (Fig. 2) of end-diastolic velocities (EDV). To date, there have been more than 1000 reported cases of either AEDV or REDV, with a cumulative perinatal mortality of 36% (Table 1). This chapter will review the pathophysiology, incidence, clinical associations, and significance of these findings, including obstetric management and short- and long-term neonatal outcome.

PATHOPHYSIOLOGY AND PLACENTAL PATHOLOGY

Changes in the umbilical flow velocity waveforms are believed to reflect primarily downstream (i.e., placental) vascular resistance, and this relationship has been clarified in a number of experimental and clinical models. Trudinger et al. (2) and McCowan et al. (3) demonstrated an obliteration of arterioles in the tertiary villi and Fok et al. (4) described intimal thickening. Arabin and coworkers (5) found that only 7% of placentas in AEDV pregnancies were normal. In 74% he noted evidence of chronic placental insufficiency, manifested by small placentas, villous fibrosis, and microfibrinous deposits. The remaining 19% showed a reduced perfusion capacity.

In a sheep model, a progressive decrease in diastolic velocities followed occlusion of the placental arterioles by embolization (6). Interestingly, increasing the resistance in the placental vascular system by infusion of angiotensin did not alter the waveforms. A full discussion of these phenomena is not within the scope of this chapter and the interested reader is referred to Chapter 9.

PHYSIOLOGIC RESPONSES ASSOCIATED WITH AEDV

In normal pregnancy, the right ventricle contributes approximately 58% of the combined ventricular output and there is low resistance in both the cerebral and peripheral vessels (7–10). In asymmetric growth retarded fetuses, the right ventricle becomes less dominant and contributed only 47% of combined ventricular output (11,12). This is associated with decreased resistance in the cerebral circulation and increased peripheral resistance, thus optimizing brain perfusion (7,13). Studies assessing the pulsatility index of the middle cerebral artery in fetuses with AEDV have shown evidence of increased blood flow to the brain, and the more hypoxemic fetuses had a more evident "brain-sparing effect" (5,14,15). This protective mechanism may explain why fetuses with AEDV exhibit normal neurobehavioral development (16). In the only study reporting cardiac flow patterns in fetuses with AEDV, Reed et al. (15) showed that the right ventricle contributed 68% of the combined ventricular output, a ratio greater than in fetuses with growth retardation and normal umbilical artery flow velocity waveforms (11,12). Arduini et al. (17) suggested that the onset of umbilical venous (UV) pulsations was associated with fetal cardiac decompensation.

D. Farine, E. N. Kelly, G. Ryan, R. J. Morrow, and J. W. Knox Ritchie: Perinatal Unit, Mount Sinai Hospital, Toronto, Ontario, Canada.

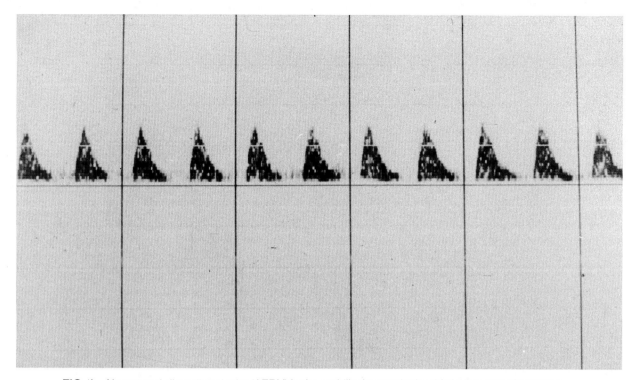

FIG. 1. Absent end-diastolic velocity (AEDV) in the umbilical artery in the third trimester of pregnancy.

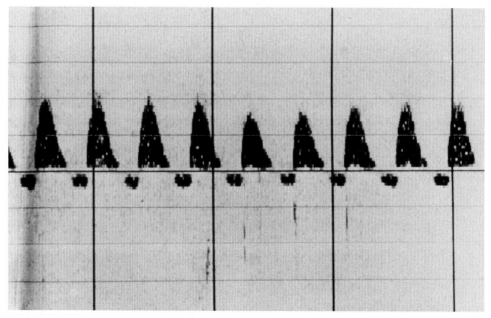

FIG. 2. Reversed diastolic velocity (REDV) in the umbilical artery in the third trimester of pregnancy.

TABLE 1. *Absent end-diastolic velocity and perinatal mortality*

Author (year)	AEDV (N)	SB (N)	NND (N)	Perinatal deaths	PNM (%)
Pattison (93)	120	34	25	59	52
Trudinger (91)	96	6	17	23	24
Ryan (89)	86	8	15	23	27
Bessis (88)	50			25	50
Weiss (92)	47			7	15
Bekedam (90)	45	2	11	13	29
Huneke (91)	38	6	7	13	34
McParland (90)	37	7	8	15	41
Arduini (93)	37	14	14	38	28
Bell (92)	33	1	7	8	24
Fairlie (91)	32	8	12	20	47
Brar (88)	31	4	2	6	50
Arabin (88)	30	3	6	9	20
Battaglia (93)	26	1	13	14	54
Malcolm (91)	25	8	1	9	48
Johnston (88)	24	1	3	4	17
Ombelet (88)	21			13	62
Pattison (93)	21			4	15
Huenke (91)	18			9	50
Tyrell (89)	17	0	4	4	24
Reuwer (87)	17			4	24
Rochelson (87)	15	6	2	8	53
Hackett (87)	15	0	7	7	27
Reed (87)	14	4	2	6	42
Divon (89)	12	0	0	0	0
Woo (87)	9	5	3	8	89
Hsieh (88)	7	8	0	8	100
Beattie (89)	6			3	50
Ashmead (93)	5	0	2	2	40
Pillai (91)	4	0	0	0	0
Freidman (85)	2			2	100
All Studies:	940			337	36

Other Studies

Rizzo (93)	192				
Wilcox (93)	39				
Gudmundsson (90)	14				
Fitzgerald (84)	13				
Wiener (90)	6				
Total	1204				

AEDV, absent end-diastolic velocity; SB, stillbirth; NND, neonatal death; PNM, perinatal mortality.

AEDV AS A NORMAL FINDING

AEDV is a normal finding in early pregnancy (18–20). End-diastolic velocities first begin to appear at 10 weeks gestation and are always present by 15 weeks (18). AEDV has also been encountered incidentally during bouts of fetal hiccups (21). These findings are not associated with any fetal pathology.

TECHNICAL ASPECTS OF DIAGNOSING AEDV

Either continuous or pulsed wave ultrasound equipment can be used for Doppler examinations. Duplex

pulsed equipment allows the operator to sample a particular area of interest and ensure that an optimal incident angle is maintained. Measurements are made with mothers in a semirecumbent position and during fetal apnea. Consecutive waveforms should be imaged and, if abnormal, confirmatory readings taken at several different sites especially if continuous-wave Doppler is employed. It is important to ensure that the lowest possible incident angle between the Doppler beam and the umbilical artery is obtained. At high angles small amounts of diastolic flow may be obscured by the wall filter (Fig. 3). With continuous wave equipment, obtaining several umbilical artery velocity samples from differing points on the maternal abdomen can eliminate this potential for the artificial appearance of AEDV. If AEDV is suspected, the wall filter should be either switched off or set as low as possible, to ensure that low-frequency flow patterns are not artificially eliminated (22).

INCIDENCE

The incidence of AEDV in the general population is low. In a screening study of 2097 *low-risk* women (23), it was concluded that there was no justification for the use of Doppler as a screening tool. In that study there were six cases of AEDV, of which three reverted to normal with good outcome, two ended in stillbirth, and one had IUGR. There were six stillbirths in all, of whom two had AEDV, two had abnormal Doppler studies, and two had normal waveforms. Johnston et al. (24) did not find any cases of AEDV in uncomplicated pregnancies.

There is a wide variation in the reported incidence of AEDV in *high-risk* populations, varying between 1% (25) and 34% (26) (Table 2), which probably reflects different study inclusion criteria.

CLINICAL ASSOCIATIONS WITH AEDV

Intrauterine Growth Retardation

The association between AEDV and IUGR is well established (Table 3). The incidence of IUGR (less than the 10th percentile) in 26 studies of 785 pregnancies with AEDV was 83%, with most birthweights being less than the 3rd percentile.

Hypertension

The majority of women whose pregnancies exhibited AEDV had chronic hypertension, preeclampsia, or both. There were 300 (57%) hypertensive patients out of 524 women in 16 studies reviewed (Table 4).

Anomalies and Chromosomal Abnormalities

In pregnancies complicated by AEDV, there was an increased incidence of fetal abnormality. The overall in-

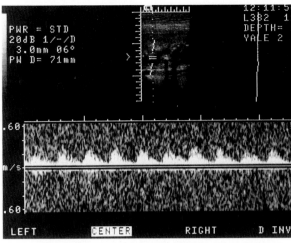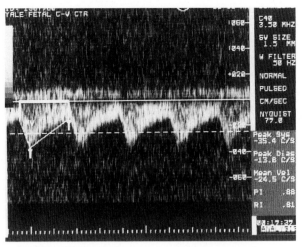

FIG. 3. Umbilical artery Doppler from a fetus with severe oligohydraminus due to renal agenesis. Left panel shows sample obtained at poor incident angle and apparent diminished end-diastolic flow. Right panel shows good end-diastolic flow when a better incident angle was obtained. Note that velocity scales are similar in both panels although different equipment was used.

cidence of structural anomalies was 11% whereas chromosomal anomalies were found in 6% (Table 5), of which trisomy 18 was the most common. Many of these conditions should be detectable at the time of the initial ultrasound assessment (27).

Amniotic Fluid Volume

A significant number of pregnancies with AEDV have oligohydramnios, most probably reflecting chronic placental insufficiency. The rates vary quite dramatically between 35% (28) and 90% (29). Arduini et al. (17) did not find that the amniotic fluid index per se correlated with outcome.

Autoimmune Disorders

Only a few patients with autoimmune disorders have been reported to have AEDV in pregnancy. Most of

TABLE 2. *Incidence (%) of absent end-diastolic velocity in high-risk pregnancies*

Author (year)	Population	Incidence
Rizzo (93)	6104	3.1
Weiss (92)	2400	2.0
Trudinger (91)	2178	4.4
Malcolm (91)	1000	2.5
Divon (89)	718	2.1
Arduini (93)	458	8.0
Johnston (88)	380	6.3
Pattison (93)	348	34.5
Ombolet (88)	260	8.1
Huneke (91)	226	16.8
Arabin (88)	137	21.9
Rochelson (87)	128	7.8

these had systemic lupus erythematosus (SLE). We could find a total of only seven cases in all the series reviewed. Many of these patients also had other problems such as IUGR, hypertension, and/or diabetes. There are two studies (30,31) suggesting that Doppler velocity measurements may be useful in monitoring pregnancies complicated by SLE and in predicting outcome. However, neither has described any cases of AEDV.

Multiple Gestations

In 89 sets of twins, Hastie et al. found that Doppler studies were not predictive of IUGR (less than the 10th percentile). However, of 11 fetuses with persistent AEDV, 1 died and 10 were growth-restricted (32).

In a series of 20 triplets, there were 9 pregnancies in which 1 or more fetuses had IUGR. In all of these cases there were abnormal umbilical Doppler findings, although not necessarily AEDV. Both of the stillborn babies had AEDV (33). Rafla (34) detected AEDV in two fetuses of a set of triplets who later developed necrotizing enterocolitis requiring major bowel resection. In contrast, five other sets of triplets who had normal umbilical flow velocities did well. These preliminary data support a role for Doppler umbilical velocimetry in multiple pregnancies.

Diabetes

There is no strong association between diabetes and AEDV. In reviewing all the articles outlined in Table 1, there were only 11 diabetic pregnancies (<1%), of which most investigators had other findings such as hypertension and/or IUGR.

TABLE 3. *Incidence of IUGR in pregnancies with absent end-diastolic velocity (AEDV)*

Author (year)	AEDV (N)	% of fetuses below: 3%	5%	10%ile	No. of fetuses below 10%ile
Pattison (93)	120			92	110
Trudinger (91)	96		72	81	78
Ryan (89)	86	77		84	72
Bessis (88)	50		50	100	50
Weiss (92)	47	47		77	36
Bell (92)	40			64	26
Wilcox (93)	39			77	30
McParland (90)	37	46		73	27
Brar (88)	31			81	25
Arabin (88)	30	70		100	30
Johnston (88)	24	92	92	92	24
Pattison (93)	21	81			17
Ombelet (88)	21			91	19
Reuwer (87)	17			100	17
Tyrell (89)	17	47		94	16
Hackett (87)	15		88		13
Rochelson (87)	15			53	8
Gudmundsson (90)	14		86		12
Reed (87)	14			78	11
Fitzgerald (84)	13			100	13
Divon (89)	12			75	9
Woo (87)	9			67	6
Beattie (89)	6			17	1
Ashmead (93)	5		20	20	1
Pillai (91)	4		100	100	4
Friedman (85)	2			50	1
Total	785			83	656 (84%)

TABLE 4. *Incidence of hypertensive disorders in pregnancies with absent end-diastolic velocity (AEDV)*

Author (year)	AEDV (N)	Hypertensive disorder
Pattison (93)	120	85
Ryan (89)	84	22
Bekedam (90)	45	31
Bell (92)	40	22
McParland (90)	37	26
Arduini (93)	37	16
Arabin (88)	30	14
Malcolm (91)	25	11
Johnston (88)	24	17
Ombelet (88)	21	14
Rochelson (87)	15	11
Gudmundsson (90)	14	10
Reed (87)	14	10
Woo (87)	9	5
Ashmead (93)	5	2
Pillai (91)	4	4
Total	524	300 (57%)

TABLE 5. *Incidence (no.) of fetal anomalies and chromosomal abnormalities in fetuses with absent end-diastolic velocity (AEDV)*

Author (year)	AEDV (N)	Malformations	Abnormal karyotype
Rizzo (93)	192		16
Pattison (93)	120	1	1
Trudinger (91)	96	9	
Ryan (89)	86	11	3
Bessis (88)	50		8
Weiss (92)	47		2
Bell (92)	40	7	2
McParland (90)	37	0	0
Arabin (88)	30	3	2
Battaglia (93)	26	0	0
Malcolm (91)	25	6	
Johnston (88)	24	0	0
Pattison (93)	21		1
Ombelet (88)	21	3	1
Reuwer (87)	17	1	1
Tyrell (89)	17	1	1
Rochelson (87)	15	1	3
Reed (87)	14	4	3
Divon (89)	12	0	0
Woo (87)	9	8	1
Hsieh (88)	8	8	4
Ashmead (93)	5	2	1
Pillai (91)	4	0	0
Total	916	65 (11%)	50 (6%)

Drug Abuse

Multiple drug abuse, including that of cocaine, has not been associated with abnormal umbilical Doppler findings (35).

Elevated MSAFP

Weiner et al. (36) described an association between elevated maternal serum α-fetoprotein (MSAFP) and abnormal umbilical flow velocity. We found (37) that only about 5% of patients with elevated MSAFP had AEDV (these patients also had preeclampsia). On the other hand, of 25 patients with AEDV in the third trimester, 6 (24%) had elevated MSAFP in the second trimester, 5 of whom had hypertensive disease.

NATURAL HISTORY OF AEDV

Once present, AEDV persists in the majority of cases and occasionally deteriorates into a pattern of reversal (REDV). In the absence of intervention, this usually leads to fetal distress and demise. The duration of AEDV does not necessarily correlate with a poor outcome (24,38,39). For example, in two series (24,38) only 1 of 11 fetuses died after AEDV of more than 14 days duration. It has also been noted that the more immature fetuses have a longer interval from time of diagnosis to onset of fetal distress (5,17,38).

IMPROVEMENT OF AEDV

An improvement in the waveform has occasionally been reported (28,40). This phenomenon should not occur if AEDV reflects irreversible damage to the arterioles in the placental bed. Bell et al. documented the return of end-diastolic velocities with maternal hydration in 11 of 33 fetuses with AEDV, all of which were admitted to hospital (28). The improvement in waveforms was not associated with an improvement in outcome, and Bell et al. were unable to predict the patients in whom waveform improvement would occur. Brar and Platt (41), on the other hand, suggested that improvement in waveforms was linked to improved outcome. Our group has never noted a permanent improvement in AEDV. It should be remembered that each of the two umbilical arteries may have a different pattern and that readings from different sites may vary as well (42).

Therapies suggested in the setting of AEDV include bed rest (28,41), antihypertensive medication (40), oxygen (43,44), and volume expansion (45). However, none of these has been tested in a prospective randomized manner.

AEDV AND FETAL ASPHYXIA

The association of AEDV with significant perinatal mortality, morbidity, fetal distress, and IUGR (Tables 1, 3, 6, and 7) has led to speculation about the role of Doppler in diagnosis of asphyxia. Fetal blood gas analysis in some IUGR fetuses has shown evidence of chronic hypoxia and acidosis (46). Fetal blood sampling (FBS) was performed prospectively to address this issue in four studies (Table 7), in which 96 fetuses had AEDV. Only 12 of these had both normal pH and pO$_2$. About 50% were acidotic, and the majority were hypoxemic; however, the authors noted a great overlap with normal values (46). Battaglia et al. (14) showed that fetuses with AEDV were also hypercapneic. In contrast, Ashmead et al. (47) found that all five fetuses with AEDV in his series had normal acid–base status, yet all went on to show evidence of fetal distress within days.

Cord gases performed at cesarean birth with no labor showed frequent acidosis and hypoxia in pregnancies complicated by AEDV (Table 7) (38,48–51). Again there was significant overlap with normal values. In the study by Fairlie et al. (52) there was no difference in the incidence of acidosis, hypoxemia, or hypercapnia between those who survived and those who died. As the incidence of abnormal gases was high, it was felt that antenatal blood gas analysis would not be beneficial for management in most cases.

Fetuses with AEDV were more susceptible to fetal distress in labor necessitating cesarean sections (Tables 6 and 7), and probably for this reason they had lower Apgar scores at birth (Table 7).

TABLE 6. *Delivery data in pregnancies with absent end-diastolic velocity (AEDV) in the umbilical artery*

Author (year)	AEDV (N)	Delivery by C/S (%)	Abnormal FH anytime (%)	Mean GA (weeks)
Trudinger (91)	96	91		31.1
Ryan (89)	86	89		31.5
Weiss (92)	51	81		32.8
Bell (92)	40	97	81	
Wilcox (93)	39			33.2
McParland (90)	37	100		
Brar (88)	31			30.1
Arabin (88)	30	96	96	33
Battaglia (93)	26	96		30.2
Johnston (88)	24	83	83	
Pattison (93)	21	100		31.4
Tyrell (89)	17			31.3
Hackett (87)	15	100	62	31.8
Rochelson (87)	15	75	92	33.5
Reed (87)	14	57		
Divon (89)	12	88		33

C/S, cesarean section; FH, fetal heart rate; GA, gestational age.

TABLE 7. *Fetal asphyxia, CSFD, and Apgar score at delivery in pregnancies complicated by absent end-diastolic velocity*

Author (year)	FBS	Cord gases	No.	Cont.	Normal	↓pH	↓pO$_2$	↑pCO$_2$	% CSFD	1'Apg % <7	5'Apg % <7
Nicolaides (88)	Y		59		7	27	47				
Weiner (90)	Y		6		0	6	6				
Battaglia (93)	Y		26				Y	Y			
Ashmead (93)	Y		5		5						69
Fairlie (91)		UV	17			15	11	16			
Pattison (93)		UA	21	Y		Y			80		
Huneke (91)		UA	18	Y		Y			100		
Gudmundsson (90)		UA/UV	14	Y			Y				
Bekedam (90)		UA/UV	45	Y		Y	Y	Y			
Brar (88)											
(reversed F1)		UA	8			4			75	75	50
Johnston (88)			24						85		
Trudinger (91)										68	27
Arabin (88)		UA	27			30				55	15
Fairlie (91)			32						70		28
Tyrell (89)		UV	17			9	15				
Weiss (92)		UA	47			21			81		

FBS, fetal blood sampling; CSFD, cesarean section for fetal distress; UA, umbilical artery; UV, umbilical vein.

Although these fetuses may be hypoxic and acidotic at time of diagnosis or at delivery, AEDV itself is not diagnostic of either and fetal condition cannot be inferred from AEDV alone. This was supported by Nicolini et al. (53) who demonstrated that fetal blood gas analysis was not useful in the clinical management of IUGR fetuses.

MANAGEMENT OF AEDV

The management of patients with AEDV in the umbilical artery is still controversial.

Reporting AEDV

Pattison et al. (54) reported or withheld the Doppler findings in a randomized manner. In the group where the results were withheld from the primary physician there were six perinatal deaths in AEDV fetuses (of which five were stillbirths) compared to one neonatal death in the group whose results were reported.

Immediate Delivery or Conservative Management

Early authors assumed that AEDV was associated with impending fetal death, and recommended immediate delivery, often with poor outcome (55,56). Most centers now adopt a much less aggressive approach and will not deliver babies for AEDV alone. Generally, admission to hospital for bed rest with treatment of any underlying maternal conditions such as hypertension is indicated. Intensive fetal monitoring is crucial to the ongoing management of such pregnancies. A trial of volume loading may be considered (45).

Fetal Karyotype

The risk of chromosomal abnormalities and fetal anomalies is often an indication for karyotyping. The clinical role of FBS in the IUGR fetus with AEDV is somewhat more controversial (43,44,47), particularly when clinical signs suggest that utero-placental insufficiency is the sole cause, and in which there are no indicators of chromosomal abnormality. These fetuses are more prone to bradycardia and fetal death secondary to the procedure (57,58), and blood gas analysis does not appear to contribute to clinical management (53).

Our approach has been to scan these fetuses carefully and to perform fetal karyotyping only in the presence of structural anomalies. In patients with AEDV, IUGR, and no obvious cause, we discuss the risks and benefits of invasive procedures in order to obtain karyotyping. In patients with preeclampsia or hypertension, or when another etiology for the AEDV is apparent, we do not suggest fetal karyotyping. This approach has failed us only once, in a chronically hypertensive mother whose fetus had trisomy 13.

Mode of Monitoring

Most series advocated an intensive scheme of monitoring for fetal well-being once (25) or twice (5) daily, whenever AEDV was detected. Most centers used nonstress tests (NSTs) for these testings with biophysical profile testing twice or more weekly as necessary (25).

The role of Doppler examinations of other vessels such as the middle cerebral artery, aorta, inferior vena cava, and umbilical vein as an aid to timing delivery is still experimental. Umbilical vein studies may have an important prognostic value, since umbilical vein pulsations in fetuses with AEDV suggest cardiac decompensation (17a). Gudmundsson et al. (59) found that six such fetuses in their series died. Weiss et al. (60) found that fetuses with resistance indices in less than the 5th percentile in the middle cerebral artery were at significant risk of poor developmental outcome, although others with similar findings were normal.

Indications for Delivery

The perinatal mortality associated with delivery after 28–30 weeks gestation is low. After this gestation delivery should be expedited once there is a maternal indication or evidence of fetal distress. The most common indications for delivery are:

1. Acute fetal distress, as evidenced by an ominous fetal heart rate tracing and/or biophysical profile ≤ 4/10
2. Worsening maternal condition, often severe preeclampsia or severe chronic hypertension unresponsive to therapy
3. Severe IUGR with no interval growth over a reasonable time period, or IUGR with proven fetal lung maturity

Some have suggested severe oligohydramnios per se as an indication for delivery (25).

Below 28–30 weeks gestation mortality is high due to the combination of prematurity and severe IUGR. The management becomes more controversial with a major factor being the neonatal facilities at hand.

Interval to Delivery

Even when expectant management is practiced, a significant number of patients are delivered soon after AEDV is detected for other obstetric indications. In several series 21–53% of patients were delivered within 24 hr of diagnosis (24,28,29). The mean duration from diagnosis of AEDV to onset of fetal distress was approximately 6–8 days (range 0–49 days) (5,15,17,24,25,62). In these studies the exact time when AEDV first appeared was unknown as most of the patients presented with established AEDV. Arduini et al. (17) followed 37 normally formed fetuses longitudinally, thus establishing the interval between appearance of AEDV and onset of fetal distress, and this ranged from 1 to 26 days (median 7 days).

Divon et al. (25) found that only 16% of patients with AEDV went into spontaneous labor in comparison to 68% of controls. The average gestational age at delivery in different studies varied between 30 and 33 weeks gestation (Table 7).

Mode of Delivery

The majority of patients in the 13 studies were delivered by cesarean section. The average cesarean section rate was 90% (range 57–100%) (Table 6). The vast majority of these deliveries were motivated by fetal distress (Table 7).

Management of Reverse End-Diastolic Flow

Reverse end-diastolic velocity (REDV) is the most extreme form of increased vascular resistance in the placental bed. In fetal embolization studies in the sheep, this pattern immediately preceded fetal death (6). Usually by the time REDV is detected in the clinical setting, severe fetal compromise is evident using more standard tests of fetal well-being. Brar and Platt (63) found this to be the case in all fetuses with REDV and all of those fetuses had IUGR. The diagnosis-to-delivery interval was 4.2 ± 1.4 days. The majority of neonates were acidotic with poor Apgar scores and the perinatal mortality was 50%. In our experience there were eight such cases resulting in two stillbirths and two neonatal deaths. However, only one of the four survivors had major long-term morbidity. The mean interval from discovery to delivery was 10.8 hr (range 1–40 hr). Divon et al. (25) had three such patients who needed to be delivered on the day of diagnosis and there were no perinatal deaths. In the Bekedam et al. (38) study only two of five fetuses with REDV survived. Ombolet et al. (29) described one survivor among three fetuses with REDV. Interestingly, this fetus was monitored *in utero* for 16 days.

It is not clear whether REDV by itself is an indication for delivery although this finding practically never occurs in isolation. Even with careful fetal monitoring it seems unlikely that the duration of pregnancy could be prolonged significantly.

SHORT-TERM PERINATAL OUTCOME

Neonatal Mortality

The finding of AEDV is associated with significant perinatal mortality, with an average reported figure of 36% (Table 1), although this rate varies greatly. Hsieh et al. (56) reported 100% mortality in all of eight malformed fetuses, whereas Divon et al. (25), in a highly selected population, had 100% survival. In these studies the majority of stillbirths weighed <500 g (61,62), while the neonatal mortality was mainly in neonates < 1000 g at birth (24,39,48,61,62), and that gestational age at ei-

TABLE 8. *Neonatal morbidity following pregnancies complicated by absent end-diastolic velocity (AEDV) and neonatal morbidity (%)*

Author (year)	NICU	IUGR <3	IUGR <5	IUGR <10	IPPV	RDS	BPD	NEC	IVH	HEM	↓Gluc	MOF
Mattice (89)				89				6	6	61	56	
Karsdorp (92)	100					60			20		30	40
Malcolm (91)								33				
Hackett (87) (aorta)			88			42		27		43		
Bessis (88)	100											
Trudinger (91)	96		72	81								
Ryan (89)	96	77	77	86	38	22	12	4	13	52	45	9
Fairlie (91)				75				11	18			
Johnstone (88)			95									
Weiss (92)		47		77	68	60			15			

NICU, neonatal intensive care unit; IPPV, intermittent positive pressure ventilation; RDS, respiratory distress syndrome; BPD, broncho-pulmonary dysplasia; NEC, necrotizing enterocolitis; IVH, intraventricular hemorrhage; MOF, multiple organ failure.

ther diagnosis (52,61) or delivery (48,61,64) was less than 28–30 weeks. Prematurity combined with IUGR, rather than AEDV per se, contributed in a major way to mortality.

Neonatal Morbidity

Admission to a neonatal intensive care unit (NICU) varied from 45% to 100% (Table 8). As expected, these babies showed many of the complications of prematurity and IUGR (Table 8) and commonly suffered from hypoglycemia (62,65), hematologic abnormalities (62,65), respiratory distress syndrome (45,50), and intracranial hemorrhage (45,65). Up to 40% of the neonates died of multiple organ failure (45). A significant association between necrotizing enterocolitis (NEC) and AEDV was reported, with an incidence of up to 33% (39,65,66). In contrast, we noted NEC in less than 5% of neonates with AEDV *in utero* (Table 8).

Pattison et al. (26,48) and Weiss et al. (50) compared the outcome of pregnancies with and without AEDV, controlling for gestational age and weight. No significant differences in neonatal outcome (lung disease, intraventricular hemorrhage, NEC, patent ductus arteriosus or septicemia) were noted. These studies suggest that the AEDV itself does not further contribute to the morbidity attributable to both prematurity and growth restriction.

LONG-TERM OUTCOME

Only two studies have reported a follow up of a year or longer (16,55) in fetuses with AEDV, and all five children were reported normal.

We assessed such 58 chromosomally normal infants at a mean age at assessment of 20 ± 6 months (67). At birth, 78% had been below the 3rd percentile for weight compared with 28% at follow-up. Similarly, 59% were less than the 3rd percentile for length at birth compared with 12 at follow-up, and 22% had head circumference less than the 3rd percentile at birth compared with 9% at follow-up. This demonstrated significant "catch-up growth" in many of these children.

Neurologic examination revealed two children (4%) with cerebral palsy. None were deaf or blind. Fifty-four children had psychometric testing, of whom 86% were normal. Three children (5%) were mentally retarded and 9% were suspect (1–2 SD below mean).

Overall, 85% of survivors were normal cognitively and neurologically and 65% were normal in terms of growth and neurologic outcome. In our experience, the long-term outcome in the majority of surviving fetuses with AEDV was normal.

SUBSEQUENT PREGNANCY

The recurrence risk, course, and outcome of subsequent pregnancies in women with AEDV was reviewed in 16 patients who had 19 subsequent pregnancies (68). The index pregnancy was invariably complicated, with a perinatal mortality of 56%, growth restriction in 94% (15/16), and prematurity in 100% (75% were born <32 weeks gestation). In contrast, the outcome of the subsequent pregnancies was much better and 74% (14/19) were uncomplicated. No perinatal deaths occurred, and none were delivered prior to 32 weeks gestation. AEDV recurred only in two pregnancies, both of which were complicated. Six women had autoantibodies and these accounted for 80% (4/5) of subsequent complicated pregnancies. We concluded that recurrence of AEDV was low. The absence of autoantibodies and normal Doppler studies were associated with improved outcome.

CONCLUSIONS

Absent end-diastolic velocity in the umbilical artery is an uncommon finding, but these fetuses are at an increased risk of perinatal mortality, growth restriction, and chromosomal and structural malformations. It is most often associated with the hypertensive disorders of pregnancy. The detection of AEDV alone is not an indication for immediate delivery but rather should be a red flag prompting admission and intensive fetal monitoring. This approach results in a high rate of premature delivery, usually by cesarean section.

AEDV was associated with a high rate of stillbirth and neonatal death especially in severely growth-restricted infants delivered before 28–30 weeks. However, in the majority of karyotypically normal survivors, the neurologic and cognitive outcome is normal, with most demonstrating significant catch-up growth.

REFERENCES

1. Fitzgerald DE, Drumm JE. Non-invasive measurement of human fetal circulation using ultrasound: A new method. *Br Med J* 1977;2:1450–1451.
2. Giles WB, Trudinger BJ, Baird PJ. Fetal umbilical artery flow velocity waveforms and placental resistance: Pathological correlations. *Br J Obstet Gynaecol* 1985;92:31–38.
3. McCowan LM, Mullen B, Ritchie K. Umbilical artery flow velocity waveforms and the placental bed. *Am J Obstet Gynecol* 1987;157:900.
4. Fok RY, Pavlova Z, Benirschke K, Paul RH, Platt LD. The correlation of arterial lesions with umbilical artery Doppler velocimetry in the placentas of small for dates pregnancies. *Obstet Gynecol* 1990;75:578–583.
5. Arabin B, Siebert M, Jimenez, Saling E. Obstetrical characteristics of a loss of end-diastolic velocities in the fetal aorta and/or umbilical artery using Doppler ultrasound. *Gynecol Obstet Invest* 1988;25:173–180.
6. Morrow RJ, Adamson L, Bull SB, Ritchie JWK. Effect of placental embolization on the umbilical arterial velocity waveform in the fetal sheep. *Am J Obstet Gynecol* 1989;161:1055–1060.
7. Wladimiroff JW, Tonge HM, Stewart PA. Doppler ultrasound assessment of cerebral blood flow in the human fetus. *Br J Obstet Gynaecol* 1986;93:471–475.
8. Allan LD, Chita SK, Al-Ghazli WH, Crawford DC, Tynan M. Doppler echocardiographic evaluation of the normal human fetal heart. *Br Heart J* 1987;57:528–533.
9. Reed KL, Meijboom EJ, Sahn DJ, Scagnelli SA, Valdescruz LM, Shenker T. Cardiac flow velocities in human fetuses. *Circulation* 1986;73:41–46.
10. Kenny JF, Plappert T, Doubilet P, et al. Changes in intracardiac blood flow velocities and right and left ventricular stroke volume with gestational age in the normal human fetus: A prospective Doppler echocardiographic study. *Circulation* 1986;74:1208–1216.
11. Al-Ghazali W, Chita SK, Chapman MG, Allan LD. Evidence of redistribution of cardiac output in asymmetrical growth retardation. *Br J Obstet Gynaecol* 1989;96:697–704.
12. Rizzo G, Arduini D, Romanini C, Mancuso S. Doppler echocardiographic assessment of atrioventricular velocity waveforms in normal and small-for-gestational age fetuses. *Br J Obstet Gynaecol* 1988;95:65–69.
13. Marsal K, Lingman G, Giles W. Evaluation of the carotid, aortic and umbilical blood flow velocity. *Proceedings of the Society of the Study of Fetal Physiology, Eleventh Annual Conference,* Oxford C33; 1984.
14. Battaglia C, Artini PG, Galli PA, D'Ambrogio G, Droghini F, Genazzani AR. Absent or reversed end-diastolic flow in umbilical artery and severe intrauterine growth retardation. An ominous association. *Acta Obstet Gynecol Scand* 1993;72:167–171.
15. Reed KL, Anderson CF, Shenker L. Changes in intracardiac Doppler blood flow velocities in fetuses with absent umbilical artery diastolic flow. *Am J Obstet Gynecol* 1987;157:774–779.
16. Pillai M, James D. Continuation of normal neurobehavioral development in fetuses with absent umbilical arterial end diastolic velocities. *Br J Obstet Gynaecol* 1991;98:277–281.
17a. Indik JH, Chen V, Reed KL. Association of umbilical venous with inferior vena cava blood velocities. *Obstet Gynecol* 1991;77:551–557.
17b. Arduini D, Rizzo G, Romanini C. The development of abnormal heart rate patterns after absent end-diastolic velocity in umbilical artery: Analysis of risk factors. *Am J Obstet Gynecol* 1993;168:43–50.
18. Arduini D, Rizzo G. Umbilical artery velocity waveforms in early pregnancy. A transvaginal color Doppler study. *J Clin Ultrasound* 1991;19:335–339.
19. Fisk NM, MacLachlan N, Ellis C, Tannirandorn Y, Tonge HM, Rodeck CH. Absent end-diastolic flow in first trimester umbilical artery. *Lancet* 1988;2:1257–1258.
20. Den Ouden M, Cohen-Overbreek TE, Wladimiroff JW. Uterine and fetal umbilical artery flow velocity waveforms in normal first trimester pregnancies. *Br J Obstet Gynaecol* 1990;97:716–719.
21. Mueller GM, Sipes SL. Isolated reversed umbilical arterial blood flow on Doppler ultrasonography and fetal hiccups. *J Ultrasound Med* 1993;12:641–643.
22. Rochelson B. The clinical significance of absent end diastolic velocity in the umbilical artery waveforms. *Clin Obstet Gynecol* 1989;32:692–702.
23. Beatty RB, Dornan JC. Antenatal screening for intrauterine growth retardation with umbilical artery Doppler ultrasonography. *Br Med J* 1989;298:631–635.
24. Johnstone FD, Haddad NG, Hoskins P, McDicken W, Chambers S, Muir B. Umbilical artery doppler flow velocity waveform: The outcome of pregnancies with absent end diastolic flow. *Eur J Obstet Gynaecol Reprod Biol;*28:171–178.
25. Divon MY, Girz BA, Lieblich R, Langer O. Clinical management of the fetus with markedly diminished umbilical artery end-diastolic flow. *Am J Obstet Gynecol* 1989;161:1523–1527.
26. Pattison RC, Odendaal HJ, Kirsten G. The relationship between absent end-diastolic velocities of the umbilical artery and perinatal mortality and morbidity. *Early Hum Dev* 1993;33:61–69.
27. Benacerraf BR. Prenatal sonography of autosomal trisomies. *Ultrasound Obstet Gynecol* 1991;1:66–75.
28. Bell JG, Ludomirsky A, Bottalico J, Weiner S. The effect of improvement of umbilical artery end-diastolic velocity on perinatal outcome. *Am J Obstet Gynecol* 1992;167:1015–1020.
29. Ombelet W, Nuradi S, Vandenberge K, Spitz B, Van Assche A. Absent or reversed end diastolic flow in the umbilical arteries: A warning sign of serious fetal compromise. *Clin Exp Pregn* 1988;B7(3):303–316.
30. Guzman E, Schulman H, Bracero L, Rochelson B, Farmakides G, Coury A. Uterine-umbilical artery Doppler velocimetry in pregnant women with systemic lupus erythematosus. *J Ultrasound Med* 1992;11:275–281.
31. Benifla JL, Tchobroutsky C, Uzan M, Sultan Y, Weill BJ, Laumond-Barny S. Predictive value of uterine artery velocity waveforms in pregnancies complicated by systemic lupus erythematosus and the antiphospholipid syndrome. *Fet Diagn Ther* 1992;7:195–202.
32. Hastie SJ, Danskin F, Neilson JP, Whittle MJ. Prediction of the small for gestational age twin fetus by Doppler umbilical artery waveform analysis. *Obstet Gynecol* 1989;74:730–733.
33. Giles WB, Trudinger BJ, Cook CM, Connelly AJ. Umbilical artery waveforms in triplet pregnancy. *Obstet Gynecol* 1990;75:813–816.
34. Rafla NM. Surveillance of triplets with umbilical artery velocimetry waveforms. *Acta Genet Med Gemellol* 1989;38:301–304.
35. Cohen LS, Sabbagha RE, Keith LG, Chasnoff IJ. Doppler umbilical velocimetry in women with polydrug abuse including cocaine. *Int J Gynaecol Obstet* 1991;36:287–290.
36. Weiner CP, Grant SS, Williamson RA. Relationship between sec-

ond trimester maternal serum alpha-fetoprotein and umbilical artery Doppler velocimetry and their association with preterm delivery. *Am J Perinatol* 1991;8:263–268.

37. Barrett JFR, Oskamp M, Farine D, et al. The relationship between elevated second trimester maternal serum alpha-fetoprotein levels (MSAFP) to abnormal third trimester doppler velocimetry. Poster presentation, Society of Obstetricians and Gynecologists of Canada, Ottawa, Ontario, June 22–26, 1993.

38. Bekedam DJ, Visser GHA, van der Zee AGJ, Snijders RJM, Poelmann-Wessjes G. Abnormal velocity waveforms of the umbilical artery in growth retarded fetuses: Relationship to antepartum late heart rate decelerations and outcome. *Early Hum Dev* 1990;24:79–89.

39. Hackett GA, Campbell S, Gamsu H, Cohen-Overbeek T, Pearce JM. Doppler studies in the growth retarded fetus and prediction of neonatal necrotising enterocolitis, haemorrhage and neonatal morbidity. *Br Med J* 1987;294:13–16.

40. Hanretty KP, Whittle MJ, Rubin PC. Reappearance of end-diastolic velocity in a pregnancy complicated by severe pregnancy induced hypertension. *Am J Obstet Gynecol* 1988;158:1123–1124.

41. Brar HS, Platt LD. Antepartum improvement of abnormal umbilical artery velocimetry: Does it occur? *Am J Obstet Gynecol* 1989;160:36–39.

42. Harper MA, Murnaghan GA. Discordant umbilical flow velocity wave forms and pregnancy outcome. *Br J Obstet Gynecol* 1989;96:1449–1450.

43. Nicolaides KH, Campbell S, Bradley RJ, Bilardo CM, Soothill PW, Gibb D. Maternal oxygen therapy for intrauterine growth retardation. *Lancet* 1987;1:942–945.

44. Arduini D, Rizzo G, Mancuso S, Romanini C. Short-term effects of maternal oxygen administration on blood flow velocity waveforms in healthy and growth-retarded fetuses. *Am J Obstet Gynecol* 1988;159:1077–1080.

45. Karsdorp VHM, van Vugt JMG, Dekker GA, van Geijn HP. Reappearance of end-diastolic velocities in the umbilical artery following maternal volume expansion: A preliminary study. *Obstet Gynecol* 1992;80:679–683.

46. Nicolaides KH, Bilardo CM, Soothill PW, Campbell S. Absence of end diastolic frequencies in umbilical artery: A sign of fetal hypoxia and acidosis. *Br Med J* 1988;297:1026–1027.

47. Ashmead GG, Lazebnik N, Ashmead JW, Stepanchak W, Mann LI. Normal blood gases in fetuses with absence of end-diastolic umbilical artery velocity. *Am J Perinatol* 1993;10:67–70.

48. Pattison RC, Hope P, Imhoff R, Manning N, Mannion V, Redman CW. Obstetric and neonatal outcome in fetuses with absent end-diastolic velocities of the umbilical artery: A case-controlled study. *Am J Perinatol* 1993;10:135–138.

49. Huneke B, Carstensen MH, Schroder HJ, Gunther M. Perinatal outcome in fetuses with loss of end-diastolic blood flow velocities in the descending aorta and/or umbilical artery. *Gynecol Obstet* 1991;32:167–172.

50. Weiss E, Ulrich S, Berle P. Condition at birth of infants with previously absent or reverse umbilical artery end-diastolic flow velocities. *Arch Gynecol Obstet* 1992;252:37–43.

51. Gudmundsson S, Lindblad A, Marsal K. Cord blood gases and absence of end-diastolic blood velocities in the umbilical artery. *Early Hum Dev* 1990;24:231–237.

52. Fairlie FM, Moretti M, Walker JJ, Sibai BM. Determinants of peri-natal outcome in pregnancy-induced hypertension with absence of umbilical artery end-diastolic frequencies. *Am J Obstet Gynecol* 1991;164:1084–1089.

53. Nicolini U, Nicolaides P, Fisk NM, et al. Limited role of fetal blood sampling in prediction of outcome in intrauterine growth retardation. *Lancet* 1990;336:768–772.

54. Pattison RC, Norman K, Odendaal HJ. The role of Doppler velocimetry in the management of high risk pregnancies: A randomized controlled trial. *J Mat Fet Investig* 1993;3:182.

55. Woo JSK, Liang ST, Lo RLS. Significance of an absent or reversed end diastolic flow in Doppler umbilical artery waveforms. *J Ultrasound Med* 1987;6:291–297.

56. Hsieh FJ, Chang FM, Ko TM, Chen HY, Chen YP. Umbilical artery flow velocity waveforms in fetuses dying with congenital abnormalities. *Br J Obstet Gynaecol* 1988;95:478–482.

57. Weiner CP, Wenstrum KD, Sipes SL, Williamson RA. Risk factors for cordocentesis and fetal intravascular transfusion. *Am J Obstet Gynecol* 1991;165:1020–1025.

58. Maxwell DJ, Johnson P, Hurley P, et al. Fetal blood sampling and pregnancy loss in relation to indication. *Br J Obstet Gynaecol* 1991;98:892–897.

59. Gudmundsson S, Tuzler G, Huhta JC, Marsal K. Venous Doppler velocimetry in fetuses with absent end-diastolic blood velocity in the umbilical artery. *J Mat–Fet Investig* 1993;3:196.

60. Weiss E, Ulrich S, Berle P. Blood flow velocity waveforms of the middle cerebral artery and abnormal neurological evaluations in live-born fetuses with absent or reverse end-diastolic flow velocities of the umbilical arteries. *Eur J Obstet Gynaecol Reprod Biol* 1992;45:93–100.

61. McParland P, Steel S, Pearce JM. The clinical implications of absent or reversed end-diastolic frequencies in umbilical artery flow velocity waveforms. *Eur J Obstet Gynaecol Reprod Biol* 1990;37:15–23.

62. Ryan G, Morrow R, Kelly E, Farine D, Ritchie JWK. Absent umbilical artery diastolic flow using doppler ultrasound: Clinical implications. *Proc. of the Ninth Annual Meeting of the Society of Perinatal Obstetricians.* New Orleans, February 1989.

63. Brar HS, Platt LD. Reverse end-diastolic flow velocity on umbilical artery velocimetry in high-risk pregnancies: An ominous finding with adverse pregnancy outcome. *Am J Obstet Gynecol* 1988;159:559–561.

64. Rochelson B, Schulman H, Farmakides G, et al. The significance of absent end-diastolic velocity in umbilical artery velocity waveforms. *Am J Obstet Gynecol* 1987;156:1213–1218.

65. Mattice K, Anderson CF, Reed KL. Neonatal outcome in fetuses with absent end diastolic velocity in the umbilical artery. *Pediatr Res* 1989;37(1):145A.

66. Malcolm G, Elwood D, Devonald K, Beilby R, Henderson-Smart D. Absent or reversed end-diastolic flow velocity in the umbilical artery and necrotising enterocolitis. *Arch Dis Child* 1991;66:805–807.

67. Kelly E, Ryan G, Farine D, Morrow R, Inwood S, Ritchie JWK. Absent end umbilical artery velocity (AEDV): Short and long term outcome. *J Mat–Fet Invest* 1993;3:203.

68. Farine D, Ryan G, Kelly EN, Morrow RJ, Laskin C, Ritchie JW. Absent end-diastolic flow velocity waveforms in the umbilical artery: The subsequent pregnancy. *Am J Obstet Gynecol* 1993;168:637–640.

Doppler Ultrasound in Obstetrics and Gynecology.
edited by Joshua A. Copel and Kathryn L. Reed.
Raven Press, Ltd., New York © 1995.

CHAPTER 21

Fetal Behavioral States

J. W. Wladimiroff, J. van Eyck, and T. W. A. Huisman

It has been demonstrated that variables such as fetal eye movements, fetal heart rate (FHR) pattern, and FHR changes associated with fetal mortality are closely related to the neurologic condition of the fetus. Behavioral states in the newborn are temporarily stable conditions of neural and anatomic fluctuations such as sleep and wakefulness. A classification of behavioral states in the full-term newborn was first introduced by Prechtl and Beintema (1) on state criteria such as eyes open/closed, respiration regular/irregular, and body movements present/absent.

In the human fetus behavioral states were studied from FHR recordings alone (2,3) and in conjunction with body movements (4,5), resulting in the description of quiet and active phases. The observations did not provide conclusive proof of the presence of true behavioral states in the human fetus since both FHR and fetal heart variability are affected by fetal motility (6). Nijhuis et al. defined four fetal behavioral states (7), with the most important ones as follows:

State 1F, representing quiescence (quiet sleep state), which can be regularly interrupted by brief gross body movements, mostly startles. Eye movements are absent. The fetal heart rate is stable, with a narrow oscillation band. Isolated FHR accelerations occur, strictly related to movements. This FHR pattern is called FHR pattern A.

State 2F (active sleep state), which comprises frequent and periodic gross body movements, mostly stretches and retroflections, and movements of the extremities. Eye movements are continuously present. FHR (pattern B) shows a wider oscillation band than pattern A. Frequent FHR accelerations occur in association with movements.

Based on the marked changes in FHR pattern and the incidence of fetal body movements between different behavioral states, it is not unlikely that these changes are associated with alterations in fetal cardiovascular performance. With the introduction of combined real-time and pulsed Doppler systems a noninvasive method became available for studying fetal hemodynamics in relation to fetal behavior.

Fetal and umbilical placental Doppler flow velocity waveform studies have demonstrated the presence of centralization of the circulation in the small-for-gestational-age (SGA) fetus (8). The clinical significance of abnormal umbilical artery waveforms in SGA fetuses is clearly reflected in the increased maternal and neonatal admission rates (neonatal intensive care unit) observed in these pathologic pregnancies (Marsal, personal communication). For a correct interpretation of recorded data it is important to establish the influence of internal fetal variables such as fetal breathing movements, FHR, fetal heart rhythm, and fetal behavioral states. An evaluation of the relationship between fetal behavioral states and fetal and umbilical placental flow velocity waveform patterns would be of interest from both the physiological and clinical points of view.

The objective of this chapter is to report on the relationship between arterial, venous, and cardiac flow velocity waveforms and fetal behavior states 1F and 2F in appropriate-for-gestational-age (AGA) and small-for-gestational-age (SGA) human fetuses.

ARTERIAL FLOW VELOCITY WAVEFORMS

Fetal Descending Aorta

In the AGA fetus at term flow velocity waveforms from the descending aorta display a clear relationship with behavioral states (9). Under standardized FHR conditions there is a statistically significant reduction in pulsatility index (PI) during behavioral state 2F compared

J. W. Wladimiroff and T. W. A. Huisman: Department of Obstetrics and Gynaecology, Academic Hospital Rotterdam-Dijkzigt, Rotterdam, The Netherlands.
J. van Eyck: Department of Obstetrics and Gynecology, Sophia Hospital, Zwolle, The Netherlands.

with PI during behavioral state 1F (Fig. 1). This behavioral state–related PI difference is nearly entirely determined by changes in end-diastolic flow velocities. The marked reduction in PI during state 2F therefore suggests a reduced peripheral vascular resistance at fetal trunk and lower extremity level with the objective to increase perfusion of the fetal skeletal musculature to meet the raised energy demands associated with motor activity during this particular behavioral state. An inverse relationship was established between PI and fetal heart rate in both behavioral states 1F and 2F (9). This inverse relationship, which was later confirmed by others (10), is mainly determined by the definition presented by Gosling and King (11) for PI calculations.

Raised PI values have been established in the descending aorta of the SGA fetus, suggesting a raised peripheral vascular resistance. As opposed to the AGA fetus in which PI values from the descending aorta are behavioral state–dependent, this phenomenon does not occur in the presence of SGA as demonstrated in Fig. 1 (12). This be-

havioral state independency may be explained by the fact that chronic hypoxia, probably present in SGA, stimulates the peripheral chemoreceptors (13,14) and subsequent release of vasoconstrictive agents such as vasopressin and catecholamines (15–17). The peripheral vasoconstriction seems to overrule state-dependent PI fluctuations. Again there was an inverse relationship between PI and FHR, which was even more pronounced than in normal growth (Fig. 1).

Since at term, FHR pattern, eye movements, and body movements align with short transition periods from combined presence to combined absence and vice versa, it is not possible to analyze whether one of these state variables is particularly associated with the observed PI changes in the descending aorta in the normal growing human fetus at term. At 27–28 weeks of gestation there are episodes of low and high FHR variability with and without eye movements and body movements. There is no proper synchronization in the cyclic appearance of these variables. Periods of coincidence often occur by chance and will result in the occurrence of eight combinations of state parameters, providing the opportunity to evaluate the relationship between these single-state parameters and PI. Using this method for analysis it has been documented that in the normal growing human fetus at 27–28 weeks of gestation, the PI in the lower thoracic part of the fetal descending aorta displays a statistically significant reduction during periods of high FHR variability compared to that during periods of low FHR variability irrespective of fetal eye or body movements (18).

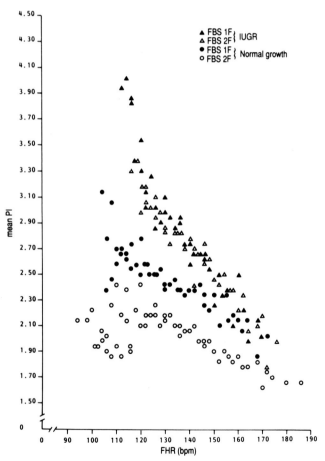

FIG. 1. Mean pulsatility index (PI) in the fetal descending aorta during fetal behavioral state (FBS) 1F and 2F relative to fetal heart rate (FHR, bpm) in normal fetal growth and intrauterine growth retardation (IUGR) at 37–38 weeks of gestation. From van Eyck et al. (12).

Fetal Intracerebral Arteries

The increase in cerebral blood flow during REM sleep (active sleep), compared with that during non-REM sleep (quiet sleep), has been shown in animals (19), human neonates (20), and adults (21). Comparison of cerebral blood flow measured by microspheres and pulsed Doppler in young piglets (22) and newborn lambs (23) demonstrated that peak systolic and end-diastolic blood flow velocities as well as the area under the velocity curve, reflecting the shape of the waveform, closely correlate with cerebral blood flow. Since the PI is determined by all three variables, the observed reduction of this index under standardized FHR conditions suggests an increase in cerebral blood flow during behavioral state 2F.

Following the introduction of Doppler ultrasound studies in fetal intracranial vessels (24), it was observed that under standardized FHR conditions in AGA fetuses there was a statistically significant reduction in PI in the internal carotid artery during behavioral state 2F compared with behavioral state 1F (Fig. 2) (25). Recent

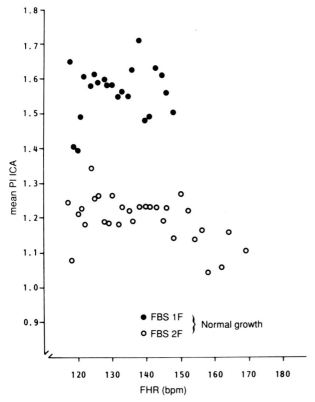

FIG. 2. Mean pulsatility index (PI) in the fetal internal carotid artery (ICA) during fetal behavioral state (FBS) 1F and 2F relative to fetal heart rate (FHR, bpm) in normal fetal growth at 37–38 weeks of gestation.

unpublished data indicate similar behavioral state–dependent changes in PI in the anterior, middle, and posterior cerebral artery (Noordam et al., unpublished data). This reduction in intracerebral arterial PI suggests a reduced peripheral vascular resistance in the fetal cerebral circulation. In both behavioral states 1F and 2F, PI is inversely related to FHR. During the last 4 weeks of pregnancy there is a fall in PI in the fetal internal carotid artery with maintenance of behavioral state dependency (26) suggesting a hemodynamic redistribution favoring blood supply to the brain during the latter weeks of gestation.

In the presence of an SGA fetus, PI showed no behavioral state dependency (Fig. 3) (27). In contrast to the marked increase in PI in the fetal descending aorta, state independency in the fetal internal carotid artery was associated with only a moderate reduction in PI, suggesting the onset of circulatory redistribution with the aim of favoring cerebral blood flow (brain-sparing effect).

Umbilical Artery

Both in the AGA fetus (25,28) and the SGA fetus at term it was shown that under standardized FHR conditions, umbilical artery PI is fetal behavioral state-independent. This is of clinical importance since it means that in term pregnancies Doppler measurements can be performed in the umbilical artery without prior fetal behavioral state determination. It also suggests that the behavioral state–dependent changes in the fetal descending aorta and fetal intracerebral arteries are of fetal origin.

CARDIAC FLOW VELOCITY WAVEFORMS

The introduction of recording techniques at ductus arteriosus (29) and foramen ovale level (30) opened the possibility of studying the influence of fetal behavioral states on cardiac hemodynamics. Ductal peak systolic

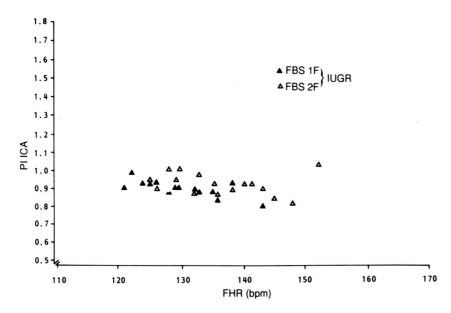

FIG. 3. Mean pulsatility index (PI) in the fetal internal carotid artery (ICA) during fetal behavioral state (FBS) 1F and 2F relative to fetal heart rate (FHR, bpm) in intrauterine growth retardation (IUGR) at 37–38 weeks of gestation.

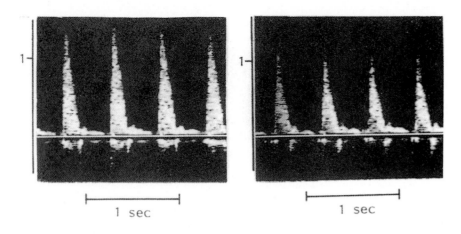

FIG. 4. Maximum flow velocity waveforms from the ductus arteriosus during fetal behavioral state (FBS) 1F (**left**) and 2F (**right**) in the normal growing fetus at 37–38 weeks of gestation. From van der Mooren et al. (31).

velocities were significantly reduced during behavioral state 2F compared to that during state 1F (Fig. 4). This suggests redistribution in left ventricular and right ventricular output in favor of the left side of the heart (31). Moreover, it was demonstrated that ductal peak systolic velocity is FHR-independent (31) and is modulated by fetal breathing movements (32). Blood flow velocity waveforms at the foramen ovale level are characterized by a typical systolic/diastolic component, as demonstrated in Fig. 5 (30). Time-average–flow velocities were statistically significantly increased in behavioral state 2F compared to that in 1F. This was mainly determined by an increase in flow velocity during the end-systolic and passive atrial filling phase, as demonstrated in Fig. 5. The increase in the time-averaged flow velocity at the foramen ovale level during behavioral state 2F suggests a redistribution of blood flow at cardiac level resulting in an increased right-to-left shunt, substantiating the behavioral state–related changes observed in the ductus arteriosus.

VENOUS FLOW VELOCITY WAVEFORMS

The documented increase in blood flow velocities at the foramen ovale level is mainly determined by the end-systolic and passive atrial filling phase of the foramen ovale flow velocity waveform, suggesting increased passive atrial filling during diastole as a result of raised preload. This could be the result of raised inferior vena cava/ductus venosus flow. Since the foramen ovale blood flow is mainly determined by well-oxygenated ductus venosus

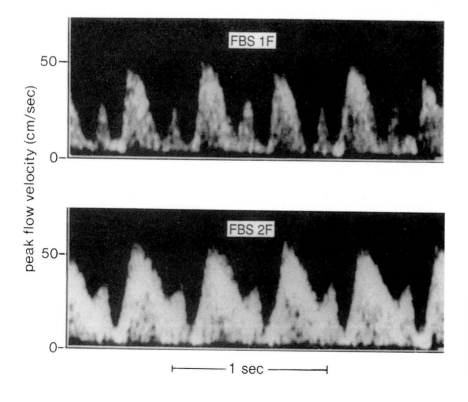

FIG. 5. Maximum flow velocity waveforms at foramen ovale level during fetal behavioral state (FBS) 1F (**top**) and 2F (**bottom**) in the normal growing fetus at 37–38 weeks of gestation. From van Eyck et al. (30).

blood flow, this mechanism could explain the behavioral state–related redistribution of blood flow at cardiac level, resulting not only in raised left ventricular cardiac output but in increased preferential streaming of well-oxygenated blood directly to the left side of the heart and subsequently to the cerebral circulation and descending aorta.

Of interest is our observation of an approximately 30% increase in peak systolic and peak diastolic flow velocity as well as time-averaged velocity in the ductus venosus during behavioral state 2F as compared with state 1F (Fig. 6) (33). The equal rise in peak systolic and peak diastolic flow velocity during fetal behavioral state 2F suggests augmented volume flow through the ductus venosus during this behavioral state. An increase in volume flow through the ductus venosus during behavioral state 2F would be consistent with the rise in volume flow at

foramen ovale (30) and mitral valve level (34) during this behavioral state.

CONCLUSIONS

In normal pregnancies, fetal neurologic development expressed by the emergence of fetal behavior and eventually resulting in well-defined fetal behavior states is clearly associated with specific hemodynamic adaptations that can be demonstrated by Doppler flow measurements. No such behavioral state dependency could be demonstrated for the umbilical artery. An increase in blood flow to the left heart is suggested with the purpose to meet raised energy demands at fetal cerebral and trunk level during the active sleep state (state 2F). This is supported by a rise in preload observed during this behavioral state.

In the SGA fetus behavioral state independency was established on the arterial side of the fetal circulation. This may be part of the process of cardiovascular adaptation in the SGA fetus, which in turn leads to centralization of the circulation with maintenance of optimal blood flow to the fetal brain, adrenals, and heart. Finally, it was established that in both behavioral states 1F and 2F, PI values obtained from the fetal descending aorta, internal carotid artery, and umbilical artery were inversely related to FHR.

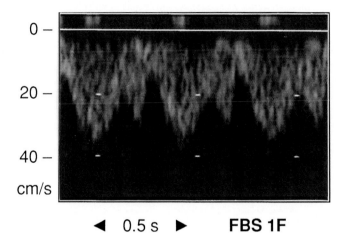

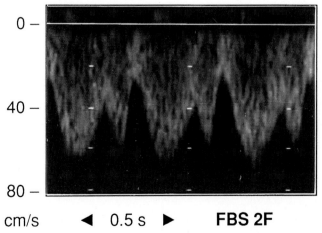

FIG. 6. Maximum flow velocity waveforms from the ductus venosus during fetal behavioral state (FBS) 1F and 2F in the normal growing fetus at 37–38 weeks of gestation.

REFERENCES

1. Prechtl HFR, Beintema DJ. The neurological examination of the full-term newborn infant. In: *Clinics in developmental medicine.* London: Heinemann; 1964;12:74.
2. Junge HD. Behavioral states and related heart rate and motor activity patterns in the newborn infant and the fetus antepartum; a comparative study. I. Technique, illustration of recordings and general results. *J Perinat Med* 1979;7:85–103.
3. Van Geijn HP, Jongsma HW, de Haan J, Eskes TKAB, Prechtl HFR. Heart rate as an indicator of the behavioral state: Studies in the newborn infant and prospects for fetal heart rate monitoring. *Am J Obstet Gynecol* 1980;136:1061–1066.
4. Timor Tritsch IE, Dierker LJ, Zador I, Hertz RH, Rosen MG. Fetal movements associated with fetal heart rate accelerations and decelerations. *Am J Obstet Gynecol* 1978;131:276–280.
5. Natale R, Nasello-Paterson C, Turliuk R. Longitudinal measurement of fetal breathing, body movement, heart rate, and heart rate accelerations and decelerations at 24 to 32 weeks of gestation. *Am J Obstet Gynecol* 1985;151:256–263.
6. Wheeler T, Guerard P. Fetal heart rate during late pregnancy. *J Obstet Gynaecol Br Commonwealth* 1974;81:348–356.
7. Nijhuis JG, Prechtl HFR, Martin CB Jr., Bots RSGM. Are there behavioural states in the human fetus? *Early Hum Dev* 1982;6:177–195.
8. Groenenberg IAL, Wladimiroff JW, Hop WCJ. Fetal cardiac and peripheral arterial flow velocity waveforms in intrauterine growth retardation. *Circulation* 1989;80:1711–1717.
9. Van Eyck J, Wladimiroff JW, Noordam MJ, Tonge HM, Prechtl HFR. The blood flow velocity waveform in the fetal descending aorta; its relationship to fetal behavioural states in normal pregnancy at 37–38 weeks of gestation. *Early Hum Dev* 1985;12:137–143.

10. Van den Wijngaard JAGW, van Eyck J, Wladimiroff JW. The relationship between fetal heart rate and Doppler flow velocity waveforms. *Ultrasound Med Biol* 1988;14:593–597.

11. Gosling RG, King DH. Ultrasound angiology. In: Harcus AW, Adamson L, eds. *Arteries and veins.* Edinburgh: Churchill Livingstone; 1975:61–98.

12. Van Eyck J, Wladimiroff JW, Noordam MJ, Tonge HM, Prechtl HFR. The blood flow velocity waveform in the fetal descending aorta; its relationship to behavioural states in the growth retarded fetus at 37–38 weeks of gestation. *Early Hum Dev* 1986;14:99–107.

13. Dawes GS, Lewis BV, Milligan IE, Roach MR, Talner NS. Vasomotor responses in the hind limbs of foetal and newborn lambs to asphyxia and aortic chemoreceptor stimulation. *J Physiol* 1968;195:55–81.

14. Itskovitz J, Goetzman BW, Rudolph AM. The mechanism of late deceleration of heart rate and its relationship to oxygenation in normoxemic and chronically hypoxemic fetal lambs. *Am J Obstet Gynecol* 1982;142:66–73.

15. Iwamoto HS, Rudolph AM, Keil LC, Heymann MA. Hemodynamic responses of the sheep to vasopressin infusion. *Clin Res* 1979;44:430–436.

16. Mott JC. Humoral control of the fetal circulation. In: Jones CT, Nathanielsz PW, eds. *The physiological development of the fetus and newborn.* London: Academic Press; 1985:113–121.

17. Oosterbaan HP. *Amniotic oxytocin and vasopressin in the human and the rat.* PhD thesis. University of Amsterdam; 1985.

18. Van Eyck J, Wladimiroff JW, Noordam MJ, Cheung KL, van den Wijngaard JAGW, Prechtl HFR. The blood flow velocity waveform in the fetal descending aorta; its relationship to fetal heart rate pattern, eye and body movements in normal pregnancy at 27–28 weeks of gestation. *Early Hum Dev* 1988;17:187–194.

19. Reivich M, Isaacs G, Evarts E, Kety S. The effect of slow wave sleep and REM sleep on regional cerebral blood flow in cats. *J Neurochem* 1968;15:301–306.

20. Mukhtar AI, Cowan FM, Stothers JK. Cranial blood flow and blood pressure changes during sleep in the human neonate. *Early Hum Dev* 1982;6:59–64.

21. Townsend RE, Prins PN, Obrist WD. Human cerebral blood flow during sleep and waking. *J Appl Physiol* 1973;35:620–625.

22. Hansen NB, Stonestreet BS, Rosenkrantz TS, Oh W. Validity of Doppler measurements of anterior cerebral artery blood flow velocity: correlation with brain blood flow in piglets. *Pediatrics* 1983;872:526–531.

23. Rosenberg AA, Narayanan V, Douglas Jones Jr. M. Comparison of anterior cerebral blood flow velocity and cerebral blood flow during hypoxia. *Pediatric Research* 1985;19:67–70.

24. Wladimiroff JW, Tonge HM, Stewart PA. Doppler ultrasound assessment of cerebral blood flow in the human fetus. *Br J Obstet Gynaecol* 1986;93:471–475.

25. Van Eyck J, Wladimiroff JW, van den Wijngaard JAGW, Noordam MJ, Prechtl HFR. The blood flow velocity waveform in the fetal internal carotid and umbilical artery; its relationship to fetal behavioural states in normal pregnancy at 37–38 weeks of gestation. *Br J Obstet Gynaecol* 1987;94:736–741.

26. Van den Wijngaard JAGW, van Eyck J, Noordam MJ, Wladimiroff JW, van Strik R. The Doppler flow velocity waveform in the fetal internal carotid artery with respect to behavioural states. A longitudinal study. *Biol Neonate* 1988;53:274–278.

27. Van Eyck J, Wladimiroff JW, Noordam MJ, van den Wijngaard JAGW, Prechtl HFR. The blood flow velocity waveform in the fetal internal carotid and umbilical artery; its relationship to fetal behavioural states in the growth-retarded fetus at 37–38 weeks of gestation. *Br J Obstet Gynaecol* 1988;95:473–477.

28. Mulders LGM, Muyser GJJM, Jongsma HW, Nijhuis JG, Hein PR. The umbilical artery blood flow velocity waveform in relation to fetal breathing movements, fetal heart rate and fetal behavioural state in normal pregnancy at 37–39 weeks. *Early Hum Dev* 1986;11:283–293.

29. Huhta JC, Moise KJ, Fisher DJ, Sharif DS, Wasserstrum N, Martin C. Detection and quantification of constriction of the fetal ductus arteriosus by Doppler echocardiography. *Circulation* 1987;75:406–412.

30. Van Eyck J, Stewart PA, Wladimiroff JW. Human fetal foramen ovale flow velocity waveforms relative to behavioral states in normal term pregnancy. *Am J Obstet Gynecol* 1990;163:1239–1242.

31. Van der Mooren K, van Eyck J, Wladimiroff JW. Human fetal ductal flow velocity waveforms relative to behavioural states in normal term pregnancy. *Am J Obstet Gynecol* 1989;160:371–374.

32. Van Eyck J, van der Mooren K, Wladimiroff JW. Ductus arteriosus flow velocity modulation by fetal breathing movements as a measure of fetal lung development. *Am J Obstet Gynecol* 1990;163:558–566.

33. Huisman TWA, Brezinka Ch, Stewart PA, Stijnen Th, Wladimiroff JW. Ductus venosus flow velocity waveforms relative to fetal behavioural states in normal term pregnancy. *Br J Obstet Gynaecol* 1994; *in press.*

34. Rizzo G, Arduini D, Valensise H, Romanini C. Effects of behavioural states on cardiac output in the healthy human fetus at 36–38 weeks of gestation. *Early Hum Dev* 1990;23:109–115.

Doppler Ultrasound in Obstetrics and Gynecology,
edited by Joshua A. Copel and Kathryn L. Reed.
Raven Press, Ltd., New York © 1995.

CHAPTER 22

The Normal Fetal Heart

Kathryn L. Reed

Doppler echocardiography was first used in the 1960s to examine human fetuses (1,2). The use of Doppler ultrasound, a noninvasive technique, has allowed obstetricians and pediatric cardiologists (among others) to study normal and abnormal fetal cardiac function. Prior to the introduction of Doppler ultrasound, knowledge about fetal cardiac function was limited to heart rate analysis, inference from two-dimensional ultrasound studies or autopsy examinations, and extrapolation of results from animal studies that used invasive techniques.

The fetal heart differs from the adult heart in several ways (3–5) (Table 1). These differences explain some of the results from Doppler studies. The placenta rather than the lungs is the major source of fetal oxygen, and intracardiac flow in the fetus includes two major shunts—the foramen ovale and the ductus arteriosus. Right-to-left shunting takes place through the foramen ovale and the ductus arteriosus, which are normally patent in the fetus. These shunts, along with the ductus venosus, allow more highly oxygenated blood to flow from the umbilical vein to the left atrium, ascending aorta, and brain. Less oxygenated blood from the superior vena cava and portions of the inferior vena cava flow into the right ventricle, across the ductus arteriosus to the descending aorta. Thus, during each cardiac cycle, both ventricles simultaneously eject blood into the systemic circulation. Branch pulmonary arteries receive relatively little flow in the fetus (7–8% of the combined cardiac output in lambs) (4), since the lungs are unnecessary to fetal life and pulmonary vascular pressures are high (4). Other major differences include a normal heart rate of 120–160 beats per minute (bpm), decreased ventricular compliance (6), increased cardiac output (and venous return) (7), and low arterial blood pressure and peripheral resis-

tance. The fetal partial pressure of oxygen is low by adult standards, although the oxygen content of systemic arterial blood is only slightly lower; oxygen extraction is approximately 30% (8).

CANDIDATES FOR FETAL ECHOCARDIOGRAPHY

Doppler echocardiography is used in fetuses with a history of relatives with congenital heart disease, fetuses of mothers with conditions that may result in the development of fetal cardiac abnormalities, fetuses of mothers who use drugs or who are exposed to teratogens known or suspected to cause fetal cardiac abnormalities, and fetuses that have abnormalities of structure or function discovered during the pregnancy (Table 2) (9).

TECHNIQUE

The Doppler examination of the fetal heart begins with an assessment of cardiac anatomy using two-dimensional ultrasound. Transvalvar flows are obtained by placing the Doppler gate just distal to the valve under investigation (Figs. 1 and 2). The Doppler beam should be as close to parallel to the estimated direction of flow as possible. If the angle is greater than 30° between the Doppler beam and the estimated direction of flow, errors in calculation of mean and peak velocities become potentially large.

Regurgitation is detected by moving the gate into the vessel or chamber from which blood is flowing. It may be most easily identified using color Doppler (Chapter 8). Flow in the direction opposite normal, of varying duration and velocity during the inappropriate time in the cardiac cycle, may indicate the presence of regurgitation.

K. L. Reed: Department of Obstetrics and Gynecology, Arizona Health Sciences Center, Tucson, AZ 85724.

TABLE 1. *Differences in cardiac function compared with adults*[a]

Anatomic differences:
Patent foramen ovale
Patent ductus arteriosus
Right ventricle larger than left
Right ventricle more hemispheric in cross-section than after birth

Physiologic differences:

Increased	*Decreased*
Mean systemic pressure	Blood pressure
Venous return	Resistance to venous return
Higher LV afterload compared with RV afterload	Systemic vascular compliance
Filling pressure	Ventricular compliance
Volume flow	Peripheral resistance
RV flow compared with LV flow	Pulmonary blood flow
Heart rate	pO_2
	O_2 saturation

RV, right ventricle; LV, left ventricle.
[a] Differences are compared with adult normals unless noted. From Reed (3).

Stenoses may restrict flow and velocities will frequently increase through the affected structure. Again, the increased velocity jet may be most easily identified using color Doppler. However, since blood flow through the fetal ventricles is in parallel, blood may simply take an alternate route and stenoses may not be identified until after delivery.

Atrioventricular valve velocities are obtained from a four-chamber view, placing the Doppler gate just distal to the valve leaflets. Both tricuspid and mitral valve velocities may be obtained from this view (Fig. 1). Regurgitation is detected by moving the gate into the respective atrium, where reverse flow may be detected if regurgitation is present.

Aortic velocities may be obtained from a variation of the four-chamber view as the aorta exits the left ventricle (Fig. 1). Pulmonary valve velocities may be obtained from the short-axis view (Fig. 1). Techniques for obtaining caval (superior and inferior vena cava) velocities are described in Chapter 29. Flows through the ductus arteriosus are discussed in Chapter 32.

Peak-velocities are measured from the zero line to the peak of the time–velocity integral (Figs. 3 and 4). Usually

TABLE 2. *Candidates for fetal echocardiography*

Family history of congenital heart disease
Predisposing maternal condition
Exposure to teratogen
Abnormal pregnancy progression

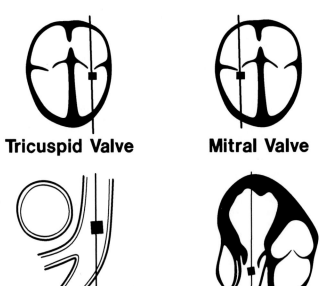

FIG. 1. Schematic of cardiac views from which to obtain Doppler flow velocity tracings. (*clockwise, from upper left*): tricuspid valve, mitral valve, aorta, pulmonary artery.

two peaks are present in atrioventricular valve velocity tracings; the initial peak during passive filling in early diastole (*E*) and the second peak during the atrial contraction in late diastole (*A*). Mean velocities are obtained by measuring the areas of a series of time–velocity inte-

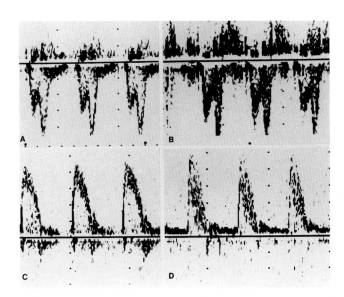

FIG. 2. Pulsed Doppler ultrasound tracings in a normal fetus. **A:** tricuspid valve; **B:** mitral valve; **C:** pulmonary artery; **D:** aortic valve. Dots are 0.5 sec apart on the horizontal axis. Direction of the peak corresponds with direction of blood flow, with flow above the line representing flow toward the transducer. Direction of peak will vary with the position of the fetus. (From Shenker et al. *Am J Obstet Gynecol,* 1988;158:1267–1973.)

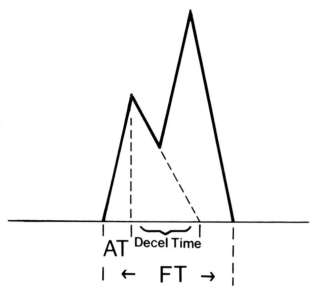

FIG. 3. Atrioventricular valve Doppler tracing. Two peaks are demonstrated: the first, which occurs during early diastole, and the second, which occurs during atrial contraction. Methods of measuring acceleration time (AT) and deceleration time (DT) are also demonstrated. Mean velocity may be calculated by digitizing the area under the curve and dividing by the time of the cardiac cycle. FT, filling time. From Reed (3).

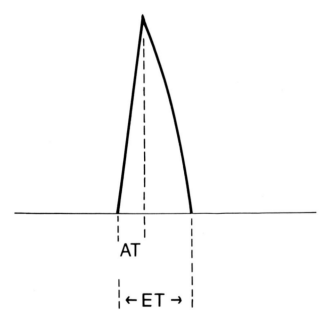

FIG. 4. Semilunar valve Doppler tracing. A single peak is present. Methods of measuring acceleration time (AT) are demonstrated. Mean velocity may be calculated by digitizing the area under the curve and dividing by the time of the cardiac cycle. ET, ejection time. From Reed (3).

TABLE 3. *Doppler measurements possible[a]*

Measurement	Method	Units
Peak or maximal velocity	Zero line to peak	cm/sec
Mean velocity	Time velocity integral/time of cardiac cycle	cm/sec
Volume flow	Mean velocity × area[b] × 60	ml/min
Acceleration time	Time from onset to peak	msec
Deceleration time	Time from peak to zero line along slope of descent	msec
A/E ratio	Peak velocity with atrial contraction (A)/peak velocity during early diastole (E)	

[a] Velocities should be measured within 30° of estimated direction of flow or be angle-corrected.
[b] Area obtained from diameters measured with two-dimensional ultrasound. From Reed (3).

grals and dividing by the time of the cardiac cycle. Acceleration times are measured from the onset of the time–velocity integral to the peak of the time–velocity integral. Deceleration times are measured from the peak of the time–velocity integral to the zero line along the slope of the deceleration. Filling and ejection times are measured from the onset to the termination of the time–velocity integral. Valve or vessel areas are measured from two-dimensional or M-mode imaging of the individual region of interest; areas are usually calculated from diameter measurements. Some of the types of measurements that can be made from the Doppler flow velocity waveforms are listed in Table 3.

The volume of blood flow (Q) may be calculated by multiplying the mean velocity (V) by the area (A) through which blood is flowing: $Q = VA$.

RESULTS

Normal fetal tricuspid, mitral, pulmonary artery, and aortic velocities are reported in Table 4. Velocities are relatively constant during the second and third trimesters. Valve measurements increase as the fetus grows, and therefore flow volumes increase. Right ventricular volume flow is greater than left ventricular volume flow by approximately 30%; however, this difference may vary widely (6). Ratios of late diastolic velocities (A) to early diastolic velocities (E) calculated from the atrioventricular transvalvar velocities decrease during gestation (10). This may be due in part to a decrease in heart rate or may result from a gradual increase in ventricular compliance with gestational age.

Measurements from normal fetuses are useful for comparison with measurements from fetuses with abnormal cardiac structure and function. These abnormalities are discussed in detail in other chapters of this book.

TABLE 4. *Normal Doppler measurements in the human fetus*

Valve	Tricuspid	Mitral	Pulmonary	Aorta
Maximal velocity (cm/sec)	51 ± 4	47 ± 4	60 ± 4	70 ± 3
Mean velocity (cm/sec)	12 ± 1	11 ± 1	16 ± 2	18 ± 2
Valve diameter (mm)[a]	8.0 ± 0.5	6.6 ± 0.4	7.6 ± 0.3	6.7 ± 0.2
Cardiac output (ml/kg/min)[a]	307 ± 30	232 ± 25	312 ± 11	250 ± 9
A/E ratio[a]	1.29 ± 0.04	1.35 ± 0.01	—	—
Deceleration time (msec)[a]	97 ± 29	110 ± 31	—	—
Acceleration time (msec)[a]	—	—	50.6 ± 12.0	46.7 ± 9.1

[a] Varies with gestational age.
From Reed (3).

SUMMARY

Studies of the fetal heart with two-dimensional Doppler ultrasound have allowed increased understanding of normal and abnormal fetal cardiac physiology and have improved the accuracy of prenatal diagnostic examinations.

REFERENCES

1. Callagan DA, Rowland TC, Goldman DE. Ultrasonic Doppler observation of the fetal heart. *Obstet Gynecol* 1964;23:637.
2. Johnson WL, Stegal HF, Lein JN, Rushmer RF. Detection of fetal life in early pregnancy with an ultrasonic Doppler flowmeter. *Obstet Gynecol* 1965;26:307.
3. Reed KL. Fetal Doppler echocardiography. *Clin Obstet Gynecol* 1989;32:728–737.
4. Rudolph AM. Distribution and regulation of blood flow in the fetal and neonatal lamb. *Circ Res* 1985;57:811–821.
5. Itskovitz J. Maternal-fetal hemodynamics. In: Maulik D, McNellis D, eds. *Reproductive and perinatal medicine. Vol. 8. Doppler ultrasound measurement of maternal fetal-hemodynamics.* Ithaca, NY: Perinatology Press, 1987:13–42.
6. Reed KL, Meijboom EJ, Scagnelli SA, Valdes-Cruz LM, Sahn DJ, Shenker L. Cardiac Doppler flow velocities in human fetuses. *Circulation* 1986;73:41–46.
7. Romero T, Covell J, Friedman WF. A comparison of pressure–volume relations of the fetal, newborn and adult heart. *Am J Physiol* 1972;222:1285.
8. Teitel DF. Physiologic development of the cardiovascular system in the fetus. In: Polin RA, Fox WW, eds. *Fetal and neonatal physiology.* Philadelphia: WB Saunders; 1992:609–619.
9. Reed KL, Sahn DJ. A Proposal for referral patterns for fetal cardiac studies. *Semin Ultrasound, CT, MR* 1984;5:249–252.
10. Reed KL, Sahn DJ, Scagnelli SA, Anderson CF, Shenker L. Doppler echocardiographic studies of diastolic function in the human fetal heart: Changes during gestation. *J Am Coll Cardiol* 1986;8:391–395.

Doppler Ultrasound in Obstetrics and Gynecology,
edited by Joshua A. Copel and Kathryn L. Reed.
Raven Press, Ltd., New York © 1995.

CHAPTER 23

The Abnormal Fetal Heart

Joshua A. Copel and Charles S. Kleinman

In contrast to the applications extensively dealt with in the other chapters of this text, much of clinical cardiac Doppler in the fetus relies on determination of flow patterns rather than comparative index measurement. Because of the unique circulation of the fetus, with the ventricles working in parallel with equal pressures normally generated in both (1), the flow patterns that occur in the presence of anatomic abnormalities differ from those seen in the neonate and older child. Extensive experience observing fetuses with structural heart disease has resulted in the current approach to the application and interpretation of both pulsed and color flow Doppler in fetal cardiac anomalies.

The normal flow patterns seen in the fetal heart are detailed in Chapter 22. The orderly progression of flow of oxygenated blood from the placenta via the ductus venosus and foramen ovale into the left atrium and ventricle (2) and then into the ascending aorta, as well as the direction of deoxygenated venous return from both the superior and inferior vena cavae across the tricuspid valve, through the right ventricle into the pulmonary artery and ductus arteriosus to the descending aorta, are the hallmarks of the normal fetal central circulation. These patterns may be influenced by cardiac pathology, and the resulting alterations can be used to confirm diagnoses suspected from the two-dimensional real-time examination. The basis of the examination must, however, be a firm understanding of the normal appearance of the fetal heart and the flow patterns typically seen.

ALTERATIONS IN FETAL FLOW

There are four major manifestations of disordered flow that may be detected in the fetus. The first is valvar regurgitation, most commonly seen at the level of the atrioventricular valves but also occurring at the semilunar valves. A second important flow perturbation is reversal of normal flow direction, typically seen in the great arteries distal to a critical semilunar valve obstruction. The third is absence of filling of a chamber, as may be seen with inflow obstruction, ventricular hypoplasia, or distal obstruction resulting in diminished ventricular compliance impeding further flow into a ventricle. Finally, malpositioned vessels may be visualized and identified based on their flow direction and pulsatile pattern.

Valvar Regurgitation

Atrioventricular valve regurgitation (Fig. 1) may be found in the presence of primary valve dysplasia (e.g., the Ebstein malformation of the tricuspid valve) or may be a secondary manifestation of pathologic damage of the papillary muscles (e.g., endocardial fibroelastosis accompanying critical aortic or pulmonic stenosis or primary cardiomyopathy). In these fetuses, biphasic diastolic flow is identified in the normal direction across the valve, and holosystolic flow is found in the reverse direction. Holosystolic regurgitation into the atrium typically results in atrial and ventricular dilation secondary to chronic volume overload. In addition to the systolic regurgitant jet, the relative noncompliance of the fetal ventricular cavities to diastolic filling (3) of the increased vascular volume imparts a significant risk of venous hypertension. Since about 92% of venous return to the fetal heart traverses the systemic veins and right atrium (1), systemic venous hypertension and consequent systemic edema and third spacing of fluid (hydrops fetalis) may

J. A. Copel: Department of Obstetrics and Gynecology, Yale University School of Medicine, New Haven, CT 06510.

C. S. Kleinman: Departments of Pediatrics, Diagnostic Imaging, and Obstetrics and Gynecology, Yale University School of Medicine, New Haven, CT 06510.

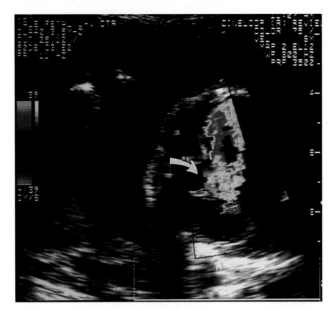

FIG. 1. Doppler color flow image of four-chamber view of fetus with Ebstein's malformation showing high-velocity regurgitant jet from right ventricle into enlarged right atrium (*curved arrow*).

accompany severe atrioventricular valve regurgitation (4).

In the fetus with Ebstein malformation the right atrium often becomes dramatically dilated due to the tricuspid valve incompetence. The asymmetrically dilated right atrium is often the cardinal sign drawing the attention of the sonographer. To establish the diagnosis of Ebstein malformation the septal leaflet of the tricuspid valve is visualized in an abnormal apically displaced location, and the anterior valve leaflet may appear thickened and sail-like in its motion. Normal biphasic diastolic flow can be seen across the tricuspid valve into the right ventricle, while the holosystolic regurgitant jet back into the atrium is usually of high velocity, often resulting in frequency aliasing if pulsed Doppler equipment is used. Using continuous wave Doppler, regurgitant velocities several meters per second may be identified.

Regurgitant velocity per se is not a barometer of disease severity since this is directly related by the Bernouilli equation ($P = 4V^2$) to the peak instantaneous pressure driving the regurgitation across the valve into the atrial cavity. A high-velocity jet may therefore suggest that there is a low atrial (venous) pressure or, conversely, could imply an elevated ventricular systolic blood pressure as might occur in the presence of an obstruction to ventricular outflow. A low regurgitant velocity may be evidence of a ventricle that is too impaired in function to generate a normal pressure. Huhta suggested that the rate of rise of the regurgitant jet (dP/dt) may be a means of assessing the rate of pressure development in the intact ventricle (5). This may serve as a means of assessing ventricular systolic pump performance. The detection of a

regurgitant velocity of >4 m/sec should raise the suspicion of a ventricular outlet obstruction (e.g., pulmonic stenosis or ductal constriction on the right side, aortic or subaortic obstruction on the left side) since fetal peak arterial pressure is not normally above 65 Torr and a regurgitant velocity of 4 m/sec implies a peak instantaneous pressure difference of 64 Torr.

The fetal heart differs from the postnatal heart because of both increased resting tension due to reduced compliance and diminished systolic contractile function due to relatively greater fibrous interstitial than muscular content (6). This limits the ability of the fetal heart to respond to changes in preload or afterload by the Frank–Starling mechanism. Although some ability exists to increase stroke volume and contractility using this mechanism, the fetal cardiovascular system is exquisitely rate-dependent for augmentation of cardiac output. The combination of structural heart disease and hydrops is frequently related to valve regurgitation, and virtually universally fatal (4). Even in the absence of hydrops, the dilated right heart associated with severe volume overload may be sufficient to compress the lung parenchyma and induce fatal lung hypoplasia (7).

Atrioventricular valve regurgitation may also occur due to papillary muscle dysfunction attending semilunar valve obstruction (8). Because a primary lesion of the tricuspid valve causing severe regurgitation and poor forward output may cause secondary pulmonic stenosis due to fused pulmonary valve leaflets (9), careful evaluation of both atrioventricular and semilunar valves is neces-

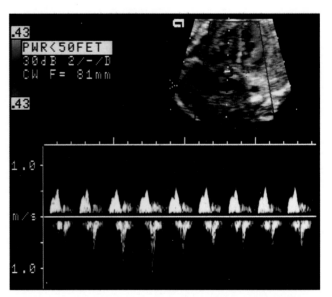

FIG. 2. Four chamber view with continuous wave Doppler of transtricuspid valve flow in a fetus with anemia secondary to parvovirus infection (fetal hematocrit 5%). Doppler sample indicated by cross-hatch on color flow map. Regurgitant flow is shown in blue at the same level. Spectral portion shows normal forward flow above baseline and early systolic regurgitation below baseline.

sary whenever regurgitation is seen. Tricuspid valve regurgitation may also be seen in severe fetal anemia, e.g., due to isoimmunization or parvovirus infection (Fig. 2), and fetuses with primary cardiomyopathies (10,11). It may also be seen in the recipient twin in the twin-to-twin transfusion syndrome (Fig. 3).

Assessment of the severity of atrioventricular valve regurgitation may be problematic. Disagreement exists regarding the grading of regurgitation in postnatal studies. While some workers have relied on color mapping of the size and depth of the regurgitant jet into the atrial cavity, others have relied on the width of the jet at the level of the atrioventricular valve leaflets (12). Certainly, marked atrial enlargement and abnormal systolic pulsations in the inferior vena cava and umbilical vein are evidence of severe atrioventricular valve regurgitation.

Atrioventricular valve regurgitation and atrial dilation may be complicated by the development of atrial tachy-arrhythmias. There appears to be a predilection for atrial flutter/fibrillation to occur in fetal hearts with dilated atria (13). Fetuses with the Ebstein malformation of the tricuspid valve may encounter a particular hazard due to their predilection for the Wolff–Parkinson–White syndrome (14).

Semilunar valve regurgitation is less common in the fetus but occurs in tetralogy of Fallot with absent pulmonary valve syndrome (15,16) (Fig. 4) and with cardiomyopathies (10). The volume overload of the fetal ventricle and the potential compromise of forward flow to the fetal body may be associated with hydrops fetalis. Marked pulmonary arterial dilation associated with the former syndrome may be associated with severe bronchial compression, bronchomalacia, and life-threatening respiratory distress in the neonate. Emmanouilides described a frequent association between tetralogy with absent pulmonary valve and congenital absence of the ductus arte-

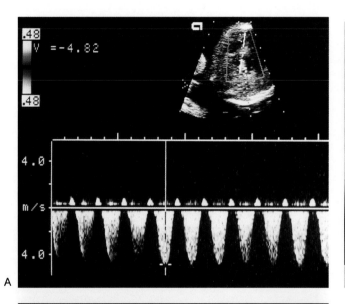

A

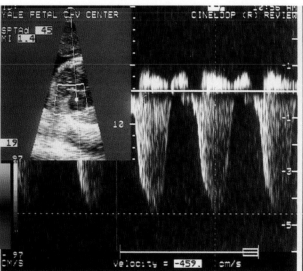

B

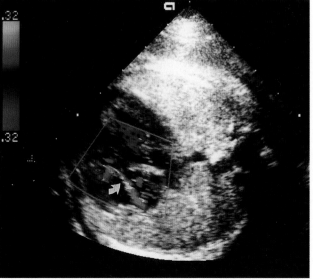

C

FIG. 3. A: Recipient twin in twin-to-twin transfusion syndrome demonstrating high-velocity tricuspid regurgitation. The continuous wave Doppler sample volume is in the regurgitant jet in the upper portion of the image, while the spectral waves are at the bottom. The peak instantaneous velocity is 4.82 m/sec. B: Same fetus 2 weeks later, with peak instantaneous velocity 4.59 m/sec. C: Same fetus 1 week later. The discrete jet of tricuspid regurgitation is seen in the right atrium (*small curved arrow*) with frequency aliasing seen as a red–yellow area in the center of the flow stream.

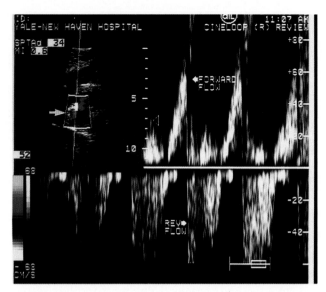

FIG. 4. Flow at the level of the pulmonary valve in a fetus with tetralogy of Fallot and absent pulmonary valve syndrome. The box in the upper left contains the two-dimensional and color flow image with the spectral Doppler sample volume. The bright blue (*arrow*) is from pulmonary valve regurgitation. Normal forward flow is seen above the spectral Doppler baseline, while the regurgitant flow (REV FLOW) is below the baseline with frequency aliasing appearing at the top of the figure.

riosus (17). It is unclear whether absence of the ductus is causative or, rather, imparts a survival advantage in avoiding the diastolic steal from the placental and systemic circulations that would occur if the aortic and pulmonary circulations were in free communication across the ductus in the presence of wide-open pulmonary valve regurgitation. In the presence of a ductus arteriosus we have documented marked negative descending aortic flow in a fetal patient with absent pulmonary valve syndrome.

Flow Reversal

The normal fetal cardiovascular system maintains forward flow in the great vessels throughout systole and diastole by means of forward pump flow and great vessel capacitance and elastic recoil. If flow into one of the great vessels is critically impaired, e.g., by obstruction of the aortic or pulmonic valve, the only access for blood into the distal vessel will be in a retrograde direction from the other great vessel, via the ductus arteriosus. Fetuses with mitral-aortic atresia or severe aortic stenosis will demonstrate retrograde filling of the aortic arch, which is generally hypoplastic secondary to low flow. The flow from the ductus arteriosus can be seen to branch as it enters the aorta, with normal flow down into the descending aorta as well as retrograde flow toward the arch and the brachiocephalic vessels (Fig. 5).

In both hypoplastic left heart syndrome (mitral-aortic

atresia with left ventricular hypoplasia) and hypoplastic right heart syndrome (tricuspid atresia with or without ventricular septal defect and small right ventricle), the great vessel downstream from the hypoplastic ventricular chamber will also become hypoplastic. It may be difficult to trace the small vessel because distortion of the usual tomographic planes obtained in fetal echocardiography may make assignment of great vessel location and assessment of whether the interventricular septum is intact somewhat difficult.

Color Doppler flow mapping can be instrumental in differentiating, for example, pulmonary atresia with a ventricular septal defect from persistent truncus arteriosus by allowing differentiation of flow into a hypoplastic main pulmonary artery vs. flow into pulmonary arteries arising directly from the truncal root. Because currently marketed color Doppler equipment is sensitive to low volumes of flow, even small volumes of flow into a hypoplastic vessel can be identified with sufficient patience and care.

Reversal of normal flow direction can also be seen in fetuses with left heart obstruction at the level of the foramen ovale (18). Whether this is a primary or a secondary lesion, fetuses with mitral and aortic obstruction, and even with coarctation of the aorta, reliably demonstrate reversal of the normal right-to-left flow pattern across the foramen (Fig. 6). More importantly, since ventricular disproportion on four-chamber screening has emerged as the single most common and important reason for referral for detailed echocardiographic study after level I sonography, it may be important to differentiate the underlying cause of right ventricular dilatation. We have

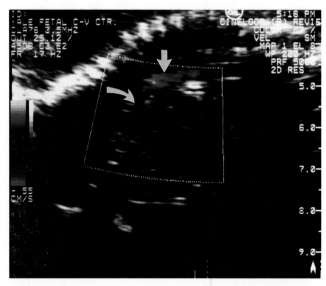

FIG. 5. Aortic arch in a fetus with mitral-aortic atresia and hypoplastic left heart syndrome. The spine is near the top of the image, and the area of red flow in the descending aorta (*straight arrow*) is derived from the ductus arteriosus. The blue flow in the narrow area of the arch (*curved arrow*) is retrograde filling, also from the ductus.

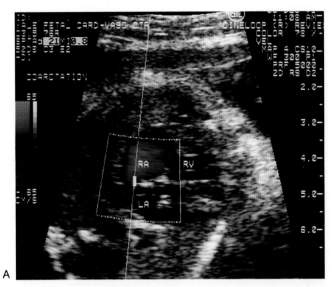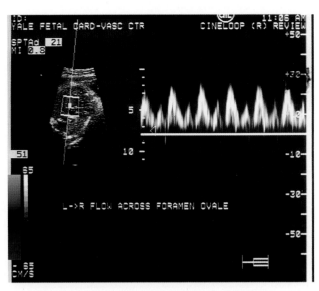

A B

FIG. 6. A: Doppler color flow mapping of four-chamber view of a fetus with coarctation of the aorta associated with Turner's syndrome (45,X). Flow from left atrium (LA) into right atrium (RA) across the foramen ovale is shown in red. RV, right ventricle. **B:** Pulsed Doppler spectral waveform of flow across the foramen ovale of the same fetus confirming the left-to-right reversal of normal flow direction.

noted that in such cases it may be difficult to distinguish primary right heart pathology from primary left heart pathology. Using Doppler color flow evaluation of foramen ovale size and flow may be critically important since small foramen ovale size and impaired or absent right-to-left shunting at this level is a highly reliable indicator of left heart obstruction/hypoplasia (18).

The importance of establishing the presence of these pathologic flow patterns is great because of the physiologic implications for the neonate. The fetus is easily able to tolerate the patterns described in this section, as opposed to the poor tolerance of the fetus for regurgitation as described in the previous section. On the other hand, the parallel circulation of the fetus is abolished in the neonate with closure of the ductus arteriosus and the foramen ovale. Advance knowledge that a ductal-dependent lesion is present permits preparations to be made for delivery at a tertiary center. Administration of prostaglandin E_1 can then be initiated soon after birth to prevent the disastrous consequences that ductal closure will have on a neonate whose systemic or pulmonary blood flow depends on persistent patency of the ductus arteriosus.

Absent Chamber Filling

Fetal cardiac disease is capable of evolving during the course of gestation. For example, fetal aortic stenosis may initially present with dilation of the left ventricle, with later progressive chamber hypoplasia due to lack of growth related to impaired flow over time even as the right ventricle continues to enlarge. The dilated chamber that is seen has little flow into it, and this can be demonstrated by color Doppler flow mapping (Fig. 7). The same

pattern may be seen in the fetus with a dilated left ventricle and echogenic myocardium due to endocardial fibroelastosis and impaired ventricular compliance and systolic emptying (19).

Before the failure of a ventricle to fill can be diagnosed with confidence, it is incumbent on the examiner to be certain that the incident angle between the Doppler beam and the stream of flow is optimal. With color Doppler flow mapping, flow into the contralateral ven-

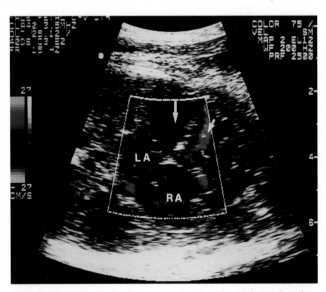

FIG. 7. Doppler color flow mapping image of four-chamber view of a fetus with interrupted aorta. Abnormal flow from the left atrium (LA) into the right atrium (RA) is seen in blue. The small arrow points to filling of the right ventricle in diastole, while the large arrow shows the absence of left ventricular filling. From Copel et al. (22).

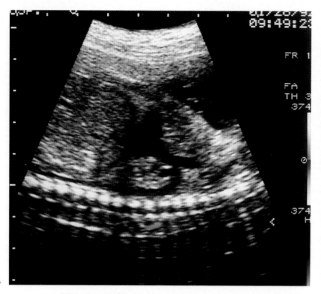
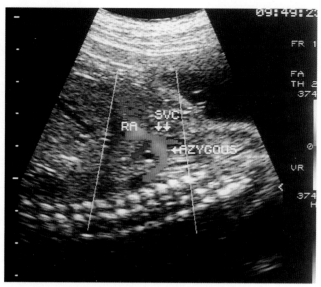

A | B

FIG. 8. (A) Two-dimensional and **(B)** Doppler color flow image of right parasagittal view of fetal thorax and abdomen in a patient with interruption of the inferior vena cava. The filling of the azygous vein with flow up toward the superior vena cava (SVC) is seen in red. The SVC then enters the right atrium (RA).

tricle can be used as a positive control (Fig. 7), since in the four-chamber view the flow streams into the two ventricles are roughly parallel.

Venous and Arterial Malpositions

Just as the course and identity of obstructed arteries may be clarified by Doppler, abnormal venous connections may also be evaluated by the combination of color and spectral Doppler. Fetuses with atrial isomerism may have complex abnormalities of the great veins. In left atrial isomerism the suprarenal portion of the inferior vena cava may be interrupted. Lower body venous return to the heart is channeled through the azygous vein, which sits posterior to the aorta, adjacent to the spine (20). Both color and spectral Doppler demonstrate venous flow toward the head in this large intrathoracic vessel, which then courses anteriorly in the upper thorax to enter the superior vena cava (Fig. 8).

Fetuses with right atrial isomerism may have complex abnormalities of pulmonary venous return, which may connect to a multitude of abnormal locations, including systemic veins below the diaphragm. Since the volume of blood flowing through the pulmonary veins of the fetus is small, less than 10% of fetal combined ventricular output (1), the veins may be hard to identify on fetal cardiac scans; nevertheless, with sufficient care the pulmonary veins can normally be seen entering the posterior wall of the left atrium (21) (see Chapter 31). In the presence of total anomalous pulmonary venous connection the posterior portion of the left atrium has not been formed and the left atrium appears hypoplastic. This apparent hypoplasia may be difficult to detect in the presence of atrial

isomerism, in which there is often the appearance of a single large atrial cavity. Whether the rare condition of partial anomalous pulmonary venous return can be correctly identified by Doppler fetal echocardiography remains to be demonstrated.

Ventricular Septal Defects

Detection of ventricular septal defects (VSDs) is important because they represent the most common cardiac anomalies. When a VSD is a part of a more com-

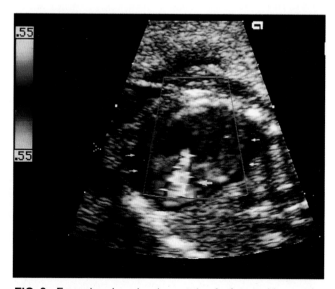

FIG. 9. Four-chamber view in systole of a fetus with an atrio-ventricular septal defect. The jet of regurgitation into the atrium is shown by the arrow. Small arrows highlight pericardial effusion.

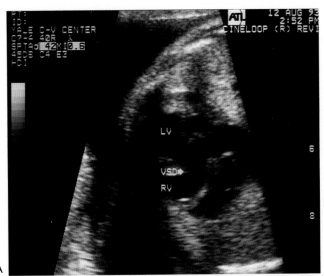
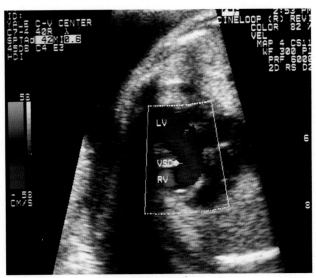

FIG. 10. (**A**) Two-dimensional and (**B**) Doppler color flow map of the four-chamber view in a fetus with tricuspid atresia and ventricular septal defect (VSD). The gap between the ventricles is clearly seen on the two-dimensional image, while the color image shows, in blue, the left-to-right flow that occurs because of the lack of flow across the tricuspid valve. The right ventricle is smaller than the left because of poor filling. LV, left ventricle; RV, right ventricle.

plex set of cardiac anomalies the issue of identification is often less pressing, since the VSDs that are present tend to be sizable and often are conotruncal defects, in which the ventricular septum and great arteries are malaligned, resulting in an easily identifiable arterial override of the VSD. The most common type of fetal cardiac anomaly encountered in our series has been the complete atrioventricular septal defect, also referred to as an endocardial cushion defect or an atrioventricular canal defect. Correct diagnosis of this abnormality rests in the identification of the common atrioventricular valve, with

valve tissue oriented on a single level, rather than the normal offset of the tricuspid valve toward the cardiac apex. Color flow mapping demonstrates a flow path across the common valve that branches as it reaches the crest of the muscular ventricular septum. The common atrioventricular valve may also display varying degrees of regurgitation, which may initially be identified as turbulent color flow regurgitation into either atrial cavity (Fig. 9). In our experience the majority (60–80%) of fetuses with atrioventricular septal defects will subsequently be found to have trisomy 21. Many of the re-

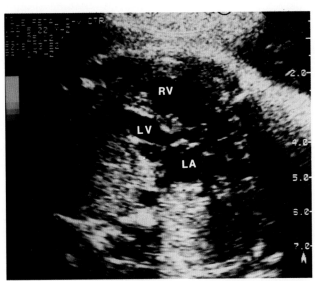
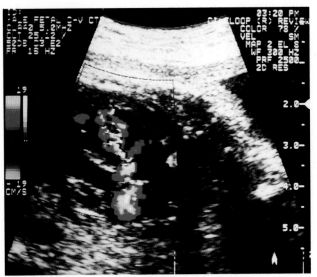

FIG. 11. (**A**) Two-dimensional and (**B**) Doppler color flow images of long axis of the left ventricle of the same fetus shown in Fig. 8. A high-velocity jet of flow is seen from the outflow portion of the left ventricle (LV) into the right ventricle (RV). The ventricular septal defect is smaller than the resolution limit of the two-dimensional image. LA, left atrium. From Copel et al. (22).

mainder will have some form of atrial isomerism. As noted above, a small jet of regurgitation is unlikely to present a critical challenge to the fetus, while holosystolic regurgitation is more problematic.

Fetuses with VSDs as part of a complex lesion that includes obstruction to flow may also demonstrate flow across the defect. For example, the fetus with tricuspid atresia and VSD will have flow from the left ventricle into the right across the defect (Fig. 10). When an outflow obstruction is present, blood will preferentially leave the ventricle through the channel with least resistance, whether that is across the stenotic valve or through a septal defect and into the contralateral great vessel (Fig. 11).

Small VSDs present a special dilemma in prenatal diagnosis. Because the pressures generated in otherwise healthy fetal ventricles are equal, there is minimal if any flow turbulence across small VSDs in the prenatal period. After birth, as a greater disparity develops between right and left ventricular pressures, the necessary pressure gradient develops for the classic high-velocity jet of flow turbulence to become apparent (23). In the absence of a concurrent downstream outflow obstruction, such small VSDs are unlikely to be associated with significant flow turbulence. For this reason small perimembranous and/or muscular ventricular septal defects, which are easily diagnosed after birth using a combination of physical findings and echocardiographic examination, may defy detection, even on exquisitely detailed fetal echocardiographic study.

UTILITY OF COLOR FLOW DOPPLER

Although there have been a number of reports on the use of color flow Doppler in fetal cardiac anomalies in the literature (24–26), there has been little critical evaluation of the utility of this expensive technology. In a retrospective analysis, we attempted to assign a relative contribution of color Doppler to the correct diagnosis of fetal cardiac disease and found that in 29% of cases it was essential to a correct diagnosis, while it was helpful in a further 47% and either not helpful or frankly misleading in the remaining 24% (22). The most striking aspect of the data was the separation of the groups based on the nature of the lesion, with an overrepresentation of fetuses with great vessel abnormalities in the group scored as "essential."

Based on this experience, we have concluded that color Doppler is an important tool for the laboratory making definitive fetal cardiac diagnoses because assignment of great-vessel patency and location has important prognostic implications and is therefore necessary for accurate patient counseling. On the other hand, the determination of the presence or absence of a fetal cardiac abnormality is rarely, if ever, solely dependent on the in-

formation provided by color Doppler flow mapping. We are unaware of any experience indicating that color flow Doppler has utility for detecting structural cardiac pathology in a screening situation in which two-dimensional screening examination has demonstrated normal four-chamber and outflow tract anatomy.

The identification of small vessels distal to obstructions or of small jets of valve regurgitation by color can be quite helpful in steering pulsed or continuous wave Doppler beams for spectral flow waveform analysis. The parallel circulation of the fetus reduces the usefulness of the Bernoulli equation for the assessment of pressure gradients because systemic pressure is maintained distal to the stenotic orifice by the other ventricle, so that a pressure drop across the stenotic valve cannot be assumed. The calculation may also not be valid when pump failure reduces the pressure difference across the stenotic valve due to low flow.

CONCLUSIONS

Two-dimensional assessment of fetal cardiac morphology and anatomy serves as the basis for the identification of fetal cardiac abnormalities. Appreciation of the specific patterns of flow can be instrumental in defining the nature of cardiac lesions and, more importantly, their functional consequences. In so doing, we can begin to understand the pathophysiology of secondary problems such as fetal hydrops, as well as the evolution of fetal heart disease. Finally, we can use the information gained to anticipate neonatal physiologic effects, such as the need for pharmacologic maintenance of ductal patency with intravenous prostaglandin E_1 in the neonate with critical valvar obstruction. This has allowed us to have a true impact on the care and outcome of fetuses affected by congenital heart disease.

REFERENCES

1. Rudolph AM. *Congenital diseases of the heart.* Chicago: Year Book; 1974.
2. Kiserud T, Eik-Nes SH, Blaas HG, Hellevik LR. Foramen ovale: An ultrasonographic study of its relation to the inferior vena cava, ductus venosus and hepatic veins. *Ultrasound Obstet Gynecol* 1992;2:389–396.
3. Romero T, Covell J, Friedman WF. A comparison of the pressure–volume relations of the fetal, newborn, and adult heart. *Am J Physiol* 1972;222:1285–1290.
4. Silverman NH, Kleinman CS, Rudolph AM, et al. Fetal atrioventricular valve insufficiency associated with nonimmune hydrops: A two-dimensional echocardiographic and pulsed Doppler ultrasound study. *Circulation* 1985;72:825–832.
5. Tulzer G, Gudmundsson S, Rotondo KM, Wood DC, Cohen AW, Huhta JC. Doppler in the evaluation and prognosis of fetuses with tricuspid regurgitation. *J Mat–Fet Invest* 1991;1:15–18.
6. Anderson PAW. Myocardial development. In: Long WA, ed. *Fetal and neonatal cardiology.* Philadelphia: WB Saunders; 1990:17–38.
7. Hornberger LK, Sahn DJ, Kleinman CS, Copel JA, Reed KL. Tricuspid valve disease with significant tricuspid insufficiency in the

fetus: Diagnosis and outcome. *J Am Coll Cardiol* 1991;17:167–173.

8. Guneroth WG, Cyr DR, Winter T, Easterling T, Mack LA. Fetal Doppler echocardiography in pulmonary atresia. *J Ultrasound Med* 1993;5:281–284.

9. Sharland GK, Chita SK, Allan LD. Tricuspid valve dysplasia or displacement in intrauterine life. *J Am Coll Cardiol* 1991;17:944–949.

10. Schmidt KG, Birk E, Silverman NH, Scagnelli SA. Echocardiographic evaluation of dilated cardiomyopathy in the human fetus. *Am J Cardiol* 1989;63:599–605.

11. Silverman NH, Schmidt KG. Ventricular volume overload in the human fetus: Observations from fetal echocardiography. *J Am Soc Echo* 1990;3:20–29.

12. Sanders SP. Echocardiography. In: Long WA, ed. *Fetal and neonatal cardiology.* Philadelphia: WB Saunders; 1990:301–329.

13. Kleinman CS, Copel JA. Electrophysiological principles and fetal antiarrhythmic therapy. *Ultrasound Obstet Gynecol* 1991;1:284–297.

14. Freedom RM, Benson LN. Ebstein's malformation of the tricuspid valve. In: Freedom RM, Benson LN, Smallhorn JF, eds. *Neonatal heart disease.* New York: Springer-Verlag; 1992:471–483.

15. Fouron J-C, Sahn DJ, Bender R, et al. Prenatal diagnosis and circulatory characteristics in tetralogy of Fallot with absent pulmonary valve. *Am J Cardiol* 1989;64:547–549.

16. Ettedgui JA, Sharland GK, Chita SK, Cook A, Fagg N, Allan LD. Absent pulmonary valve syndrome with ventricular septal defect: Role of the arterial duct. *Am J Cardiol* 1990;66:233–234.

17. Emmanouilides GC, Thanopoulos B, Siassi B, Fishbein M. "Agenesis" of ductus arteriosus associated with the syndrome of tetralogy of Fallot and absent pulmonary valve. *Am J Cardiol* 1976;37:403–409.

18. Feit LR, Copel JA, Kleinman CS. Foramen ovale size in the normal and abnormal human fetal heart: An indicator of transatrial flow physiology. *Ultrasound Obstet Gynecol* 1991;5:313–319.

19. Carceller AM, Maroto E, Fouron JC. Dilated and contracted forms of primary endocardial fibroelastosis: A single fetal disease with two stages of development. *Br Heart J* 1990;65:311–313.

20. Belfar HL, Hill LM, Peterson CS, et al. Sonographic imaging of the fetal azygous vein: Normal and pathologic appearance. *J Ultrasound Med* 1990;9:569–573.

21. DiSessa TG, Emerson DS, Felker RE, Brown DL, Cartier MS, Becker JA. Anomalous systemic and pulmonary venous pathways diagnosed in utero by ultrasound. *J Ultrasound Med* 1990;9:311–317.

22. Copel JA, Morotti R, Hobbins JC, Kleinman CS. The antenatal diagnosis of congenital heart disease using fetal echocardiography: Is color flow mapping necessary? *Obstet Gynecol* 1991;78:1–8.

23. Ortiz E, Robinson PJ, Deanfield JE, Franklin R, Macartney FJ, Wyse RKH. Localisation of ventricular septal defects by simultaneous display of superimposed colour Doppler and cross sectional echocardiographic images. *Br Heart J* 1985;54:53–60.

24. Devore GR, Hornstein J, Siassi B, Platt LD. Doppler color flow mapping: Its use in the prenatal diagnosis of congenital heart disease in the human fetus. *Echocardiography* 1985;2:551–557.

25. Sharland GK, Chita SK, Allan LD. The use of colour Doppler in fetal echocardiography. *Int J Cardiol* 1990;28:229–236.

26. Chiba Y, Kanzaki T, Kobayashi H, Murakami M, Yutani C. Evaluation of fetal structural heart disease using color flow mapping. *Ultrasound Med Biol* 1990;16:221–229.

Doppler Ultrasound in Obstetrics and Gynecology,
edited by Joshua A. Copel and Kathryn L. Reed.
Raven Press, Ltd., New York © 1995.

CHAPTER 24

The Evolution of Fetal Heart Disease

Mary Jo Rice, Robert W. McDonald, and David J. Sahn

Two-dimensional echocardiography revolutionized the diagnosis of congenital heart disease in the 1970s with a significant impact on the treatment and outcome of affected infants and children. Pulsed and continuous wave Doppler echocardiography came into wide use in the early 1980s and added considerable information regarding cardiac hemodynamics to the structural information from two-dimensional echocardiography that previously could only be obtained by invasive means. Color flow Doppler's introduction and later wide dissemination in the 1980s added further information about spatial distribution of flow as well as hemodynamic information about cardiac function and disease. An echocardiogram today is not a comprehensive assessment of the cardiac status without the use of all Doppler echocardiographic modalities.

The use of Doppler techniques in fetal echocardiography to improve definition of normal and abnormal fetal cardiac anatomy and physiology is therefore a logical step to a better understanding of the morphology and function of the fetal heart. The presence of congenital heart disease can be detected from a two-dimensional echocardiographic four-chamber view 85–95% of the time when performed by an experienced fetal echocardiographer (1,2) and can be detected 69% of the time on routine ultrasonography as early as 14–16 weeks gestation (3). Doppler echocardiography not only aids diagnosis of certain cardiac defects but can also provide a complete cardiac diagnosis and assess the cardiac status. Though there has been some concern about the higher energy exposure with the use of Doppler, the information obtained about normal and abnormal fetal cardiac flow has been invaluable in understanding human fetal cardiac work, flow related growth, and fetal cardiac function. Much information regarding fetal cardiac hemodynamics has been obtained from invasive work on animal

models but not all of these data may pertain to the human fetal heart and fetal echocardiography offers the only comprehensive noninvasive window to the human fetal heart.

METHOD OF FETAL DOPPLER

To use Doppler to assess the fetal heart, a thorough knowledge of two-dimensional echocardiographic cardiac structure is needed. The Doppler study can usually be performed in conjunction with the two-dimensional study since the same transducer is generally used. All two-dimensional echocardiographic exams of the fetal heart should undergo Doppler evaluation if there is suspected structural disease, rhythm abnormalities, or abnormal cardiac function.

Since normal flow velocities in the fetal heart are rarely greater than 1 m/sec, pulsed Doppler can be used to interrogate each valve (tricuspid, mitral, pulmonary, and aortic) as well as the ductus arteriosus and umbilical vessels (Fig. 1). The mitral and tricuspid valves are best evaluated from the four-chamber view, the pulmonary artery from the short-axis view, the ascending aorta from the five-chamber view (or aortic arch view), and the ductus arteriosus from the ductal arch view (Fig. 2). Color flow Doppler can aid in ascertaining the correct position of the Doppler sample volume. By obtaining quality waveforms across the cardiac valves, just distal to the valves themselves, normal and abnormal hemodynamic patterns can be evaluated.

Color flow Doppler can be used in a survey mode to detect abnormal or turbulent flow, which can then be further evaluated with pulsed or continuous wave Doppler as needed. This will keep the energy exposure from Doppler to a minimum, exposing only the fetuses with abnormal flow patterns to the higher energy pulsed and continuous wave modes and limiting the area of the fetal heart to which they are applied. Doppler flow velocities

M. J. Rice, R. W. McDonald, and D. J. Sahn: Oregon Health Sciences University, School of Medicine, Portland, OR 97201.

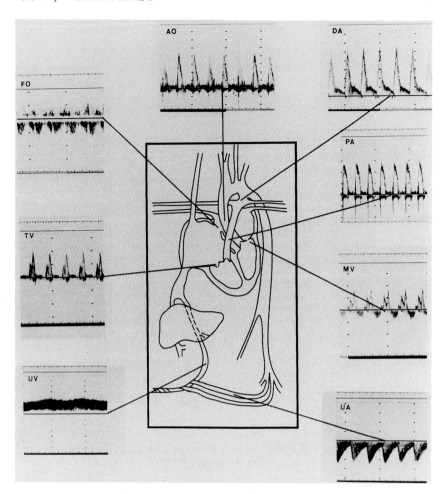

FIG. 1. Normal Doppler flow in the human fetus: pulmonary artery (PA), ascending aorta (AO), foramen ovale (FO), ductus arteriosus (DA), tricuspid valve (TV), mitral valve (MV), umbilical vein (UV), umbilical artery (UA).

should be obtained as parallel to flow as possible, keeping within 30° of the direction of blood flow.

For assessing ventricular output, the diameter of the atrioventricular valves are measured in diastole in the four-chamber view. The diameter of the aorta and pulmonary artery are measured just distal to the semilunar valves. By obtaining mean temporal flow velocities by planimetering Doppler waveforms, volume flow can be estimated through valves or vessels using the formula Vol = mean velocity × area × 60, where area = $\pi(d/2)^2$.

NORMAL FETAL DOPPLER PARAMETERS

To understand abnormal fetal Doppler measurements found in heart disease, the fetal echocardiographer must first be able to obtain normal fetal Doppler data and understand how fetal cardiac flow physiology changes during fetal life.

Doppler evaluation of the fetal heart was first attempted by Abelson and Balin (4). Maulik et al. (5) evaluated the Doppler tracing obtained in the pulmonary artery and with the pulmonary artery diameter calculated right ventricular stroke volume. They also noted changes in flow in the pulmonary and umbilical arteries during atrial extrasystoles. Several authors (6–8) noted that Doppler flow velocities through the atrioventricular

valves show a dominant A wave (Fig. 3) suggesting the increased importance of atrial systole in the fetus and implying decreased diastolic compliance. In addition, the A/E ratio decreases with increasing gestational age (7).

Tricuspid valve peak flow velocities are greater than mitral valve flow velocities (7,9) and calculated right ventricular output is about 1.3 times left ventricular output (8,9). Both these Doppler results confirm M-mode and two-dimensional as well as fetal animal studies that show there to be right ventricular dominance in the fetal heart.

Pulmonary artery peak flow velocities are lower than aortic flow velocities despite higher pulmonary artery flow volume (8,10). The ductus arteriosus has the highest normal flow velocities in the fetal circulation. Peak ductal velocities can be as high as 200 cm/sec during the last 4 weeks of pregnancy, which is thought to reflect increased right ventricular output secondary to decreased placental resistance through a fixed ductal diameter that has an active muscular tone that is hormonally maintained (11). Machado et al. (12) found the acceleration time (Fig. 4) in the pulmonary artery to be shorter than in the aorta, suggesting that pulmonary artery pressure or resistance may be higher than aortic. The right ventricle, with its larger output and preload, may also be less mechanically efficient than the left ventricle. Reed et al.

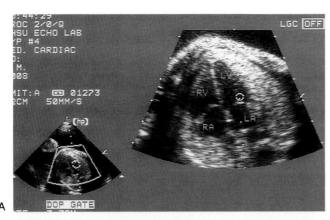
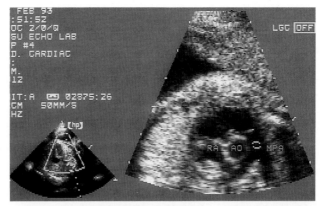
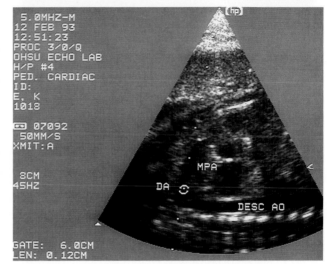
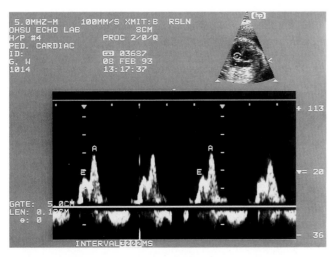

FIG. 2. Positioning of pulsed Doppler in fetal heart to obtain best flow profiles. **A:** Mitral and tricuspid flows are obtained from four-chamber view just beyond valve leaflets. **B:** Pulmonary flow is obtained from short-axis view in the main pulmonary artery. **C:** Aortic flow is obtained from five-chamber view in the ascending aorta. **D:** Ductal flow is obtained from ductal arch view at the aortic end of the ductus arteriosus. AO, ascending aorta; DA, ductus arteriosus; DESC AO, descending aorta; LA, left atrium; LV, left ventricle; MPA, main pulmonary artery; RA, right atrium; RV, right ventricle.

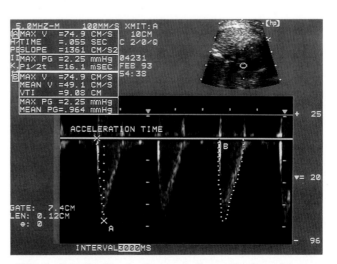

FIG. 3. Doppler flow velocity profile across tricuspid and mitral valves showing prominent A wave and *A/E* ratio greater than 1.

FIG. 4. Doppler flow in the ascending aorta (or pulmonary artery) demonstrating how acceleration time (AT) is measured. (A). Mean temporal velocity can be calculated by taking the area under the model velocity curve (B) and dividing by the ejection time (ET).

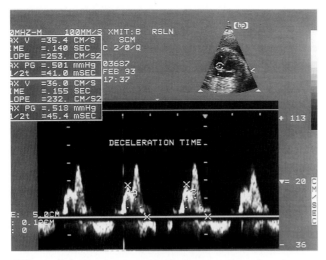

FIG. 5. Doppler flow across the mitral valve (or tricuspid valve) demonstrating how deceleration time (DT) is measured. Mean velocity can be calculated by taking the area under the curve and dividing by the filling time (FT).

(13) found tricuspid and mitral deceleration times (Fig. 5) to increase with increasing gestational age, suggesting an increase in ventricular compliance. Normal Doppler measurements are listed in Table 1.

EVOLUTION OF FETAL HEART DISEASE

Not only is echocardiography helpful in establishing a correct diagnosis of congenital heart disease, but the fetal cardiac structures can be followed over time to determine the natural history and progression of congenital heart disease *in utero*. Doppler techniques have been able to add to this assessment by documenting normal and abnormal hemodynamic changes with gestational age.

The normal changes in the fetal heart throughout gestation have been determined in several studies (7,8, 11,13–16). Allan et al. (17) were the first to describe progression in severity of a congenital heart defect during fetal life. In their case, a fetal echocardiogram at 21 weeks gestation showed an apparently normal aortic arch with a discrete coarctation. By 34 weeks the arch could not be completely visualized and postnatally severe arch and isthmic hypoplasia was found. Pulsed and color flow Doppler could have aided in demonstrating these changes by demonstrating changes in direction and patterns of flow.

Progression of semilunar valve stenosis, particularly pulmonary stenosis, has been shown in fetuses with tricuspid valve disease, presumably from lack of forward flow (18,19) and in tetralogy-like defects (20,21) as a part of the progression of these defects that has been seen postnatally as well. Doppler evaluation has been important in documenting this progression by showing increasing pulmonary flow velocities with progressive pulmonary stenosis and lack of retrograde pulmonary flow when pulmonary atresia occurs (Fig. 6). In two studies of fetuses with tricuspid valve disease, progression of right ventricular outflow tract obstruction (RVOT) was seen. In the study by Hornberger (18), 4 of 27 fetuses initially had normal forward flow in the pulmonary artery. On subsequent fetal echoes there was retrograde pulmonary artery and ductal flow with development of pulmonary stenosis in 1 and pulmonary atresia in 3. In the study by Sharland et al. (19), 5 of 38 fetuses had progression of RVOT from the prenatal to the postnatal study. In 2 fetuses, pulmonary stenosis was found prenatally but pulmonary atresia was present postnatally, and in 3 fetuses no pulmonary stenosis was detected prenatally but was found postnatally. There have also been two studies showing progression of RVOT in fetuses with tetralogy-like defects. In the study by Allan and Sharland (20), the pulmonary artery in 3 fetuses failed to grow with the fetus and therefore became relatively smaller. Similar findings were found by Rice et al. (21) in 2 fetuses (Fig. 7).

Bharati et al. (22) demonstrated *in utero* closure of the foramen ovale secondary to left heart disease. Doppler flow interrogation in their case documented normal patency of the foramen ovale and normal right-to-left atrial flow initially; later in gestation lack of flow across the foramen ovale suggested its closure.

Several authors raised the important issue of progressive disease by describing cases where they had seen normal cardiac anatomy on initial evaluation only to document heart disease later in pregnancy. In three studies, fetuses with normal examinations at 18–21 weeks gestation developed severe right ventricular inflow obstruction and right ventricular hypoplasia (2) or severe RVOT (23,24). In a study by Schmidt et al. (25), two of six fetuses that developed a dilated cardiomyopathy at or beyond 30 weeks gestation initially had a normal exam at 20 weeks gestation. There was also one fetus that had only tricuspid regurgitation at 26 weeks, but had developed a cardiomyopathy at 30 weeks gestation. Fetuses of

TABLE 1. *Normal Doppler flow velocities in the fetus (cm/sec)*

	Tricuspid	Mitral	Pulmonary	Aorta	Ductus	Foramen ovale
Maximal velocity	51 ± 4	47 ± 4	60 ± 4	70 ± 3	<150 Systolic <40 Diastolic	41±12 (Systolic)
Mean velocity	12 ± 1	11 ± 1	16 ± 2	18 ± 2	— —	

Data from Refs. 15,38, and 39.

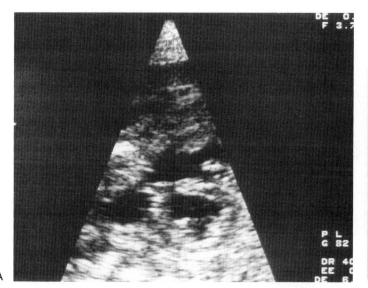

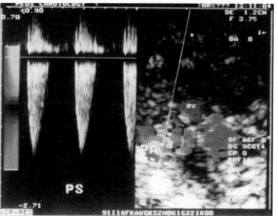

FIG. 6. Doppler flow in fetus with pulmonary stenosis showing pulmonary flow velocity (140 cm/sec) to be greater than aortic flow velocity (65 cm/sec), which is the opposite of normal.

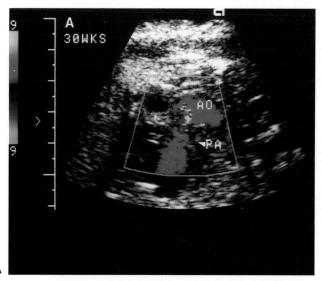

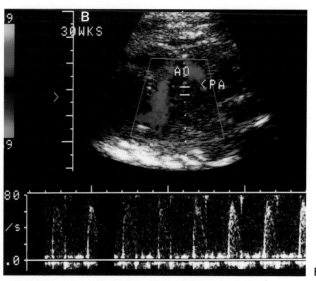

FIG. 7. At 30 weeks gestation in a fetus with a single ventricle, color Doppler (**A**) shows normal forward flow in the aorta (AO) and only a small amount of forward flow in the pulmonary artery (PA). Pulsed Doppler (**B**) also demonstrates forward flow in the pulmonary artery. At 38 weeks gestation, there was only retrograde flow in the pulmonary artery, suggesting development of pulmonary atresia.

diabetic women who have early normal echocardiographic exams can develop hypertrophic cardiomyopathy, particularly if the mother's diabetes is not well controlled. Anderson and Brown (26) described a fetus with a normal exam at 20 weeks gestation that had hypoplastic left heart syndrome at birth. Groves et al. (27) described a fetus with a normal exam at 18 weeks that had multiple tumors seen at 22 weeks gestation. Clearly, echocardiographic exams done at 18–22 weeks gestation can be normal and yet the fetus can develop severe cardiac defects later in gestation. This has prompted many centers to offer a second examination 6–8 weeks

later, particularly in cases where there is a family history of outflow obstruction or cardiomyopathy. In addition, Doppler echocardiography has helped to demonstrate progressive atrioventricular valve regurgitation (Fig. 8) often later associated with fetal hydrops (28) and subsequent deterioration of cardiac hemodynamics measured by Doppler.

Resolution or improvement in congenital heart defects has also been documented. Silverman and Golbus (29) first described a fetus with ventricular septal defect at 18 weeks gestation. On serial echocardiograms the defect decreased in size and was not present at birth. More

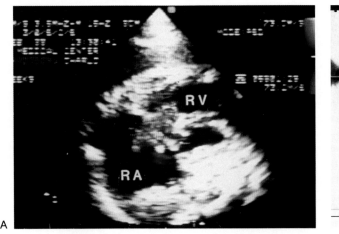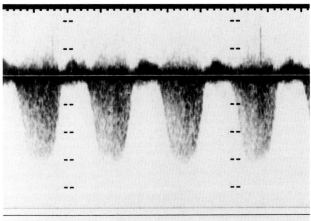

A   B

FIG. 8. Tricuspid regurgitation in a fetus with Ebstein anomaly by color flow Doppler (**A**) and pulsed Doppler (**B**). Flow velocity of the tricuspid regurgitation in 3 m/sec. LV, left ventricle; RA, right atrium; RV, right ventricle; TR, tricuspid regurgitation.

recently, Orie et al. (30) described a ventricular septal defect in 21 fetuses. The ventricular septal defects closed *in utero* in 15 (71%) and remained present at birth in 6. Recently, 2 fetuses with echocardiographic measurements, including Doppler studies, consistent with some degree of left heart hypoplasia have shown changes toward normal in echocardiographic measurements as pregnancy progressed and were subsequently found to have significantly less severe forms of left heart disease after birth (31).

Because fetal heart disease can change during pregnancy, these fetuses need close and repeated fetal echocardiographic evaluation to document the *in utero* natural history of fetal congenital heart disease and to detect changes in cardiac hemodynamics that can effect the fetus pre- or postnatally.

IMPORTANCE OF DOPPLER IN DIAGNOSIS OF CONGENITAL HEART DISEASE

Pulsed Doppler echocardiography has played an increasing role in the diagnosis of congenital heart disease. Doppler can not only help to identify disease and determine cardiac hemodynamics but allows a more accurate and comprehensive understanding of complex fetal congenital heart disease. The first cardiac abnormality detected by Doppler was atrioventricular valve regurgitation and it was found that this was often associated with fetal hydrops (28,32,33). Doppler has also been used to document abnormal ventricular output in fetuses with heart failure and in those with arrhythmias. Huhta et al. (32) showed decreased ventricular stroke volume with ectopic beats and suggested the technique of placing the

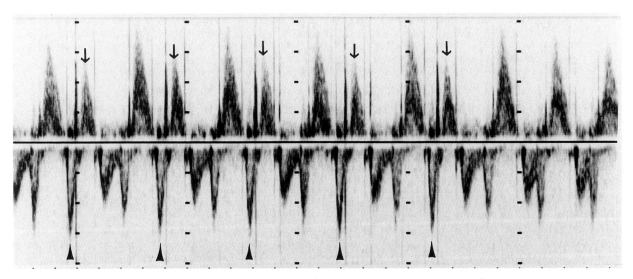

FIG. 9. Simultaneous Doppler inflow and outflow demonstrating premature atrial contractions (*arrowhead*) causing decreased ventricular output (*arrow*).

TABLE 2. *Changes in Doppler flow velocities with cardiac anomalies*

	Tricuspid valve	Mitral valve	Pulmonary artery	Aorta
Hypoplastic right ventricle	Decreased	Increased	Decreased	Increased
Hypoplastic left ventricle	Increased	Absent	Increased	Absent
Tricuspid atresia	Absent	Increased	Decreased	Increased
Ebstein's anomaly	Increased[a]	Increased	Decreased	Increased
Pulmonary atresia	Increased[a]	Increased	Absent	Increased
Tetralogy of Fallot	Unchanged	Unchanged	Decreased	Increased
Transposition of the great vessels	Unchanged	Unchanged	Unchanged	Unchanged
Double-outlet right ventricle	Increased	Decreased	Varies	Varies
Atrioventricular canal defect	Increased[a]	Increased[a]	Varies	Varies

Data from Ref. 15.
[a] Regurgitant flow may be present.

Doppler sample volume between the inflow and outflow tracts so that atrial and ventricular flow activity can be demonstrated simultaneously to aid in rhythm determination (Fig. 9). Maulik et al. (33) also showed decreased ventricular stroke volume with ectopic beats and, in addition, demonstrated increased ventricular stroke volume in congenital heart block.

Reed et al. (8,15) looked at several congenital heart defects and determined the abnormal Doppler flow velocities across the heart valves in the various defects (Table 2). As is seen postnatally, valve atresia can be demonstrated by no flow through the valve or retrograde flow in the associated great artery (34,35), valve stenosis can be associated with turbulent flow and increased flow velocities (Fig. 10), and valve regurgitation is demonstrable by turbulent retrograde flow when the valve should be closed (34,36,37). In a study by Allan et al. (38), Doppler helped to identify cases of coarctation or interrupted aortic arch, which can be difficult to diagnose by two-dimensional echocardiography, by showing decreased blood flow in the ascending aorta. Two cases thought to have a coarctation by two-dimensional exam were found to have normal Doppler flows and no coarctation postnatally. There were four false-positive cases with an abnormal two-dimensional and Doppler exam prenatally. Doppler can also aid in the evaluation of ventricular competence with outlet obstruction. In a study by Joulk and Rambaud (39), the fetal left ventricle was able to generate a flow velocity of 3.5 m/sec across a stenotic aortic valve suggesting, as is true postnatally, that there was adequate ventricular filling and systolic function.

Doppler echocardiography has been essential in identifying ductal constriction from prostaglandin synthetase inhibitors. Recently, Tulzer et al. (40) showed that increased systolic and diastolic flow velocities across the ductus arteriosus are only found with ductal constriction. An increase in only systolic ductal flow velocities can be seen with increased right ventricular output in fe-

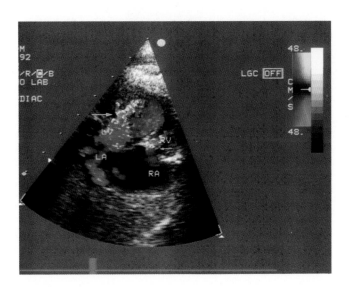

FIG. 10. Fetus with hypoplastic right ventricle and tricuspid stenosis showing turbulent flow across the tricuspid valve (*small arrow*). There is also turbulent flow across the mitral valve (*large arrow*) secondary to increased flow across this valve. LA, left atrium; LV, left ventricle; RA, right atrium; RV, right ventricle.

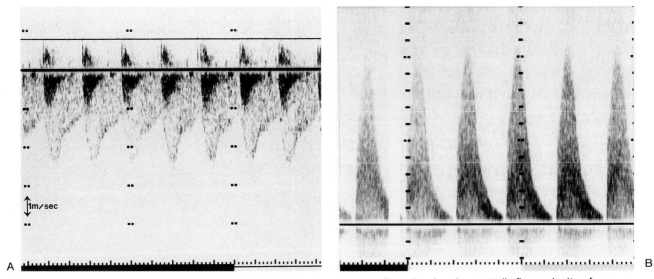

FIG. 11. **A:** Ductal constriction assessed by continuous wave Doppler showing systolic flow velocity of 240 cm/sec (normal <150 cm/sec) and diastolic flow velocity of 120 cm/sec (normal <40 cm/sec). **B:** Pulsed Doppler flow velocity in a fetus of 38 weeks gestation showing increased systolic flow velocity, 210 cm/sec, but normal diastolic flow velocity. Scale = 20 cm/sec.

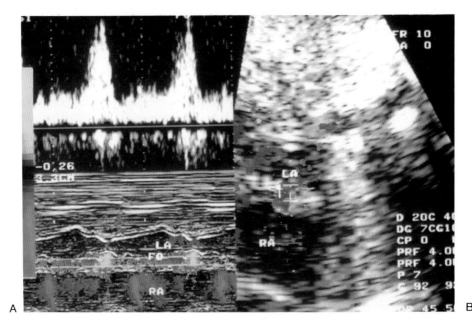

FIG. 12. Restrictive foramen ovale in fetus with a hypoplastic left heart showing **(A)** turbulent color flow Doppler jet from left atrium (LA) to right atrium (RA) and **(B)** increased flow velocity by pulsed Doppler, 100 cm/sec (normal 41 ± 12 cm/sec).

tuses exposed to terbutaline or in those with a hypoplastic left heart (Fig. 11).

The foramen ovale has also been studied by Doppler. Wilson et al. (41) defined normal two-dimensional and Doppler parameters of the foramen ovale so that restriction of the foramen ovale can be identified (42) (Fig. 12). Doppler, especially color flow Doppler, has also been able to help confirm the presence or absence of ventricular septal defects (43) (Fig. 13). Doppler can also identify whether echo free spaces are vascular and/or whether there is arterial or venous flow present (44–46). In a study by Maulik et al. (33), Doppler showed pulsatile flow in an echo-free space and an aneurysmal main pulmonary artery was identified in a fetus with tetralogy of Fallot.

Two groups (47–49) used Doppler during transvaginal examinations as early as 11 weeks gestation. There is of course more concern about using Doppler in the first trimester, but Doppler is the only way to study cardiac hemodynamics in the human fetus. Kurjak et al. (49) found that color flow Doppler facilitates detection of abnormalities on transvaginally performed studies and decreases the time of the exam in fetuses less than 12 weeks

gestation. Four-chamber and short-axis views as well as Doppler flows can be obtained and normal flow patterns determined. A fetus with atrioventricular canal was shown to have atrioventricular valve regurgitation by Doppler but also had outflow obstruction not appreciated on the two-dimensional exam alone.

Color flow Doppler can make a significant difference in the assessment of the fetal heart by Doppler. As a survey mode it can quickly identify normal and abnormal flow patterns in the fetal heart which then can be investigated further by pulsed or continuous wave Doppler as needed (Fig. 14). Color flow Doppler can also help to better align pulsed and continuous wave Doppler. The use of color flow Doppler was first reported in the fetal heart by DeVore et al. (50,51) to evaluate tricuspid regurgitation and atrial and ventricular septal defects. It was also found to be useful in assessing normal and abnormal inflow and outflow tracts. Gembruch et al. (52) found color flow Doppler helpful in identifying transposition of the great arteries and flow through the foramen ovale and ductus arteriosus. Chiba et al. (53) found color flow Doppler necessary for a complete diagnosis in 19

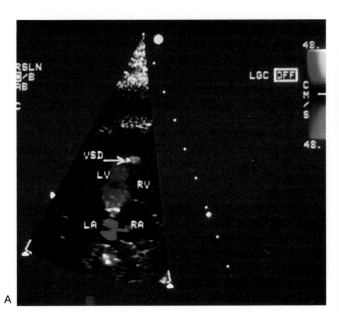

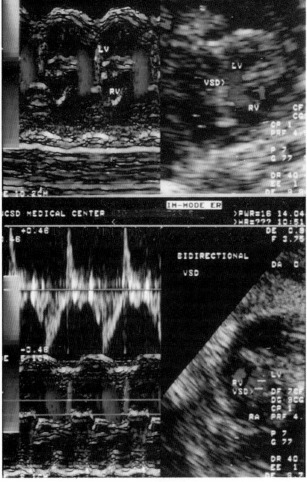

FIG. 13. Color flow Doppler demonstrating (**A**) a small muscular ventricular septal defect with a left-to-right shunt and (**B**) a perimembranous ventricular septal defect with a bidirectional but predominately right-to-left shunt. LA, left atrium; LV, left ventricle; RA, right atrium; RV, right ventricle; VSD, ventricular septal defect.

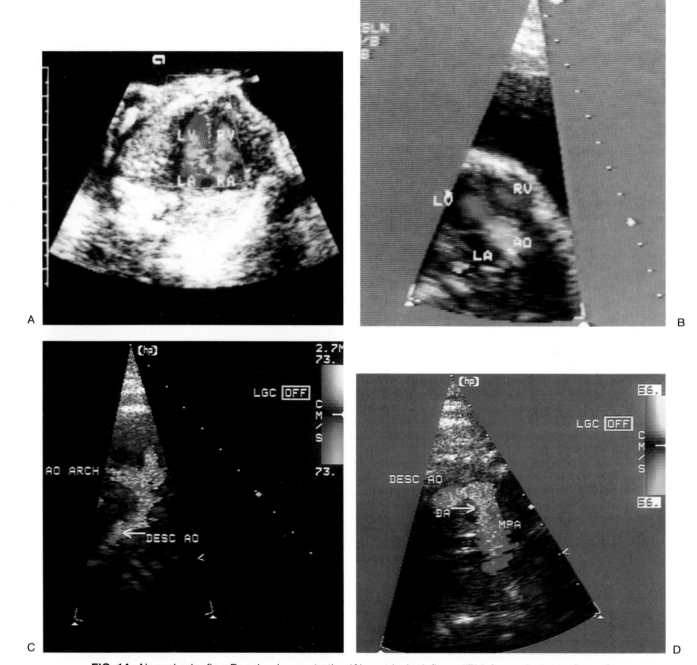

FIG. 14. Normal color flow Doppler demonstrating (**A**) ventricular inflows, (**B**) left ventricular outflow, (**C**) aortic arch, and (**D**) ductal arch. AO, ascending aorta, AO ARCH, aortic arch; DA, ductus arteriosus; DESC AO, descending aorta; LA, left atrium; LV, left ventricle; MPA, main pulmonary artery; RA, right atrium; RV, right ventricle.

cases of fetal congenital heart disease and 76% effective in detecting the presence of congenital heart disease. They demonstrated a "single blood flow stream" in defects such as atrioventricular canal and tricuspid atresia. They were also able to pick up more septal defects and functional abnormalities. Color flow Doppler can also help to identify the aortic and ductal arches and the direction of blood flow across cardiac communications (54).

In a study by Copel et al. (55), color flow Doppler was essential to a correct diagnosis in 29% of fetuses, primarily in showing the course and flow direction in the great arteries with obstruction or transposition and abnormal flow across the foramen ovale. It was helpful but not essential in 47% where it identified small jets of atrioventricular valve regurgitation and trivial septal defects. It added little to the diagnosis of congenital heart disease in 24%.

OTHER USES FOR FETAL DOPPLER

Doppler flow has been used to assess other fetal diseases and abnormalities that can affect the fetal heart. Its use to evaluate cardiac function in intrauterine growth retardation is addressed in Chapter 28.

In erythroblastosis fetalis, right and left ventricular output has been determined before and after transfusion by Doppler (56) as well as monitoring umbilical venous and arterial flows to avoid complications of cordocentesis (57).

Inferior vena caval flow has been studied and found to be abnormal in fetuses with arrhythmias and intrauterine growth retardation (58). There can be reversal of inferior vena caval flow with tachy- and bradyarrhythmias and increased forward flow in congenital heart block.

Doppler cardiac output has been used to assess the hemodynamic status in twin–twin transfusion (58). The cardiac output of the twins can distinguish the donor from the recipient as well as determine the risk of progressive circulatory compromise. The development of atrioventricular valve regurgitation by Doppler can also be an early indicator of compromised fetal cardiac functions.

Extracardiac vascular abnormalities with cardiac effects have also been diagnosed by Doppler. Cerebral arteriovenous malformations (32,60) and a cavernous hemangioma (61) have been identified.

Finally, perinatal changes in the normal fetal circulation have been evaluated by Doppler (62). The increase in left ventricular output that occurs postnatally appears to be secondary to increased stroke volume, not increased heart rate. The increase in stroke volume appears to be secondary to increased left ventricular size and contractility.

SUMMARY

Clearly Doppler evaluation of the fetal heart adds significant understanding of normal fetal cardiac hemodynamics as well as improving the understanding of fetal congenital heart disease. It can also document the progression of fetal cardiac disease during fetal life, which can affect prenatal and postnatal outcome. An abnormal fetal echocardiogram is no longer complete without a Doppler evaluation of the fetal heart.

Doppler echocardiography has already had a major impact on fetal cardiac diagnosis and management.

ACKNOWLEDGMENT

The authors thank Deborah Donaldson for manuscript preparation.

REFERENCES

1. Sherman FS, Sahn DJ. Pediatric Doppler echocardiography 1987: Major advances in technology. *J Pediatr* 1987;110:333–342.
2. Copel JA, Pilu G, Green J, Hobbins JC, Kleinman CS. Fetal echocardiographic screening for congenital heart disease: The importance of the four-chamber view. *Am J Obstet Gynecol* 1987;157:648–655.
3. Cullen S, Sharland GK, Allan LD, Sullivan ID. Potential impact of population screening for prenatal diagnosis of congenital heart disease. *Arch Dis Child* 1992;67:775–778.
4. Abelson D, Balin H. Analysis of the Doppler signals from the fetal heart. *Am J Obstet Gynecol* 1972;112:796–801.
5. Maulik D, Nanda NC, Saini VD. Fetal Doppler echocardiography: Methods and characterization of normal and abnormal hemodynamics. *Am J Cardiol* 1984;53:572–578.
6. Reed KL, Meijboom EJ, Sahn DJ, Scagnelli SA, Valdes-Cruz LM, Shenker L. Cardiac Doppler flow velocities in human fetuses. *Circulation* 1986;73:41–46.
7. Reed KL, Sahn DJ, Scagnelli S, Anderson CF and Shenker L. Doppler echocardiographic studies of diastolic function in human fetal heart: Changes during gestation. *J Am Coll Cardiol* 1986;8:391–395.
8. Reed KL. Fetal and neonatal cardiac assessment with Doppler. *Semin Perinatol* 1987;11:347–356.
9. Maulik D, Saini VD, Nanda NC, Rosenzweig MS. Doppler evaluation of fetal hemodynamics. *Ultrasound Med Biol* 1982;8:705–710.
10. Reed KL, Anderson CF, Shenker L. Fetal pulmonary artery and aorta: Two-dimensional Doppler echocardiography. *Obstet Gynecol* 1987;69:175–178.
11. van der Mooren K, Barendregt LG, Wladimiroff JW. Flow velocity wave forms in the human fetal ductus arteriosus during the normal second half of pregnancy. *Pediatr Res* 1991;30:487–490.
12. Machado MVL, Chita SC, Allan LD. Acceleration time in the aorta and pulmonary artery measured by Doppler echocardiography in the midtrimester normal human fetus. *Br Heart J* 1987;58:15–18.
13. Reed KL, Appleton CP, Sahn DJ, Anderson CF. Human fetal tricuspid and mitral deceleration time: changes with normal pregnancy and intrauterine growth retardation. *Am J Obstet Gynecol* 1989;161:1532–1535.
14. Kenny JF, Plappert T, Doubilet P, et al. Changes in intracardiac blood flow velocities and right and left ventricular stroke volumes with gestational age in the normal human fetus: A prospective Doppler echocardiographic study. *Circulation* 1986;74:1208–1216.
15. Reed KL. Fetal Doppler echocardiography. *Clin Obstet Gynecol* 1989;32:728–737.
16. van der Mooren K, Barendregt LG, Wladimiroff JW. Fetal atrioventricular and outflow tract flow velocity waveforms during normal second half of pregnancy. *Am J Obstet Gynecol* 1991;165:668–674.
17. Allan LD, Crawford DC, Tynan M. Evolution of coarctation of the aorta in intrauterine life. *Br Heart J* 1984;52:471–473.
18. Hornberger LK, Sahn DJ, Kleinman CS, Copel JA, Reed KL. Tricuspid valve disease with significant tricuspid insufficiency in the fetus: Diagnosis and outcome. *J Am Coll Cardiol* 1991;17:167–173.
19. Sharland GK, Chita SK, Allan LD. Tricuspid valve dysplasia or displacement in intrauterine life. *J Am Coll Cardiol* 1991;17:944–949.
20. Allan LD, Sharland GK. Prognosis in fetal tetralogy of Fallot. *Pediatr Cardiol* 1992;13:1–4.
21. Rice MJ, McDonald RW, Reller MD. Progressive pulmonary obstruction in the fetus: Two case reports. *Am J Perinatol* 1993;10:424–427.
22. Bharati S, Patel AG, Varga P, Husain AN, Lev M. In utero echocardiographic diagnosis of premature closure of the foramen ovale with mitral regurgitation and large left atrium. *Am Heart J* 1991;122:597–600.
23. Todros T, Presbitero P, Gaglioti P, Demarie D. Pulmonary stenosis with intact ventricular septum: Documentation of development of the lesion echocardiographically during fetal life. *Int J Cardiol* 1988;19:355–360.

24. Allan LD. Development of congenital lesions in mid or late gestation. *Int J Cardiol* 1988;19:361–362.
25. Schmidt KG, Birk E, Silverman NH, Scagnelli SA. Echocardiographic evaluation of dilated cardiomyopathy in the human fetus. *Am J Cardiol* 1989;63:599–605.
26. Anderson NG, Brown J. Normal size left ventricle on antenatal scan in lethal hypoplastic left heart syndrome. *Pediatr Radiol* 1991;21:436–437.
27. Groves AMM, Fagg NLK, Cook AC, Allan LD. Cardiac tumours in intrauterine life. *Arch Dis Child* 1992;67:1189–1192.
28. Silverman NH, Kleinman CS, Rudolph AM, et al. Fetal atrioventricular valve insufficiency associated with nonimmune hydrops: A two-dimensional echocardiographic and pulsed Doppler ultrasound study. *Circulation* 1985;72:825–832.
29. Silverman NH, Golbus MS. Echocardiographic techniques for assessing normal and abnormal fetal cardiac anatomy. *J Am Coll Cardiol* 1985;5:20S–29S.
30. Orie JD, Flotta DL, Sherman FS. To be or not to be a ventricular septal defect. *J Am Coll Cardiol* 1993;21:190A.
31. Marasini M, De Caro E, Pongiglione G, Ribaldone D, Caponnetto S. Left heart obstructive disease with ventricular hypoplasia: Changes in the echocardiographic appearance during pregnancy. *J Clin Ultrasound* 1993;21:65–68.
32. Huhta JC, Strasburger JF, Carpenter RJ, Reiter A, Abinader E. Pulsed Doppler fetal echocardiography. *J Clin Ultrasound* 1985;13:247–254.
33. Maulik D, Nanda NC, Moodley S, Saini VD, Thiede HA. Application of Doppler echocardiography in the assessment of fetal cardiac disease. *Am J Obstet Gynecol* 1985;151:951–957.
34. Yeager SB, Parness IA, Sanders SP. Severe tricuspid regurgitation simulating pulmonary atresia in the fetus. *Am Heart J* 1988;115:906–908.
35. Allan LD, Crawford DC, Tynan MJ. Pulmonary atreisa in prenatal life. *J Am Coll Cardiol* 1986;8:1131–1136.
36. Marasini M, Cordone M, Zampatti C, Pongiglione G, Bertolini A, Ribaldone D. Prenatal ultrasound detection of truncus arteriosus with interrupted aortic arch and truncal valve regurgitation. *Eur Heart J* 1987;8:921–924.
37. Fouron JC, Sahn DJ, Bender R, et al. Prenatal diagnosis and circulatory characteristics in tetralogy of Fallot with absent pulmonary valve. *Am J Cardiol* 1989;64:547–549.
38. Allan LD, Chita SK, Anderson RH, Fagg N, Crawford DC, Tynan MJ. Coarctation of the aorta in prenatal life: An echocardiographic, anatomical, and functional study. *Br Heart J* 1988;59:356–360.
39. Jouk PS and Rambaud P. Prediction of outcome by prenatal Doppler analysis in a patient with aortic stenosis. *Br Heart J* 1991;65:53–54.
40. Tulzer G, Gudmundsson S, Sharkey AM, Wood DC, Cohen AW, Huhta JC. Doppler echocardiography of fetal ductus arteriosus constriction versus increased right ventricular output. *J Am Coll Cardiol* 1991;18:532–536.
41. Wilson AD, Rao PS, Aeschlimann S. Normal fetal foramen flap and transatrial Doppler velocity pattern. *J Am Soc Echo* 1990;3:491–494.
42. Chobot V, Hornberger LK, Hagen-Ansert S, Sahn DJ. Prenatal detection of restrictive foramen ovale. *J Am Soc Echo* 1990;3:15–19.
43. Yagel S, Hochner-Celnikier D, Hurwitz A, Palti Z, Gotsman MS. The significance and importance of prenatal diagnosis of fetal cardiac malformations by Doppler echocardiography. *Am J Obstet Gynecol* 1988;158:272–277.
44. Maulik D, Nanda NC. Doppler echocardiography part IV: Fetal Doppler echocardiography. *Echocardiography* 1985;2:377–391.
45. Benacerraf BR, Sanders SP. Fetal echocardiography. *Radiol Clin North Am* 1990;28:131–147.
46. Schmidt KG, de Araujo LMD, Silverman NH. Evaluation of structural and functional abnormalities of the fetal heart by echocardiography. *Am J Card Imag* 1988;2:55–76.
47. Gembruch U, Knopfle G, Chatterjee M, Bald R, Hansmann M. First-trimester diagnosis of fetal congenital heart disease by transvaginal two-dimensional and Doppler echocardiography. *Obstet Gynecol* 1990;75:496–498.
48. Wladimiroff JW, Huisman TWA, Stewart PA. Fetal cardiac flow velocities in the late first trimester of pregnancy: A transvaginal Doppler study. *J Am Coll Cardiol* 1991;17:1357–1359.
49. Kurjak A, Crvenkovic G, Salihagic A, Zalud I, Miljan M. The assessment of normal early pregnancy by transvaginal color Doppler ultrasonography. *J Clin Ultrasound* 1993;21:3–8.
50. DeVore GR, Hornstein J, Siassi B, Platt LD. Doppler color flow mapping: its use in the prenatal diagnosis of congenital heart disease in the human fetus. *Echocardiography* 1985;2:551–557.
51. DeVore GR, Horenstein J, Siassi B, Platt LD. Fetal echocardiography: VII. Doppler color flow mapping: A new technique for the diagnosis of congenital heart disease. *Am J Obstet Gynecol* 1987;156:1054–1064.
52. Gembruch U, Hansmann M, Redel DA, Bald R. Fetal two-dimensional Doppler echocardiography (colour flow mapping) and its place in prenatal diagnosis. *Prenat Diagn* 1989;9:535–547.
53. Chiba Y, Kanzaki T, Kobayashi H, Murakami M, Yutani C. Evaluation of fetal structural heart disease using color flow mapping. *Ultrasound Med Biol* 1990;16:221–229.
54. Sharland GK, Chita SK, Allan LD. The use of colour Doppler in fetal echocardiography. *Int J Cardiol* 1990;28:229–236.
55. Copel JA, Morotti R, Hobbins JC, Kleinman CS. The antenatal diagnosis of congenital heart disease using fetal echocardiography: Is color flow mapping necessary? *Obstet Gynecol* 1991;78:1–8.
56. Rizzo G, Nicolaides KH, Arduini D, Campbell S. Effects of intravascular fetal blood transfusion on fetal intracardiac Doppler velocity waveforms. *Am J Obstet Gynecol* 1990;1163:1231–1238.
57. Rotmensch S, Liberati M, Luo JS, Hobbins JC. Monitoring of intravascular fetal transfusions with Doppler velocimetry. *Am J Obstet Gynecol* 1992;167:1314–1316.
58. Reed KL, Appleton CP, Anderson CF, Shenker L, Sahn DJ. Doppler studies of vena cava flows in human fetuses: Insights into normal and abnormal cardiac physiology. *Circulation* 1990;81:498–505.
59. Achiron R, Rabinovitz R, Aboulafia Y, Diamant Y, Glaser J. Intrauterine assessment of high-output cardiac failure with spontaneous remission of hydrops fetalis in twin–twin transfusion syndrome: Use of two-dimensional echocardiography, Doppler ultrasound, and color flow mapping. *J Clin Ultrasound* 1992;20:271–277.
60. Dan U, Shalev E, Greif M, Weiner E. Prenatal diagnosis of fetal brain arteriovenous malformation: The use of color Doppler imaging. *J Clin Ultrasound* 1992;20:149–151.
61. Battaglia C, Artini PG, D'Ambrogio G, Droghini F, Genazzani AR. Fetal abdominal cavernous hemangioma diagnosed by duplex Doppler velocimetry. *Acta Obset Gynecol Scand* 1992;71:476–478.
62. Agata Y, Hiraishi S, Oguchi K, et al. Changes in left ventricular output from fetal to early neonatal life. *J Pediatr* 1991;119:441–445.

Doppler Ultrasound in Obstetrics and Gynecology,
edited by Joshua A. Copel and Kathryn L. Reed.
Raven Press, Ltd., New York © 1995.

CHAPTER 25

Fetal Heart Failure

Norman H. Silverman

The remarkable advances in fetal cardiac ultrasound in the past 10 years now provide the opportunity to define not only the natural history of cardiac disorders prenatally from the time of fetal development, but also developmental morphology and function from as early as the sixteenth week of gestation. This chapter examines the ultrasound findings associated with fetal heart failure, techniques for measuring left and right ventricular output and its regional distribution, and the mechanisms identifiable by cardiac ultrasound that contribute to fetal cardiac failure.

METHODS

Cross-Sectional (Two-Dimensional) Methods

The fundamental modality of ultrasound for fetal cardiac assessment is the B-mode real-time scan. Imaging the fetal heart is attempted from as many planes as possible in order to define the morphology and for interrogation with the other modalities of ultrasound (1). Current equipment enables appropriate magnification of the cross-sectional image for definition and reduces measurement errors. Multiple-plane imaging also provides a better opportunity for alignment of the Doppler ultrasound and M-mode cursors. The fetal heart is imaged in long-axis, short-axis, and four-chamber views as described previously (2). To reduce measurement errors in small images, the images of the atrioventricular (AV) and semilunar valves as well as the descending aorta and umbilical vein are magnified 1.5–3.0 times. Measurement of the annulus size of the atrioventricular and semilunar valves and the corresponding velocity–time interval are used to calculate the cardiac output.

Measurement of the regional distribution of cardiac output can be calculated by cross-sectional echocardiography and pulsed Doppler techniques. Cross-sectional echocardiography and Doppler ultrasound have been used in the fetus to measure the flow across the cardiac valves and to determine the regional cardiac output. More recently, experimental validations of ultrasound measurements have been made. Measurement of fetal ventricular volume of both the left and right ventricles has been achieved in fetal lamb models (3). This technique can be applied to calculating volume from images of the human fetal left and right ventricles. Long-axis views are used; for the left ventricle, the orthogonal views—the equivalent of the apical two- and four-chamber views of the left ventricle—and the orthogonal views for the right ventricle, the equivalent of the subcostal coronal and sagittal views. For the latter pair of right ventricular images, the common long axis is the line drawn between the pulmonary valve and the midpoint of the diaphragmatic surface of the left ventricle. The technique requires biplane orthogonal views. In addition, experimental studies in the lamb fetus have shown the possibility of defining fetal cardiac output and its regional distribution (Figs. 1–4). The dimensions of the cardiac chambers and vessels and wall thicknesses can be measured from the cross-sectional images (4–6) (Figs. 5–13).

Doppler Ultrasound Methods

Numerous studies have been performed in the fetus (7–18). As in the postnatal examination, volume flow is determined from the velocity–time integral (systolic for aortic or pulmonary valve, diastolic for the tricuspid and mitral valve). The transvalvar flow (Q) may then be calculated from the formula:

$$Q \text{ (ml/min)} = \text{VTI} \cdot \pi \cdot \frac{D^2}{4} \cdot \text{HR}$$

N. H. Silverman: Departments of Pediatrics and Radiology (Cardiology), University of California, San Francisco 94143.

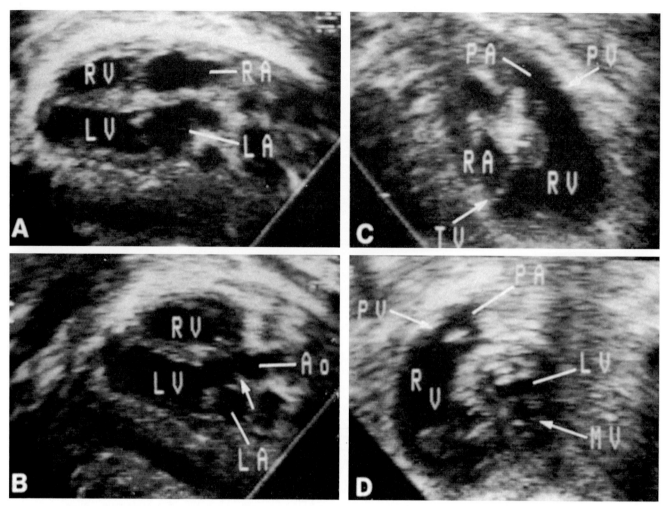

FIG. 1 Two-dimensional echocardiographic images of the left (A, B) and right (C, D) ventricle in fetal lambs. **A:** The left ventricle (LV) is shown in an equivalent of an apical four-chamber view; the right ventricle (RV), the right atrium (RA), and the left atrium (LA) are also seen. **B:** In an equivalent of an apical two-chamber view, the left ventricular outflow tract and the aortic valve (*arrow*) as well as the proximal ascending aorta (Ao) are seen. **C:** This frame depicts the right ventricle in an equivalent of a subcostal coronal view, where the tricuspid valve (TV) bordering the right atrium as well as the pulmonary valve (PV) and the proximal pulmonary artery (PA) are seen. **D:** In the equivalent of a subcostal sagittal view of the right ventricle, the left ventricle and the mitral valve (MV) within it are imaged in cross-section. From Schmidt et al. (3).

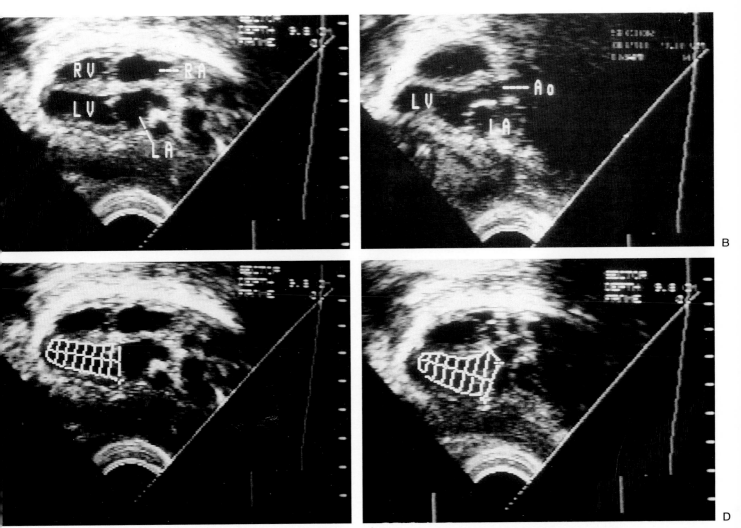

FIG. 2. Calculation of end-diastolic left ventricular volume in a fetal lamb from area outlines in two perpendicular planes using Simpson's rule. In the four-chamber view, the left ventricular endocardium is traced (**A**) and the long axis is placed between the apex and the center of the mitral valve (**B**). In the two-chamber view (**C, D**), the same procedure is performed; the ventricular volume is equal to the sum of volumes of the eight slices. From Schmidt et al. (3).

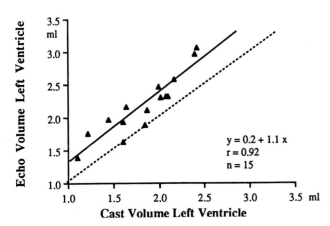

FIG. 3. Plot of right ventricular end-diastolic volumes determined by cast measurements (x axis) compared with those calculated from echocardiographic images (y axis). Solid line is the regression line; broken line is the line of identity. From Schmidt et al. (3).

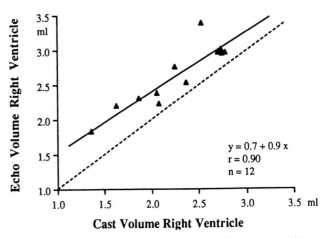

FIG. 4. Plot of left ventricular end-diastolic volumes determined by cast measurements (x axis) compared with those calculated from echocardiographic images (y axis). Solid line is the regression line; broken line is the line of identity. From Schmidt et al. (3).

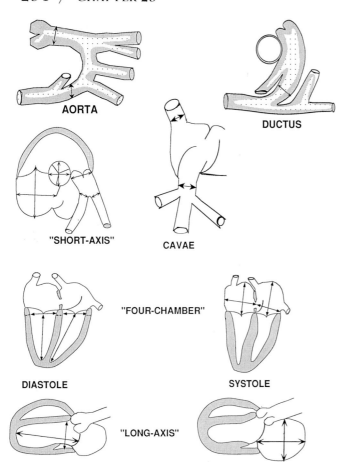

FIG. 5. Graphic representation of the views obtained and the dimensions (*arrows*) that were measured. **Top row:** On the left, measurements made in the ascending and aortic isthmic region, and on the right, measurement of the ductus dimension. **Second row:** From the "short-axis" view (*left*), measurements of the right atrial, aortic root, pulmonary arterial, and branch left and right pulmonary arterial dimensions. The superior and inferior caval veins were measured (*right*) at the entrance of each cava into the right atrium. **Third row:** In the "four-chamber" view during diastole (*left*), the ventricular dimensions were measured just below the opposed tips of the atrioventricular valve leaflets; the ventricular lengths were also measured, as well as wall and septal thickness. In systole (*right*), the atrial dimensions were measured. **Bottom row:** On the left, measurements of the left heart in diastole obtained from "long axis" equivalent and the left ventricular minor and major axis, and on the right, the left atrial dimensions from this view measured in systole. The arch of the aorta shown in the top left of the diagram was often seen from this plane. From Tan et al. (5).

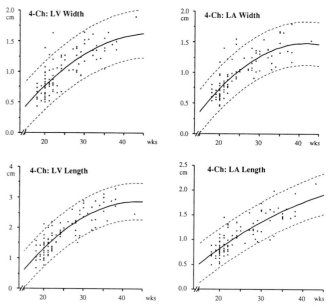

FIG. 6. Left heart measurements from the four-chamber view (4-Ch). LV, left ventricular; LA, left atrial. *Note:* In each graph in this and the following figures, gestational age, in weeks, is displayed on the ordinate measurement, and ultrasound dimension, in centimeters, on the abscissa. Likewise, all graphs show the line of regression as a bold, continuous line, the 95% confidence intervals as dotted lines, and the data points for each fetus. From Tan et al. (5).

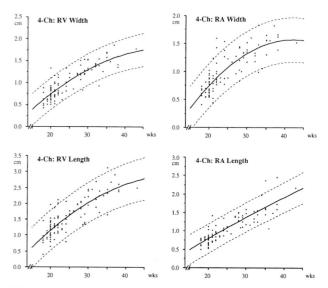

FIG. 7. Right heart measurements from the four-chamber view (4-Ch). RV, right ventricular dimensions; RA, right atrial dimensions. From Tan et al. (5).

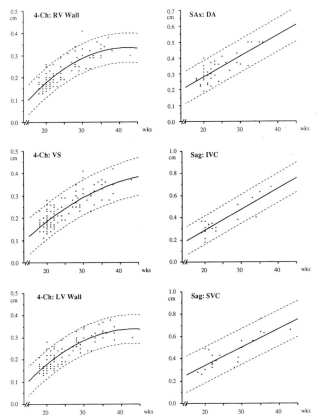

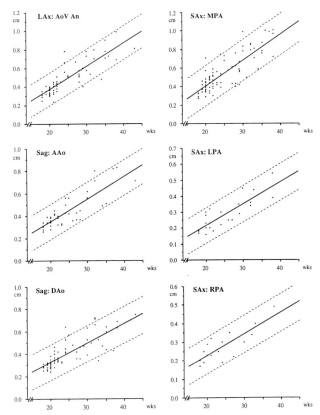

FIG. 8. Left: From the four-chamber view (4-Ch), the dimensions of the right ventricular (RV) wall, ventricular septum (VS), and left ventricular (LV) wall. **Right:** From the short-axis view (SAx), the dimensions of the ductus arteriosus (DA), and from the sagittal view (Sag), the inferior vena cava (IVC) and superior vena cava (SVC). From Tan et al. (5).

FIG. 9. Measurements of the aortic and pulmonary arteries. **Left:** From the long-axis view (LAx), the diameter of the aortic valve annulus (AoV An), and from the sagittal view (Sag), the diameters of the ascending aortic root (AAo) and the descending aortic root (DAo). **Right:** From the short-axis view (SAx), the diameter of the main pulmonary artery (MPA), left pulmonary artery (LPA), and right pulmonary artery (RPA). From Tan et al. (5).

where D is the diameter of the valve annulus, VTI is the velocity–time integral (Fig. 14), and HR represents heart rate.

Left ventricular output is calculated from the aortic annulus or the mitral annulus cross-sectional area and the mean temporal velocity through the aorta or mitral valve, respectively (18). The right ventricular output is calculated from the pulmonary annulus cross-sectional area or the tricuspid annulus cross-sectional area and the respective mean temporal velocity of the pulmonary or the tricuspid valve (19). The sample volume is kept as small as possible (1–2 mm) and placed just distal to the valve for recording the Doppler signal (19).

It is necessary to consider correction for angle between interrogation and flow. It is my practice to correct for intercept angles greater than 20°. The corollary of this dictum is to try always to keep the intercept angle less than 20°, but this is extremely difficult in the fetus unless the lie is perfect. The reason not to correct for angles less than 20° related to the cosine of the intercept angle is that this deviation reduces the flow computation by only 6%. For an intercept angle of 30° the underestimate is ap-

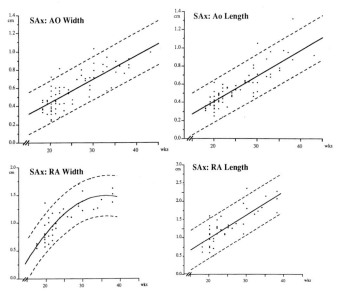

FIG. 10. Measurements made from the short axis (SAx). Top graphs show the dimension of the aorta (AO) from the horizontal plane (Width) on the left, and on the sagittal plane (Length) on the right. Bottom graphs show corresponding right atrial measurements (RA). From Tan et al. (5).

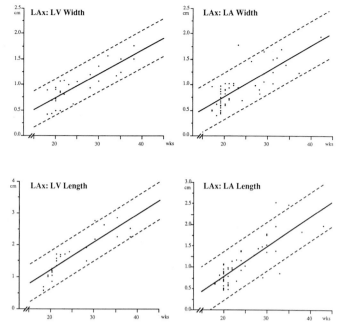

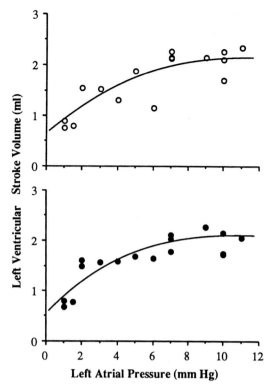

FIG. 11. Left heart dimensions from the long-axis view (LAx). Left-hand graphs show the diastolic left ventricular (LV) minor axis (Width) and major axis (Length), while the graphs on the right show the left atrial (LA) anteroposterior dimension (Width) and superoinferior dimension (Length). From Tan et al. (5).

FIG. 13. Plot of left ventricular stroke volumes (*y* axis) against left atrial pressures (*x* axis) as observed in one animal. Upper graph shows measurements by the electromagnetic flow transducer (○), whereas lower graph shows the simultaneous echocardiographic calculations (●). Note that the shapes of the left ventricular function curves are similar. From Schmidt et al. (3).

proximately 13%. For an intercept angle of 40° the underestimate is 24%.

Certain assumptions are made about the dimension of the atrioventricular valve annuli (mitral and tricuspid), which might affect the calculation of flow adversely. These annuli are not circular, nor is the orifice through which blood is flowing of a uniform, constant dimension throughout the period of flow. Nevertheless, regardless of these assumptions, reasonable estimates of ventricular

output have been achieved in human fetuses as well as experimentally in fetal animal models (8,9,11–13,19).

Regional Blood Flow

Determination of regional blood flow has been determined within the lower abdominal aorta and the intraabdominal portion of the umbilical vein (Fig. 15). The umbilical vein within the abdomen may be interrogated by Doppler or Doppler color flow and the diameter measured. The mean velocity may be measured by integrating the profile of the forward velocity tracing throughout systole and diastole because there is usually forward flow throughout the cardiac cycle. Umbilical flow is determined from the product of the mean velocity (*V*) and the vessel cross-sectional area ($\pi/4 \cdot D^2$) [according to the method of Eik-Nes et al. (10)] whereby

$$Q \text{ (ml/min)} = \bar{V} \cdot \frac{\pi}{4} \cdot D^2 \times 60$$

The difference in these calculations relates to the use of mean velocity (*V*), which is the integral of forward flow throughout the cardiac cycle or over unit time expressed in cm³/sec. To convert this value to ml/min one

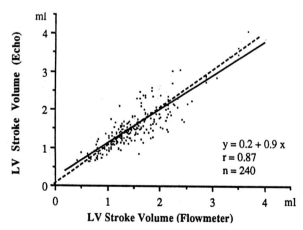

$$y = 0.2 + 0.9 \, x$$
$$r = 0.87$$
$$n = 240$$

FIG. 12. Plot of left ventricular (LV) stroke volumes at different levels of preload measured by an electromagnetic flow transducer (*x* axis) compared with those calculated from echocardiographic images (*y* axis). Solid line is the regression line; broken line is the line of identity. From Schmidt et al. (3).

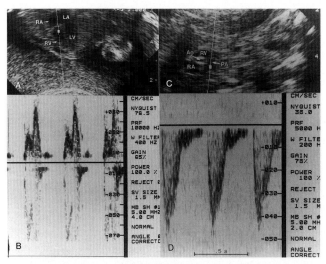

FIG. 14. Normal fetal Doppler flow profiles across an atrioventricular and a semilunar valve are shown. **Left:** In a four-chamber view (*top*) the left atrium (LA), the right atrium (RA), the left ventricle (LV), and the right ventricle (RV) are seen. The sample volume lies below the tricuspid valve. The Doppler display (*bottom*) shows the diastolic inflow into the right ventricle above the baseline, indicating its direction towards the transducer. A biphasic signal is seen with a smaller v-component resulting from rapid venous filling, followed by a larger *a* component (*black arrowheads*) resulting from atrial contraction. This pattern with predominant *a* waves is typical for the fetus. The mirror-like display below the baseline is an artifact caused by too high a gain setting. **Right:** In a fetal short axis view (*top*), the right atrium (RA), right ventricle (RV), pulmonary artery (PA), and aorta (Ao) are seen. The sample volume lies distal to the pulmonary valve within the pulmonary artery. The characteristic arterial Doppler flow signal below the baseline is directed away from the transducer (*bottom*). Volume flow is the product of the vessel cross-sectional area, the velocity–time interval, and the heart rate. From Schmidt et al. (2).

has to multiply by the number of seconds per minute. Descending aortic flow is calculated from the mean temporal velocity within the aorta and the product of the descending aortic vessel diameter ($\pi/4 \cdot D^2$). We have validated this technique in the fetal lamb model (20) (Figs. 16 and 17).

Color Flow Methods

Currently, atrioventricular valve insufficiency is best recognized using Doppler color flow mapping. The Doppler color flow method, particularly in the fetus, is the method of choice for defining jets, minor flow disturbances, and the direction of blood flow and for setting up the cursor for examination with the other Doppler ultrasound modalities, such as measuring the intercept angle (Fig. 18) (21). The Doppler color flow method facilitates the rapid detection of stenotic or regurgitant jets, thereby diminishing the time required for Doppler interrogation. Techniques different from postnatal echocardiography are used to define the low-velocity signals found in many fetal chambers and vessels. The wall filter should be set at low levels, the Nyquist limit should be set to the lowest levels, and the gain should be increased. The color flow map we prefer for all echocardiography displays variations of both velocity and flow toward the transducer in warm colors (red to yellow) and flow away from the transducer in cool colors (blue and turquoise). These setting alterations allow one to display the low-velocity signals seen in the fetus. By expanding the scale in such a manner, the lower velocities found in the fetus become easier to display. Using color flow we have been able to define tricuspid regurgitation, particularly in a

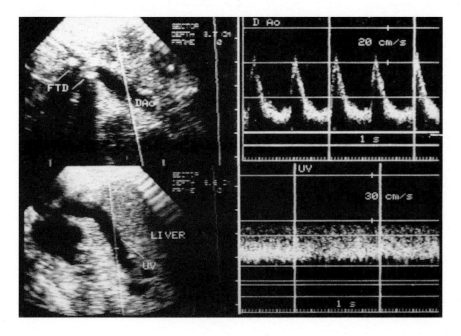

FIG. 15. Doppler echocardiographic assessment of blood flow in descending aorta (*top*) and umbilical vein (*bottom*) of a fetal lamb. **Top left:** Distal descending aorta (DAo) and two electromagnetic flow transducers (FTD). Sample volume of pulsed Doppler system is placed centrally within vessel. **Top right:** Spectral display of Doppler shift indicates blood velocity; vertical scale markers relate to velocity, and horizontal scale markers relate to time. **Bottom left:** Umbilical vein (UV) at its intraabdominal course surrounded by liver tissue. **Bottom right:** Spectral display shows typical uniform velocity pattern with little changes throughout cardiac cycle within UV. From Schmidt et al. (7).

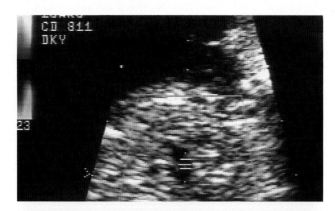

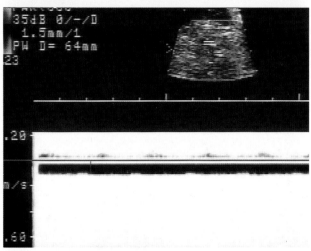

FIG. 16. Top: Magnified view of the umbilical vein running through the undersurface of the liver in an 18-week-old fetus. The dimension of the vein is 0.25 cm as judged from the electronic caliper measurement between the sample volume gate. **Bottom:** The resulting sample volume. This velocity reads 10 cm/sec (0.1 m/sec).

number of fetuses in which this would have been impossible prior to the incorporation of this technique, simply because the regurgitant jet was small or eccentrically directed.

M-Mode Methods

M-mode echocardiography has been established as a means of quantitating fetal heart dimensions (2,4,5,22–28). This technique has in the past been the standard for measurement of the fetal cardiac dimensions. The difference between this technique before and after birth is the lack of ability to standardize the planes of examination in the fetus by defining the internal and external reference points. After birth most M-mode measurements are made from the standardized precordial position. *In utero* no such standardization is possible. Nevertheless, the technique remains a useful and rapid means of assessing some cardiac dimensions and ventricular performance.

CONDITIONS

Hydrops Fetalis

Hydrops fetalis was initially related to Rh isoimmunization (29). Diamond et al. attributed the mechanisms for the edema to chronic congestive heart failure and chronic hypoxia (secondary to anemia and hypoproteinemia). One or all of these factors is responsible for this syndrome. The ultrasound diagnosis comprises serous effusions including pericardial effusion and skin edema (30) (Fig. 19).

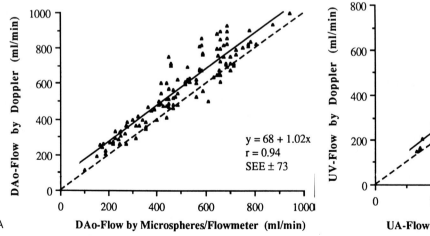

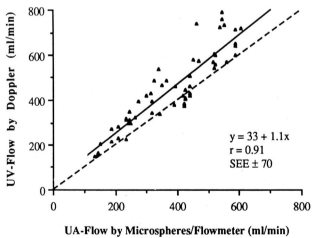

FIG. 17. A: Scatterplots of regression analysis correlating descending aortic (DAo) flow measured invasively by radionuclide-labeled microspheres and an electromagnetic flow transducer (*x* axis) and by Doppler echocardiography (*y* axis). Solid line is regression line; broken line is line of identity. **B:** Scatter plots of regression analysis correlating umbilical flow measured invasively by radionuclide-labeled microspheres and an electromagnetic flow transducer at umbilical artery (UA, *x* axis) and by Doppler echocardiography at umbilical vein (UV, *y* axis). Solid line is regression line; broken line is line of identity. From Schmidt et al. (7).

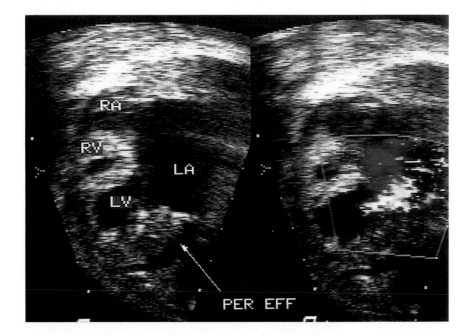

FIG. 18. The left frame shows the appearance of a markedly enlarged left atrium (LA) and left ventricle (LV) and pericardial effusion (PER EFF) in a case of cardiomyopathy associated with mitral regurgitation. The right atrium (RA) and right ventricle (RV) are seen in this four-chamber view for comparison and are of normal size for gestational age. The right frame, taken in systole, demonstrates the regurgitant jet from the mitral regurgitation. Note that from this frame it would not be possible to obtain an accurate estimate of the velocity because of the direction of the color flow image.

There are six determinants of fetal edema (31), namely, alterations in

1. Hydrostatic pressure, most likely resulting from heart failure or impedance of venous return
2. Colloid osmotic pressure
3. Membrane permeability
4. Interstitial gel
5. Lymphatic drainage
6. Water homeostasis of fetoplacental–amniotic fluid compartments

Cardiac failure may occur without hydrops and vice versa. I feel that the when nonimmune hydrops occurs, it is a severe expression of heart failure akin to the anasarca or the old description of "dropsy" arising from the same etymologic root.

Hutchinson has classified hydrops as follows (31):

1. *Due to increased hydrostatic pressure:* tachyarrhythmias, tumors with a large vascular supply, i.e., neuroblastoma, placental chorioangioma, sacrococcygeal teratoma, pulmonary sequestration, parasitic fetus
2. *Due to low cardiac output failure:* bradyarrhythmias, structural cardiac anomalies, i.e., ventricular hypoplasia, valvar disease, premature closure of the ductus arteriosus and venosus, myocardial dysfunction, isch-

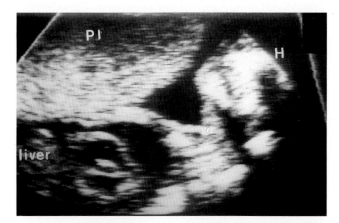

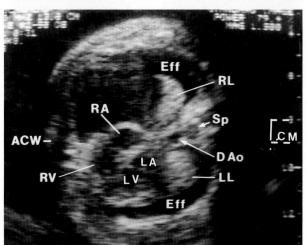

FIG. 19. Top: In this example of hydrops, marked placental thickening (Pl) is seen. The viscera, the heart (H) seen above the diaphragm, and the liver, below the diaphragm, are evident, and large pleural effusions are present. **Bottom:** Taken with transverse scanning, this frame demonstrates the position of the heart, which is enlarged, lying within the thorax, large, bilateral pleural effusions (Eff), and compressed lungs on the left (LL) and right (RL). The spine (Sp) and descending aorta (DAo) are seen. The four chambers of the heart are identified—right atrium (RA), left atrium (LA), right ventricle (RV), and left ventricle (LV). There is scleroderma, evidenced by the thickening of the skin overlying the anterior chest wall (ACW). From Schmidt and Silverman (68).

emic or cardiomyopathic tumors, increased peripheral resistance (arterial calcification), venous obstruction such as cystic adenomatoid malformation of the lung, diaphragmatic hernia, cystic hygroma, lymphangiectasia, gastrointestinal malformations, venous thrombosis

3. *Due to decreased osmotic pressure:* hepatic dysfunction, renal dysfunction

4. *Due to altered capillary endothelium permeability,* resulting either from intrinsic causes such as chromosomal disorders, inborn metabolic errors, acquired causes such as hypoxia/ischemia, infections, or from neoplasia.

There are many overlapping causes from one group or another.

Nonimmune hydrops also has many causes. Holzgreve and colleagues have determined that only 16% of cases in their series of 50 pregnancies were idiopathic. The rest had some recognizable cause (32). Some report an incidence of idiopathic hydrops as high as 28.4% (33). Nonimmune hydrops has been reported to be cardiac in origin in 16.5% to 22.0% of cases (32,33). The association of nonimmune hydrops and cardiac failure *in utero* was first reported by Moller et al. (34). Kleinman et al. first recognized this *in utero* using ultrasound (30). Several other examples and mechanisms for nonimmune hydrops have been defined above, but the recognition of nonimmune hydrops has been an important feature of

the definition of cardiac failure *in utero.* In many cases described in the literature, hydrops was associated with a cardiac lesion (32,35–50).

There have been some attempts to define hydrops as a cause of heart failure. In atrioventricular valve insufficiency, for example, many mechanisms described above act in concert (51). The atrioventricular valve regurgitation acts to increase the venous pressure. This phenomenon, together with the low oncotic pressure in the fetal capillaries related to low serum albumin, possible mild tissue hypoxia, and diminished myocardial performance, acts to produce hydrops. The chronic venous congestion leads to liver malfunction, further fueling the cycle that causes fluid to seep out into the tissues and serous cavities, producing fetal hydrops (51–53). As this example shows, the classification of the causes of cardiac failure into one group or another, just as for the classification of hydrops, is somewhat arbitrary with many factors contributing whenever a particular primary cause is operative.

From the classification of Hutchinson (31), the causes of fetal heart failure may be presented as in Table 1.

Low-Output Cardiac Failure

Low-output cardiac failure is probably responsible for the majority of fetuses presenting with cardiac failure. Many factors lead to diminution of cardiac output, e.g.,

TABLE 1.

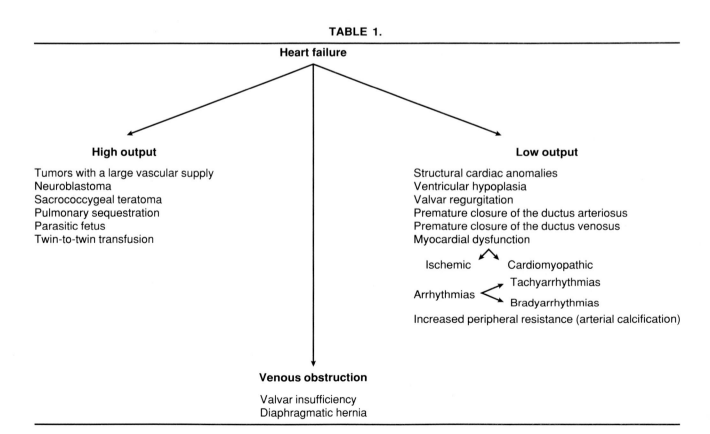

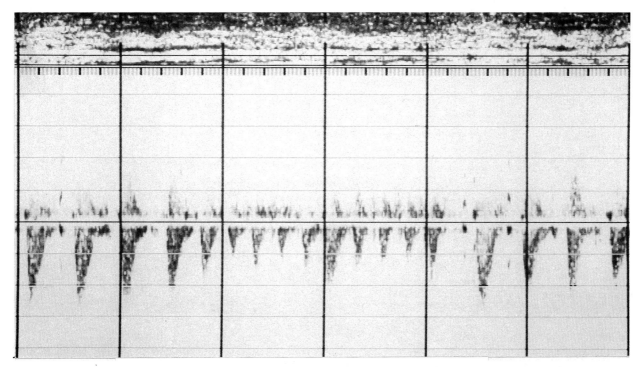

FIG. 20. Pulsed Doppler interrogation within the pulmonary artery of a fetus with short runs of supraventricular tachycardia. Note the reduction in stroke volume at the onset of tachycardia after the first four regular beats. Ten beats in tachycardia are followed by a pause and resumption of normal sinus rhythm. Horizontal lines are markers of velocity shift (0.25 m/sec); vertical lines are time markers (1 sec). From Schmidt and Silverman (68).

structural cardiac abnormalities, such as ventricular hypoplasia, valvar regurgitation, premature closure of the ductus arteriosus and foramen ovale, myocardial dysfunction due to ischemic or cardiomyopathic causes, or increases in vascular resistance.

From observations of heart failure before the ultrasound era, it was determined that fetal heart failure occurs with abnormalities of heart rate. Fetal tachyarrhythmias have long been known to be associated with hydrops (54–58). In tachycardias, the flow caused by atrial contraction is absent or diminished. As the contribution of atrial contraction to adequate ventricular filling is large in the fetus, cardiac output is likely to be compromised, although Lingman and Marsal stated that cardiac output is not decreased (58). Our own experience shows a diminution of the velocity–time interval with the initiation of tachycardia (Fig. 20). With the bradycardia associated with heart block, hydrops can occur re-

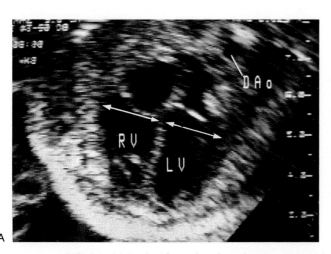
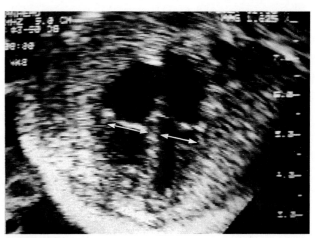

A   B

FIG. 21. Magnified four-chamber view in a normal fetus of 31 weeks gestation illustrating how measurements of ventricular cavity dimensions were made. **A** is at end diastole and **B** is at end systole. Ao, aorta; LV, left ventricle; RV, right ventricle. From Schmidt et al. (27).

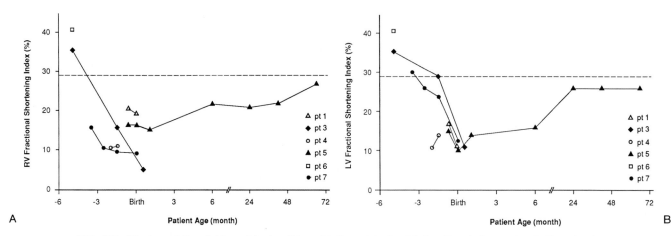

FIG. 22. Display of the right ventricular (**A**) and left ventricular (**B**) fractional shortening indices in six fetuses with congestive cardiomyopathies. Dotted lines indicate two standard deviations below the mean. From Schmidt et al. (27).

lated solely to rate. In our experience this occurs either when the ventricular rate has been less than 55/min or in association with slow atrial rates (59).

In situations where there is an abnormality of myocardial performance, such as that occurring in fetal cardiomyopathy, heart failure manifested as hydrops also occurs (27). The hydrops is associated with features

indicating diminished cardiac performance. This could be the fractional shortening index measured by M-mode, or from the real-time B scan directly (Figs. 21 and 22), or it may be assessed from volume measurements of the left and right ventricles (Fig. 23). The heart failure occurred either with or without atrioventricular valve insufficiency (27) (Fig. 24). An important feature of familial

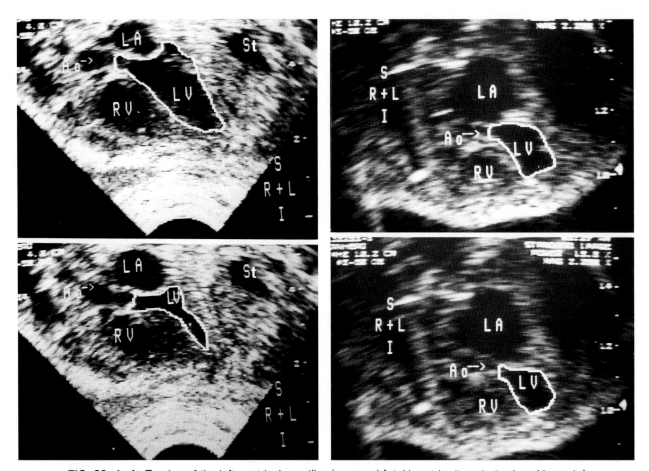

FIG. 23. Left: Tracing of the left ventricular outline in normal fetal heart in diastole (*top*) and in systole (*bottom*). **Right:** For comparison, the change in ventricular size at end diastole and end systole in a patient with a primary left-sided cardiomyopathy. From Silverman (1).

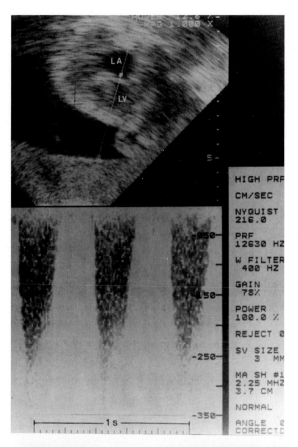

FIG. 24 Top: A patient with cardiomyopathy in whom the Doppler sample volume has been placed in the left atrium (LA) just proximal to the mitral valve. The left ventricle (LV) is seen below this. Bottom: High pulse repetition frequency Doppler signal shows the peak velocity = 250 cm/sec, consistent with a regurgitant pressure difference between the left ventricle and left atrium of 25 mm Hg. From Schmidt et al. (2). Demonstration of atrioventricular valve regurgitation by pulsed Doppler ultrasound in a fetus with dilated cardiomyopathy. A: Sample volume is placed just above the mitral valve in the left atrium (LA). B: High pulse repetition frequency Doppler displays a holosystolic mitral regurgitant (MR) signal with a peak velocity of 2.3 m/sec. C: In the same fetus the sample volume is placed within the right atrium (RA) just above the tricuspid valve. D: The spectral display of the Doppler shift demonstrates a similar signal with a peak velocity of 2.15 m/sec, consistent with tricuspid regurgitation (TR). From Schmidt et al. (27).

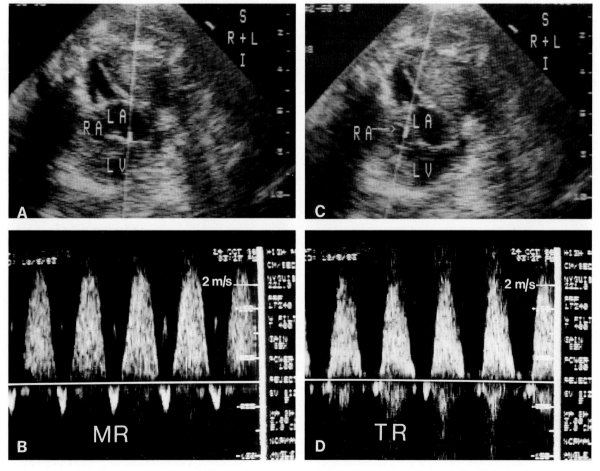

cardiomyopathy to remember, as for many of the genetically linked cardiomyopathies, is that the expression of the genetic deficiency may only manifest itself some time after birth. We have found that some fetal patients with cardiomyopathy occasionally have predominantly right-sided expressions of their cardiomyopathy (Figs. 25 and 26).

High-Output Cardiac Failure

Fewer lesions *in utero* produce high-output cardiac failure. These include neuroblastoma, tumors with a large vascular supply such as sacrococcygeal teratomas, pulmonary sequestrations, and parasitic twin and twin-to-twin transfusion.

We have investigated a group of fetuses who presented with high-output cardiac failure due to large sacrococcy-geal teratomas. Most presented in the second trimester, from 21 to 27 weeks of gestation with large sacrococcy-geal teratomas (Fig. 27) (19,53), either with or developing hydropsa in the course of our observations (Table 2). The tumors contained cystic and solid elements. Some of the cystic elements were found to be vascular by color flow examination, and the base of the tumor had numerous feeding arterial vessels from which pulsed Doppler signals were obtained. In this group of fetuses we obtained numerous measurements of dimensions and flow (Fig. 28; Table 2).

In one previable fetus presenting at 21 weeks that we were able to follow with serial ultrasound measurements, we intervened surgically to remove the teratoma. Pulsed Doppler assessment of the teratoma as well as the descending aortic and umbilical arteries showed high-amplitude signals in the abdominal aorta and the arterial

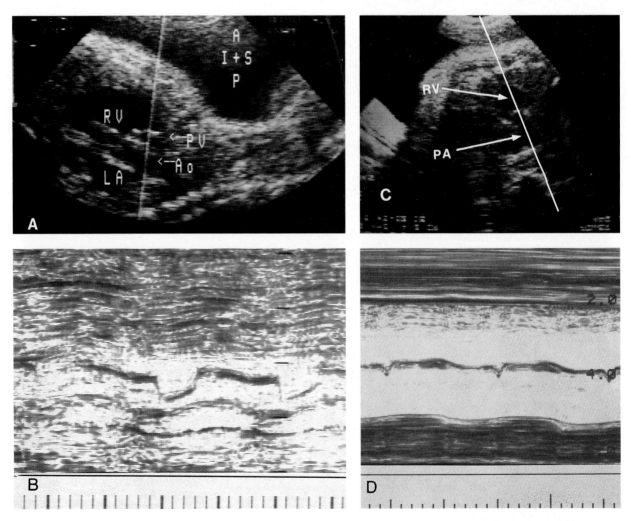

FIG. 25. This is a series of images (**top**) taken through the pulmonary valve with cross-sectional imaging and duplex M-mode imaging in a fetus with (**bottom**) a predominately right ventricular myopathy. The cross-sectional image is used as a reference to direct the M-mode cursor. At 20 weeks (*left*), the pulmonary valve motion is vigorous and of the usual character whereas by later gestation (*right*), as the ventricular myopathy became evident, the motion of the pulmonary valve is reduced to a sinusoidal wave with very limited excursion during systole. From Schmidt et al. (27).

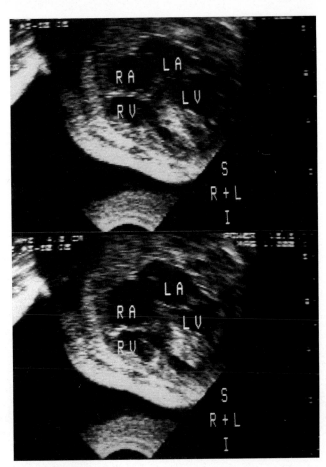

FIG. 26. Four-chamber views in the same fetus as that shown in the previous panel, i.e., a 32-week fetus with familial right-sided cardiomyopathy (**top**) and a 31-week fetus with cardiomyopathy, severe mitral regurgitation, and hydrops (**bottom**). The top frame, taken in end diastole, shows that the right-sided chambers are enlarged. In the bottom end-systolic frame, the left atrium (LA) and the left ventricle (LV) are not enlarged, whereas the right atrium (RA) and right ventricle (RV) are enlarged and contract poorly. From Silverman (1).

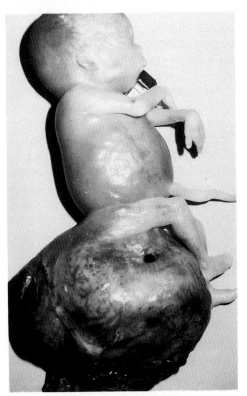

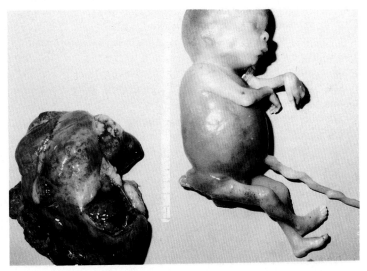

FIG. 27. Left: Example of a 27-week fetus with a sacrococcygeal teratoma that died *in utero* with hydrops fetalis. Note the distended abdomen and large sacrococcygeal teratoma below the lower limb. **Middle and right:** Pictures of the type of surgical resection that separates the teratoma and the fetus, which was successfully employed in one of our patients.

TABLE 2. *Fetal hydrops and AV regurgitation*

Gestational age (wks)	Hydrops	Atrioventricular regurgitation	Structural abnormality	Outcome
33	yes	TR	DORV, VSD	fetal death at 34 wks
20	yes	Severe TR	Ebstein's	born at 35 wks, died on day 1
36	yes	AVR	L-ISOM, AVSD, PS[a]; born at 36 wks, died on day 1	
21	yes	Severe TR	PA, IVS	premature labor 24 wks, stillborn
34	yes	TR	HLH	born at 34 wks, died on day 1
25	yes	TR	none[a]	fetal death at 29 wks
21	yes	Severe AVR	L-ISOM, AVSD, PA[a]	pregnancy terminated
25	yes	AVR	AVSD, PA	born at term, died on day 1
26	yes	Severe TR	Ebstein's	born at term, died on day 4
30	yes	TR	PA, IVS	stillborn at 37 wks
26	yes	TR	Ebstein's	fetal death at 36 wks
33	yes	TR	Ebstein's	born at term, died on day 4
33	yes	Mild TR	none	stillborn at 34 wks
23	yes	Severe TR	none	pregnancy terminated
37	yes	TR	PA, IVS	born at term, died at 1 wk
26	yes	Mild TR	none	stillborn at 32 wks
33	yes	TR	TA, TS, HLV	fetal death at 35 wks
28	yes	MR	AS, EFE	born at term, died 10 hr after birth and 3 hr after aortic valvotomy

From Silverman and Schmidt (18).
AS, aortic stenosis; AVR, atrioventricular regurgitation; AVSD, atrioventricular septal defect; DORV, double-outlet right ventricle; EFE, endocardial fibroelastosis; HLH, hypoplastic left heart; HLV, hypoplastic left ventricle; IVS, intact ventricular septum; L-ISOM, left isomerism; MR, mitral regurgitation; PA, pulmonary atresia; PS, pulmonary stenosis; TA, truncus arteriosus; TR, tricuspid regurgitation; TS, truncal stenosis.
[a] Complete heart block.

vessels in the teratoma (Figs. 29 and 30). The systolic-to-diastolic velocity ratios indicated low vascular resistance in the teratoma with a somewhat lower ratio in the placenta, suggesting a "steal" phenomenon similar to that found in patent ductus arteriosus and other causes of diastolic runoff in the abdominal aorta (Fig. 31).

We were able to obtain serial measurements on one fetus that showed progressive deterioration in the measured indices, increasing ventricular volume overload, and the appearance of worsening cardiac function (Fig. 32). The heart was structurally normal in all of these fetuses, but the ventricles were enlarged greater than 2 SD above the mean for gestation in all. A relatively normal fractional shortening index was maintained in these, confirming the large stroke volume from each ventricle. Pericardial effusions, other serous cavity effusions, and skin edema were manifestations of the nonimmune hydrops, representing heart failure. The inferior vena cava diameter was enlarged, reflecting the increased venous return from the lower body in all the fetuses in this group (Fig. 33).

This fetus showed a progressive increase in combined ventricular output, increasing flow to the descending aorta and placenta (Fig. 32). The levels fell after the teratoma was removed. The tumor weighed 0.6 kg, which approximated the weight of the rest of the fetus at the time of surgery. The combined ventricular output and placental and descending aortic flow diminished only slightly until the fourth postoperative day, when fetal cord blood sampling under ultrasonic guidance demonstrated that the hematocrit was only 16%. After transfusion via the umbilical cord of 33 ml of washed, packed red cells, the abnormal indices fell further toward the expected normal levels. Although there was still an increase in the descending aortic flow comprising a marked increase of placental blood flow and descending aortic blood flow (tumor blood flow), the fetus showed spontaneous resolution of the fetal hydrops on the ultrasound examinations. Unfortunately, 2 weeks after fetal surgery, despite all efforts at tocolysis, spontaneous rupture of membranes occurred, and a cesarean section was performed to deliver a premature infant weighing 0.8 kg, who died of respiratory distress despite intensive postnatal management.

Doppler assessment of flow indicated that the combined ventricular output was markedly increased (Table 3). Mean values were 1280 ml/min/kg, range 757–1600 ml/min/kg [normal range = 553 ± 153 ml/min/kg (9)]. The abdominal aortic flow was also increased, ranging from 549 to 1151 ml/min/kg (normal = 184 ± 20 ml/min/kg) (16). Placental flow was calculated to be markedly increased, ranging from 260 to 600 ml/min/kg (normal placental flow = 110 ± 26 ml/min/kg) (10). The percentage of placental flow to the descending aortic flow is

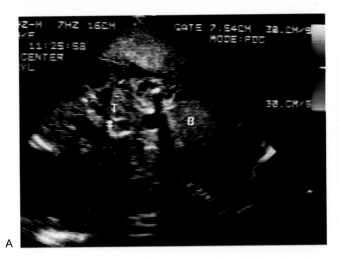

A

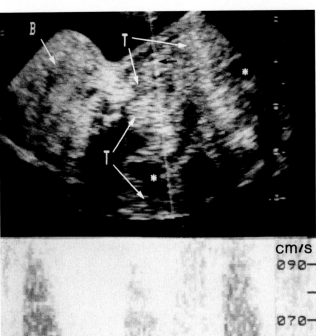

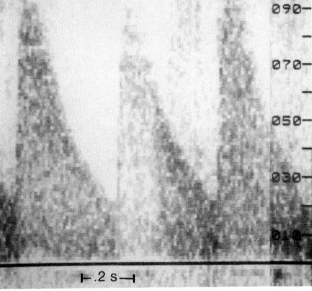

B

FIG. 28. A: In this example, taken at 23 weeks, blood flow is identified in the sacrococcygeal teratoma at the junction of the tumor with the body. A number of cystic areas that do not contain blood are identified. **B:** In this frame Doppler signals from feeding vessel at the base of teratoma are displayed. Sample volume within a vessel is identified by *arrow*. Cystic, nonvascular spaces are identified by asterisks. Resulting pulsatile arterial flow within teratoma demonstrates high-velocity flow to about 95 cm/sec in systole and diastolic flow to 20 cm/sec in diastole. B, fetal body; T, teratoma. From Silverman and Schmidt (18).

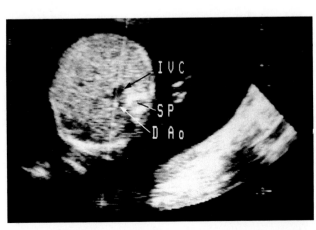

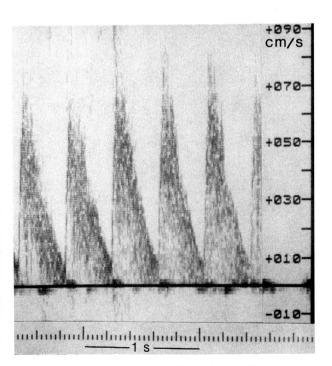

FIG. 29. Cross-sectional scan demonstrating the position of the inferior vena cava (IVC), the descending aorta (DAo), and the spine (Sp), and a Doppler sample obtained within the abdominal aorta demonstrates the systolic-to-diastolic ratio. The sample volume is placed within the aorta. Arterial signal demonstrates high velocity of flow and relatively low diastolic runoff despite the poor angle. From Silverman and Schmidt (18).

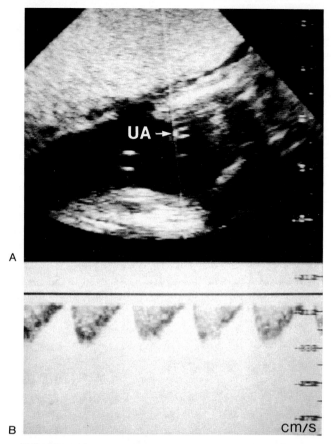

A

B

cm/s

FIG. 30. A: Sector scan showing Doppler sample volume (*arrow*) placed within umbilical artery (UA). **B:** Doppler flow signal demonstrating very blunted attenuated signal, with the diastolic velocity below the 400-Hz level. At other times, when the wall filter was turned as low as possible, the diastolic signal returned to baseline. From Silverman and Schmidt (18).

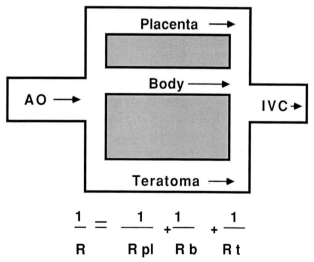

$$\frac{1}{R} = \frac{1}{R\,pl} + \frac{1}{R\,b} + \frac{1}{R\,t}$$

FIG. 31. Relationship of vascular resistances from the body, umbilical circulation, and the teratoma in parallel. The reciprocal of the total vascular resistances equals the sum of the reciprocals of the separate resistances. Therefore, the greater the teratoma vascular bed, the greater the flow through this area and the less the flow through the placenta and the body. From Silverman and Schmidt (18).

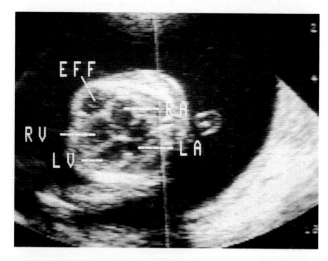

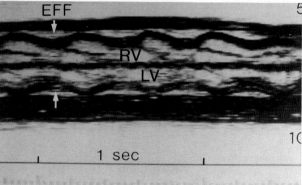

1 sec

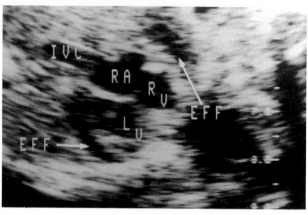

FIG. 32. Top: Cardiomegaly equal almost to the entire thoracic diameter. A pericardial effusion (EFF) is present. The M-mode cursor line is shown. **Middle:** Resultant M-mode demonstrates the dimensions of the ventricles and the presence of a pericardial effusion (EFF). **Bottom:** Large pericardial effusion (EFF) surrounding the heart, and a dilated inferior vena cava (IVC) 5 mm in diameter. RA, right atrium; RV, right ventricle; LV, left ventricle. From Silverman and Schmidt (18).

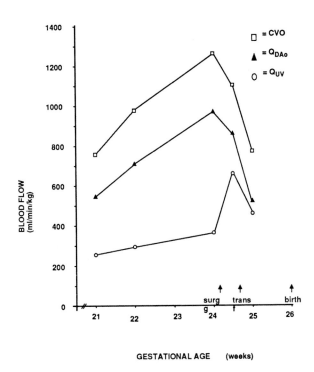

FIG. 33. Serial flow calculations in the third patient with a sacrococcygeal teratoma. Symbols used to indicate the placental flow (Q_{UV}), descending aortic flow (Q_{DAo}), and combined ventricular output (CVO) are shown. Following fetal surgery (surg) combined ventricular output and descending aortic flow decreased, but placental flow increased. After fetal transfusion (transf), placental flow decreased as well. From Schmidt et al. (52).

usually 60–70%. In two of the three fetuses it accounted for less, suggesting a relative steal of flow from the placenta by the tumor, although flow to both organs was increased.

Because the tumor mass was as large as the fetus, greater than twice the normal cardiac output would be expected. This was indeed the case. The regional output was also increased, with the majority of the flow directed to the placenta and the teratoma, with a relatively greater component directed to the tumor. The autopsy demonstrated that complete removal of the tumor had been achieved. The ability to recognize ventricular volume overload in the instance of the teratomas offers a potential for surgical relief of this profound circulatory disorder in the *previable* human fetus and indicates the importance of prenatal circulatory measurement by ultrasound for decisions to be made regarding therapy.

The high cardiac output places demands on the ventricles, which appear to fail at about twice the estimated normal range. The low fetal colloidal pressure and elevated hydrostatic pressure tend to lead to the accumulation of fluid in the tissues, which eventually expresses itself as hydrops. This may be aggravated by decreased hepatic albumin formation, and in regard to the teratomas, by the increased substrate utilization by tumor growth and blood loss into the tumor itself.

It is of interest to consider how the regional distribution of the cardiac output is altered in the fetuses with teratomas. Clearly the increase in absolute and regional distribution is to the teratoma and the placenta (which was markedly thickened in all of these pregnancies). De-

scending aortic flow accounted for 68–77% of the combined ventricular output, compared with normal levels of about 55%.

Conventional opinion held that fetal cardiac output is at its zenith with respect to the Frank–Starling relationship because only slight increases in the combined ventricular output have occurred with acute volume expansion (60,61). Recent experimental studies (62) indicate that if preload is increased at the same time as afterload is decreased (tumor growth), a similar increase in cardiac output can be observed.

Although we have seen large cerebral arteriovenous malformations *in utero*, none of these fetuses has presented with cardiac failure, presumably because the relatively small size of these tumors in comparison to the sacrococcygeal tumors (63,64).

Venous Obstruction

Venous obstruction occurs as part of the other forms of failure in large part, but can occur as a direct effect, e.g., in diaphragmatic hernia or atrioventricular valve regurgitation. Because the parallel nature of the fetal circulation permits bypass of obstructions by redirecting flow, atrioventricular valve insufficiency will affect the fetal circulation by producing systemic venous hypertension because the foramen ovale provides free communication between the atria regardless of which atrioventricular valve is leaking.

The fetuses that presented with atrioventricular valve

TABLE 3. *Ultrasonographic findings in three fetuses with large sacrococcygeal teratomas*

A. M-Mode Findings

Patient/study	Gestational age (wks)	Weight (kg)	LVEDD[b] (mm)	LV FS (%)	RVEDD[b] (mm)	RV FS (%)	PT[b] (mm)	IVC (mm)	PE
1	21	0.45	10.7 [6.8]	35	12.0 [8.1]	34	40 [20]	5.8	+
2	27	0.9	13.1 [9.4]	29	14.1 [11.0]	28	51 [28]	8.3	+
3a	21	0.4[a]	9.1 [6.8]	34	9.4 [8.1]	34	36 [22]	4.5	−
3b	22	0.45[a]	10.1 [7.2]	36	10.2 [8.6]	34	37 [23]	5.1	−
3c	24	0.6[a]	12.1 [8.1]	40	12.8 [9.6]	39	51 [25]	6.9	+
3d	24.5	0.65[a]	12.4 [8.4]	29	13.2 [9.9]	31	63 [25.5]	5.8	+
3e	25	0.7[a]	12.2 [8.6]	34	12.8 [10.1]	34	62 [26]	5.8	−

B. Doppler Ultrasound Flow Calculations

Patient/study	CVO[c] (ml/min/kg)	Q_{DAo}[d] (ml/min/kg)	Q_{DAo}/CVO (%)	Q_{UV}[e] (ml/min/kg)	Q_{UV}/Q_{DAo} (%)
1	1600	1151	72	600	52
2	987	672	68	489	73
3a	757	549	73	260	47
3b	984	704	72	296	42
3c	1262	972	77	358	37
3d	1109	869	78	660	76
3e	787	524	67	460	88

From Silverman and Schmidt (18).

CVO, combined ventricular output; GA, gestational age; LVEDD, left ventricular end-diastolic diameter; LV FS, left ventricular fractional shortening index [nl: 34 ± 3% (mean ± SD)]; IVC, inferior vena cava [nl: 2.9–4.1 mm in fetuses of 21–28 weeks GA]; PE, pericardial effusion; PT, placental thickness; Q_{DAo}, descending aortic flow; Q_{UV}, umbilical venous flow; RVEDD, right ventricular end-diastolic diameter; RV FS, right ventricular fractional shortening index [nl: 34 ± 3%].

[a] Extrapolated from birthweight.
[b] Normal mean for gestational age is shown in brackets; flows are related to estimated fetal weight.
[c] Normal: 553 ± 153 ml/min/kg (mean ± SD) (9).
[d] Normal: 184 ± 20 ml/min/kg (8).
[e] Normal: 110 ± 26 ml/min/kg (10).

regurgitation had associated heart disease. The qualitative finding of tricuspid regurgitation, mitral regurgitation, or regurgitation through a common atrioventricular valve in association with cardiac structural lesions also produces ventricular volume overload. When this reaches a certain level, hydrops develops, reflecting a profound nature of the disorder. These fetuses had either Ebstein's anomaly (51,65–67) or other atrioventricular valve regurgitation leading to the presence of hydrops on a hydrostatic basis. The findings of fetal hydrops in fetuses with congenital heart disease are shown in Table 2. These fetuses had atrioventricular valve regurgitation as a common association, be it through a tricuspid, mitral, or common atrioventricular valve. Almost all patients in this group died in the perinatal period, indicating the profound nature of the disorder as well as the advanced nature of the finding of hydrops (27).

REFERENCES

1. Silverman NH. Prenatal recognition of cardiac abnormalities. In: *Pediatric echocardiography.* Baltimore, MD: Williams and Wilkins; 1993:553–596.
2. Schmidt KG, de Araujo LML, Silverman NH. Evaluation of the fetal heart by echocardiography. I. Structural and functional abnormalities. *Am J Cardiac Imag* 1988;2:57–76.
3. Schmidt KG, Silverman NH, Van Hare GF, Hawkins JA, Cloez JL, Rudolph AM. Two-dimensional echocardiographic determination of ventricular volumes in the fetal heart. Validation studies in fetal lambs. *Circulation* 1990;81:325–333.
4. Shime J, Gresser CD, Rakowski H. Quantitative two-dimensional echocardiographic assessment of fetal cardiac growth. *Am J Obstet Gynecol* 1986;154:294–300.
5. Tan J, Silverman NH, Hoffman JIE, Villegas M, Schmidt KG. Cardiac dimensions in the human fetus from 18 weeks to term: A cross-sectional echocardiographic study. *Am J Cardiol* 1992;70:1459–1467.
6. Hornberger LK, Weintraub RG, Pesonnen E, et al. Echocardiographic study of the morphology and growth of the aortic arch in the human fetus: Observations related to the prenatal diagnosis of coarctation. *Circulation* 1992;86:741–747.
7. Schmidt KG, Di Tommaso M, Silverman NH, Rudolph AM. Doppler echocardiographic assessment of fetal descending aortic and umbilical blood flows—validation studies in fetal lambs. *Circulation* 1991;83:1731–1737.
8. Meijboom EJ, Horowitz S, Valdes-Cruz LM, Sahn DJ, Larson DF, Lima CO. A Doppler echocardiographic method for calculating volume flow across the tricuspid valve: Correlative laboratory and clinical studies. *Circulation* 1985;71:551–557.
9. De Smedt MCH, Visser GHA, Meijboom EJ. Fetal cardiac output estimated by Doppler echocardiography during mid- and late gestation. *Am J Cardiol* 1987;60:338–342.
10. Eik-Nes SH, Brubakk AO, Ulstein MK. Measurement of human blood flow. *Br Heart J* 1980;280:283–285.
11. Reed KL, Meijboom EJ, Sahn DJ, Scagnelli SA, Valdez-Cruz LM,

Shenker L. Cardiac velocities in human fetuses. *Circulation* 1986;73:41–46.

12. St. John Sutton M, Theard MA, Bhatia SJS, Plappert T, Salzman DH, Doubilet P. Changes in placental blood flow in the normal human fetus with gestational age. *Pediatr Res* 1990;28:383–387.

13. Maulik D, Nanda NC, Saini VD. Fetal Doppler echocardiography: Methods and characterization of normal and abnormal hemodynamics. *Am J Cardiol* 1984;53:572–578.

14. Allan LD, Chita SK, Al-Ghazali W, Crawford DC, Tynan M. Doppler echocardiographic evaluation of the normal human fetal heart. *Br Heart J* 1987;57:528–533.

15. Huhta JC, Moise KJ, Fisher DJ, Sharif DS, Wasserstrum N, Martin C. Detection and quantitation of constriction of the fetal ductus arteriosus by Doppler echocardiography. *Circulation* 1987;75:406–412.

16. Eldridge MW, Berman W, Greene ER. Serial echo-Doppler measurements of human fetal abdominal aortic blood flow. *J Ultrasound Med* 1985;4:453–458.

17. Barss VA, Doubilet PM, St. John-Sutton M, Cartier MS, Frigoletto FD. Cardiac output in a fetus with erythroblastosis fetalis: Assessment using pulsed Doppler. *Obstet Gynecol* 1987;70:442–444.

18. Silverman NH, Schmidt KG. Ventricular volume overload in the human fetus: observations from fetal echocardiography. *J Am Soc Echo* 1990;3:20–29.

19. Shiraishi H, Silverman NH, Rudolph AM. Accuracy of right ventricular output estimated by Doppler echocardiography in the sheep fetus. *Am J Obstet Gynecol* 1993;168:947–953.

20. Schmidt KG, Di Tommaso M, Silverman NH, Rudolph AM. Evaluation of changes in umbilical blood flow in the fetal lamb by Doppler waveform analysis. *Am J Obstet Gynecol* 1991;164:1118–1126.

21. Sharland GK, Chita SK, Allan LD. The use of colour Doppler in fetal echocardiography. *Int J Cardiol* 1990;28:229–236.

22. Sahn DJ, Lange LW, Allen HD, Goldberg SJ, Anderson C, Giles H, Haber K. Quantitative real-time cross-sectional echocardiography in the developing normal human fetus and newborn. *Circulation* 1980;62:588–597.

23. Allan LD, Joseph MC, Boyd EGC, Campbell S, Tynan M. M-mode echocardiography in the developing human fetus. *Br Heart J* 1982;47:573–583.

24. Azancot A, Caudell TP, Allen HD, et al. Analysis of ventricular shape by echocardiography in normal fetuses, newborns, and infants. *Circulation* 1983;68:1201–1211.

25. St. John Sutton MG, Gewitz MH, Shah B, et al. Quantitative assessment of growth and function of the cardiac chambers in the normal human fetus: A prospective longitudinal echocardiographic study. *Circulation* 1984;69:645–654.

26. DeVore GR, Siassi B, Platt LD. Fetal echocardiography. IV. M-mode assessment of ventricular size and contractility during the second and third trimesters of pregnancy in the normal fetus. *Am J Obstet Gynecol* 1984;150:981–988.

27. Schmidt KG, Birk E, Silverman NH, Scagnelli SA. Echocardiographic evaluation of dilated cardiomyopathy in the human fetus. *Am J Cardiol* 1989;63:599–605.

28. Veille JC, Sivakoff M, Nemeth M. Accuracy of echocardiography measurements in the fetal lamb. *Am J Obstet Gynecol* 1988;158:1225–1232.

29. Diamond LK, Blackfan KD, Batty JM. Erythroblastosis fetalis and its associations with universal edema of the fetus, icterus gravis neonatorum, and anemia of the newborn. *J Pediatr* 1932;1:269–309.

30. Kleinman CS, Donnerstein RL, DeVore GR, et al. Fetal echocardiography for evaluation of in utero congestive heart failure. *Engl J Med* 1982;306:568–575.

31. Hutchinson AA. Pathology of hydrops fetalis. In: Long WA, ed. *Fetal and neonatal cardiology.* Philadelphia: WB Saunders; 1990:197–210.

32. Holzgreve W, Curry CJR, Golbus MS, Callen PW, Filly RA, Smith C. Investigation of nonimmune hydrops fetalis. *Am J Obstet Gynecol* 1984;150:805–812.

33. Chescheir NC, Seeds JW. Management of hydrops fetalis. In: Long WA, ed. *Fetal and neonatal cardiology.* Philadelphia: WB Saunders; 1990:211–219.

34. Moller JH, Lynch RP, Edward JE. Fetal cardiac failure resulting from congenital anomalies of the heart. *J Pediatr* 1966;68:699–703.

35. Carlson DE, Platt LD, Medearis AL, Horenstein J. Prognostic indicators of the resolution of nonimmune hydrops fetalis and survival of the fetus. *Am J Obstet Gynecol* 1990;163:1785–1787.

36. Castillo RA, Devoe LD, Hadi HA, Martin S, Geist D. Nonimmune hydrops fetalis: Clinical experience and factors related to a poor outcome. *Am J Obstet Gynecol* 1986;155:812–816.

37. Crawford DC, Chita SK, Allan LD. Prenatal detection of congenital heart disease: Factors affecting obstetric management and survival. *Am J Obstet Gynecol* 1988;159:352–356.

38. Cyr DR, Guntheroth WG, Nyberg DA, Smith JR, Nudelman SR, Ek M. Prenatal diagnosis of an intrapericardial teratoma. A cause of nonimmune hydrops. *J Ultrasound Med* 1988;7:87–90.

39. DeVore GR, Donnerstein RL, Kleinman CS, Platt LD, Hobbins JC. Fetal echocardiography. II. The diagnosis and significance of a pericardial effusion in the fetus using real-time-directed M-mode ultrasound. *Am J Obstet Gynecol* 1982;144:693–700.

40. Guereta LG, Burgueros M, Elorza MD, Alix AG, Benito F, Gamallo C. Cardiac rhabdomyoma presenting as fetal hydrops. *Pediatr Cardiol* 1986;7:171–174.

41. Jeanty P, Romero R, Hobbins JC. Fetal pericardial fluid: a normal finding of the second half of gestation. *Am J Obstet Gynecol* 1984;149:529–532.

42. Koivu MK, Nuutinen EM. Large placental chorioangioma as a cause of congestive cardiac failure in newborn infants. *Pediatr Cardiol* 1990;11:221–224.

43. Leake RD, Strimling B, Emmanouilides GC. Intrauterine cardiac failure with hydrops fetalis. Case report in a twin with the hypoplastic left heart syndrome and review of the literature. *Clin Pediatr* 1973;12:649–651.

44. Mahony BS, Filly RA, Callen PW, Chinn DH, Golbus MS. Severe nonimmune hydrops fetalis: Sonographic evaluation. *Radiology* 1984;151:757–761.

45. Pesonen E, Haaavisto H, Ammala P, Teramo K. Intrautrine hydrops fetalis caused by premature closure of the foramen ovale. *Arch Dis Child* 1983;58:1015–1016.

46. Sahn DJ, Shenker L, Reed K, Valde-Cruz L, Sobonya R, Anderson RC. Prenatal ultrasound diagnosis of hypoplastic left heart syndrome in utero associated with hydrops fetalis. *Am Heart J* 1982;104:1368–1372.

47. Sharf M, Abinader EG, Shapiro I, Rosenfeld T, Eibschitz I. Prenatal echocardiographic diagnosis of Ebstein's anomaly with pulmonary atresia. *Am J Obstet Gynecol* 1983;147:300–303.

48. Thomas CS, Leopold GR, Hilton S, Key T, Coen R, Lynch F. Fetal hydrops associated with extralobar pulmonary sequestration. *J Ultrasound Med* 1986;5:668–671.

49. Weinberg PM, Peyser K, Hackney JR. Fetal hydrops in a newborn with hypoplastic left heart syndrome: Tricuspid valve "stopper." *J Am Coll Cardiol* 1985;6:1365–1369.

50. Younis JS, Granat M. Insufficient transplacental digoxin transfer in severe hydrops fetalis. *Am J Obstet Gynecol* 1987;157:1268–1269.

51. Silverman NH, Kleinman CS, Rudolph AM, et al. Fetal atrioventricular valve insufficiency associated with nonimmune hydrops: A two-dimensional echocardiography and pulsed Doppler ultrasound study. *Circulation* 1985;72:825–831.

52. Schmidt KG, Silverman NH, Harrison MR, Callen PW. High-output cardiac failure in fetuses with large sacrococcygeal teratoma: Diagnosis by echocardiography and Doppler ultrasound. *J Pediatr* 1989;114:1023–1028.

53. Alter DN, Reed KL, Marx GR, Anderson CF, Shenker L. Prenatal diagnosis of congestive heart failure in a fetus with a sacrococcygeal teratoma. *Obstet Gynecol* 1988;71:978–981.

54. Kesson CW. Foetal paroxysmal auricular tachycardia. *Br Heart J* 1958;20:552–556.

55. Allan LD, Anderson RH, Sullivan ID, Campbell S, Holt DW, Tynan M. Evaluation of fetal arrhythmias by echocardiography. *Br Heart J* 1983;50:240–245.

56. Allan LD, Crawford DC, Anderson RH, Tynan M. Spectrum of congenital heart disease detected echocardiographically in prenatal life. *Br Heart J* 1985;54:523–526.

57. Maxwell DJ, Crawford DC, Curry PVM, Tynan MJ, Allan LD.

Obstetric importance, diagnosis, and management of fetal tachycardias. *Br Med J* 1988;297:107–110.

58. Lingman G, Marsal K. Circulatory effects of fetal cardiac arrhythmias. *Pediatr Cardiol* 1986;7:67–74.

59. Schmidt KG, Ulmer HE, Silverman NH, Kleinman CS, Copel JA. Perinatal outcome of fetal complete atrioventricular block: A multicenter experience. *J Am Coll Cardiol* 1991;17:1360–1366.

60. Gilbert RD. Control of fetal cardiac output during changes in blood volume. *Am J Physiol* 1980;238:H80–H86.

61. Thornburg KL, Morton MJ. Filling and arterial pressures as determinants of RV stroke volume in the sheep fetus. *Am J Physiol* 1983;244:H656–H663.

62. Hawkins J, Van Hare GF, Schmidt KG, Rudolph AM. Effects of increasing afterload on left ventricular output in fetal lambs. *Circ Res* 1989;65:127–134.

63. Ciricillo SF, Schmidt KG, Silverman NH, et al. Serial ultrasonographic evaluation of neonatal vein of Galen malformations to assess the efficacy of interventional neuroradiological procedures. *Neurosurgery* 1990;27:544–548.

64. Ciricillo SF, Edwards MS, Schmidt KG, et al. Interventional neuroradiological management of vein of Galen malformations in the neonate. *Neurosurgery* 1990;27:22–27.

65. Roberson DA, Silverman NH. Ebstein's anomaly: Echocardiographic and clinical features in the fetus and neonate. *J Am Coll Cardiol* 1989;14:1300–1307.

66. Silverman NH, Golbus MS. Echocardiographic techniques for assessing normal and abnormal fetal cardiac anatomy. Bethesda Conference #14. *J Am Coll Cardiol* 1985;5:20S–29S.

67. Silverman NH, Birk E. Ebstein's malformation of the tricuspid valve: cross-sectional echocardiography and Doppler. In: Anderson RH, Neches WH, Park SC, Zuberbuhler JR, eds. *Perspectives in pediatric cardiology.* Mount Kisco, NY: Futura; 1988:113–125.

68. Schmidt KG, Silverman NH. Prenatal recognition of cardiac abnormalities. In: Harrison MR, Golbus MS, Filly RA, eds. *The unborn patient: Prenatal diagnosis and treatment.* Philadelphia: WB Saunders; 1980:269–284.

69. Schmidt KG, Silverman NH. Evaluation of the fetal heart by ultrasound. In: Callen PW, ed. *Ultrasonography in obstetrics and gynecology.* Philadelphia: WB Saunders; 1988:165–206.

Doppler Ultrasound in Obstetrics and Gynecology,
edited by Joshua A. Copel and Kathryn L. Reed.
Raven Press, Ltd., New York © 1995.

CHAPTER 26

Fetal Arrhythmias

Charles M. McCurdy, Jr. and Kathryn L. Reed

Fetal rhythm disturbances are diagnosed in approximately 1–2% of gestations (1,2). The vast majority of these disturbances will result in no adverse sequelae during gestation or the immediate neonatal period. However, approximately 10% of fetal cardiac arrhythmias can result in significant morbidity or mortality. As an indication for referral, fetal arrhythmias may account for 15–20% of referrals to tertiary centers for suspected antenatal congenital heart disease (3,4). Fetal arrhythmias can be subdivided into tachyarrhythmias (rate > 180 bpm), bradyarrhythmias (rate < 100 bpm), and irregular rhythms. Of arrhythmias, 80–85% are irregularly/irregular rhythms caused by extrasystolic beats and are of no consequence in at least 95% of fetuses (3). As in the adult, disturbances affecting the cardiac conduction system result in fetal arrhythmias. However, unique to the fetus, the cardiac conduction system is developing in concert with the embryo/fetus and subject to additional congenital and environmental influences. In addition, the fetal heart is developing throughout early gestation, and maintains physiologic and anatomic differences from the mature adult cardiovascular system into the immediate neonatal period in the normal case, and even longer in many cases of congenital heart disease.

In the past, diagnosis of fetal arrhythmias has relied on fetal electrocardiograms, two-dimensional ultrasound, and M-mode ultrasound. Doppler ultrasound provides a means to evaluate fetal cardiovascular physiology in the normal and diseased state. The role of Doppler ultrasound in the evaluation of fetal rhythm disturbances has emerged as a valuable adjunct in diagnosing and monitoring the progression of disease, or in assessing response to therapy. Study of velocity waveforms in the heart, arterial vessels, and major venous supply to the heart can assist in diagnosis and management.

Management and prognosis are specific to the abnormal rhythm present. Management options can include observation, *in utero* therapy via maternal administration of antiarrhythmic agents, direct fetal infusion of antiarrhythmic agents via intravascular or umbilical venous administration, early delivery, and cardiac pacing (5). As with all fetal abnormalities the gravida should be apprised of the condition of the fetus and counseled with regard to possible etiologies, the range of associated cardiac and extracardiac anomalies, associated maternal conditions, and the range of expected outcomes. Only through this process can the gravida make the decisions that will ultimately affect outcome.

In this chapter we will review the embryology of the fetal heart and conduction system including the unique physiologic and anatomic differences that exist during fetal life. The role of ultrasound, and specifically pulsed Doppler ultrasound, in evaluation and management will be described. Finally, fetal arrhythmias will be discussed based on rate and rhythm disturbance with emphasis on etiology, diagnosis, prognosis, and management options.

THE DEVELOPING FETAL HEART

The recognizable embryology of the fetal heart begins with the fusion of paired endothelium-lined heart tubes on embryologic days 18–19 (6). Formation of the two cardiac tubes in a more cephalic (relative to the ultimate intrathoracic location) position in the trilaminar embryo occurs as a result of migration and proliferation of mesenchymal angioblastic tissue. Subsequent canalization results in paired tubes. The primitive heart tube will ultimately become the endocardium of the mature heart. Rapid and disproportionate growth results in folding and convolution of the heart tube. Structures first recognized in this process are the bulbis cordis, common ventricle, and common atrium. Concurrently in the fourth week, the development of the head fold results in ventral and

C. M. McCurdy, and K. L. Reed: Department of Obstetrics and Gynecology, University of Arizona Health Sciences Center, Tucson, Arizona 85724.

caudal migration of the evolving cardiac tube. Convolution leads to an anterior and cephalad displacement of the atrium and the now-formed sinus venosus. The sinus venosus, initially a separate chamber, fuses with the right atrium leaving the coronary sinus and a portion of the atrial wall as mature remnants. Similarly, the ventricles and bulbus cordis (continuous with the truncus arteriosus at this time) migrate caudally and ventrally. Mesenchymal induction results in migration and formation of the myocardial mantle, the progenitor of the myocardium. Septation of the atrioventricular (AV) canal begins with the formation of endocardial cushions in the fourth embryologic week. Completion of the AV separation into right- and left-sided structures of atria and ventricles separated by midline structures occurs by the seventh week with completion of the membranous portion of the interventricular septum. Atrial separation is accomplished by the end of the fifth week with the formation of the valve of the foramen ovale (remainder of the septum primum) over a persistent caudal defect in the septum secundum, the foramen ovale (6,7).

Truncal ridges first appear in the bulbus cordis in the fifth embryologic week. A spiraling of the truncal ridges separates the bulbus cordis and truncus arteriosus into the aortic outflow tract and the concentrically spiraling pulmonary outflow tract. The semilunar aortic and pulmonic valves are formed from endocardial thickenings in the bulbus cordis in a fashion similar to that of the atrioventricular valves. The septation of the great vessels is completed as the membranous interventricular septum fuses with the interatrial septum and the aorticopulmonary septum in the seventh week (6).

Circulation of blood begins on approximately day 21 with cells of extraembryonal origin in vessels derived from the primitive yolk sac and allantois, making the fetal cardiovascular system the first within the embryo to function (6,8,9). At this time, three sets of primordial veins drain to the primitive fetal heart: the vitelline veins (draining the yolk sac), the cardinal veins (draining the caudal and cephalad portions of the embryo), and the umbilical veins (draining the embryonic placenta). The primitive structures are mostly resorbed with portions of the cardinal veins incorporated into venous drainage of the fetal head and neck, and the left umbilical vein persisting until birth. The aortic arch and descending aorta result from persistence of the left fourth aortic arch. Derivatives of the third through sixth aortic arches supply the head, neck, and pulmonary vasculature including the ductus arteriosus (6).

Anatomic differences in the fetus with respect to the infant include a series of shunts and a right ventricular dominance, which persist until birth or the early neonatal period in the normal case. Right ventricular dominance is manifested by approximately 55% of the cardiac output (307 ml/kg/min) exiting the right ventricular outflow tract (10). Ultrasonographically, a slight disparity in ventricular size may be appreciated. The ductus arteriosus, a remnant of the distal left sixth aortic arch, allows shunting of the right ventricular output past the fetal lungs to the caudal fetal body secondary to a pressure gradient of 2–3 mm Hg, with systemic pressure less than pulmonary pressure (11). The foramen ovale allows shunting of blood from the right atrium to the left-sided circulation and ultimately to the cranial vessels. The last and singularly important fetal shunt is that of the ductus venosus that allows shunting of approximately 60% of the oxygenated umbilical venous return to the right atrium bypassing the microcirculation of the fetal liver (12).

DEVELOPMENT OF THE CONDUCTION SYSTEM AND AUTONOMIC INNERVATION

The vast majority of studies regarding the fetal heart and its function are derived from nonprimate (e.g., chick, porcine embryo) models (13–15). However, the few studies utilizing the human model provide corroboration for many, but not all, of the earlier studies in animals (10,16). Many of the developmental aspects of the innervation of the fetal heart remain speculative. Earliest automaticity in the fetal heart begins in the ventricular myocyte on about day 21 (7,8). Subsequent convolution of the fetal heart tube and caudal fusion of the atrial and ventricular components results in a directional peristalsis of blood through the fetal heart. Even before AV valve formation, accumulation of tissue in the area of the AV junction provides some degree of obstruction to retrograde flow such that directional flow through the immature heart is accentuated (6,17).

The sinoatrial (SA) node has its origin in the sinus venosus after fusion of this structure with the atrium. This density of cells in the anteromedial portion of the junction of the cavum and atrium and its supplying artery are recognizable by the seventh embryologic week (6,18). Of note, in the fourth embryologic week, the sinus venosus, atria, and ventricle each have intrinsic pacemaker activity with rates that decrease respectively (5,17). The earliest *in vivo* evidence of intrinsic cardiac activity reveals a mean heart rate of 90 bpm at four embryologic weeks increasing 35% during the fifth week to a mean of 124 bpm (9). This increase continues until a maximum of 180 bpm is reached at 8–10 embryologic weeks with a subsequent progressive decline to term (8).

Internodal preferential pathways differentiate from atrial myocardium and the AV node develops as a result of the septation of the fetal atria and ventricles. The AV node develops from primitive myocytes within the SA ring, the septum primum, anterior aspect of the AV ring, and, to some extent, the primitive atrium. The specialized conducting tissue of the ventricle most likely develops from the bulboventricular ring as a differentiation of ventricular myocytes, and does so concomitant with the above-described interatrial and junctional conduction system development. The AV node and the junctional pathway to the ventricles appear intact by the tenth to twelfth week (19).

The neural control over the fetal rate is primarily via sympathetic and parasympathetic innervation. Sympathetic innervation of the fetal heart is mediated by α_1- and β_1-adrenergic receptors that release norepinephrine at the myocyte cell membrane. Parasympathetic innervation is provided by muscarinic-cholinergic receptors primarily at the SA and AV nodes. The ventricular myocardium also contains histochemical evidence of muscarinic receptors; however, the density of these receptors is much less than in the specialized nodal areas of the atrium (20). Papp demonstrated responsiveness of the fetal heart at 4 weeks to the pacemaker inhibition of acetylcholine (21). At approximately 4–5 postconceptional weeks, these authors and others demonstrated a positive chronotropic response to norepinephrine (20,22).

The maturation of autonomic nerves in the fetal heart lags behind the demonstrable presence of receptors for their respective neurotransmitters. Parasympathetic fibers are demonstrable cytochemically by 6 postconceptional weeks, and sympathetic fibers by 10 weeks (20). Histochemical evidence of receptor presence and cytologic evidence of intact neural tissue are not evidence of intact function of the autonomic system. Clinical evidence in the human fetus exists for intact parasympathetic inhibition of pacemaker activity by 12–17 weeks gestational age and intact sympathetic stimulatory effect by 22–23 completed gestational weeks (21,23). The autonomic effect on the AV node and the ventricle is less relative to the SA node.

METHODS OF ASSESSMENT

Fetal ECG

In the neonatal period, the electrocardiogram (ECG) provides the most useful information in diagnosing fetal arrhythmias. However, the fetal ECG is much less useful than its neonatal counterpart. Transabdominal fetal ECG typically yields its best results if utilized in the late second or third trimester. Even in advanced gestation with a normal gravid habitus, external fetal ECG fails to allow discrimination of atrial activity (p wave) secondary to insufficient voltage to measure above background "noise" in a majority of cases. In addition, maternal cardiac electrical impulses interfere with assessment of the fetal QRS complex. Once fetal scalp electrode placement is possible the problem of maternal electrical interference is reduced but identification of atrial activity remains limited. Fetal scalp electrode application is significantly limited to assessing only cases of fetal arrhythmia complicating labor. Fetal ECG obtained by

scalp electrode may be interpreted generally as for an adult ECG (24). Because of these limitations, the fetal ECG has been of little value as a diagnostic tool in the antenatal differentiation of fetal arrhythmias.

Two-Dimensional Echocardiography

Two-dimensional echocardiography can be used to evaluate the fetal heart for abnormalities associated with fetal arrhythmias, yet is of limited value in identifying the individual arrhythmia. A systematic approach to evaluating the fetal heart for anomalies consists of a series of sonographic views that focus on symmetry and changes throughout the cardiac cycle with respect to the heart chambers, AV valves, foramen ovale, and cardiac wall and septum movement (25). The heart should appear in the ventral aspect of the chest with the cardiac axis to the fetal left at 35–55°. The transverse sonographic view through the fetal chest that images the heart in the four-chamber view is optimal for comparing chambers for symmetry in size and function and for assessing valvular function in real time (26). In the four-chamber view of the fetal heart anomalous return of pulmonary veins can be a clue to atrial isomerism and concomitant complete AV block (27). In addition, the presence of cardiomegaly or pericardial effusions can be detected with the four-chamber view and suggest the various possibilities of complete AV dissociation, supraventricular tachycardia, or other arrhythmic causes of heart failure (28). The outflow tracts can be imaged best with minimal manipulation from the transverse four-chamber view. The ventricular outflow tracts should be imaged with a focus on proximal dilation in the case of obstruction or atresia, and function and presence of semilunar valves. Great vessels can be interrogated as they enter the heart in a parasagittal plane (long axis) and an oblique plane (short axis) through the right side of the fetal heart. The long- and short-axis views of the great vessels can be used to identify transposition or other conotruncal abnormalities. Finally, two-dimensional ultrasound is of greatest value in differentiating fetal arrhythmias, as it allows directing the M-mode or pulsed Doppler interrogation of the heart.

M-Mode Echocardiography

It is with M-mode, or time–motion mode, ultrasound that the fetal echocardiographer has the greatest experience in diagnosing fetal arrhythmias. Structures interrogated by a narrow ultrasound beam are displayed vs. time as a variable on the horizontal axis. M-mode echocardiography has been utilized with great success in determining physiologic consequences (excitation–contraction coupling) of abnormal electrophysiology in the adult heart (28,29). In obstetrics, M-mode was initially used to detect and document the presence of fetal cardiac activity (8,9). In addition, M-mode sonography can be used to accurately measure chamber size and valvular area, calculate fractional shortening, and document the presence and extent of pericardial effusions (30,31). Currently, two-dimensional sonography is used to guide M-mode interrogation of the fetal heart.

M-mode evaluation of fetal arrhythmias must target a structure or structures that move discriminantly with atrial and ventricular wall movement (32). A view slightly oblique from the apical four-chamber view that places the M-mode cursor across an atrial and ventricular wall (and includes the interventricular or interatrial septum) is valuable to discern most types of fetal arrhythmia. Atrial wall motion and ventricular motion can be compared for timing and conduction of atrial events. This view of the atria and ventricles may be of limited usefulness in cases of dilated cardiomyopathy, endocardial fibrosis, and other abnormalities that result in reduced cardiac wall motion. Additional views that target AV or semilunar valves can also provide useful information regarding the timing of atrial and ventricular events.

Doppler Echocardiography

Doppler ultrasound has been used to study most of the fetal cardiovascular system, placental–umbilical circulation, and uterine circulation as well (33–35). Pulsed Doppler interrogation of the fetal heart and fetal vasculature has provided insight into normal and abnormal physiology in the human fetus (10,35,36,37). This

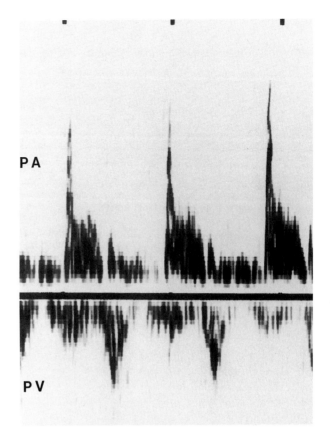

FIG. 2. Pulsed Doppler simultaneous interrogation of pulmonary artery (PA) and pulmonary vein (PV) with normal sinus rhythm. Heart rate is 130 bpm.

method of study has been utilized to corroborate animal model–implied physiologic determinants (10,12). Original *in vivo* studies utilized continuous wave Doppler to interrogate structures that fell within the ultrasound beam. Subsequently, pulsed Doppler interrogation has added the ability to image the area of interest and gate the vessel, or structure, to be studied individually. The addition of color flow mapping to the armamentarium of the sonographer furthers the ability to assess cardiac anatomy and physiology (38). Currently, the major usefulness of color Doppler is as a guide to placement of the cursor for pulsed Doppler insonation of a particular area of interest.

Rate and rhythm disturbances can be detected in the peripheral placental–umbilical circulation. Pulsed Doppler interrogation of the umbilical circulation may assist in the initial detection of an arrhythmia (5). Umbilical artery waveforms provide insight into ventricular systolic events. Ventricular systole-to-systole variation can be assessed analogous to the R-R segment electrophysiologic variation that occurs in physiologic and pathologic conditions (e.g., sinus arrhythmia, extrasystoles, AV block). Systolic-to-diastolic ratios of umbilical arterial waveforms appear to be rate-dependent and are of little or no value in assessing fetal well-being. How-

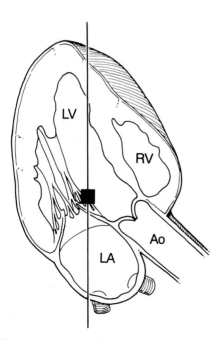

FIG. 1. Doppler gate placed simultaneously over left ventricular inflow and outflow tracts, left atrium (LA), left ventricular (LV), right ventricle (RV), and aorta (Ao).

ever, absent or reversed flow may represent fetal decompensation and impending demise. Use of umbilical venous waveforms allows insight into inferior vena cava and right heart events that when compared to umbilical arterial waveforms can assist in sequencing AV dynamics (37).

Intracardiac pulsed Doppler studies have been performed since the early 1980s. The Doppler gate is placed distal to the mitral, tricuspid, pulmonic, or aortic valve (Chapter 22). Insonated in this fashion, Doppler waveforms not only assess sequential activity in the atria and ventricles, but also assess the effect of anomalous anatomy or fetal dysrhythmia on the cardiovascular physiology. Normal intracardiac Doppler values have been ascertained and are included elsewhere in this text (Chapter 22).

Additional cursor placements have been suggested in diagnosing fetal arrhythmias. A sample volume of 2–5 mm over the left ventricular inflow and outflow tracts allows simultaneous imaging of atrial and ventricular waveforms and events. Atrial rate can further be assessed by placing the Doppler gate over the interatrial septum at the level of the foramen ovale (39) (Fig. 1).

Chan and coworkers advocate simultaneous velocimetry on the abdominal aorta and inferior vena cava. Vena cava waveforms represented right atrial activity and ventricular activity was estimated by aorta velocimetry. With the addition of this method of analysis, these authors were able to diagnose all arrhythmias correctly in this small series, including a case of heart block at 13 weeks gestation (40). Additionally, simultaneous interrogation of the pulmonary artery and a pulmonary vein can yield information pertinent to ventricular and atrial events, respectively (Fig. 2). The value of vena caval velocimetry in evaluating fetal arrhythmias and fetal cardiac function and subsequent perinatal morbidity in growth-retarded fetuses and gestations affected by fetal arrhythmias has been demonstrated (36). Table 1 lists

TABLE 1. *Ultrasound in evaluation of arrhythmias*

Two-dimensional	Fetal anatomy
	Fetal biophysical profile
	Cardiac anatomy
	Chamber dilation, pericardial effusion
	Hydrops (ascites, tissue edema, and polyhydramnios)
M-mode	Timing of atrial and ventricular events
	Effusions
	Chamber dilation or wall hypertrophy
Pulsed Doppler	Timing of atrial and ventricular events
	Cardiac function
	Serial examination
	Valvular regurgitation
Color Doppler	Pulsed Doppler gate placement
	Flow disturbances (turbulence)
	Cardiac function in complex cardiac defects

TABLE 2. *Classification of arrhythmias*

Irregular rhythms
  Sinus arrhythmia
  Extrasystoles
    Premature atrial contractions
    Premature ventricular contractions
  Tachyarrhythmias with blocked conduction
Tachyarrhythmias
  Sinus tachycardia
  Supraventricular tachycardia
  Atrial flutter
  Atrial fibrillation
  Ventricular tachycardia
Bradyarrhythmias
  Sinus bradycardia
  Heart block
    Second-degree heart block
    Atrioventricular dissociation
  Nonconducted supraventricular extrasystoles

the advantages of two-dimensional, M-mode, pulsed, and color Doppler ultrasound in the evaluation of arrhythmias.

ARRHYTHMIAS

Fetal arrhythmias cover a broad range of electrophysiologic abnormalities in addition to probable variants of normal. The extent is analogous to those found in the neonate or the adult. However, the consequences of these arrhythmias in the fetus, and subsequently in the newborn, are variable and unique. A categorization of fetal arrhythmias based on auscultatory or fetal heart rate monitor findings is presented in Table 2. This classification is most cogent in that it relates to the method originally responsible for detection and referral of the fetal arrhythmia for definitive diagnosis.

IRREGULAR RHYTHMS

Sinus Arrhythmias

Irregular rhythms account for up to 85% of all fetal arrhythmias (1,41). Most of these arrhythmias are of little or no consequence in the fetus or neonate. The incidence of sinus arrhythmias is unknown. Though these arrhythmias originate in the SA node, the etiology for each arrhythmia is diverse. Fetal state and maternal drug administration (e.g., scopolamine, meperidine, morphine, diazepam, and atropine) can affect fetal heart rate or variability. Increased variability of R-R segments is commonly attributed to a healthy and intact sympathetic–parasympathetic interaction at the level of the fetal heart. Increases in this variability may be a prodromal indicator of a prolonged hypoxic state and degenerate to a sinus tachycardia (42).

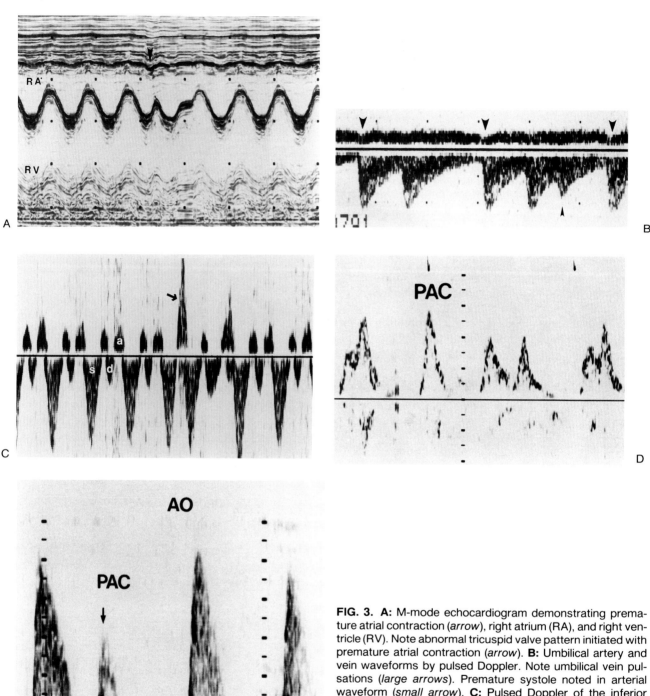

FIG. 3. A: M-mode echocardiogram demonstrating premature atrial contraction (*arrow*), right atrium (RA), and right ventricle (RV). Note abnormal tricuspid valve pattern initiated with premature atrial contraction (*arrow*). **B:** Umbilical artery and vein waveforms by pulsed Doppler. Note umbilical vein pulsations (*large arrows*). Premature systole noted in arterial waveform (*small arrow*). **C:** Pulsed Doppler of the inferior vena cava (IVC). Systolic (s) and diastolic (d) waveforms are denoted; atrial contraction (a) is evident as reversal of flow. PAC (*arrow*) is remarkable for pronounced reversal of flow. **D:** Mitral valve velocimetry with PAC noted. Passive ventricular diastolic filling is obscured during the conducted PAC with only atrial contraction waveform evident. Note postextrasystolic prolongation of diastolic flow. **E:** PAC recorded with velocimetry in the proximal aorta (AO); note pause following PAC prior to next aortic systolic waveform, which is larger than normal. (**B** and **D** from ref. 35.)

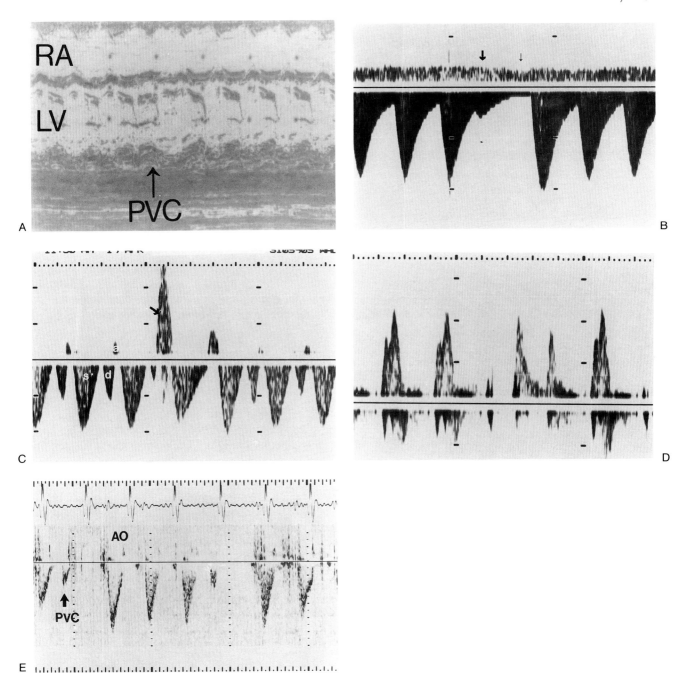

FIG. 4. A: M-mode through right atrium (RA), atrioventricular valve, and left ventricle (LV). Premature ventricular contraction (PVC) marked with arrow. Note that ventricular wall is first structure to move. **B:** PVC (*large arrow*) noted at umbilical vessel pulsed Doppler evaluation. Note decreased diastolic flow in umbilical waveform following PVC with associated umbilical vein pulsation (*small arrow*). **C:** IVC velocimetry with PVC (*arrow*) illustrated by accentuated reversal of flow interrupting the diastolic portion of the waveform. Systolic wave (s), diastolic wave (d), and atrial contraction (a) are labeled. **D:** Intracardiac Doppler across tricuspid valve. First two waveforms are normal. PVC occurs before third waveform and is remarkable for absence of flow across the tricuspid valve. Diastolic filling flow is prolonged following PVC. **E:** PVC on intracardiac Doppler across aortic valve (AO). Compensatory pause between first waveform and waveform immediately following PVC is evident, with increased velocity–time integral compared with normal. (From ref. 35.)

Evaluation of the fetus with a sinus arrhythmia relies on the M-mode demonstration of sequential atrial and ventricular activity. Rate may be determined by this method as well. Prognosis for sinus arrhythmia is almost uniformly good. In the cases where this arrhythmia is ultimately a predictor of poor outcome (with continuous fetal monitoring), ominous and recognizable fetal patterns will ensue (e.g., sinus tachycardia, decreased variability, and severe fetal heart rate decelerations).

Extrasystoles

Extrasystoles are the most common individual class of arrhythmia diagnosed (1,41). Incidence in otherwise healthy neonates may approach 1% and is estimated to be higher in otherwise normal fetuses by some authors (43). As a group, extrasystoles are rarely associated with structural heart disease (1–2%). Atrial septal aneurysms have been found with increased frequency in fetuses with atrial extrasystoles (1,41,44).

Premature atrial contractions (PACs) are the most commonly observed arrhythmia in the fetus and account for over 70% of all arrhythmias (41). The etiology of PACs is usually an ectopic focus in the atria or a preferential pathway. Hypothetically, fetal exposure to stimulatory substances could result in PACs. The most commonly attributed causes are maternal stimulant ingestion, maternal thyroid disease, fetal or maternal catecholamine secretion, or intrinsic fetal cardiac abnormality. Prognosis of this arrhythmia is good, with resolution common pre- or postnatally. However, in 1–2% these arrhythmias will degenerate to supraventricular tachycardia (SVT) (41). SVT with blocked AV conduction will be addressed further with other tachyarrhythmias.

Pulsed Doppler interrogation of the umbilical circulation can delineate the presence of early ventricular systoles; however, umbilical arterial waveforms alone cannot be used to differentiate reliably between premature atrial and ventricular activity. The possibility of umbilical vein waveforms being used to differentiate these and other forms of arrhythmia exists and deserves further study. Simultaneous pulsed Doppler interrogation of vena caval and aortic flows may be used to discriminate between conducted atrial premature beats and nonconducted beats. Inferior vena cava waveforms during PACs are remarkable for increased reversal of flow with atrial contraction immediately preceding the systolic portion of the next waveform (36).

Intracardiac Doppler assessment of extrasystoles is of greatest value in differentiating not only atrial from ventricular activity, but diagnosing conducted and nonconducted ectopic atrial activity as well. Intracardiac Doppler velocimetry on fetuses affected with premature atrial systoles first allowed the demonstration of an intact

Frank–Starling mechanism in the fetus and the existence of a postextrasystolic potentiation of flow (35). With the cursor placed distal to the mitral or tricuspid valve, flow attributable to ventricular early diastole, atrial contraction (late diastole), and ventricular contraction can be identified. Conducted premature atrial contractions will be identified as early forward flow across the AV valve followed by systolic ejection.

Management of these arrhythmias concerns the exclusion of concurrent cardiac anomalies and monitoring for degeneration to a supraventricular tachycardia with the possibility of fetal hydrops ensuing. In addition, in the case of frequent nonconducted atrial activity, AV node dysfunction or degeneration to fetal heart block should be considered. Fetuses with extrasystoles tolerate labor well and should be managed based on routine obstetric practice. Continuous fetal monitoring is encouraged with the use of realtime, M-mode, and Doppler ultrasound to evaluate the onset of a more complex arrhythmia (Figs. 3 and 4).

TACHYARRHYTHMIAS

Sinus Tachycardia

Sinus tachycardias can represent normal variants in the preterm fetus; however, at or near term, maternal or fetal disease must be excluded. The ausculted or monitored fetal heart rate is regular and greater than 160 bpm but almost always less than 200 bpm. Maternal factors leading to fetal sinus tachycardia include fever, β-agonist therapy, significant infection or illness, thyroid disease, and endogenous catecholamine production. Fetal or pregnancy-related etiologies include hypoxia (chronic), anemia, intrauterine infection, endogenous β-agonists, and congestive heart failure (1,45–48).

Evaluation of the fetus with a sinus tachycardia relies on the M-mode demonstration of sequential atrial and ventricular activity and fetal heart rate. A combination of real-time ultrasound, M-mode, and pulsed Doppler can assess for other signs of decompensation or fetal well-being to provide useful information as to the etiology of the tachycardia. Initially, biophysical assessment with two-dimensional ultrasound can assess the fetal condition. In addition, evidence of hydrops (much more common in rates associated with SVT) or other organ system involvement is best determined in this fashion.

Prognosis for sinus tachycardia is determined by the underlying etiology. In the case of fetal compromise, the degree of compensation of the fetus and timing of delivery correlate with fetal outcome. Delivery should be based on obstetric parameters including fetal heart rate monitoring (the presence or absence of decreased variability and decelerations) and the maternal condition.

Supraventricular Tachycardia

Tachyarrhythmias are the most common sustained arrhythmias found in the fetus. They account for about half of sustained arrhythmias and have been reported to be detected in 7–8% of all fetuses with arrhythmia (1,40). Classically, SVT can be distinguished from sinus tachycardia by the typical rate of 220–240 bpm, which exceeds that seen with sinus tachycardia (170–200 bpm). The onset and cessation of SVT is often abrupt in contrast to the more gradual onset and resolution in sinus tachycardia. The electrophysiologic subtypes of SVT include reentrant, excitable secondary ectopic focus, or a variant of atrial flutter or fibrillation. The etiologies of SVT include degeneration from frequent atrial extrasystoles or atrial flutter/fibrillation, cardiac structural disease in 0–37% (e.g., Ebstein's anomaly, pulmonary atresia, cardiac tumors), viral infection (e.g., cytomegalovirus, coxsackie B virus), defective cardiac conduction system, and dilated cardiomyopathy (5,40,49). The significance of this rhythm abnormality lies in the development of congestive heart failure associated with untreated SVT in 40–80% of fetuses (40,49). The subsequent occurrence of hydrops fetalis carries a poorer prognosis (40,49,50). Conversely, 20% of all etiologies and 30% of cardiac causes of nonimmune hydrops may be secondary to SVT (51).

Evaluation of this rhythm disturbance includes an overall fetal assessment with two-dimensional ultrasound. A focus on the presence of cardiac anomalies, effusions, and associated anomalies is emphasized. The fetal biophysical state should be assessed. Two-dimensional ultrasound may be used to identify atrial or ventricular enlargement, which may be an early sign of developing heart failure. M-mode evaluation can accurately determine rate, measure cardiac wall thickness and chamber diameter, as well as establish a one-to-one atrial and ventricular contraction rate. In the case of SVT with blocked AV conduction, M-mode can be useful in identification of blocked beats. Intracardiac pulsed Doppler interrogation can provide information about cardiac output (44). In addition, intracardiac simultaneous left ventricular inflow and outflow insonation, or simultaneous great vessel assessment, can also identify blocked beats in SVT with incomplete conduction. Serial evaluations in fetuses with SVT can further assess the fetus for decompensation or improvement, while expectant or interventional therapy is ongoing.

Some controversy exists over the appropriate therapy for SVT (40,49). In the absence of fetal hydrops, expectant therapy has been advocated (40). However, in the case of the hydropic fetus with SVT, transplacental or direct fetal therapy with antiarrhythmic agents has been used with a subsequent good outcome (40,49,50,51). Antiarrhythmic therapy is not without risk (i.e., the potentiation of AV conduction in SVT leading to tachycardic ventricular response) (40). Ultimately, the decision to treat any SVT is based on the presence or absence of associated fetal anomalies, heart rate, and degree of hemodynamic compensation. Labor in fetuses with SVT can be difficult to manage secondary to the difficulty in assessing fetal well-being by conventional fetal heart rate monitoring. M-mode and pulsed Doppler ultrasound can be used to confirm persistent SVT and assess for change in the fetal rhythm. Resolution of the SVT should allow a trial of labor. In the setting of fetal hydrops and lung maturity, *in utero* fetal therapy may still be recommended to resolve the heart failure prior to delivery as possibly providing the optimal outcome (40,51). Hansmann and coworkers retrospectively reported excellent results treating all SVT regardless of the presence of hydrops (49).

Transplacental or direct fetal administration of antiarrhythmic agents via cordocentesis provides the mainstay of therapy in SVT. The majority of reports since 1980 comment on the use of digoxin therapy in fetal SVT. Maternal administration of digoxin in doses of 0.25–0.75 mg every 8 hr should result in "therapeutic" maternal serum levels of 0.5–2.0 ng/ml (51–54). Onset of therapeutic effect is slow. A recent meta-analysis of reported cases of SVT treated with digoxin revealed an average duration from initiation of therapy to conversion of 11 days. In this series 16 of 29 patients responded to digoxin therapy with 60% of responders converting within 10 days (54). Absence of response or evidence of fetal decompensation should lead to use of a second agent or cordocentesis to provide vascular access for direct fetal therapy (49). Other drugs utilized in the treatment of SVT with heart failure include propranolol, quinidine, verapamil, procainamide, amiodorone, and, recently, adenosine (5,40,49,55–58). Some authors advocate direct fetal therapy as an initial therapeutic alternative (48).

Prognosis of uncomplicated SVT without structural cardiac disease is good. Refractory hydrops fetalis and SVT with initial diagnosis prior to lung maturity carries a dismal prognosis (38,49). Later onset disease and successful conversion of the SVT with resolution of the hydrops carries a significantly improved prognosis with most of these fetuses surviving (40,49,52). The overall survival ultimately reflects the underlying etiology.

Atrial Flutter/Fibrillation

Atrial flutter or fibrillation in the fetus accounts for approximately 15% of sustained arrhythmias. These two arrhythmias are uncommon in the fetus, yet are even less stable in the neonate and extremely uncommon. Shenker reviewed the literature and reported a 21% incidence of structural congenital heart disease associated

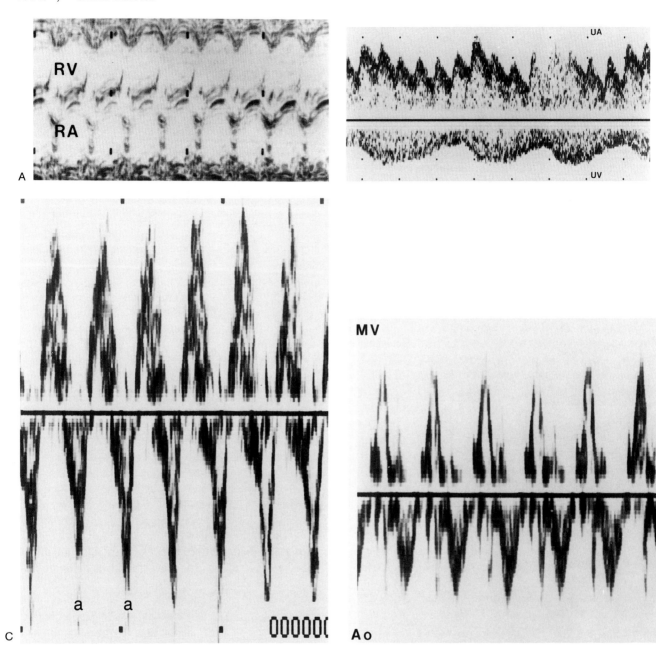

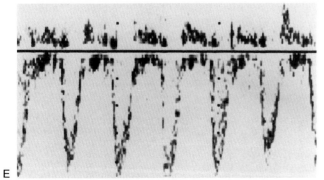

FIG. 5. A: M-mode through right atrium (RA), tricuspid valve, and right ventricle (RV) in fetus with SVT and heart rate of 240 bpm. **B:** Umbilical vessel velocimetry in same fetus. Rate is 240 bpm. UA, Umbilical artery; UV, umbilical vein. Note fetal breathing evidenced in UV pattern. **C:** IVC Doppler flow waveforms in fetus with SVT and rate of 240 bpm. Note fused diastolic and systolic waves and prominent atrial contraction (a). **D:** Simultaneous Doppler waveforms across left ventricular inflow (MV) and outflow (Ao) in fetus with SVT and rate of 270 bpm. Note fusion of a and e waves in mitral valve waveform. **E:** Doppler insonation of the aorta in fetus with rate of 240 bpm and SVT.

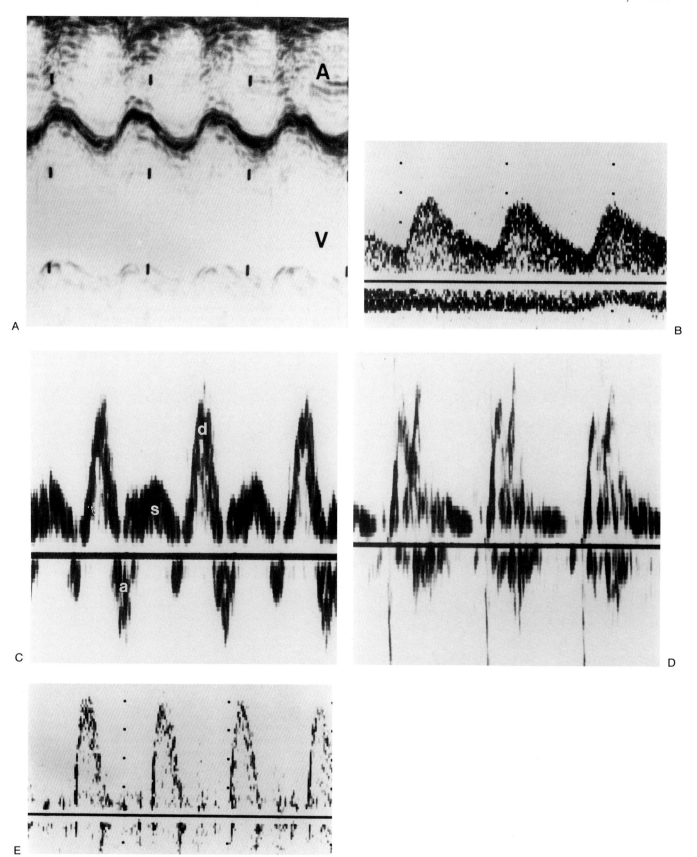

FIG. 6. A–E. M-mode (**A**) with atrium (A) and ventricle (V) labeled, umbilical artery and vein (**B**), IVC (**C**), mitral valve (**D**), and aorta (**E**) pulsed Doppler in fetus with SVT following conversion to sinus rhythm with a heart rate of approximately 130 bpm. On IVC tracing note the unusual appearance of the systolic wave (s) and diastolic wave (d) in this fetus following conversion from SVT; atrial systole (a).

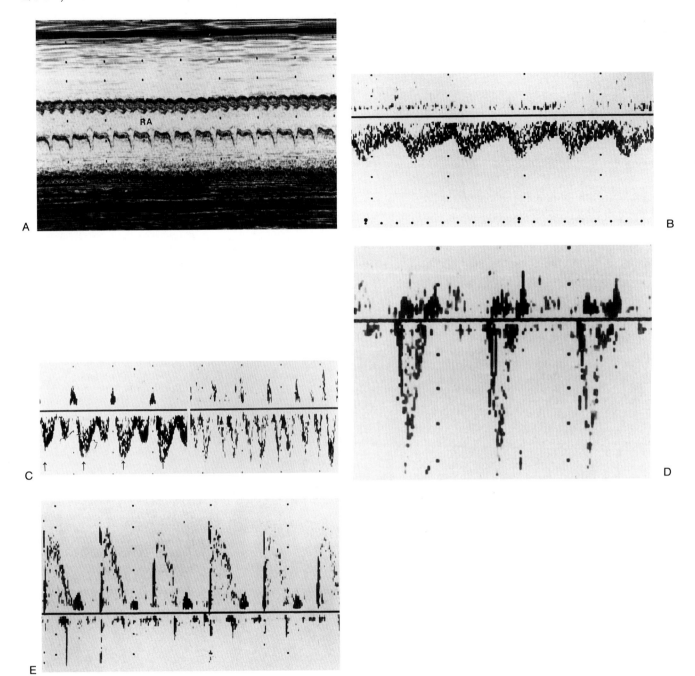

FIG. 7. A: M-mode interrogation of fetus with atrial flutter. Atrial rate (RA) at 360 bpm with 2:1 block and ventricular rate approximately 180 bpm (as estimated by tricuspid valve motion). **B:** Umbilical artery waveform with ventricular rate of 180 bpm in fetus with atrial flutter. **C:** Interrogation of a fetus in sinus rhythm (*arrows*) followed by episode of atrial flutter with an atrial rate of 360 bpm (From reference 36). **D:** Mitral valve intracardiac Doppler velocimetry in fetus with an atrial rate of 360 bpm and ventricular response of 180 bpm (2:1 block). **E:** Velocimetry across aortic valve in same fetus as 7D, with ventricular response of 180 bpm. (**C** from ref. 36.)

with atrial flutter or fibrillation (1). Kleinman et al. reported two of three cases of atrial flutter complicated by hydrops fetalis with perinatal loss of both cases (41). The overall incidence of hydrops complicating either atrial flutter or fibrillation appears to range from 11% to 40% (1,41,59). The atrial rate with atrial flutter can range from 300 to 460 bpm. A variable AV block results in a varying ventricular response of ratios ranging from 1:2 to 1:4, which accounts for the irregularity of this arrhythmia. Intermittently, complete conduction can ensue, or SVT can periodically be present in these arrhythmias, theoretically placing the fetus at risk of congestive heart failure and hydrops.

Neonatal ECG can detect the sawtooth pattern of atrial activity associated with atrial flutter. M-mode diagnosis relies on the detection of atrial wall or AV valve activity at a rate consistent with flutter. Simultaneous imaging of the left atrial wall and the aortic valve can be valuable. Fibrillation is characterized by an undulating atrial wall but is difficult to discern by M-mode ultrasound. Doppler imaging distal to the tricuspid or mitral valve, or at the mitral and aortic roots, allows diagnosis by this method. Again, fibrillation is extremely difficult to assess by velocimetry.

The decision to treat these fetuses is made in the same manner as other supraventricular tachycardias. Digoxin and quinidine or procainamide appear to provide the best results (either individually or in combination) in the small number of patients treated in the literature. In the neonatal period, cardioversion may provide optimal outcomes (1,39,40,58,59). Operative delivery may be required in fetuses with persistent atrial fibrillation or flutter because standard monitoring techniques are unreliable and fetal vagal stimulation in labor may cause extreme degrees of AV block (Figs. 5–7).

Ventricular Tachycardias

Antenatal diagnosis of ventricular tachycardia is rare (1,61). The importance of diagnosing these lesions lies in the potential coexistence of ventricular tumors or ventricular dysfunction (4). Secondary to the extremely uncommon nature of this lesion prognosis and antenatal therapy are limited to neonatal experience.

Ventricular activity unrelated to atrial events characterizes this arrhythmia. M-mode and pulsed Doppler can distinguish these events. If retrograde conduction occurs, this lesion may be indistinguishable from SVT (4).

BRADYARRHYTHMIAS

Sinus Bradycardia

Sinus bradycardias can occur in relationship to fetal head stimulation (e.g., cervical examination, ultrasound evaluation, and malpresentation of the fetal head in labor) (62). An acute parasympathetic discharge or, more ominously, an acute response by the fetus to hypoxia or hypoperfusion can result in sinus bradycardia (63). Characteristically, the final stages of decompensation in the stressed fetus result in sinus bradycardia, which precedes fetal demise (64). Cameron and coworkers reported on six cases of sinus bradycardia (14% of sustained arrhythmias) with a 60% incidence of associated structural heart disease (65). Prolonged QT syndrome can also result in fetal bradycardia with the additional risk of degeneration to a ventricular tachyarrhythmia (66). A case report of sinus bradycardia in the absence of discernible pathophysiology or stimulating factors has been reported with an excellent outcome (67).

Diagnosis of sinus bradycardia can be made with a fetal heart rate less than 100–110 bpm and the appearance of synchronous activity in the atria and ventricles. M-mode and Doppler ultrasound can identify this arrhythmia. The prognosis of fetal sinus bradycardia is variable and related to the underlying etiology of the rhythm disturbance. Cameron reported a 60% mortality associated with sinus bradycardia (65). Second-trimester onset and coexistent structural heart disease were poor prognostic factors in this study (65).

Heart Block

A prolonged PR segment on electrocardiogram characterizes the first-degree block, which is rarely diagnosed antenatally. Second-degree block occurs more commonly, with incomplete conduction of atrial events through the AV perinodal area to the ventricle. Complete dissociation of atrial and ventricular events with an autonomous ventricular rate of 45–90 bpm (depending on proximity to or involvement of the AV node in the automaticity) accounts for the most commonly diagnosed antenatal form of fetal heart block. The failure of the AV node and the proximal ventricular conduction system (i.e., bundle of His) to fuse by 10–12 weeks, or subsequent injury to the conduction system, has been proposed as the primary etiology of this arrhythmia (19,68,69).

The incidence of congenital complete heart block (CHB) is roughly 0.5–1/10,000 births (70). Though idiopathic forms exist, 40–60% are associated with structural cardiac disease (1,71,72). Left atrial isomerism, AV inversion, transposition, and AV septal defects are the most common cardiac lesions identified (1,5,71,72). In 1977 an original series of neonates with uncomplicated CHB reported a 64% incidence of serologic evidence of maternal connective tissue disorder (73). Since this report, the association of fetal or neonatal CHB with maternal autoimmune disease has been thoroughly documented (74–77). The birth of a neonate with CHB in the absence of structural heart disease should prompt a maternal investigation for autoimmune connective tissue disorders (e.g., lupus erythematosis, Sjogren's syndrome, and rheumatoid arthritis) (74,78). The presence of fetal CHB without discernible structural heart disease is associated with maternal anti-Ro and anti-La antibodies with or without a positive antinuclear antibody (74–78).

Diagnosis of heart block relies on identification of dysynchronous atrial and ventricular beats. After a targeted evaluation of the fetal cardiac system with two-dimensional ultrasound, M-mode interrogation can be used to depict the characteristic 2:1 atrial-to-ventricular wall movement seen with second-degree block. Intracardiac velocimetry across the mitral valve, tricuspid valve, or at left outflow and inflow tracts can be of value as well. Simultaneous great vessel interrogation will also allow indirect timing of atrial and ventricular events. CHB is characterized by dissociation of the atrial and ventricular rhythms with ventricular automaticity relying on the proximity of the origin of the autonomous electrical impulse to the AV node. Atrial rates should fall within normal ranges specific for gestational age, and slow or rapid rhythms should suggest the possibility of tachyarrhythmias with blocked conduction (e.g., SVT, atrial flutter, atrial fibrillation) or of fetal decompensation with hypoperfusion leading to atrial tachycardia. Doppler ultrasound can be of additional value in estimating cardiac output in the affected fetus.

Antenatal treatment for heart block is dependent on the atrial and ventricular rates, the degree of fetal compensation, and the suspected underlying etiology. Atrial tachycardia or bradycardia with absence of otherwise reassuring fetal heart tracing parameters may best be dealt with by delivery. Likewise, at maturity, severe ventricular bradycardia (<55 bpm) with the absence of reassuring fetal findings by conventional electronic methods, or with evidence of decompensation by ultrasound, would best be managed by delivery with postnatal pacing of the neonatal ventricle (71). Digoxin and furosemide have been utilized antenatally in the setting of hydrops fetalis and CHB with measured success (79). In the gestation complicated by positive serology for Ro and La, dexamethasone suppression of both the maternal and fetal immune system has been reported to have a positive result in a limited number of patients with resolution of the hydrops, but not resolution of the CHB (74,80). Plasmapheresis has been attempted with success in cases refractory to steroid therapy (71,74). Our experience agrees with the published data regarding delivery of these gestations (27). Delivery may be vaginal utilizing monitoring of atrial events by conventional continuous wave Doppler devices for recognizable signs of fetal well-being (i.e., normal baseline, absence of pathologic decelerations, and presence of heart rate variability). In the presence of nonreassuring fetal atrial monitoring or significant slowing of the ventricular rate during labor (as assessed by direct electronic means), operative delivery may provide the best outcome. Neonatal therapy may include either transvenous or surgical pacing of the ventricle (71, 74,78).

Prognosis for CHB associated with congenital structural cardiac disease is poor (27,71,78). Schmidt et al. reported 55 gestations complicated by CHB (71). Survival of affected neonates with associated structural disease was 14% compared to 89% survival of those neonates without structural disease. The presence of hydrops is associated with adverse outcome (71). CHB with maternal autoimmune disease, or idiopathic CHB, has a much more favorable perinatal survival (71,78,79). These neonates may also require pacemaker therapy depending on ventricular rate and degree of compensation (Figs. 8 and 9).

Insights into Fetal Physiology Provided by Doppler Ultrasound

Use of Doppler ultrasound to measure time–velocity integrals during abnormal fetal heart rates or rhythms has provided some evidence that the fetal heart can alter cardiac output in specific circumstances. After the pause that follows the premature beat, during which time the ventricle fills more than normal, the time–velocity integral with ejection is greater than that during a normal heart rhythm (Fig. 3D,E and 4D,E). Thus the ventricle ejects more if filled more, consistent with the Frank–Starling mechanism (35). Fetuses with increases of heart rate following acoustic stimulation had decreases in stroke volume (80). The ability of the fetal heart rate to adjust cardiac output with rate changes is also demonstrated by the intact survival of fetuses with complete heart block, with sustained heart rates in the 50–60 bpm range.

Studies of the inferior vena cava during fetal heart rate abnormalities have also yielded information of interest. The time–velocity integral of reverse flow in the inferior vena cava with atrial contraction is usually less than 10% of the combined time–velocity integrals during forward flow, i.e., during systole and early diastole (3,6). Fetuses with heart rates increasing above 160 bpm or decreasing below 120 bpm have increases in the percentage of reverse flow with atrial contraction in the inferior vena cava (see Chapter 29). An interesting exception to this phenomenon is the fetus with complete heart block. Fetuses with complete heart block have normal reversals of blood flow in the inferior vena cava with atrial contraction, unless the atrial contraction occurs during ventricular systole. A cannon wave is produced when the atrium contracts against closed atrioventricular valves. It can be inferred that the fetus with complete heart block has forward flow patterns that more closely resemble normal (i.e., reverse flow with atrial contraction is in the normal

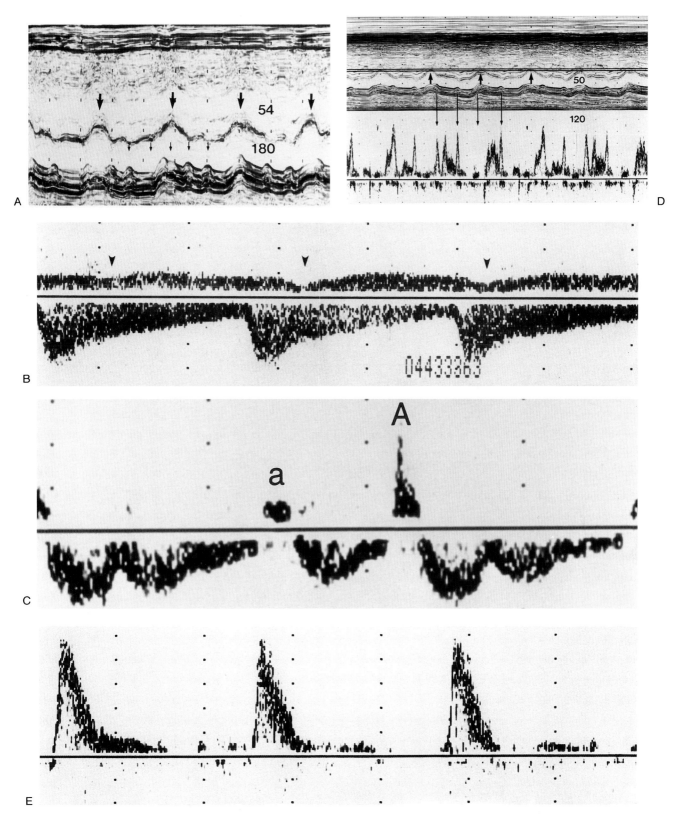

FIG. 8. A: M-mode evaluation in fetus with complete atrioventricular dissociation. Atrial rate is 180 bpm and atrial wall movement is marked by small arrows. Ventricular rate is 54 bpm and atrioventricular movement is marked by large arrows. **B:** Umbilical velocimetry in fetus with complete heart block (CHB). Pulsations in the umbilical vein are illustrated (*arrows*). Ventricular rate as estimated by umbilical artery waveform is 50 bpm. **C:** IVC waveforms in fetus with CHB. Normal atrial systole (a) seen and compared to cannon a wave (A), which occurs when atrial contraction occurs concomitant with ventricular systole and atrioventricular valve closure. **D:** Simultaneous tricuspid valve Doppler waveform and M-mode tracing in a fetus with CHB. Atrial rate is 120 bpm (*long arrows*) and ventricular rate is 50 bpm (*short arrows*). **E:** Pulmonary artery Doppler velocity waveform in fetus with CHB and ventricular rate of 55 bpm. (**A** and **D** from Reed KL, et al. *Fetal Echocardiology: An Atlas,* Wiley/Liss, NY, 1988; **C** from ref. 36.)

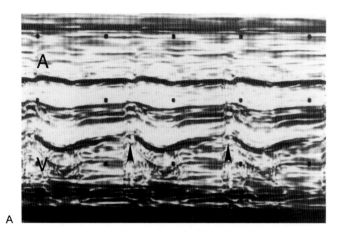

FIG. 9. A: M-mode of fetal sinus bradycardia. Atrial (A) and ventricular (V) events are synchronous. Ventricular rate (*arrows*) is 80 bpm. **B:** Umbilical arterial and venous Doppler velocities in sinus bradycardia. As rate slows from 85 to 70 bpm, umbilical vein pulsations become more prominent. Note the decreased diastolic flow prior to the systolic portion of the arterial waveform. **C:** IVC velocity waveform in fetus with normal rate of 150 bpm with subsequent bradycardia to 100 bpm (*arrows*). Note increased reverse flow in IVC with slowing of heart rate (a). **D:** Left ventricular inflow (MV) and outflow (Ao) waveforms in sinus bradycardia with a heart rate of 80 bpm. (**B** from ref. 37; **C** from ref. 36.)

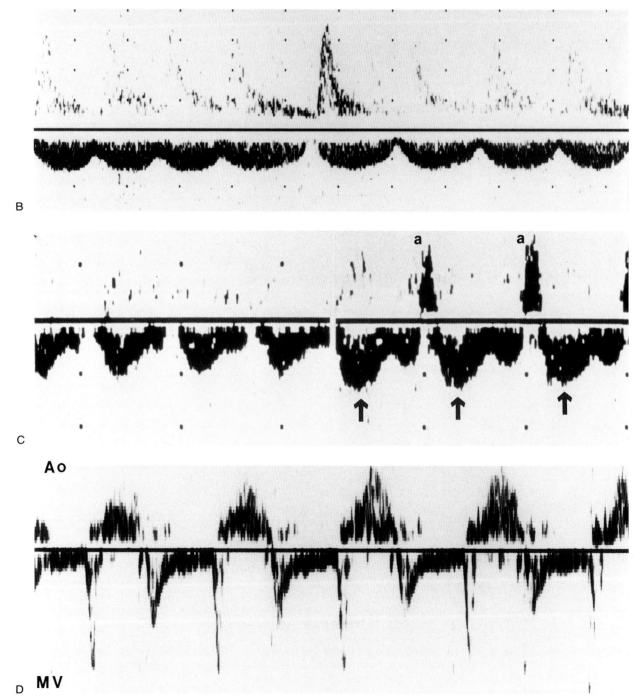

range). The continued filling of the ventricle with the normal rate of atrial contractions may explain in part a fetus's ability to tolerate complete heart block, whereas a fetus with the same ventricular rate and a single atrial beat (sinus bradycardia) is unlikely to survive if the slow rate is sustained.

SUMMARY

Fetal arrhythmias bring a significant number of patients to evaluation at a tertiary center. Rhythm disturbances may be associated with structural congenital heart disease and may result in fetal hydrops. Correct diagnosis in the past has relied heavily on fetal electrocardiography as well as two-dimensional and M-mode ultrasound. The addition of pulsed Doppler ultrasound has added to the ability to diagnose fetal rhythm disturbances (e.g., incomplete conduction at the atrioventricular node). Furthermore, assessment of cardiac physiology by intracardiac velocimetry allows the investigator additional insight into the state of the affected fetus. In addition, the use of Doppler ultrasound to monitor the response to therapy or to screen for progression of a specific arrhythmia is invaluable in the treatment of these gestations. Finally, the ultimate goal in the diagnosis of fetal arrhythmias is to provide the optimal surveillance followed by a coordinated perinatal–neonatal effort to optimize the circumstances surrounding delivery.

REFERENCES

1. Shenker L. Fetal cardiac arrhythmias. *Obstet Gynecol Surv* 1979;34:561–572.
2. Elkayham U, Gleicher N. *Cardiac problems in pregnancy. Diagnosis and management of maternal and fetal disease.* New York: Alan R. Liss; 1982:535–564.
3. Copel JA, Kleinman CS. The impact of fetal echocardiography on perinatal outcome. *Ultrasound Med Biol* 1986;12:327–335.
4. Fyfe DA, Meyer KB, Case CL. Sonographic assessment of fetal cardiac arrhythmias. *Sem Ultrasound CT MR* 1993;14:286–297.
5. Reed KL. Fetal arrhythmias: Etiology, diagnosis, pathophysiology, and treatment. *Sem Perinatol* 1989;13:294–304.
6. Moore KL. The cardiovascular system. In: *The developing human: Clinically oriented embryology.* 4th Ed. Philadelphia: WB Saunders; 1988:286–333.
7. Sissman NJ. Developmental landmarks in cardiogenic morphogenesis: Comparative chronology. *Am J Cardiol* 1970;25:141–148.
8. Robinson HP, Shaw-Dunn J. Fetal heart rates as determined by sonar in early pregnancy. *J Obstet Gynaecol Br Commonw* 1973;80:805–809.
9. Shenker L, Astle C, Reed KL, Anderson C. Embryonic heart rates before the seventh week of pregnancy. *J Reprod Med* 1986;31:333–335.
10. Reed KL, Meijboom EJ, Sahn DJ, et al. Cardiac flow velocities in human fetuses. *Circulation* 1986;73:41–46.
11. Heymann MA. Fetal cardiovascular physiology. In: Creasy RK, Resnick R, eds. *Maternal–fetal medicine: Principles and practice.* 2nd Ed. Philadelphia: WB Saunders; 1989:288–302.
12. Rudolph AM. Distribution and regulation of blood flow in the fetal and neonatal lamb. *Circ Res* 1985;57:811–821.
13. Manasek FJ. Embryonic development of the heart. I. A light and electron microscopy study of myocardial development in the early chick embryo. *J Morphol* 1968;125:329–365.
14. Clark EB, Hu N. Developmental hemodynamic changes in the chick embryo from stages 18 to 27. *Circ Res* 1982;51:810–815.
15. Clark EB, Hu N, Dummett JL, et al. Ventricular function and morphology in chick embryo from stages 18 to 29. *Am J Physiol* 1986;250:H407–413.
16. Krechmer N. Enzymatic patterns during development: An approach to a biochemical definition of immaturity. *Pediatrics* 1959;23:606–617.
17. St. John Sutton M, Gill T, Plappert T. Functional anatomic development in the fetal heart. In: Polin RA, Fox WW, eds. *Fetal and neonatal physiology.* Philadelphia: WB Saunders; 1992:598–610.
18. Van Meirop LHS. Location of the pacemaker in chick embryo heart at the time of initiation of heart beat. *Am J Physiol* 1967;212:407–415.
19. Anderson RH, Becker AE, Arnold CG, Wenink MD, Janse MJ. The development of the cardiac specialized tissue. In: Wellens HJJ, Lie KI, Janse MJ, eds. *The conduction system of the heart.* Philadelphia: Lea and Febiger; 1976:3–28.
20. Long WA, Henry GW. Autonomic and central neuroregulation of fetal cardiovascular function. In: Polin RA, Fox WW, Eds. *Fetal and neonatal physiology.* Philadelphia: WB Saunders; 1992:629–645.
21. Papp JG. Autonomic responses and neurohumoral control in the human early antenatal heart. *Basic Res Cardiol* 1988;83:2–9.
22. Papp JG. Age-related changes in cardiac responsiveness to positive ionotropic agents. In: Patron W, et al., eds. *Symposium on Cardiac Ionotropic Agents.* IUPHAR 9th International Congress of Pharmacology. London: Macmillan; 1984:21–27.
23. Wolfson RN, Sorokin Y, Rosen MG. Autonomic control of fetal cardiac activity. In: Elkayam U, Gleicher N, eds. *Cardiac problems in pregnancy.* New York: Alan R. Liss; 1982:365–379.
24. Beall MH, Paul RH. Artifacts, blocks, and arrhythmias: Confusing nonclassical heart rate tracings. *Clin Obstet Gynecol* 1986;29:83–94.
25. Reed KL. Fetal echocardiography. *Semin Ultrasound CT MR* 1991;12:2–10.
26. McCurdy CM, Reed KL. Basic technique of fetal echocardiography. *Semin Ultrasound CT MR* 1993;14:267–276.
27. Shenker L, Reed KL, Anderson CF, et al. Congenital heart block and cardiac anomalies in the absence of maternal connective tissue disease. *Am J Obstet Gynecol* 1987;157:248–253.
28. D'Cruz IA, Prabhu R, Cohen HC, Glick G. Echocardiographic features of second degree atrioventricular block. *Chest* 1977;72:459–463.
29. Fujii J, Foster JR, Mills PG, Moos S, Craig E. Dual echocardiographic determination of atrial contraction sequence in atrial flutter and other related atrial arrhythmias. *Circulation* 1978;58:314–337.
30. DeVore GR, Donnerstein RL, Kleinman CS, Platt LD, Hobbins JC. Fetal echocardiography. II. The diagnosis and significance of a pericardial effusion in the fetus using real-time-directed M-mode ultrasound. *Am J Obstet Gynecol* 1982;144:693–700.
31. DeVore GR, Donnerstein RL, Kleinman CS, Platt LD, Hobbins JC. Fetal echocardiography. I. Normal anatomy as determined by real-time-directed M-mode ultrasound. *Am J Obstet Gynecol* 1982;144:249–260.
32. Crowley DC, Dick M, Rayburn WF, Rosenthal A. Two-dimensional and M-mode echocardiographic evaluation of fetal arrhythmia. *Clin Cardiol* 1985;8:1–10.
33. McCallum WD, Williams CS, Napel S, et al. Fetal blood velocity waveforms. *Am J Obstet Gynecol* 1978;132:425–429.
34. Schulman H. The clinical implications of Doppler ultrasound analysis of the uterine and umbilical arteries. *Am J Obstet Gynecol* 1987;156:889–893.
35. Reed KL, Sahn DJ, Marx GR, Anderson CF, Shenker L. Cardiac Doppler flows during fetal arrhythmias: Physiologic consequences. *Obstet Gynecol* 1987;70:1–6.
36. Reed KL, Appleton CP, Anderson CF, Shenker L, Sahn DJ. Doppler studies of vena cava flows in human fetuses. Insights into normal and abnormal cardiac physiology. *Circulation* 1990;81:498–505.
37. Indik JM, Chen J, Reed KL. Association of umbilical venous with inferior vena cava blood flow velocities. *Obstet Gynecol* 1991;77:551–557.

38. Copel JA, Morotti R, Hobbins JC, Kleinman CS. The antenatal diagnosis of congenital heart disease using fetal echocardiography: Is color flow mapping necessary? *Obstet Gynecol* 1991;78:1–8.

39. Strasburger JF, Huhta JC, Carpenter RJ, Garson A, McNamara DG. Doppler echocardiography in the diagnosis and management of persistent fetal arrhythmias. *JACC* 1986;7:1386–91.

40. Chan FY, Woo SK, Ghosh A, Tang M, Lam C. Prenatal diagnosis of congenital fetal arrhythmias by simultaneous pulsed Doppler velocimetry of the fetal abdominal aorta and inferior vena cava. *Obstet Gynecol* 1990;76:200–204.

41. Kleinman CS, Copel JA, Weinstein EM, Santulli TV, Hobbins JC. In utero diagnosis and treatment of fetal supraventricular tachycardia. *Semin Perinatol* 1985;9:113–29.

42. Hammacher K, Huter KA, Bokelmann J, Werners PH. Foetal heart rate frequency and perinatal conditions of foetus and newborn. *Gynaecologia* 1968;166:349–360.

43. Van der Mooren K, Wladimiroff JW, Stijnen T. Fetal atrioventricular and outflow tract flow velocity waveforms during conducted and blocked supraventricular extrasystoles. *Ultrasound Obstet Gynecol* 1992;2:182–189.

44. Stewart PA, Wladimiroff JW. Fetal atrial arrhythmias associated with redundancy/aneurysm of the foramen ovale. *J Clin Ultrasound* 1988;16:643–650.

45. Ferrer PL. Arrhythmias in the neonate. In: Roberts NK, Gelbrand H, eds. *Cardiac arrhythmias in the neonate, infant, and child.* New York: Appleton-Century-Crofts; 1977:265–316.

46. Odendaal HJ, Crawford JW. Fetal tachycardia and maternal pyrexia during labor. *S Afr Med J* 1975;49:1873–1875.

47. Cohn HE, Piasecki GJ, Jackson BT. The effect of beta-adrenergic stimulation on fetal cardiovascular function during hypoxemia. *Am J Obstet Gynecol* 1982;144:810–816.

48. Cohn HE, Sacks EJ, Heymann MA, Rudolph AM. Cardiovascular responses to hypoxemia and acidemia in fetal lambs. *Am J Obstet Gynecol* 1974;120:817–824.

49. Hansmann M, Gembruch U, Bald R, Manz M, Redel DA. Fetal tachyarrhythmias: Transplacental and direct treatment of the fetus: A report of 60 cases. *Ultrasound Obstet Gynecol* 1991;1:162–170.

50. Wiggins JW, Bowes W, Clewell W, et al. Echocardiographic diagnosis and intravenous digoxin management of fetal tachyarrhythmias and congestive heart failure. *Am J Dis Child* 1986;140:202–204.

51. Kleinman CS, Donnerstein RL, DeVore GR, et al. Fetal echocardiography for evaluation of in utero congestive heart failure. A technique for study of nonimmune hydrops. *N Engl J Med* 1982;306:568–574.

52. Pinsky WW, Rayburn WF, Evans MI. Pharmacologic therapy for fetal arrhythmias. *Clin Obstet Gynecol* 1991;34:304–309.

53. Harrigan JT, Kangos JJ, Sikka A, et al. Successful treatment of fetal congestive heart failure secondary to tachycardia. *N Engl J Med* 1981;304:1527–1529.

54. Lasser DM, Laxmi B. Fetal response time to transplacental digoxin therapy for supraventricular tachyarrhythmia: A meta-analysis. *J Mat–Fet Med* 1993;2:70–74.

55. Cowan RH, Waldo AL, Harris HB, Cassady G, Brans YW. Neonatal paroxysmal supraventricular tachycardia with hydrops. *Pediatrics* 1975;55:428–430.

56. Rae AP, Webb CR. Management of supraventricular tachycardia. *Cardiol Pract* 1984;10:197–205.

57. Garson A Jr. Supraventricular tachycardia. In: Gillette PC, Garson A, eds. *Pediatric cardiac dysrhythmias.* Orlando: Grune and Stratton; 1981:77–120.

58. Reder RF, Rosen MR. Basic electrophysiology principles. Application to treatment of dysrhythmias. In: Gillette PC, Garson A, eds. *Pediatric cardiac dysrhythmias.* Orlando: Grune and Stratton; 1981:121–144.

59. Moller JH, Davachi F, Anderson RC. Atrial flutter in infancy. *J Pediatr* 1969;75:643–651.

60. Allan LD, Crawford DC, Anderson RH, Tynan M. Evaluation and treatment of fetal arrhythmias. *Clin Cardiol* 1984;7:467–473.

61. Lingman G, Lundstrom N, Marsal K, Ohrlander S. Fetal cardiac arrhythmias. Clinical outcome in 113 cases. *Acta Obstet Gynecol Scand* 1986;65:263–267.

62. Young BK, Katz M, Klein SA, Silverman F. Fetal blood and tissue pH with moderate bradycardia. *Am J Obstet Gynecol* 1979;135:45–52.

63. Gilstrap LC III, Hauth JC, Hankins GDV, Beck AW. Second stage fetal heart rate abnormalities and type of neonatal acidemia. *Obstet Gynecol* 1987;70:191–195.

64. Herbert CM, Boehm FM. Prolonged end-stage fetal heart rate deceleration: A reanalysis. *Obstet Gynecol* 1981;57:589–593.

65. Cameron A, Nicholson S, Nimrod C, Harder J, Davies D, Fritzler M. Evaluation of fetal cardiac dysrhythmias with two-dimensional, M-mode, and pulsed Doppler ultrasonography. *Am J Obstet Gynecol* 1988;158:286–290.

66. Green DW, Ackerman NB, Lund G, Wright D. Prolonged QT syndrome presenting as fetal bradycardia. *J Mat–Fet Med* 1992;1:202–205.

67. Minagawa Y, Akaiwa A, Hidaka T, et al. Severe fetal supraventricular bradyarrhythmia without fetal hypoxia. *Obstet Gynecol* 1987;70:454–456.

68. Carter JB, Bleiden LC, Edwards JE. Congenital heart block: Anatomic correlations and review of the literature. *Arch Pathol* 1974;97:51–57.

69. James TN. Cardiac conduction system: Fetal and postnatal development. *Am J Cardiol* 1970;25:213–226.

70. Gochberg SH. Congenital heart block. *Am J Obstet Gynecol* 1964;88:238–241.

71. Schmidt KG, Ulmer HE, Silverman NA, et al. Perinatal outcome of fetal complete atrioventricular block: A multicenter experience. *J Am Coll Cardiol* 1991;17:1360–1366.

72. Kleinman CS and Copel JA. Fetal cardiac dysrhythmias. In: Creasy RK, Resnick R, eds. *Maternal–fetal medicine: Principles and practice.* 2nd Ed. Philadelphia: WB Saunders; 1989:344–356.

73. McCue CM, Mantakas ME, Tinglestad JB, Ruddy S. Congenital heart block in newborns of mothers with connective tissue disease. *Circulation* 1977;56:82–90.

74. Buyon JP, Winchester R. Congenital complete heart block. A human model of passively acquired autoimmune injury. *Arthritis Rheum* 1990;33:609–614.

75. Silverman ED, Mamula MJ, Hardin JA, Laxer RM. The association of the congenital heart block of neonatal lupus erythematosus and both anti-Ro and anti-La antibodies (abstract). *Arthritis Rheum* 1989;32:S104.

76. Buyon JP, Ben-Chetrit E, Karp S, et al. Acquired congenital heart block: pattern of maternal antibody response to biochemically defined antigens of the SSA/Ro–SSB/La system in neonatal lupus. *J Clin Invest* 1989;84:627–634.

77. Taylor PV, Taylor KF, Norman A, Griffiths S, Scott JS. Prevalence of maternal Ro (SS-A) and La (SS-B) autoantibodies in relation to congenital heart block. *Br J Rheumatol* 1988;27:128–132.

78. Olah KS, Gee, H. Fetal heart block associated with maternal anti-Ro (SS-A) antibody: Current management. A review. *Br J Obstet Gynaecol* 1991;98:751–755.

79. Harris JP, Alexson CG, Manning JA, Thompson HO. Medical therapy for the hydropic fetus with congenital complete atrioventricular block. *Am J Perinatol* 1993;10:217–219.

80. Kenny J, Plappert T, Doubilet P, Salzman D, St. John Sutton. Effects of heart rate on ventricular size, stroke volume, and output in the normal human fetus: A prospective Doppler echocardiographic study. *Circulation* 1987;76:52–58.

Doppler Ultrasound in Obstetrics and Gynecology,
edited by Joshua A. Copel and Kathryn L. Reed.
Raven Press, Ltd., New York © 1995.

CHAPTER 27

Fetal Cardiac Output Measurement in Normal and Pathologic States

Domenico Arduini, Giuseppe Rizzo, and Carlo Romanini

Much of today's knowledge of fetal hemodynamics is derived from animal studies. Such studies employing radionuclide-labeled microspheres or electromagnetic flow transducers have allowed measurement of blood flow in different vascular beds under both normal and abnormal situations. Because this involves the measurement of absolute volumetric flow rate (i.e., the amount of blood passing per minute across a vascular structure), the most direct means of evaluating blood flow, the majority of investigations had quantified this parameter.

Recent developments of Doppler technique have permitted the noninvasive study of fetal hemodynamics. On the basis of previous experience with animals, several attempts were performed a decade ago to quantify absolute volume flow in the human fetus. These attempts were directed not only to fetal cardiac regions but also to peripheral and placental vessels. In fact, volume flow measurements of umbilical venous or descending aortal flow were among the first to be made in the fetus (1,2). Difficulties and inaccuracies in these measurements (3) resulted in attention to qualitative indices derived from relative ratios between systolic, diastolic, and mean velocities. These indices (e.g., S/D, resistance index, and pulsatility index) are independent of the absolute velocity values and of the angle of insonation between the Doppler beam and the direction of blood flow, and are therefore more easily obtained with an acceptable level of reproducibility. As a consequence, these latter indices are commonly used in obstetrics at the level of fetal peripheral vessels.

During the last few years technological advances in ultrasound resolution have made possible detailed anatomic studies of the human fetal heart, and the use of pulsed and color Doppler techniques has allowed the examination of fetal cardiac flows. Thus volumetric studies have once again been attempted at the level of the fetal heart under normal and abnormal conditions (4,5).

In this chapter we will outline the principles and the limits of fetal Doppler echocardiography in the measurement of absolute cardiac output. Furthermore, we will review the results of human fetal cardiovascular research using Doppler measurements of cardiac output.

GENERAL PRINCIPLES

The calculation of volume flow is based on two measurements: the cross-sectional area of the valve and the length of the column of blood passing through the valve. This latter parameter is represented by the instantaneous flow velocity obtained by the fast Fourier transformation of the Doppler signal. Since the velocity of blood passing through a valve is not constant but changes with the cardiac cycle, the integral of the velocity waveforms over the cardiac cycle [time–velocity integral, (TVI)] is considered to be a measure of the length of the column of blood. The product of TVI by the cross-sectional area of the valve (A) provides the measurement of the stroke volume (SV). Multiplication of this value by heart rate (HR) gives the absolute flow per minute (Q). Q per minute may be therefore calculated by the following formula:

$$Q = \text{TVI} \times \text{HR} \times A$$

where TVI (cm) = mean velocity ($\bar{V}$) (cm/sec)/duration of cardiac cycle (sec) and HR = 60/duration of cardiac cycle. Alternatively, Q can be calculated by the following formula:

D. Arduini: Department of Obstetrics and Gynecology, Università di Ancona, Italy.

G. Rizzo and C. Romanini: Department of Obstetrics and Gynecology, Università di Roma "Tor Vergata," Italy.

$$Q = \bar{V} \times 60 \times A$$

With both formulas it is necessary to obtain the Doppler spectrum of the blood flow passing through the valve and the cross-sectional area of the valve. The reliability of Q measurement depends on the degree of accuracy with which the above-mentioned measurements were performed. Crucial factors are as follows:

1. *Quality of Doppler spectrum.* The first important assumption is that the characteristics of flow are laminar. Under this condition the Doppler spectrum is "flat" (i.e., plug flow) (6) and the maximum frequency envelope of the flow velocity waveform is considered equivalent to the mean velocity. Studies on adults have demonstrated that near the cardiac valves the flow is laminar (6) and that this characteristic is lost more distally. There is no direct evidence regarding the characteristics of flow in the human fetus but the presence of flat Doppler velocity profile obtained immediately distal to the cardiac valve strongly suggests a laminar flow also in the human fetus. On the other hand, recordings not performed immediately distal to the valve may be misleading as the loss of a flat profile may lead to erroneous measurement of the mean velocity or TVI.

The second important assumption is that the Doppler spectrum reflects all velocities inside the vessel (or valve). Among all possible methods of obtaining such data the so-called even insonation method has been mainly used in the fetus (5). With this method the entire volume of blood whose flow rate is to be assessed must be insonated uniformly by the Doppler beam. As a consequence the sample volume has to be sufficiently wide to sample the entire vessel. Finally, as the cardiac valves are extremely close to each other in the human fetus, real-time two-dimensional ultrasound of the exact position of the sample volume is necessary to check its proper position.

2. *Angle of insonation.* According to Doppler equation the blood flow velocities are directly related to the cosine of the angle of incidence between the Doppler beam and the direction of blood flow. Measurements of absolute flow velocities therefore require the knowledge of the angle of insonation, which may be difficult to obtain with accuracy. The error in the estimation of the absolute velocity resulting from the uncertainty of angle measurement is strongly dependent on the magnitude of the angle itself. For angles less than about 20° the error will be reduced to practical insignificance. For larger angles the cosine term in the Doppler equation changes the small uncertainty in the measurement of the angle in a large error in velocity equations (7). As a consequence, recordings should be obtained with the Doppler beam as parallel as possible to the estimated direction of blood flow and all the recordings with an estimated angle greater than 20° should be rejected. Color Doppler may solve many of these problems by showing in real time the flow direction, thus allowing the proper alignment of the Doppler beam in the direction of the blood flow.

3. *Valve cross-sectional area.* The valve area may be measured directly by planimetering the valve orifice and this method should be preferred at the level of atrioventricular valves (7). In the fetus most investigators assume a circular symmetry of all cardiac valves and therefore measure a single diameter. Because area is calculated on the basis of one half the diameter squared, the percentage error in diameter measurement may greatly affect the reliability of flow measurements. For example, a 0.5-mm uncertainty in the measurement of a 4-mm valve will produce a 25% variation in the flow calculation. To reduce this source of error multiple measurements are required and the results obtained must be averaged.

4. *Simultaneous recording of velocities and valve area.* Since the dimensions of velocities and vessels may change with time, a simultaneous recording of both parameters should be performed (7). Several technical difficulties limit this approach because the views used to measure velocities usually differ from those used to measure valve dimensions. However, in contrast to peripheral vessels, it is assumed that no significant changes occur at the level of cardiac valves dimensions in short time intervals, thus minimizing this factor.

TECHNIQUE

Cardiac output may be measured either at the level of atrioventricular valves or at the outflow tract. Measurements obtained from mitral or aortic valves reflect the left cardiac output (LCO) whereas measurements from tricuspid or pulmonary valves reflect the right cardiac output (RCO). From these two values it is possible to calculate the combined cardiac output (CCO = LCO + RCO) and the ratio between right and left ventricular outputs (RCO/LCO).

As reported above, to obtain reliable recordings it is necessary to follow these general rules:

1. Verify in real time and color flow imaging the correct position of the sample volume before, during, and after each Doppler recording.
2. Check the presence of a flat profile of the velocity waveforms suggestive of laminar flow.
3. Minimize the angle of insonation between Doppler beam and the direction of flow, and reject all the recordings with an angle greater than 20°.
4. Limit Doppler recordings to period of fetal rest and apnea, as behavioral states greatly influence the measurements (8).
5. Perform multiple measurements of the valve sizes in order to reduce the inaccuracies.

The detailed technique for calculating cardiac output follows:

Atrioventricular Valve

1. *Doppler recordings.* The ultrasound transducer is oriented in a transverse plane of the fetal thorax in order to obtain an apical four-chamber view of the fetal heart (Fig. 1A). The color flow mapping function is then superimposed and the ventricular inflow during diastole visualized. The sample volume of the pulsed Doppler is placed in one of the two ventricles just inferior of the atrioventricular leaflets (9) (Fig. 1B). Care is taken with small movements of the transducer to optimize the angle of insonation of the Doppler beam with the direction of flow as estimated by color imaging. Velocity waveforms are then recorded and ten consecutive uniform waveforms are considered for velocity measurements. Measurements are performed on frozen images with a digitizing tablet linked to a computer, planimetering the maximum frequency envelope of the waveforms. The averaged value obtained from the different waveforms is used for the calculation of the cardiac output. The same technique is followed for both tricuspid and mitral valves.

2. *Valve measurements.* The diameter of the atrioventricular orifice is measured from a four-chamber view showing the largest diameters of each valve. Images are recorded on videotape and later played back with the frame-by-frame function. Measurement are performed during the diastolic phase (when the leaflets are opened and are parallel to each other) just apical to the insertion of the valves (Fig. 1C). The reflections of the fibrous skeleton of the atrioventricular valve helps in identifying the annulus. At least five measurements on different cardiac cycles are required. The superimposition of color function must be avoided. In fact, measurement of the width

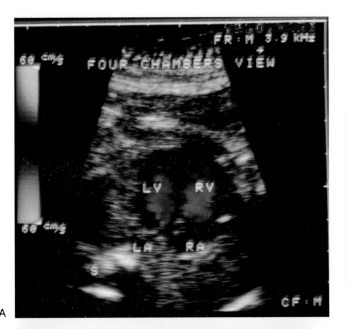

A

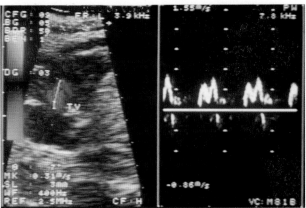

B

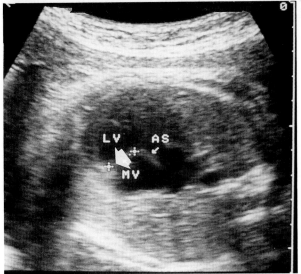

C

FIG. 1. Real-time image with color flow mapping superimposed showing an apical four-chamber view of the fetal heart during diastole (**A**), blood flow velocity waveforms from the tricuspid valve (**B**) (note the flat flow profile and the angle of insonation near zero), and four-chamber view of the fetal heart illustrating measurement of the mitral valve (**C**) (*arrow*).

of the color column passing across the valve does not reflect the valve dimension as the spatial resolution of the color function is substantially inferior to that of real-time image, and most of the machines employ a great deal of cosmetic processing to allow a good appearance of color images. Furthermore several machine control functions such as the pulse repetition frequency, the high-pass filter, the color threshold, and the color gain may change the apparent lumen size of one valve (3).

Outflow Tracts

1. *Doppler recordings.* Flow velocity waveforms from aortic valve are obtained from a five-chamber view of the fetal heart (Fig. 2A) while pulmonary waveforms are recorded from the short axis of the right ventricle (Fig. 3A) (10). With these view it is possible to keep the angle of insonation near zero. The sample volume of the pulsed Doppler is placed immediately distal to valve leaflets and velocity waveforms are recorded (3A,B). The following procedures of analysis are similar to those described for atrioventricular valves.

2. *Valve measurements.* The outlet valves are imaged with the roots of the aorta or pulmonary artery viewed in long axis. Similar to atrioventricular valves, images are videorecorded and then reanalyzed. Diameters are measured from inner wall to inner wall at the level of valve insertion immediately after valve opening (Figs. 2C, 3C). Multiple measurements on different cardiac cycle are required and the superimposition of color function must be avoided.

There is controversy among authors on the choice to measure the cardiac output from either atrioventricular or outflow tracts (Table 1). Some authors prefer the former situation as it is easy to obtain an apical four-chamber view. Furthermore velocities from atrioventric-

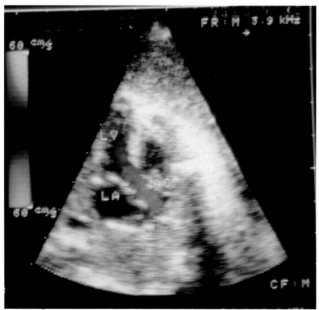

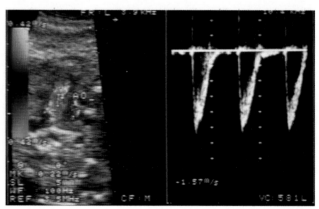

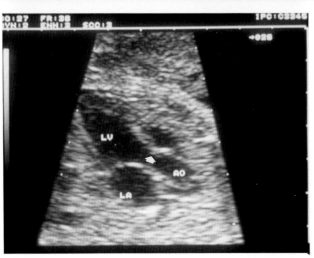

FIG. 2. Real-time image with color flow mapping superimposed showing a five-chamber view of the fetal heart during systole (**A**), blood flow velocity waveforms from aortic valve (**B**) (note the flat flow profile and the angle of insonation near zero), and long-axis view of the fetal heart illustrating measurement of the aortic valve (*arrow*) (**C**).

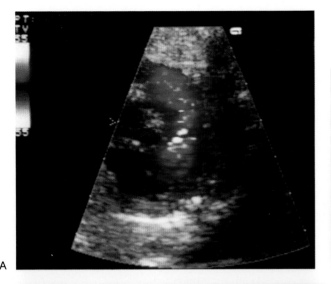

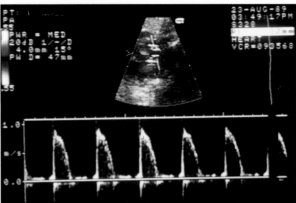

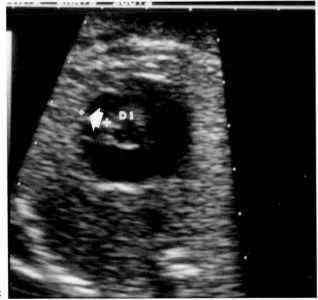

FIG. 3. Real-time image with color flow mapping superimposed showing a short-axis view of the fetal heart during systole (**A**), blood flow velocity waveforms from pulmonary valve (**B**) (note the flat flow profile and the angle of insonation near zero), and short-axis view of the fetal heart illustrating measurement of the pulmonary valve (*arrow*) (**C**).

TABLE 1. *Reported values of volume flow estimations of left cardiac output (LCO), right cardiac output (RCO), and combined cardiac output (CCO) corrected for fetal weight*

Author	Site of recording	LCO (ml/m)			RCO (ml/m)			CCO (ml/m/kg)
		19–21	29–31	36–40	19–21	29–31	36–40	
Reed	AV valves	—	—	—	—	—	—	539
Kenny	Outflow tracts	118	282	676	132	302	692	—
De Smedt	AV valves	84	333	820	105	372	915	553
Allan	Outflow tracts	70	269	647	93	361	886	450
Allan	AV valves	109	333	686	140	428	883	—
Copel	AV valves	—	—	—	—	—	—	644
Rizzo	Outflow tracts	78	284	670	100	390	866	525
Rizzo	AV valves	91	320	693	134	435	890	546

ular valves are lower than those from outflow tracts, thus avoiding problems in velocity aliasing. However, measurements of the cross-sectional area of the atrioventricular valves seem to be less accurate and a higher variability in values has been reported (11). On the other hand, the higher accuracy in the measurement of the outflow tracts dimensions is associated with more laborious acquisition of Doppler signals.

Our approach is to measure cardiac output always from both atrioventricular and arterial valves. The comparison of the value obtained in the two regions is a useful internal check of the quality of the measurements (see next section).

REPRODUCIBILITY

A major concern in obtaining measurements of cardiac output is their reproducibility. Following a technique of analysis as rigorous as that previously described is the essential prerequisite to obtain reproducible recordings. As a consequence, successful recordings may not be obtained in all subjects but in a percentage varying from 60% to 78% (11,12). The intra- and interobserver coefficients of variation differ between studies and are usually higher for valve measurements than for Doppler recordings, but several authors have reported values below 10% (13–15).

As reported above, an easy internal check of the quality of the measurements may be obtained by comparing the values obtained at the atrioventricular valves with those obtained at the level of the corresponding great artery. In Fig. 4 the correlation between the two measurements is shown in 234 healthy fetuses free from structural cardiac disease. Slightly higher values are usually achieved at the level of atrioventricular valves, probably because of the difficulties in valve measurements, but a good relationship between measurements exists. We consider adequate only the measurements in which the variation between the two sites of recording is lower than 10% and feel this adds certainty about the reliability of the recordings.

Finally, as the most difficult and error-prone measurement is the valve area, several authors and we have avoided this parameter under particular conditions simply by calculating the cardiac output by the product TVI × HR (16–18). This is possible in longitudinal observations over a short period of time in which the valve dimensions are assumed to remain constant. Furthermore it is also possible to use this approach to calculate the relative ratio between RCO and LCO (RCO/LCO), since the relative dimensions of the right and left valves remain constant through gestation in the absence of cardiac structural disease (19), and therefore their omission in the calculation of RCO/LCO does not affect the final value.

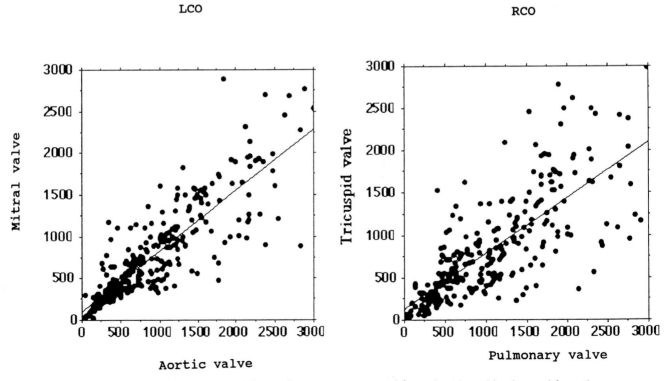

FIG. 4. Relationships between right cardiac output measured from the tricuspid valve and from the pulmonary valve (**right**) and between left cardiac output measured from the mitral valve and from the aortic valve (**left**).

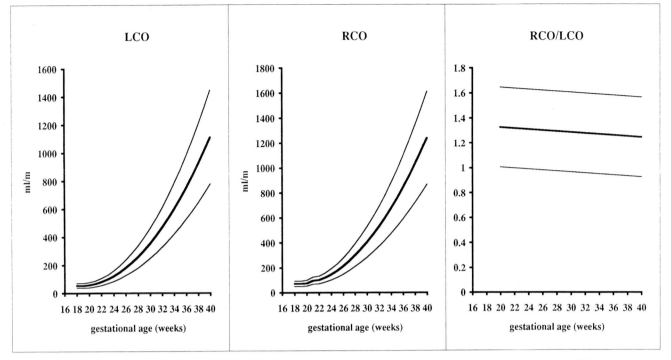

FIG. 5. Normal values for gestation (median and 95% confidence limits) of left cardiac output (LCO), right cardiac output (RCO), and RCO/LCO ratio obtained from atrioventricular valve in 284 healthy fetuses studied cross-sectionally.

NORMAL VALUES

Cardiac output has been measured as early as 15 weeks gestation (12). There is an exponential increase of CCO with advancing gestation with values of about 120 ml/min at 15 weeks of gestation; up to 1800 ml/min at term (Fig. 5). However, when corrected for fetal weight the CCO is constant through gestation with values of 500–600 ml/min/kg (Table 1). The RCO is slightly higher than the LCO resulting in a RCO/LCO ratio of 1.3, which is constant during the second and third trimesters (12,13,20,21). The dominance of the RCO was also found in the fetal lamb (24). However, in this species the ratio found is much larger (1.8) than in the human fetus. This may be explained on the basis of the output of the left ventricle being directed through the ascending aorta to upper body organs, thus perfusing preferentially the brain while the right ventricle through the patent ductus arteriosus and the descending aorta mainly perfuses the lower body and placenta. The larger brain mass of humans with respect to sheep may explain the higher LCO in the human fetus and therefore the lower RCO/LCO ratio. This concept is validated by the data obtained in anencephalic fetuses where the RCO/LCO is higher than that in normal human fetuses (25).

The use of transvaginal ultrasound has also allowed the study of cardiac flows as early as 11 weeks gestation (see Chapter 10). At this gestational age the small dimensions of valve orifices preclude absolute measurements but an estimation of the ratios between the right to left products of TVI × HR may be obtained. It is noteworthy that from 11 to 20 weeks of gestation there is a significant increase in this ratio measured either at the level of both great vessels or atrioventricular valves, suggesting a preferential streaming of blood to the right heart with advancing gestation (26). This is consistent with the selective modifications of cardiac afterload occurring in early gestation and supports the high relationship of this index to variations in cardiac afterload.

CARDIAC DOPPLER FINDINGS IN ABNORMAL GESTATIONS

Congenital Heart Disease

Although the prenatal diagnosis of congenital heart disease is based on conventional two-dimensional ultrasound and is completed by pulsed and color Doppler (27), the measurement of cardiac output may add some pathophysiologic information regarding the severity of disease. This may be the case with outflow obstructions in which the calculation of the output from the contralateral side may be performed. Figure 6 reports our experience in fetuses with either right-sided obstruction (tetralogy of Fallot, N = 6; pulmonary stenosis or atresia, N = 4) or left obstruction (hypoplastic left ventricle, N = 7). The clinical significance of these measurements remains to be established.

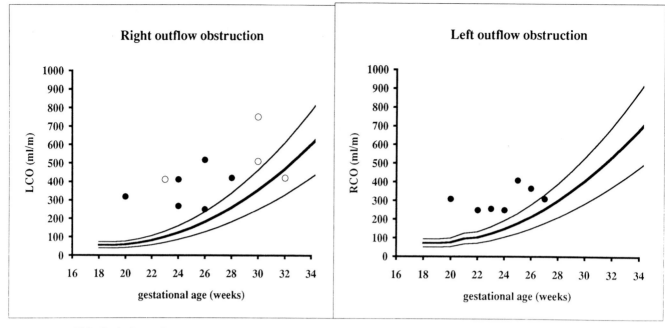

FIG. 6. Left cardiac output in fetuses with right outflow obstruction [tetralogy of Fallot (*filled circles*)] and pulmonary atresia (*empty circles*) and right cardiac output in fetuses with left outflow obstruction (hypoplastic left heart).

Growth-Retarded Fetuses

Intrauterine growth-retarded (IUGR) fetuses secondary to uteroplacental insufficiency are characterized by selective changes of peripheral vascular resistances (i.e., the so-called brain-sparing effect) that influence cardiac hemodynamics (28). Due to the brain-sparing condition, changes occur in cardiac afterload, with a decreased left ventricle afterload due to the cerebral vasodilation and an increased right ventricle afterload due to the systemic vasoconstriction. As a consequence IUGR fetuses show a relative increase of LCO associated with decreased RCO (14,18). These hemodynamic intracardiac changes are compatible with a preferential shift of cardiac output in favor of the left ventricle leading to improved perfusion to the brain. Thus in the first stages of the disease, the supply of substrates and oxygen can be maintained at near-normal levels despite any absolute reduction of placental transfer. The absolute CCO may be maintained at a first stage of disease and there is some evidence that when corrected for fetal weight it may be even higher than in normal fetuses (18).

Longitudinal studies of progressively deteriorating IUGR fetuses have shown that the RCO/LCO ratio remains stable during serial recordings, suggesting the absence of significant changes in cardiac output redistribution after the establishment of the brain-sparing mechanism (18). However, cardiac output gradually declines with progression of gestation and there is evidence of a temporal association between the fall of CCO and the onset of late heart rate decelerations (18) (Fig. 7).

The study of cardiac output should therefore be suggested as a useful tool for longitudinal monitoring of fetal condition in pregnancies complicated by IUGR. However, the modifications of CCO are closely associated with changes in blood flow parameters inside the heart (e.g., peak velocities at outflow tracts) or in the venous circulation (e.g., % reverse flow in inferior vena cava), which are easier to obtain and have an higher reproducibility, thus limiting the volumetric applications (29–31).

Fetal Anemia

Red cell isoimmunization results in a progressive destruction of fetal red cells leading to fetal anemia. Furthermore, intravascular fetal blood transfusion by cordocentesis represents the standard treatment for fetal anemia and this procedure leads to rapid injection of large amounts of blood with respect to fetoplacental volume.

The measurement of CCO has made it possible to elucidate the hemodynamic response of the human fetus to anemia and its rapid correction (16,22,23).

Before transfusion (in a condition of anemia), the left and right cardiac outputs are significantly higher than normal and a significant relationship is present between the severity of fetal anemia and cardiac output (16, 22,23). The fetal cardiac output is increased presumably to maintain adequate oxygen delivery to organs. Although the mechanisms causing the increase of cardiac output remain unclear, two main factors have been sug-

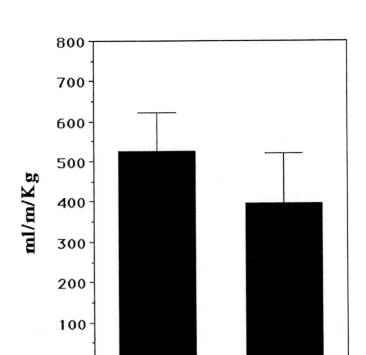

FIG. 7. Serial change of absolute cardiac output in IUGR fetuses preceding the onset of heart late decelerations (**left**) and cardiac output corrected for fetal weight obtained at the last recording close to the onset of heart late decelerations (**right**). From Rizzo and Arduini (18).

gested (32): first, decreased blood viscosity leading to increased venous return and cardiac preload, and second, peripheral vasodilation due to a fall in blood oxygen content and therefore reduced cardiac afterload.

There is no evidence for a redistribution of cardiac output similar to that described in hypoxic IUGR fetuses (brain-sparing effect) since the RCO/LCO ratio is normal in anemic fetuses (23). This is in agreement with the normal values of the pulsatility index present in peripheral vessels of anemic fetuses (33). These findings suggest that in the red cell isoimmunization the changes in fetal cardiac function are mainly related to the low blood viscosity leading to a hyperdynamic situation.

After intravascular transfusion, there is a significant temporary fall in right and left cardiac outputs (16,23). The decrease of cardiac output may be secondary to four different factors (heart rate, preload, myocardial contractility, or afterload). The first factor may be excluded as cardiac output decreases in the absence of any significant changes in fetal heart rate (16). Preload should be decreased to support the decrease of cardiac output, but the high values of the early to active (*E/A*) filling of the ventricle found in Doppler recordings from the atrioventricular valves suggest an increase of preload rather than a decrease (23). Similarly, an impaired myocardial con-

tractility seems unlikely on the basis of the velocity waveforms in the aorta and the pulmonary artery (16). Therefore an increase in cardiac afterload seems to offer the best explanation for the decrease in cardiac output (16). This hypothesis is consistent with experimental animal studies showing an evident increase of mean arterial pressure and therefore of cardiac afterload after transfusion (34).

It is noteworthy that the fall of cardiac output in the human fetus is significantly related to the amount of expansion of the fetoplacental volume (23). Moreover, within 2 hr of transfusion all the echocardiographic parameters return to the normal range suggesting a rapid possibility of recovery of the fetal circulation to volume expansion (23). Studies performed 24 hr after the transfusion failed to demonstrate any change (22).

Effects of Maternal Pharmacologic Treatment on Cardiac Function

Several of the agents used in the treatment of pregnancy complications may cross the placenta and affect fetal cardiac output. So far, a paucity of data has been reported.

β Agonists (ritodrine, terbutaline) used to treat premature labor have an inotropic effect on the fetal heart by increasing cardiac contractility. As a consequence, a significant increase of TVI $\times$ HR has been reported with short-term treatment (17). The long-term effects of such treatments remain to be investigated.

Indomethacin similarly used in the treatment of premature labor may induce a constriction of the ductus arteriosus (35). Under these circumstances it is logical to predict a shift of cardiac output to the left ventricle but no direct evidence has yet been provided.

No data are available on antihypertensive drugs commonly used in pregnancy (e.g., calcium antagonists, β antagonists) that may affect fetal cardiac function.

CONCLUSION

The measurement of cardiac output is possible in the human fetus under rigorous techniques of recording. This limits its applicability and its practical use in routine clinical work. Moreover, under experimental conditions its assessment has allowed us to clarify the pathophysiology of different conditions of pregnancy, allowing a better understanding of the hemodynamic mechanisms occurring in the human fetus.

REFERENCES

1. Gill RW. Pulsed Doppler with B-mode imaging for quantitative blood flow measurement. *Ultrasound Med Biol* 1979;5:223–235.
2. Eik-Nes SH, Brubaak AO, Ulstein MK. Measurement of human fetal blood flow. *Br Med J* 1980;280:283–284.
3. Burns PN. Measuring volume flow with Doppler ultrasound. An old nut. *Ultrasound Obstet Gynecol* 1992;2:238–241.
4. Maulik D, Nanda NC, Saini VD. Fetal Doppler echocardiography: Methods and characterization of normal and abnormal hemodynamics. *Am J Cardiol* 1984;53:572–577.
5. Maulik D, Nanda NC, Moodley S, Saini VD, Thiede HA. Application of Doppler echocardiography in the assessment of fetal cardiac disease. *Am J Obstet Gynecol* 1985;151:951–957.
6. Lynch PR, Bove AA. Patterns of blood flow through the intact heart and valves. In: Brewer LA, ed. *Prosthetic heart valves.* Springfield, IL: Charles C Thomas; 1968:24–42.
7. Burns PN. Doppler flow estimations in the fetal and maternal circulations: principles, techniques and some limitations. In: Maulik D, McNellis D, eds. *Doppler ultrasound measurement of maternal-fetal hemodynamics.* Ithaca, NY: Perinatology Press; 1987:43–78.
8. Rizzo G, Arduini D, Valensise H, Romanini C. Effects of behavioural states on cardiac output in the healthy human fetus at 36–38 weeks of gestation. *Early Hum Dev* 1990;23:109–115.
9. Rizzo G, Arduini D, Romanini C, Mancuso S. Doppler echocardiographic assessment of atrioventricular velocity waveforms in normal and small for gestational age fetuses. *Br J Obstet Gynaecol* 1988;95:65–69.
10. Rizzo G, Arduini D, Romanini C, Mancuso S. Doppler echocardiographic evaluation of time to peak velocity in the aorta and pulmonary artery of small for gestational age fetuses. *Br J Obstet Gynaecol* 1990;97:603–607.
11. Beeby AR, Dunlop W, Hunter S. Reproducibility of ultrasonic measurement of fetal cardiac haemodynamics. *Br J Obstet Gynaecol* 1991;98:807–814.
12. De Smedt MCH, Visser GHA, Meijboom EJ. Fetal cardiac output estimated by Doppler echocardiography during mid- and late gestation. *Am J Cardiol* 1987;60:338–342.
13. Reed KL, Meijboom EJ, Sahn DJ, Scagnelli SA, Valdes-Cruz LM, Skenker L. Cardiac Doppler flow velocities in human fetuses. *Circulation* 1986;73:41–56.
14. Al-Ghazali W, Chita SK, Chapman MG, Allan LD. Evidence of redistribution of cardiac output in asymmetrical growth retardation. *Br J Obstet Gynaecol* 1989;96:697–704.
15. Groenenberg IAL, Hop WCJ, Wladimiroff JW. Doppler flow velocity waveforms in the fetal cardiac outflow tract; reproducibility of waveform recording and analysis. *Ultrasound Med Biol* 1991;17:583–587.
16. Moise KJ, Mari G, Fisher DJ, Hutha JC, Cano LE, Carpenter RJ. Acute fetal hemodynamic alterations after intrauterine transfusion for treatment of severe red blood cell alloimmunization. *Am J Obstet Gynecol* 1990;163:776–784.
17. Sharif DS, Hutha JC, Moise KJ, Morrow RW, Yoon GY. Changes in fetal hemodynamics with terbutaline treatment and premature labor. *J Clin Ultrasound* 1990;18:85–89.
18. Rizzo G, Arduini D. Fetal cardiac function in intrauterine growth retardation. *Am J Obstet Gynecol* 1991;165:876–882.
19. Comstock CH, Riggs T, Lee W, Kirk J. Pulmonary to aorta diameter ratio in the normal and abnormal fetal heart. *Am J Obstet Gynecol* 1991;165:1038–1043.
20. Kenny JF, Plappert T, Saltzman DH, et al. Changes in intracardiac blood flow velocities and right and left ventricular stroke volumes with gestational age in the normal human fetus: A prospective Doppler echocardiographic study. *Circulation* 1986;74:1208–1216.
21. Allan LD, Chita SK, Al-Ghazali W, Crawford DC, Tynan M. Doppler echocardiographic evaluation of the normal human fetal heart. *Br Heart J* 1987;57:528–533.
22. Copel JA, Grannum PA, Green JJ, et al. Fetal cardiac output in the isoimmunized pregnancy: A pulsed Doppler–echocardiographic study of patients undergoing intravascular intrauterine transfusion. *Am J Obstet Gynecol* 1989;161:361–364.
23. Rizzo G, Nicolaides KH, Arduini D, Campbell S. Effects of intravascular fetal blood transfusion on fetal intracardiac Doppler velocity waveforms. *Am J Obstet Gynecol* 1990;163:1231–1238.
24. Rudolph AM. Distribution and regulation of blood flow in the fetal and neonatal lamb. *Circ Res* 1985;57:811–821.
25. Rizzo G, Arduini D. Cardiac output in anencephalic fetuses. *Gynecol Obstet Invest* 1991;32:33–35.
26. Rizzo G, Arduini D, Romanini C. Fetal cardiac and extra-cardiac circulation in early gestation. *J Mat–Fet Invest* 1991;1:73–78.
27. Copel JA, Morotti R, Hobbins JC, Kleinmann CS. The antenatal diagnosis of congenital heart disease using fetal echocardiography: Is color flow mapping necessary? *Obstet Gynecol* 1991;78:1–8.
28. Groenenberg IAL, Wladimiroff JW, Hop WCJ. Fetal cardiac and peripheral arterial flow velocity waveforms in intrauterine growth retardation. *Circulation* 1989;80:1711–1717.
29. Indik JH, Chen V, Reed KL. Association of umbilical venous with inferior vena cava blood flow velocities. *Obstet Gynecol* 1991;77:551–557.
30. Rizzo G, Arduini D, Romanini C. Inferior vena cava flow velocity waveforms in appropriate and small for gestational age fetuses. *Am J Obstet Gynecol* 1992;166:1271–1280.
31. Arduini D, Rizzo G, Romanini C. The development of abnormal heart rate patterns after absent end diastolic velocity in umbilical artery: Analysis of risk factors. *Am J Obstet Gynecol* 1993;168:50–53.
32. Fumia FD, Edelstone DI, Holzman IR. Blood flow and oxygen delivery as functions of fetal hematocrit. *Am J Obstet Gynecol* 1984;150:274–282.
33. Copel JA, Grannum PA, Belanger K, Green J, Hobbins JC. Pulsed Doppler flow velocity waveforms before and after intrauterine intravascular transfusion for severe erythroblastosis fetalis. *Am J Obstet Gynecol* 1988;158:768–774.
34. Chestnut DH, Pollack KL, Weiner CP, Robillard JE, Thompson CS, DeBruyn CS. Does furosemide alter the hemodynamic response to rapid intravascular transfusion of the anemic lamb fetus? *Am J Obstet Gynecol* 1989;161:1571–1575.
35. Moise KJ, Huhta JC, Sharif DF, et al. Indomethacin in the treatment of premature labor. Effects on fetal ductus arteriosus. *N Engl J Med* 1988;319:327–331.

Doppler Ultrasound in Obstetrics and Gynecology,
edited by Joshua A. Copel and Kathryn L. Reed.
Raven Press, Ltd., New York © 1995.

CHAPTER **28**

Fetal Cardiovascular Dynamics in Intrauterine Growth Retardation

Jean-Claude Fouron and Susan Pamela Drblik

One of the major problems involved with analyzing the impact of intrauterine growth retardation (IUGR) on the fetal cardiovascular system is the diversity of the etiologic factors (1–3). Lack of fetal growth may be genetically determined, the result of various insults either to the fetus or to the umbilicoplacental circulation, or related to maternal afflictions. Obviously, the underlying etiology will determine the degree to which the basic determinants of fetal cardiovascular dynamics will be compromised.

Another confounding element is the gestational age at which the onset of growth retardation occurs. It is generally accepted that an insult during the first 16 weeks of gestation will impair fetal cellular hyperplasia and will cause a proportionate decrease in the size of all organs (4). This is referred to as symmetric IUGR. On the other hand, if the problem occurs between the 16th and 32nd week of gestation, it will interfere with increases in cell size and number and result in a disproportionate decrease in the dimension of the fetal abdomen relative to the head. This form of development is referred to as asymmetric IUGR, which represents as much as 70% of all IUGR fetuses (5). Asymmetric fetal growth is usually a direct result of an impairment in the uteroplacental circulation as reflected by an increase in placental vascular resistance. Fetal cardiovascular adjustments cannot be expected to be the same in the presence or absence of changes in resistance to placental blood flow. In this chapter, therefore, efforts will be made to discuss, whenever possible, growth-retarded fetuses on the basis of their umbilicoplacental circulatory condition, giving to the resistance of the placental vascular bed a dominant role in the final circulatory patterns of these infants.

J.-C. Fouron and S. P. Drblik: Fetal Cardiology Unit, Service of Cardiology and Pulmonary Medicine, Department of Pediatrics, Sainte-Justine Hospital, University of Montreal, Montreal, Quebec, Canada.

No significant change in heart rate has been described in IUGR fetuses unless advanced stages of hypoxia with acidosis are reached causing deceleration patterns. Heart rate therefore will not be considered in this chapter as a significant element in the cardiovascular changes observed during fetal growth impairment.

VENTRICULAR AFTERLOAD AND PRELOAD IN IUGR

During fetal life, the two ventricles work in parallel. Consequently, discussion of any changes in ventricular loading should always specify which ventricle is being primarily affected. This information is important in terms of our ability to understand the behavioral characteristics of each ventricle.

Changes in Afterload

Left Ventricular Afterload

During fetal life, 70% of the blood ejected by the left ventricle perfuses the upper body (arms and head) (6). Therefore, any changes of resistance and pressure in these vascular beds will specifically influence the afterload of the fetal left heart. In particular, the effects on the cerebral circulation due to changes in left ventricular afterload have been the focus of most investigations owing to the potential risk of brain damage.

There is a scarcity of information on left ventricular afterload changes in growth-retarded fetuses with normal placental vascular resistance (7). The condition of the cerebral vascular network in this group of fetuses shall in all likelihood be dependent on factors that have an impact on the cerebral circulation such as carbon dioxide, hydrogen ions, and blood oxygen delivery (8,9). Among these factors, impairment of oxygen delivery to the fetus is theoretically possible during pregnancy under maternal conditions such as cyanotic heart disease, pulmonary insufficiency, and high altitude, which could all lead to IUGR with normal placental resistance. Vasodilatation of the cerebral arteries therefore is possible under these conditions whereas umbilical blood flow has not been shown to change in relation to arterial O_2 content (8). On the other hand, in IUGR fetuses with structural or chromosomal abnormalities oxygen delivery to the brain should be normal and no change in left ventricular afterload would be expected. Doppler flow velocities of the carotid arteries have confirmed this point (7).

In asymmetric IUGR left ventricular afterload has been better investigated both experimentally and clinically during an increase in resistance of the placental vascular bed. Although it is accepted that fetal arterial PO_2 decreases because of placental insufficiency, this relation is not linear. It is important to keep in mind that an increase in placental vascular resistance and changes in the Doppler flow velocity waveforms do not necessarily mean fetal hypoxemia. Contrary to what is observed in IUGR with normal placental perfusion, however, PCO_2 tends to rise with placental insufficiency. Similarly, acid metabolites have less of a chance to cross the placental barrier and tend to accumulate in the fetus. Consequently, for the same level of hypoxemia, respiratory and metabolic acidemia should develop earlier in these cases compared to those with normal placental vascular resistance. Vasodilatation of the cerebral arteries should therefore be expected owing to the presence of both hypoxemia and hypercarbia. Indeed, such a phenomenon has been demonstrated experimentally by many investigators (10–12). The drop in cerebral vascular resistance and left ventricular afterload in IUGR human fetuses has been confirmed by Doppler echocardiography where an increase of the diastolic component of the cerebral arteries flow velocity waveforms has been repeatedly recorded (13–16).

The state of the other vascular beds perfused by the left ventricle (heart, upper body) has not been the specific subject of investigations in IUGR with normal placental circulation. On the other hand, vasodilatation of the coronary arteries has been reported in a few studies that experimentally reproduced the conditions that lead to IUGR with an increase in placental vascular resistance (10,17).

Right Ventricular Afterload

During fetal life, the right ventricular outlet consists of a large main pulmonary artery from which smaller left and right arteries branch off at very sharp angles. The widely patent ductus arteriosus forms a natural prolongation of the main pulmonary artery toward the descending thoracic aorta. Ninety percent of the blood ejected by the right ventricle goes with minimal resistance through the ductus arteriosus into the descending thoracic aorta (6). Because of this arrangement, fetal right ventricular afterload is essentially dictated by the resistances of the various vascular beds distal to the descending aorta. The significantly lower resistance and higher volume flow (more than 50% of the combined ventricular output) of the umbilical circulation confer to the placental vessels a dominant role in establishing the level of right ventricular afterload.

The few Doppler investigations performed on fetuses with symmetric IUGR showed persistence of the normal flow velocity pattern of the umbilical artery characterized by a significant forward diastolic flow (7,18). It can be assumed, therefore, that growth deficiency caused by an impairment of cellular hyperplasia that occurs early in gestation is not necessarily associated with any significant alteration in placental vascular resistance. To our knowledge, what actually takes place in other vascular beds such as the mesenteric and renal circulations in IUGR with normal placental resistance and normal arterial O_2 content has not been the subject of any reports. Right ventricular afterload is not expected to increase in most of these cases. On the other hand, as previously mentioned, IUGR without uteroplacental insufficiency can be associated with fetal chronic hypoxemia. In these cases, blood flow redistribution comparable to what is described in chronic fetal hypoxemia can be expected, characterized by a decrease in flow to the kidneys, the gut, and the carcass (8,19).

There has been a proliferation of reports on Doppler flow velocity investigations of the umbilical artery confirming that IUGR fetuses with uteroplacental insufficiency have an increased resistance to their placental blood flow (13,20–25). This observation alone is sufficient to expect an increase in right ventricular afterload in these cases. The response of the remaining arterial network will vary according to the presence or absence of hypoxemia. It has been shown that the pulsatility index rises in the fetal femoral artery during an increase in placental vascular resistance (26). The same phenomenon has also been described in the renal artery of a similar group of fetuses, suggesting an increase in resistance to renal perfusion and explaining the occurrence of oligohydramnios (27).

Despite these increases in peripheral resistance, experimental studies failed to demonstrate any significant change in descending aorta pressure during an increase in resistance to placental flow, probably because of a concomitant decrease in right ventricular output (28,29). However, a clinical study suggested an increase in diastolic blood pressure of IUGR fetuses with chronic impairment of umbilical circulation (30). This last study was based on pulsatile diameter changes of the fetal descending aorta.

It can be concluded, therefore, that one of the fundamental hemodynamic differences between IUGR fetuses with and without placental circulatory insufficiency is the consistent presence of a significant increase in right ventricular afterload in the former group. This differential feature must play a crucial role both in peripheral blood redistribution described in asymmetric IUGR and individual ventricular outputs. This last point will be discussed later.

Balance Between the Afterloads of the Two Fetal Vascular Systems: Importance of the Isthmus

Since the afterloads of the two ventricles are modified in opposite fashion in IUGR fetuses with placental insufficiency, a ratio between velocimetric indices of cerebral and umbilical circulations has been derived for this group of fetuses (18,31–33). This logical approach has resulted in an index proven to be more sensitive than individual indices recorded at either the cerebral or the umbilical level.

With the same rationale in mind, we recently investigated the blood flow velocity behavior within the aortic isthmus of IUGR fetuses. The isthmus is indeed the only arterial segment linking the two vascular systems perfused by both the left and right ventricles. The flow pattern within the isthmus should therefore be very sensitive to afterload changes in either the cerebral or the placental vascular network. Normally, because of the lower resistance of the placental circulation, forward diastolic flow is constantly recorded in the aortic isthmus (34). An increase in resistance to placental flow, severe enough to create a reversal of diastolic velocities in the umbilical circulation, has been shown also to cause a reverse diastolic flow in the aortic isthmus—a pattern that has been demonstrated both experimentally (28) and clinically (35). More recently, an acute experimental increase in resistance to umbilical flow in fetal lambs showed that changes in flow patterns in the isthmus precede those usually observed in the umbilical artery (36). Here again, these experimental observations have been confirmed in the human fetus (Fig. 1) (37). Furthermore, in fetal lambs, when placental resistance was mechanically and progressively increased to the point of equalization in af-

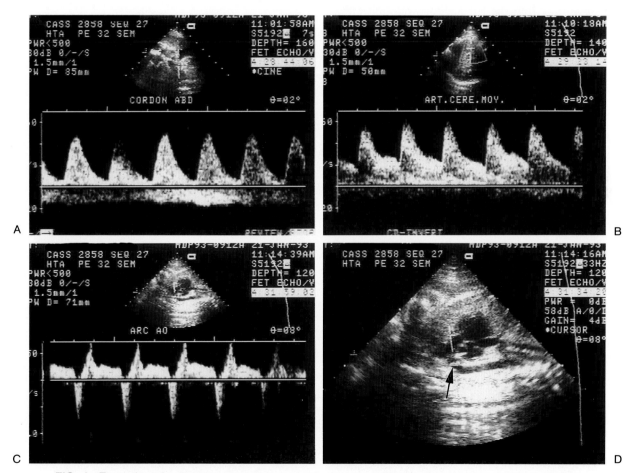

FIG. 1. Examples of a Doppler blood flow velocity study in a 32-week fetus with growth retardation illustrating a more severe alteration in the flow profile of the aortic isthmus compared to the umbilical artery. **A:** In the umbilical artery a moderate decrease in the forward diastolic flow is observed. **B:** Velocity waveform in the middle cerebral artery showing an increase in diastolic forward flow. **C:** Flow velocity profile through the aortic isthmus where a significant reverse diastolic flow is recorded. **D:** Point of localization of the Doppler sample volume in the aortic isthmus (*arrow*).

terloads of the cerebral and umbilical circulatory systems, blood flow through the isthmus was negligible (38). The two ventricles were then ejecting blood into two arterial systems completely independent of each other. Further clinical investigations are warranted to assess the value of aortic isthmus flow velocity recordings as a fetal monitoring tool.

Changes in Preload

Preload is usually assessed clinically by measuring the end-diastolic pressure or volume of the ventricles. Analysis of factors influencing fetal ventricular preload is complicated by the fact that even though the ventricles perfuse two parallel vascular systems, their respective venous returns do not follow a similar parallel arrangement but a more complex pattern. Seventy percent of the blood ejected by the left ventricle returns, through the superior vena cava, entirely to the right ventricle (6). The blood ejected by the right ventricle returns to the heart via the inferior vena cava whereupon it divides into two unequal parts, one part crossing the foramen ovale (approximately 40%) into the left atrium while the other flows into the right atrium and ventricle. In a normal fetus, therefore, left ventricular preload will be greatly influenced not only by the size of the foramen ovale but also by the volume flow from the inferior vena cava. Under physiologic conditions, the pulmonary venous return represents approximately 7% of the total venous return and plays a minor role in left ventricular preload. On the other hand, right ventricular volume load is made up not only of superior vena cava blood but also of the fraction of the inferior vena cava return that did not go through the foramen ovale. It is apparent that the redistribution of the venous return will also be influenced by any change in the respective ventricular diastolic filling characteristics.

Left Ventricular Preload in IUGR

To our knowledge, investigation of left ventricular preload in symmetric IUGR has been limited. Since a normal umbilical flow and normal inferior vena cava return can be expected in the majority of these cases, volume flow into the left ventricle should be preserved. However, this speculation remains to be confirmed.

On the other hand, asymmetric IUGR caused by an increase in placental resistance is associated with a fall in umbilical flow (22,39,40) and, as a consequence, a decrease in inferior vena cava venous return. Theoretically, a decrease in inferior vena cava blood flow should result in a reduction of volume flow toward both ventricles and a decrease in combined cardiac output. However, experimental (29) as well as clinical (41,42) reports have shown that the left ventricular output is less affected than

the right. We recently made the same observation in a group of fetal lambs in whom increase in resistance to placental flow was created by progressive compression of the umbilical vein (Fig. 2). This observation could be explained by an increase in the proportion of inferior vena cava blood that crosses the foramen ovale, a rise in pulmonary venous return, or a combination of the two. A relative increase in the proportion of the more oxygenated inferior vena cava blood through the foramen ovale was indeed observed in fetal lambs where resistance to placental flow was acutely increased (10,43). Despite this inferior vena cava blood redistribution, a significant increase in left ventricular output has not been reported (44) suggesting that in absolute value the same amount of blood was being shunted through the foramen ovale. On the other hand, the possibility of a rise in pulmonary venous return is not unrealistic in the presence of an elevated placental resistance. Indeed, in these circumstances a secondary increase in pressure of the descending aorta and presumably main pulmonary artery would direct more blood through the pulmonary circulation. This could be an explanation for the reports of a higher incidence of persistent pulmonary hypertension in newborns with asymmetric IUGR (45,46). In addition, secondary changes in ventricular diastolic function resulting from an elevated placental resistance may modify the normal redistribution of venous return between the two ventricles. This could occur since the adaptive response to changes in afterload has been shown to be different between the ventricles (47). This point will be discussed in the next section on myocardial performance.

Right Ventricular Preload in IUGR

Our knowledge of the preloading parameters of the right side of the heart in IUGR with or without an in-

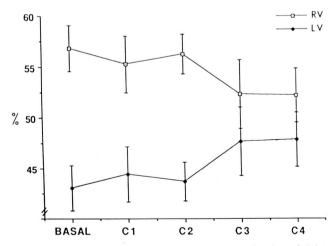

FIG. 2. Percent change in the respective contribution of right (RV) and left (LV) ventricles to the combined cardiac output in five fetal lambs during graded compression (from C_1 to C_4) of their umbilical vein.

crease in placental resistance is more speculative than factual. One important difference between the left and right fetal ventricular preloading conditions is the role played by the superior vena cava return. As previously mentioned, under normal conditions, superior vena cava blood returns in its entirety to the right ventricle. Some symmetric IUGR fetuses with normal placental vascular resistance could be chronically hypoxemic and have a secondary cerebral vasodilatation. Under these circumstances volume flow through the superior vena cava would be increased, resulting in an elevated right ventricular preload. This could be a possible explanation for the isolated right ventricular dilatation reported in some cases of IUGR (48). On the other hand, in IUGR with an elevated placental resistance, there is a decrease in venous return coming from the inferior vena cava. As previously stated, a greater proportion of this decreased inferior vena cava blood probably goes through the foramen ovale. Another important hemodynamic element associated with an increase in placental resistance is the fall in the forward flow normally observed through the aortic isthmus (37). In severe cases, isthmic flow becomes negligible (38). This means that a greater proportion of the left ventricular output remains available for upper body tissue perfusion (mainly the brain) and is drained through the superior vena cava toward the right ventricle. It becomes apparent that right ventricular preload of IUGR fetuses with placental insufficiency could be influenced by two divergent elements. On the one hand, a decrease in the proportion of inferior vena cava blood going in the right atrium would favor a lower preload. On the other hand a greater venous return through the superior vena cava would have the opposite effect. Further studies are obviously needed to determine what actually happens to right ventricular preload in this situation.

MYOCARDIAL PERFORMANCE IN IUGR

From the preceding discussion, it appears that an alteration in cardiac function in IUGR fetuses can be expected because of significant changes observed in the loading conditions of the heart. Experimental studies have indeed shown that the fetal ventricles are sensitive, albeit differently, to both preload and afterload modifications (49–51). On the other hand, during fetal growth impairment, factors such as chronic hypoxemia, acidemia, and a fall in essential amino acids (52) could directly impair myocardial performance even in the absence of ventricular loading disturbances. Report of histologic lesions in the myocardium of infants dying from severe IUGR (53) could also be considered as pathologic evidence of intrinsic myocardial damage. Irrespective of its origin, the functional myocardial impairment in IUGR could manifest itself during both diastole and systole.

Myocardial Diastolic Function

With the advent of Doppler ultrasound technology, it is possible to study the blood flow velocity patterns through the fetal atrioventricular valves. The diastolic flow profile is made of two waves corresponding to the early ventricular filling (E wave) and the atrial contraction late in diastole (A wave). While in extrauterine life the E wave is predominant, it is now well known that the fetal profile is characterized by a higher peak A than E wave. This has been interpreted as an indication of low compliance of the fetal myocardium. The fact that the E/A ratio increases progressively and approaches unity toward the end of gestation has also been considered as a sign of progressive improvement in myocardial compliance. It is now known, however, that throughout pregnancy the peak velocity of the A wave does not significantly change while that of the E wave steadily increases (54). This observation would support the concept of a progressive maturational change involving almost exclusively the active process of ventricular relaxation.

At least two reports have shown that in growth-retarded fetuses the E/A ratio is abnormally higher than that of normal controls for the same gestational age (55,56). The same observation has also been made in our unit in fetuses with abnormal flow velocity profiles in the umbilical artery (Fig. 3). All fetuses reported in these studies had absent diastolic flow in their umbilical arteries suggesting an increase in placental resistance and, as a result, a decrease in venous return from the inferior vena cava. The alteration in the E/A ratio could therefore be, at least in part, related to preload changes without necessarily involving impairment in fetal myocardial diastolic function (57,58).

Another noninvasive measurement of the ventricular relaxation process has been the assessment of the deceleration time of the E wave across the atrioventricular valve (59), impairment in relaxation being reflected by an increase in deceleration time. In IUGR, an increase in deceleration time relative to normals has indeed been reported (60). However, the same authors observed in normal fetuses a prolongation of the deceleration time with an increase in gestational age. This latter finding would appear to contradict the accepted notion that ventricular diastolic function improves with gestation. Obviously, consideration must be given to the interrelationship that exists between atrial and ventricular pressures, volume, and functions on the diastolic filling pattern of the ventricles. Unfortunately, the noninvasive nature of current ultrasound fetal investigation does not permit absolute measurement of these variables, which renders difficult, if not impossible, the interpretation of an isolated finding.

In IUGR fetuses with abnormal flow velocities in the umbilical artery, studies of the flow profile of the inferior vena cava close to the heart have consistently demon-

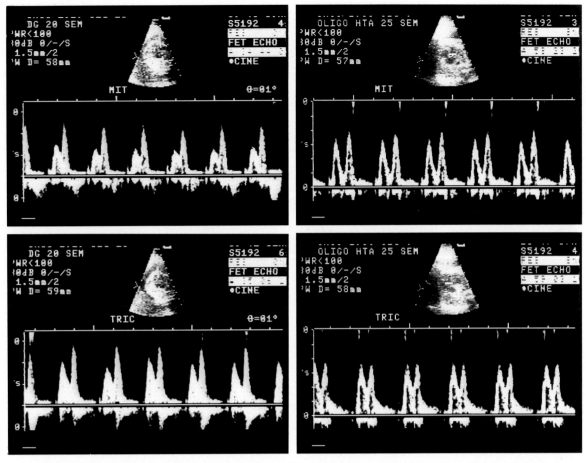

FIG. 3. Comparison of Doppler flow velocity profiles through the mitral (**top**) and tricuspid (**bottom**) valves. On the left-hand side are recordings taken from a normal 20-week fetus, and on the right from a 25-week growth-retarded fetus with absent diastolic flow in the umbilical artery. Note the A wave dominance in the normal and the equalization of A and E waves in the IUGR fetus.

strated a significant accentuation of the reverse flow that normally occurs during atrial contraction (61,62). Here again the possibility of abnormal diastolic function, characterized by a lack of myocardial compliance, has been raised on the basis that a stiffer myocardium would be less easy to stretch and would cause a greater reflux of blood toward the inferior vena cava during atrial contraction.

Myocardial diastolic function in symmetric IUGR with normal umbilical artery velocimetry has to our knowledge never been reported. In theory there would be no reason to expect changes in the diastolic function of these infants unless hypoxemia was present.

Myocardial Systolic Function

Ventricular Outputs

There is limited information on the relative ventricular outputs in IUGR with normal placental resistance. In one report, 15 such fetuses were studied and 12 were found to have a normal cardiac output (42). Right ven-

tricular preponderence, in a range comparable to normal controls, was also found in all but one.

Conversely, in asymmetric IUGR with placental circulatory insufficiency, a significant drop in combined cardiac output has been reported (41,42). Longitudinal studies have shown that this decline increases proportionally with the duration of the disease (41). With the exception of one study (55), these fetuses showed a greater decrease in right ventricular output. This is in accordance with observations made in animal studies designed to increase placental vascular resistance, in which not only a reduction in cardiac output was observed but a significantly greater drop in right compared to left output flow was demonstrated (Fig. 2) (29). These results support the widespread concept that in the presence of hypoxemia there is a redistribution of fetal blood flow resulting in what is commonly referred to as the brain-sparing effect. However, there is evidence to suggest that hypoxemia is not the only responsible factor. Indeed, under experimental conditions, isolated hypoxemia did not affect the normal fetal right ventricular dominance (63). Furthermore, as previously mentioned, fetuses with symmetric growth retardation with a normal placental circulation did not reveal intracardiac redistribution of their blood flow patterns (42). These data suggest, therefore, that an increase in placental resistance (ventricular afterload) is a determining factor in the decline of the right ventricular output. Studies on fetal lambs have shown that for a similar increase in afterload, a significantly greater reduction in right ventricular stroke volume was observed compared to the left (47). This may be explained by the difference in the morphology of the two fetal ventricles, the difference in impedance of the aorta and pulmonary artery (50,64), or a combination of the two. It is interesting to note that this proportionally greater fall in right ventricular output observed in IUGR fetuses has not been found to influence the diameter of the pulmonary artery (65), as is generally seen in congenital malformations associated with low right ventricular output.

The relative size of the heart within the thoracic cavity has also been the subject of investigation (66,67). An abnormally elevated cardiothoracic ratio has been reported in infants with IUGR. It is somewhat surprising, however, to see cardiomegaly reported in cases with low cardiac output. These observations could be the reflection of either myocardial damage related to chronic hypoxemia and polycythemia or, as previously suggested, the result of a normal-sized heart in a smaller thoracic cavity. Unfortunately, in none of the reported cases with elevated cardiothoracic ratio was myocardial function assessed nor was the type of growth retardation clearly identified.

M-Mode Echocardiography

Myocardial contractility using M-mode echocardiography has been studied in human fetuses with chronic placental insufficiency (68). Right ventricular fractional shortening was decreased, and the ratio of right over left ventricular end-diastolic diameters was increased. The left ventricular size and myocardial contractility did not differ from that of normal fetuses. These data are in accordance with observations made on right and left ventricular function of fetal sheep exposed to long-term

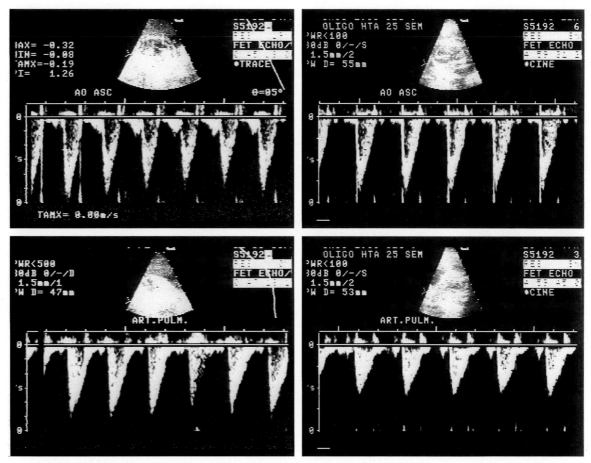

FIG. 4. Examples of lower peak systolic velocities in both aortic (65 mm/sec) (**upper right**) and pulmonary artery (43 mm/sec) (**bottom right**) flow profiles of a growth-retarded fetus with absent diastolic flow in the umbilical artery. On the left are examples of a normal aortic (1.2 m/sec) (**top**) and pulmonary artery (1.0 m/sec) (**bottom**) flow velocity waveform. The angle of insonation is less than 20° for all recordings.

high-altitude hypoxemia (63); an elevation of their mean arterial pressure was associated with a reduction in right ventricular function. In contrast, the left ventricular function curve was not significantly different from control values. These observations would lend further support to the concept that the fetal right ventricle is more sensitive to afterload than the left (47). However, a chronic increase in afterload has been shown to improve right ventricular function in fetal sheep possibly by an increase in wall thickness and secondary decrease in cavity size (50).

Doppler Indices

Velocity and acceleration of blood flow in the ascending aorta have been used in the assessment of left ventricular systolic function (69). In IUGR infants with decreased placental blood flow, peak velocities in both ascending aorta and main pulmonary artery have been found to be decreased (13,41,42). Figure 4 is an example of such changes in velocities. However, since aortic flow velocity has been shown to be inversely related to afterload (70), these low peak velocities may not only reflect an impairment in myocardial contractility but could also be due to the associated increase in placental vascular resistance. Another possible explanation could be the fall in ventricular outputs. It is interesting to note that growth-retarded fetuses with normal flow velocities in their umbilical arteries also have normal peak velocities in both the aorta and pulmonary artery (42).

Time to peak velocity, or acceleration time, of both the aorta and pulmonary artery has also been studied in IUGR. In normal fetuses, acceleration time is known to be shorter in the pulmonary artery than in the aorta (71). This finding has been explained by the higher resistance of the pulmonary vascular bed in the fetus. However, as previously mentioned, the right ventricle is pumping toward the placenta through a widely patent ductus arteriosus. The possibility that in normal fetuses the shorter acceleration time is due to a better right ventricular performance (higher stroke volume, lower afterload) deserves investigation (72). In IUGR fetuses with an increase in placental vascular resistance, a further decrease in acceleration time in the pulmonary artery has been reported (73).

CONCLUSION

Our understanding of the cardiovascular changes associated with fetal growth impairment is still limited especially in the so-called symmetric IUGR. Most of the available experimental data reproduced fetal retardation in a relatively short period of time, which is in contrast to the chronic situation observed in the human fetus. Moreover, these studies rarely focus on myocardial func-

tion. In addition, the clinical studies based on Doppler echocardiography do not allow a complete assessment of all dynamic parameters such as arterial and venous pressures. Despite these limitations, it is nevertheless apparent that one inherent element that will constantly determine the cardiovascular dynamics of the growth-retarded fetus is the status of the placental circulation. An increase in placental resistance should indeed significantly modify the cardiac loading conditions and output.

Knowledge of alterations in the cardiovascular system of IUGR is important not only for a better understanding of the pathophysiology of this condition, but also in the search of variables that could be used to determine the severity of the pathologic process. This would benefit the clinician by providing more accurate information on the growth-retarded fetus, which should reduce the conjecture and strengthen the rationale in any decision-making process.

REFERENCES

1. Pollack RN, Divon MY. Intrauterine growth retardation: Definition, classification, and etiology. *Clin Obstet Gynecol* 1992;35(1): 99–107.
2. Longo LD. Intrauterine growth retardation: A "mosaic" hypothesis of pathophysiology. *Semin Perinatol* 1984;8(1):62–72.
3. Brar HS, Rutherford SE. Classification of intrauterine growth retardation. *Semin Perinatol* 1988;12(1):2–10.
4. Winick M. Cellular changes during placental and fetal growth. *Am J Obstet Gynecol* 1971;109:166–176.
5. Campbell S. Fetal growth. *Clin Obstet Gynaecol* 1974;1:41–65.
6. Rudolph AM, Heymann MA. Circulatory changes during growth in the fetal lamb. *Circ Res* 1970;26:289–299.
7. Wladimiroff JW, Tonge HM, Stewart PA. Doppler ultrasound assessment of cerebral blood flow in the human fetus. *Br J Obstet Gyneacol* 1986;93:471–475.
8. Peeters LLH, Sheldon RE, Jones MD, Makowki EL, Meschia G. Blood flow to fetal organs as a function of arterial oxygen content. *Am J Obstet Gynecol* 1979;135:637–646.
9. Jones MD, Hudak ML. Regulation of the fetal cerebral circulation. In: Polin RA, Fox WW, eds. *Fetal and neonatal physiology.* Philadelphia: WB Saunders; 1992;1:682–690.
10. Itskovitz J, La Gamma F, Rudolph AM. Effects of cord compression on fetal blood flow distribution and O_2 delivery. *Am J Physiol* 1987;252:H100–H109.
11. Bocking AD, Gagnon R, White SE, Homan J, Milne KM, Richardson BS. Circulatory responses to prolonged hypoxemia in fetal sheep. *Am J Obstet Gynecol* 1988;159:1418–1424.
12. Sonesson SE, Teyssier G, Bonnin P, Fouron JC. The effect of elevated placental resistance on changes in fetal carotid artery blood velocities induced by maternal oxygen administration. *J Mat–Fet Invest* 1993;34:796–800.
13. Groenenberg IAL, Wladimiroff JW, Hop WCJ. Fetal cardiac and peripheral arterial flow velocity waveforms in intrauterine growth retardation. *Circulation* 1989;80:1711–1717.
14. Marsal K, Lingman G, Giles W. Evaluation of the carotid, aortic and umbilical blood velocity. In: *Proceedings of the Eleventh Annual Conference of the Society for the Study of Fetal Physiology.* Oxford: 1984; abstract C33.
15. Arbeille PH, Roncin M, Patat F, Pourcelot L. Exploration of the fetal cerebral blood flow by duplex Doppler linear array system in normal and pathological pregnancies. *Ultrasound Med Biol* 1987;13:329–332.
16. Mari G, Deter RL. Middle cerebral artery flow velocity waveforms in normal and small-for-gestational-age fetuses. *Am J Obstet Gynecol* 1992;166:1262–1270.

17. Block BSB, Llanos AJ, Creasy RK. Responses of the growth-retarded fetus to acute hypoxemia. *Am J Obstet Gynecol* 1984; 148:878–885.

18. Wladimiroff JW, Wijngood JACW, Degani S, et al. Cerebral and umbilical arterial and growth retarded pregnancies. *Obstet Gynecol* 1987;69:705–709.

19. Cohn HE, Sacks EJ, Heymann MA, Rudolph AM. Cardiovascular responses to hypoxemia and acidemia in fetal lambs. *Am J Obstet Gynecol* 1974;120:817–824.

20. McCowan LM, Mullen BM, Ritchie K. Umbilical artery flow velocity waveforms and the placental vascular bed. *Am J Obstet Gynecol* 1987;157:900–902.

21. Bracero LA, Beneck D, Kirshenbaum N, Peiffer M, Stalter P, Schulman H. Doppler velocimetry and placental disease. *Am J Obstet Gynecol* 1989;161:388–393.

22. Laurin J, Lingman G, Marsal K, Persson PH. Fetal blood flow in pregnancies complicated by intrauterine growth retardation. *Obstet Gynecol* 1987;69:895–902.

23. Giles WB, Trudinger GJ, Baird PJ. Fetal umbilical artery flow velocity waveforms and placental resistance: Pathological correlation. *Br J Obstet Gynaecol* 1985;92:31–38.

24. Fok RY, Pavlova Z, Benirschke K, Paul RH, Platt LD. The correlation of arterial lesions with umbilical artery Doppler velocimetry in the placentas of small-or-dates pregnancies. *Obstet Gynecol* 1990;75:578–583.

25. Divon MY, Hsu HW. Maternal and fetal blood flow velocity waveforms in intrauterine growth retardation. *Clin Obstet Gynecol* 1992;35:156–171.

26. Mari G. Arterial blood flow velocity waveforms of the pelvis and lower extremities in normal and growth-retarded fetuses. *Am J Obstet Gynecol* 1991;165:143–151.

27. Arduini D, Rizzo G. Fetal renal artery velocity waveforms and amniotic fluid volume in growth-retarded and post-term fetuses. *J Obstet Gynecol* 1991;77(3):370–373.

28. Fouron JC, Teyssier G, Maroto E, Lessard M, Marquette G. Diastolic circulatory dynamics in the presence of elevated retrograde diastolic flow in the umbilical artery: A Doppler echographic study in lambs. *Am J Obstet Gynecol* 1991;164(1):195–203.

29. Goodwin JW. The impact of the umbilical circulation on the fetus. *Am J Obstet Gynecol* 1968;100(4):461–471.

30. Stale H, Marsal K, Gennser G, Benthin M, Dahl P, Lindstrom K. Aortic diameter pulse waves and blood flow velocity in the small, for gestational age fetus. *Ultrasound Med Biol* 1991;17(5):471–478.

31. Arduini D, Rizzo G, Romanini C, Mancuso S. Fetal blood flow waveforms as predictors of growth retardation. *Obstet Gynecol* 1987;70:7–10.

32. Arbeille P, Patat F, Tranquart F, et al. Exploration Doppler des circulations artérielles ombilicale et cérébrale du foetus. *J Gynecol Obstet Biol Reprod* 1987;16:45–51.

33. Gramellini D, Folli MC, Raboni S, Vadora E, Merialdi A. Cerebral–umbilical Doppler ratio as a predictor of adverse perinatal outcome. *Obstet Gynecol* 1992;79:416–420.

34. Fouron JC, Zarrelli M. Flow velocity profile through the fetal aortic isthmus. *J Mat–Fet Invest* 1992;2:122.

35. Fouron JC, Teyssier G, Shalaby L, Lessard M, van Doesburg NH. Fetal central blood flow alterations in human fetuses with umbilical artery reverse diastolic flow. *Am J Perinatol* 1993;10:197–207.

36. Teyssier G, Fouron JC, Bonnin P, Sonesson SE, Skoll A, Lessard M. Blood flow velocity profile in the fetal aortic isthmus: A sensitive indicator of changes in systemic peripheral resistance I-Experimental studies. *J Mat–Fet Invest* 1993;3:213–218.

37. Fouron JC, Teyssier G, Bonnin P, Sonesson SE, Skoll A, Lessard M. Blood flow velocity profile in the fetal aortic isthmus: A sensitive indicator of changes in systemic peripheral resistance II-Clinical observations. *J Mat–Fet Invest;* in press.

38. Bonnin P, Fouron JC, Teyssier G, Sonesson SE, Skoll A. Quantitative assessment of circulatory changes in the fetal aortic isthmus during progressive increase of resistance to placental blood flow. *Circulation* 1993;88:216–222.

39. Gill RW, Kossoff G, Warren PS, et al. Umbilical venous flow in normal and complicated pregnancy. *Ultrasound Med Biol* 1984;10:349.

40. Jouppila P, Kirkinen P. Umbilical vein blood flow as an indicator of fetal hypoxia. *Br J Obstet Gynaecol* 1984;91:107.

41. Rizzo G, Arduini D. Fetal cardiac function in intrauterine growth retardation. *Am J Obstet Gynecol* 1991;165:876–882.

42. Al-Ghazali W, Chita SK, Chapman MG, Allan LD. Evidence of redistribution of cardiac output in asymmetrical growth retardation. *Br J Obstet Gynaecol* 1989;96:697–704.

43. Dawes GS, Mott WA. Changes in O_2 distribution and consumption in foetal lambs with variations in umbilical blood flow. *J Physiol* 1964;170:524–540.

44. Block BS, Schlafer DH, Wentworth RA, Kreitzer LA, Nathanielsz PW. Regional blood flow distribution in fetal sheep with intrauterine growth retardation produced by decreased umbilical placental perfusion. *J Dev Physiol* 1990;2:81–85.

45. Soifer SJ, Kaslow D, Roman C, Heymann MA. Umbilical cord compression produces pulmonary hypertension in newborn lambs: A model to study the pathophysiology of persistent pulmonary hypertension in the newborn. *J Dev Physiol* 1987;9:239–252.

46. Siassi B, Naves E, Starck C, Cabal LA. Normal and abnormal transitional circulation in the neonates with intrauterine growth retardation (IUGR). *Pediatr Res* 1988;23(1416):437A.

47. Reller MD, Morton MJ, Reid DL, Thornburg KL. Fetal lamb ventricles respond differently to filling and arterial pressures and to in utero ventilation. *Pediatr Res* 1987;22:621–626.

48. Devore GR. Examination of the fetal heart in the fetus with intrauterine growth retardation using M-Mode echocardiography. *Semin Perinatol* 1988;12(1):66–79.

49. Hawkins J, Van Hare GF, Klaus G, Schmidt KG, Rudolph AM. Effects of increasing afterload on left ventricular output in fetal lambs. *Circ Res* 1989;65:127–134.

50. Pinson CW, Morton MJ, Thornburg KL. Mild pressure loading alters right ventricular function in fetal sheep. *Circ Res* 1991;68:947–957.

51. Gilbert RD. Effects of afterload and baroreceptors on cardiac function in fetal sheep. *J Dev Physiol* 1982;4:299–309.

52. Cetin I, Corbetta C, Sereni LP, et al. Umbilical amino acid concentrations in normal and growth-retarded fetuses sampled in utero by cordocentesis. *J Obstet Gynecol* 1990;162:253–261.

53. Naeye RL. Cardiovascular abnormalities in infants malnourished before birth. *Biol Neonat* 1965;8:104–113.

54. Fouron JC, Carceller AM. Determinants of the Doppler flow velocity profile through the mitral valve of the human fetus. *Br Heart J* 1993;70:457–460.

55. Reed KL, Anderson CF, Shenker L. Changes in intracardiac Doppler blood flow velocities in fetuses with absent umbilical artery diastolic flow. *Am J Obstet Gynecol* 1987;157:774–779.

56. Rizzo C, Arduini D, Romanini C, Mancuso S. Doppler echocardiographic assessment of atrioventricular velocity waveforms in normal and small-for-gestational-age fetuses. *Br J Obstet Gynaecol* 1988;95:65–69.

57. Berk MR, Gongyuan X, Kwan OL, et al. Reduction of left ventricular preload by lower body negative pressure alters Doppler transmitral filling patterns. *J Am Coll Cardiol* 1990;16:1387–1392.

58. Courtois M, Vered Z, Barzilai B, Ricciotti N, Pérez JE, Ludbrook PA. The transmitral pressure-flow velocity relation: Effect of abrupt preload reduction. *Circulation* 1988;78:1459–1468.

59. Appleton CP, Hatle LK, Popp RL. Relation of transmitral flow velocity patterns to left ventricular diastolic function: New insights from a combined hemodynamic and Doppler echocardiographic study. *J Am Coll Cardiol* 1988;12:426–440.

60. Reed KL, Appleton CP, Sahn DJ, Anderson CF. Human fetal tricuspid and mitral deceleration time: Changes with normal pregnancy and intrauterine growth retardation. *Am J Obstet Gynecol* 1989;161:1532–1533.

61. Reed KL, Appleton CP, Anderson CF, Shenker L, Sahn DJ. Doppler studies of vena cava flows in human fetuses. *Circulation* 1990;81:498–505.

62. Rizzo G, Arduini D, Romanini C. Inferior vena cava flow velocity waveforms in appropriate- and small-for-gestational-age fetuses. *Am J Obstet Gynecol* 1992;166:1271–1280.

63. Kamitomo M, Longo LD, Gilbert RD. Right and left ventricular function in fetal sheep exposed to long-term high-altitude hypoxemia. *Am J Physiol* 1992;262:H399–H405.

64. Noble MM. Left ventricular load, arterial impedance and their interrelationship. *Cardiovasc Res* 1979;13:183–198.

65. Cartier MS, Doubilet PM. Fetal aortic and pulmonary artery di-

ameters: Sonographic measurements in growth-retarded fetuses. *AJR* 1988;151:991–993.

66. Bozynski MEA, Hanafy FH, Hernandez RJ. Association of increased cardiothoracic ratio and intrauterine growth retardation. *Am J Perinatol* 1991;8(1):28–30.

67. Edwards DK, Higgins CB, Gilpin EA. The cardiothoracic ratio in newborn infants. *AJR* 1981;136:907–913.

68. Rasanen J, Kirkinen P, Jouppila P. Right ventricular dysfunction in human fetal compromise. *Am J Obstet Gynecol* 1989;161:136–140.

69. Bennet ED, Barclay SA, Davis AL, Mannering D, Netha N. Ascending aortic blood velocity and acceleration using Doppler ultrasound in the assessment of left ventricular function. *Cardiovasc Res* 1984;18:632–638.

70. Harrison MR, Clifton GD, Berk MR, DeMaria AN, Carter A, Burns D. Effect of blood pressure and afterload on Doppler echocardiographic measurements of left ventricular systolic function in normal subjects. *Am J Cardiol* 1989;64:905–908.

71. Machado MVL, Chita SC, Allan LD. Acceleration time in the aorta and pulmonary artery measured by Doppler echocardiography in the midtrimester normal human fetus. *Br Heart J* 1987;58:15–18.

72. Alverson DC, Blomquist T, Eldridge MW, Berman W. Assessment of myocardial contractility in dogs using pulsed-Doppler ultrasound. *J Cardiovasc Ultrason* 1987;6:77–83.

73. Rizzo G, Arduini D, Romanini C, Mancuso S. Doppler echocardiographic assessment of time to peak velocity in the aorta and pulmonary artery of small for gestational age fetuses. *Br J Obstet Gynaecol* 1990;97:603–607.

Doppler Ultrasound in Obstetrics and Gynecology,
edited by Joshua A. Copel and Kathryn L. Reed.
Raven Press, Ltd., New York © 1995.

CHAPTER **29**

The Fetal Venous System

Kathryn L. Reed

The fetal venous vasculature plays an important role during fetal life. Since the placenta is the source of oxygen and nutrition in the fetus, blood flow through the umbilical vein is key to survival. In adults, approximately 75% of the blood volume in the systemic circulation is contained in the venous system (1); in the fetus, there is proportionately less blood in the pulmonary circulation and there is the additional component of the highly vascular placenta.

Venous blood flows have been examined in some detail in animal fetuses and, more recently, in human fetuses. Blood flows from the placenta through the umbilical vein into the ductus venosus, left lobe of the liver, and portal vein. Approximately 45% of umbilical venous blood flows into the left lobe of the liver and portal veins and 55% into the ductus venosus; the percentages may change with fetal condition (2). Portal blood flows through the right lobe of the liver and then, through the hepatic veins, joins with inferior vena cava blood returning to the heart. Blood flowing through the ductus venosus also joins the blood flowing through the inferior vena cava, although the extent of actual mixture at the site of joining and in the right atrium is a subject of investigation (see Chapter 30).

Blood streams through the region of the right atrium from the inferior vena cava, the superior vena cava, and the ductus venosus. Blood in the inferior vena cava flows both into the right ventricle and into the left atrium; it appears that the portion of the blood flowing in the inferior vena cava contributed by the ductus venosus preferentially flows through the foramen ovale into the left atrium (2).

Blood that has flowed into the branch pulmonary arteries [7–8% of the combined ventricular output in the fetal sheep (2)] returns to the left atrium through the pulmonary veins.

TECHNIQUE

Umbilical venous blood flow velocities may be obtained from various sites in the umbilical cord (near the placental insertion, near the fetal insertion, or in a free-floating loop). The umbilical vein continues for some distance in the fetal abdomen, and velocities may also be obtained in this location. The umbilical vein can usually be readily identified on two-dimensional ultrasound due to its size. Simultaneous velocity measurements in the venous and arterial umbilical vessels may be useful for interpretation.

Ductus venosus velocities may be obtained from either a transverse or longitudinal (fetal) view, since the ductus venosus curves as it traverses the fetal abdomen between the umbilical vein and the inferior vena cava and right atrium. Velocities are relatively high in the ductus venosus, and color Doppler may be useful for identification of the ductus venosus, since its diameter is often small and more difficult to identify with two-dimensional ultrasound.

Blood flow velocities in the inferior vena cava have been measured at multiple sites, including immediately distal to the right atrium and below the diaphragm. Superior vena cava velocities may be obtained either from the fetal long axis, as the superior vena cava enters the right atrium, or from a more transverse plane of the fetus, adjacent to the ascending aorta. Pulmonary venous blood flow is identified by locating and sampling the veins as they enter the left atrium.

K. L. Reed: Department of Obstetrics and Gynecology, Arizona Health Sciences Center, 1501 N. Campbell Ave, Tucson, AZ 85724.

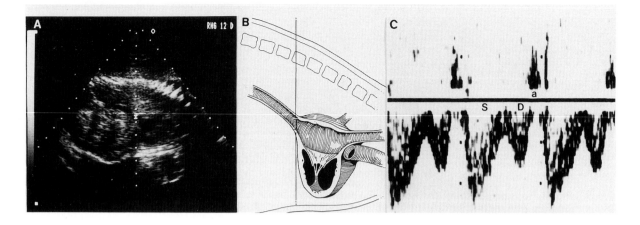

FIG. 1. Two-dimensional ultrasound (**A**), schematic (**B**), and Doppler flow velocity waveform (**C**) of the fetal inferior vena cava. Velocities are greatest during systole (S); a second peak occurs during diastole (D), and reverse flow is seen during atrial contraction (a). From Reed et al. (3).

WAVEFORM MEASUREMENT

Velocities may be analyzed quantitatively or qualitatively. If the angle between the Doppler beam and the direction of blood flow is known, mean velocity can be measured. Changes in blood flow velocity in the umbilical vein from one cardiac cycle to the next may be noted, if present. Since blood flow directions are often difficult to ascertain, percentage changes (independent of blood flow direction) in velocity are often employed. In caval blood flow analysis, peak velocities or time–velocity integrals at different times in the cardiac cycle can be measured and compared (Fig. 1) (3). Reverse flow with atrial contraction may be expressed as a percentage of forward flow during other parts of the cardiac cycle.

Ductus venosus blood flow usually consists of two velocity peaks and a prominent slowing (or less frequently reversal) of blood flow at the time of atrial contraction. Again, peak velocities or time–velocity integrals during systole and diastole may be measured and compared, and diastolic flow velocities may be used to create ratios of flow velocities for comparison of blood flow velocity changes over time or between fetuses (see Chapter 30).

Analysis of blood flow velocities in the pulmonary veins may be performed in a similar fashion, although the pulmonary venous blood flow may have three peak velocities and may not completely reverse with atrial contraction (Fig. 2).

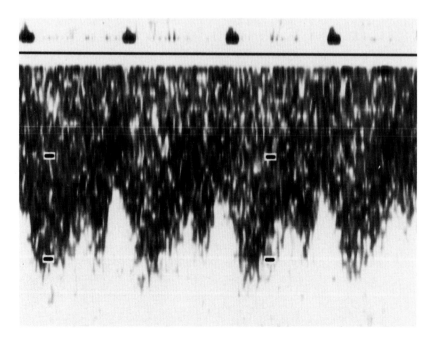

FIG. 2. Normal pulmonary venous velocities in a human fetus at 38 weeks gestation.

RESULTS

Normals

Umbilical Vein

Umbilical venous velocities are usually monophasic in the normal second- or third-trimester fetus that is not active and not breathing. Volume flows are reported to be 120 ml/kg/min; they are relatively constant until late gestation when they decrease to 90 ml/kg/min (4).

Early in gestation, umbilical venous velocities vary with the arterial velocities, i.e., the velocities "pulsate" until 13 weeks gestation (5). Persistent pulsations after this gestational age may indicate that abnormal blood flow is present (6).

Breathing

Blood flow velocities in the fetal umbilical vein vary during fetal breathing activity (7). The timing of variations in velocity has been found to correlate with the timing of variations in arterial velocity, which suggests an interconnection between umbilical venous and arterial hemodynamics (7).

Venae Cavae

Inferior and superior vena cava velocities are usually triphasic (Fig. 1). Velocities, and time–velocity integrals, are usually greatest during ventricular systole, immediately following atrial contraction (and therefore during atrial relaxation). A second blood flow velocity peak occurs during early diastole, when the atrioventricular valves open to allow blood flow from the atrium to the ventricle. At this point, the atrium and cavae are acting as a conduit of blood flow from the body and umbilical vein into the ventricle. A third period of blood flow occurs with atrial contraction, in the reverse direction into the superior and inferior vena cava. This is usually the smallest time–velocity integral of the three.

The ratio of blood flow velocity during systole and diastole is between 3.5 and 3.7, and in a serial study has been reported to be constant during gestation (8). The percentage of the time–velocity integral of reverse flow during atrial contraction relative to the time–velocity integral during "forward flow" (systole and early diastole combined) is usually less than 10% in the normal fetus (3,8,9). Reverse flow is most readily detectable near the right atrium.

Ductus Venosus

Ductus venosus blood flow velocities are the highest venous velocities in the fetus, ranging from 65 to 75 cm/sec (10–12). Flow velocities are highest during ventricular systole and lower during ventricular diastole. Blood flow is usually continuously forward, even during atrial contraction, when the lowest velocities occur (30–40 cm/sec) (11). Ductus venosus blood flow is discussed in more detail in Chapter 30.

Pulmonary Veins

Pulmonary venous flow has been examined in fetuses with cardiac anomalies such as hypoplastic left heart, truncus arteriosus, pulmonary atresia, and anomalous pulmonary venous return. Abnormal pulmonary venous flow patterns were found to be helpful in further defining the cardiac physiology in these fetuses (13). Pulmonary venous flow is further described in Chapter 31.

Abnormals

Changes in umbilical venous flow, ductus venosus, caval, and pulmonary venous blood flow velocities have been identified in human fetuses with abnormalities of growth, cardiac anatomy, or cardiac function.

Abnormal Umbilical Artery Flow/IUGR

Early studies of umbilical venous blood flow consisted of volume flow measurements. Fetuses with intrauterine growth retardation (IUGR) had decreases in the volume of blood flowing through the umbilical vein (4).

More recently, persistent rhythmic decreases in venous velocities have been identified. These decreases in venous velocity occur in end diastole in fetuses with regular heart rates and have been termed *venous pulsations.* Venous pulsations are seen in some fetuses with abnormal umbilical arterial velocities (specifically absence of end-diastolic velocities) and are associated with increases in reverse flow velocities in the inferior vena cava with atrial contraction (Fig. 3) (6). In fetuses followed serially for IUGR, the development of venous pulsations was associated with development of an abnormal fetal heart rate pattern (14). Fetuses with umbilical venous pulsations have a higher morbidity and mortality, even in the setting of normal umbilical arterial blood flow (6).

The most significant Doppler flow velocity abnormality in fetuses followed for IUGR was the development of increased reversal of blood flow velocity in the inferior vena cava with atrial contraction (15). Similar changes in the inferior vena cava blood flow were reported in hypoxic sheep fetuses (16). The mechanism of this increase is not known at present but is currently attributed to abnormal ventricular filling characteristics, abnormal ventricular chamber or wall compliance, or abnormal end-diastolic pressures (3).

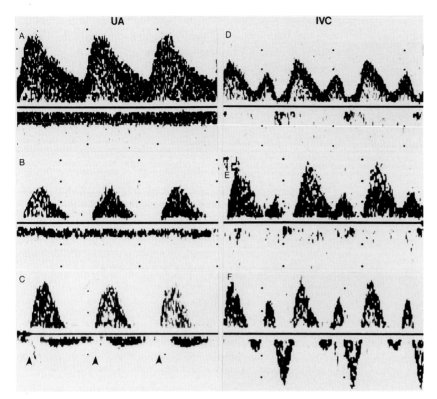

FIG. 3. Umbilical arterial, venous, and inferior vena cava velocities in a normal 38-week fetus and in two fetuses (one a 28-week fetus, one a 34-week fetus) with absent end-diastolic velocities in the umbilical artery. **A:** Umbilical arterial and venous velocity in the normal fetus. **B:** Umbilical arterial and venous velocity in the fetus with absent end-diastolic velocity in the umbilical artery and no venous pulsations. **C:** Umbilical arterial and venous velocity in the fetus with absent end-diastolic velocities in the umbilical artery and (marked) umbilical venous pulsations. **D:** Inferior vena cava waveform from the fetus in A. **E:** Inferior vena cava waveform from the fetus in B. **F:** Inferior vena cava waveform from the fetus in C. Note the increase in reverse flow in E, the fetus with umbilical venous pulsations. Dots are 0.5 s apart. From Indik et al. (6).

Hydrops

Similar associations between reverse flow in the inferior vena cava, umbilical venous pulsations, and increases in fetal morbidity have been reported in fetuses with hydrops. In a study by Gudmundsson, fetuses with hydrops could be separated into two groups: those with umbilical venous pulsations and those without (9). The group with umbilical venous pulsations was felt to have functional cardiac abnormalities (heart failure), while the group without umbilical venous pulsations had a different etiology for hydrops, such as a viral infection. Increases in reverse flow in the inferior vena cava during atrial contraction were also noted in those fetuses with umbilical venous pulsations that had examinations of the inferior vena cava waveform performed.

Ductus venosus flows in fetuses with "failure" were also abnormal, having increased reversals of flow velocities during atrial contraction (10,11,17).

Arrhythmias

Fetuses with arrhythmias also have abnormal caval, ductus venosus, and umbilical venous blood flows. It was noted that as heart rates decreased below 120 bpm or increased above 160 bpm, the reverse flow velocity with atrial contraction increased as a percentage of forward flow (Fig. 4). Fetuses with sustained tachycardias or sinus

bradycardias have increases in reverse flow in the inferior vena cava with atrial contraction and umbilical venous pulsations (6). Abnormalities of ductus venosus flows have been reported in fetuses with supraventricular tachycardias (10,11,17).

Fetuses with complete heart block have increased reversal of inferior vena cava blood flow velocities (and umbilical venous pulsations) during "cannon a waves" produced when the atrium contracts against atrioventricular valves that are closed during ventricular systole (Fig. 5).

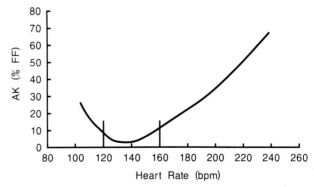

FIG. 4. Reverse flow in the inferior vena cava during atrial contraction (AK) as a percentage of forward flow (FF) at different heart rates. Reverse flow is lowest between heart rates of 120 and 160 bpm. From Reed et al. (3).

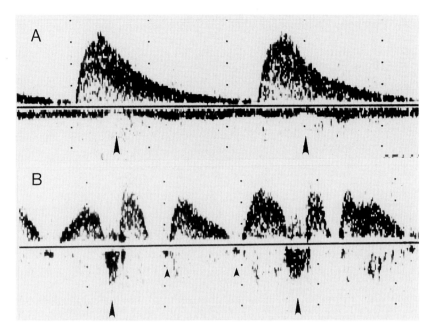

FIG. 5. Umbilical venous and arterial waveforms (**A**) and inferior vena cava waveforms (**B**) in a fetus with complete heart block. The umbilical venous velocity decreases coincide with atrial contractions that occur against closed atrioventricular valves during ventricular systole. From Indik et al. (6).

SUMMARY

A correlation between reverse flow in the inferior vena cava and the development of intermittent decreases in umbilical venous blood flow has been suggested by the results of several studies. The presence of umbilical venous pulsations in fetuses with abnormal umbilical arterial flow velocities was associated with an increase in fetal morbidity and mortality. Umbilical venous pulsations were also seen in fetuses with supraventricular tachycardia, bradycardia, and premature atrial or ventricular contractions; these fetuses also had increases in reverse flow in the inferior vena cava with atrial contraction.

Blood flow through the venous system in the human fetus can be examined with Doppler ultrasound, and information derived from these studies provides insights into fetal cardiovascular physiology. Abnormal blood flow through the fetal heart, from abnormal filling or abnormal pressures, may result in increases in reverse blood flow through the inferior (or superior) vena cava with atrial contraction. It appears that this abnormal reverse flow is associated with the development of pulsations in umbilical venous velocities that can be readily identified with a relatively simple Doppler ultrasound examination.

REFERENCES

1. Guyton AC. Overview of the circulation, and medical physics of pressure, flow and resistance. In: Guyton AC, ed. *Textbook of medical physiology.* 8th Ed. Philadelphia: WB Saunders; 1991:150–158.
2. Rudolph AM. Distribution and regulation of blood flow in the fetal and neonatal lamb. *Circ Res* 1985;57:811–821.
3. Reed KL, Appleton CP, Anderson CF, Shenker L, Sahn DJ. Doppler studies of vena cava flows in human fetuses. *Circulation* 1990;81:498–505.
4. Gill RW, Warren PS. Doppler measurement of umbilical blood flow. In: Sanders RC, James AE, eds. *The principles and practice of ultrasonography in obstetrics and gynecology.* 3rd Ed. Norwalk, CT: Appleton-Century-Crofts; 1985:87–97.
5. Rizzo G, Arduini D, Romanini C. Umbilical vein pulsations: A physiologic finding in early gestation. *Am J Obstet Gynecol* 1992;167:675–677.
6. Indik JH, Chen V, Reed KL. Association of umbilical venous with inferior vena cava velocities. *Obstet Gynecol* 1991;77:551–557.
7. Indik JH, Reed KL. Variation and correlation in human fetal umbilical Doppler velocities with fetal breathing: Evidence of the fetal-cardiac connection. *Am J Obstet Gynecol* 1990;163:1792–1796.
8. Huisman TWA, Stewart PA, Wladimiroff JW. Flow velocity waveforms in the fetal inferior vena cava during the second half of normal pregnancy. *Ultrasound Med Biol* 1991;17:679–682.
9. Gudmundsson S, Huhta JC, Wood DC, Tulzer G, Cohen AW, Weiner S. Venous Doppler ultrasonography in the fetus with non-immune hydrops. *Am J Obstet Gynecol* 1991;164:33–37.
10. Kiserud T, Eik-Nes SH, Blaas HK, Hellevik LR. Ultrasonographic velocimetry of the fetal ductus venosus. *Lancet* 1991;338:1412–1414.
11. Kiserud T, Eik-Nes SH, Hellevik LR, Blaas HG. Ductus venosus: A longitudinal Doppler velocimetric study of the human fetus. *J Mat-Fet Invest* 1992;2:5–11.
12. Huisman TWA, Stewart PA, Wladimiroff JW. Ductus venosus blood flow velocity waveforms in the human fetus: A Doppler study. *Ultrasound Med Biol* 1992;18:33–37.
13. Cartier MS, Emerson DS, Felker RE, et al. Color flow Doppler for evaluation of abnormal fetal pulmonary blood flow. *J Ultrasound Med* 1993;12:S54.
14. Arduini D, Rizzo G, Romanini C. The development of abnormal heart rate patterns after absent end-diastolic velocity in the umbilical artery: Analysis of risk factors. *Am J Obstet Gynecol* 1993;168:43–50.
15. Rizzo G, Arduini D, Romanini C. Inferior vena cava flow velocity waveforms in appropriate- and small-for-gestational age fetuses. *Am J Obstet Gynecol* 1992;166:1271–1280.
16. Reuss ML, Rudolph AM, Dae MW. Phasic blood flow patterns in the superior and inferior venae cavae and umbilical vein of fetal sheep. *Am J Obstet Gynecol* 1983;145:70–78.
17. Kiserud T, Eik-Nes SH, Hellevik LR, Blaas H-G. Ductus venosus blood velocity changes in fetal cardiac diseases. *J Mat-Fet Invest* 1993;3:15–20.

Doppler Ultrasound in Obstetrics and Gynecology,
edited by Joshua A. Copel and Kathryn L. Reed.
Raven Press, Ltd., New York © 1995.

CHAPTER 30

The Fetal Ductus Venosus

Torvid Kiserud and Sturla H. Eik-Nes

The ductus venosus (venous duct, ductus Arantii) is one of the three specific shunts in fetal circulation. Together with the foramen ovale and the ductus arteriosus, the ductus venosus constitutes the main circulatory adaptation for intrauterine life. Although the ductus venosus has long been recognized to be of significance for fetal circulation (1–3), it is only during the last few years that this vessel has been brought into diagnostic application (4,5).

DEVELOPMENT AND ANATOMY

During the early embryonic period, the venous inlet below the liver is a paired arrangement (6–8). At week 7 it has developed into one main axis formed by the left umbilical vein, which leads into the umbilical sinus and communicates with the portal system to the right. At this stage, the ductus venosus forms a rather broad continuation of the umbilical vein into the inferior vena cava.

Toward the end of the embryonic period the ductus venosus develops a trumpet-like shape with the smallest diameter at its entrance. For the rest of the pregnancy the ductus venosus retains this shape and remains a narrow isthmian structure, hardly exceeding a diameter of 2 mm, in contrast to the surrounding vessels, which continue their rapid growth (4,6).

During the second and third trimester the branchless ductus venosus connects the intraabdominal umbilical vein (portal sinus, umbilical sinus) directly to the inferior vena cava (Fig. 1). The ductus venosus leaves the umbilical sinus where the sinus starts turning right to join the portal vein. The ductus venosus itself points posterior and upward, slightly toward the left side to join the inferior vena cava in a steep course (9–11). It enters the left

side of the inferior vena cava together with the left and median hepatic vein just below the heart. An unusual and rare course of the ductus venosus has been described as a connection to a lower level of the abdominal inferior vena cava (12).

The narrow portion of the ductus venosus has been described, often disputedly, as a sphincter (2,3,6,13–16). Neural elements and muscular fibers have been reported to be identified in the area (17). Adrenergic response has been discussed, and it is assumed that a prostaglandin-mediated relaxation maintains the patency (18–27). Much in the same way as with the ductus arteriosus, a cytochrome P450 system seems to mediate the closure of the ductus venosus during postnatal life. Blood flow has, however, been traced in the ductus venosus until 2–3 weeks after birth in healthy babies (28).

PHYSIOLOGY

Despite its modest size, the ductus venosus early attracted the interest of physiologists (29–33). Under normal conditions a considerable proportion of the oxygenated blood flowing through the umbilical vein is delivered through the ductus venosus directly to the inferior vena cava to form the preferential bloodstream across the foramen ovale (34–36). Such an arrangement ensures that the coronary and cerebral arteries are given highest priority regarding oxygen supply. This concept is experimentally well founded and has recently been confirmed by ultrasound studies in the human fetus (37,38). The ductus venosus delivers a high-velocity jet crossing the left side of the inferior vena cava directly to enter the foramen ovale (Fig. 1) (4,11). By ultrasound it can be shown that the jet follows a well-defined pathway into the left atrium (11), thus avoiding an extensive mixture with the deoxygenated blood in the inferior vena cava and right atrium.

The ductus venosus–foramen ovale pathway addition-

T. Kiserud and S. H. Eik-Nes: Department of Obstetrics and Gynecology, National Center for Fetal Medicine, Trondheim University Center, Trondheim, Norway.

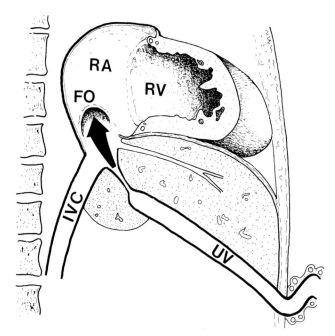

FIG. 1. Sagittal section of the lower central venous inlet in the fetus. The umbilical vein (UV) continues into the narrow, trumpet-shaped ductus venosus. The ductus venosus projects a high-velocity stream (*arrow*) towards the foramen ovale (FO) and the left atrium. The inferior vena cava (IVC) points slightly forward to direct its blood into the right atrium (RA) and right ventricle (RV) in a plane immediately anterior and to the right of the ductus venosus blood stream. From Kiserud et al. (4).

ally receives blood from the left and medial hepatic vein (11,32). A probably modest oxygen extraction in the left half of the liver makes these hepatic veins an important additional source of oxygenated blood for the preferential bloodstream through the foramen ovale.

In fetal sheep 50% of the umbilical blood is shunted through the ductus venosus (32,34). During induced hypoxia or hypovolemia the proportion shunted directly through the ductus venosus mounts to 70% of the umbilical blood flow, indicating that this small vessel plays a key role in the central venous blood distribution (39–43).

Occlusion of the ductus venosus increases umbilical vein pressure and the hepatic blood flow in the fetal sheep, but seems otherwise not to cause any major change in regional blood distribution (44). An absent or abnormal ductus venosus has been described in the live neonate (12). Such information indicates that the fetus has several mechanisms for regulating oxygen supply.

The ductus venosus is not an isolated regulator of oxygenated blood flow. Rather it should be appreciated as part of a larger unit: the umbilical vein with its sinus, and the ductus venosus joined closely together with the liver and its portal system (29–36,45). This unit regulates the total oxygenated venous return from the placenta. Thus the blood flow in the ductus venosus depends on the pressure in the umbilical sinus, the resistance in the duc-

tus venosus, the resistance in the liver parenchyma, and the pressure in the inferior vena cava. An increased resistance of the liver parenchyma may increase direct shunting through the ductus venosus. The increased liver resistance causes a raised pressure in the umbilical sinus and a higher pressure gradient across the ductus venosus. Correspondingly, a larger blood volume is directed to the foramen ovale at a high velocity.

On the other hand, a contraction of a ductus venosus sphincter would increase the resistance as well. The effect would be a reduced blood volume through the ductus venosus and a corresponding increased blood flow in the direction of the liver parenchyma.

Both the circulation through the liver and through the ductus venosus seem to respond to vasoactive transmitters and local hormones (19,20,26). The dynamics and regulatory ability of the whole unit should be kept in mind when ductus venosus velocimetry is employed to evaluate clinical problems.

ULTRASOUND IMAGING

Two-Dimensional Ultrasound Imaging

In conventional two-dimensional ultrasound imaging, the ductus venosus can regularly be visualized in a sagittal section as a continuation of the umbilical vein toward the proximal portion of the inferior vena cava (Fig. 2) (4,9–11,37). The course is rather steeply posterior toward the left portion of the inferior vena cava, which widens considerably at the level of the ductus venosus outlet.

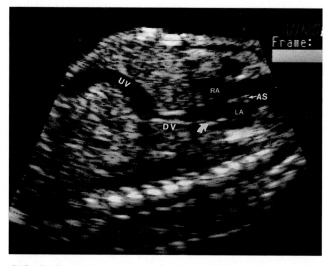

FIG. 2. Sagittal sonogram of a fetus of 18 weeks exposing the umbilical vein (UV) connected to the ductus venosus (DV), which is directed to the left side of the atrial septum (AS). At this stage the trumpet shape of the ductus seems well established. Note that the abdominal inferior vena cava situated slightly to the right of the present section is not exposed. LA, left atrium; RA, right atrium. Foramen ovale flap (*arrow*).

The ductus venosus inclination increases by 7° to fuse with the inferior vena cava at an angle of 48° (11). This makes it appear slightly bowed (Fig. 3). The narrow isthmic entrance of the ductus venosus hardly exceeds a diameter of 2 mm at any time during the pregnancy (4). The next portion widens smoothly, much like a trumpet (Fig. 3). This profile is found from week 17 onward (Fig. 2), but is probably present in the early second trimester as well.

The entrance of the ductus venosus into the inferior vena cava is closely related to the entrance of the left and medial hepatic veins. Together with the ductus venosus these two hepatic veins have a more or less common inlet into the inferior vena cava. At the corresponding level, the inferior vena cava widens to include a left-sided recess that guides the oxygenated blood flow toward the foramen ovale (11). When identifying the ductus venosus with two-dimensional ultrasound one should consider the proximity to the hepatic veins as a possible source of errors. Visualization of the narrow ductus venosus as a communication between two wider lumina (the umbilical vein and the inferior vena cava) in the very same image, however, is dependable (Fig. 3).

Although the anterior or posterior sagittal insonation gives the best visualization of the ductus venosus, an oblique transection of the upper fetal abdomen is also good (37,38).

Color Doppler Imaging

The small dimensions of the ductus venosus sometimes make it difficult to identify, especially in cases of maternal obesity, polyhydramnios, or in multiple preg-

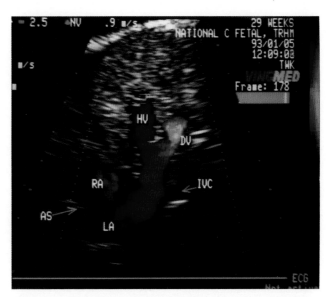

FIG. 4. Color Doppler image in a sagittal section of a normal fetus of 29 weeks showing the preferential stream from the ductus venosus (DV) and left hepatic vein (HV). Note the increased intensity of signals signifying the isthmic portion of the ductus venosus and the flow direction. AS, atrial septum; IVC, inferior vena cava; LA, left atrium; RA, right atrium.

nancy. The identification is greatly enhanced by color Doppler (4,11). The high velocity in the ductus venosus is normally easily traced and signifies the location of the vessel as well as the flow direction (Fig. 4). Since the ductus venosus produces the highest venous velocities in the area, this is a reliable method. In complicated pregnancies, however, when the velocity patterns are altered, both two-dimensional imaging and color Doppler should be applied to ensure the differentiation between the ductus venosus and the neighboring hepatic veins.

PULSED DOPPLER VELOCIMETRY TECHNIQUE

Insonation Technique

Once the ductus venosus is identified by two-dimensional imaging and color Doppler, the blood velocity can be measured by the Doppler technique. Insonation from below in the sagittal section is preferred. In this section, the umbilical vein is visualized and a good color Doppler image of the ductus venosus is obtained at a small angle of insonation. Whenever applicable, a transthoracic insonation in a paravertebral plane from the back often gives the best Doppler signals (Fig. 5). The oblique transection of the abdomen is sometimes the only accessible plane of examination. This insonation is, however, less suitable for estimating the angle of interrogation since the ductus venosus has its steepest course in the sagittal plane.

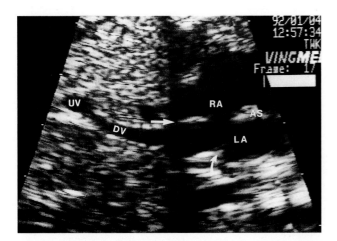

FIG. 3. Oblique sagittal sonogram of a fetus of 30 weeks showing the ductus venosus (DV) as a slightly bowed communication between the umbilical vein (UV) and the inferior vena cava. The inlet of the ductus venosus remains narrow and the outlet points to the left of the atrial septum (AS) and the Eustachian valve (straight arrow). LA, left atrium; RA, right atrium. Insertion of the foramen ovale flap (bowed arrow).

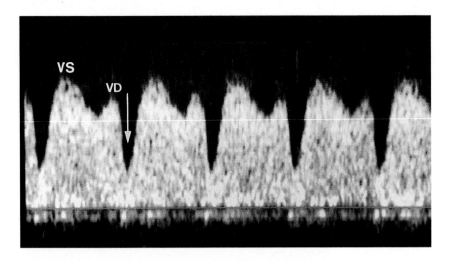

FIG. 5. Normal pulsed Doppler velocimetry of the ductus venosis in a fetus of 18 weeks. The velocity is high and has a typical profile reflecting the heart cycle: a peak during ventricular systole (VS), a peak during the passive filling during ventricular diastole (VD), and a minimum during the atrial contraction (*arrow*).

In early pregnancy (before week 12) the transvaginal examination seems superior to the abdominal and gives a high rate of successful velocity recordings (46).

Standard Conditions

To avoid interference from neighboring vessels, the pulsed Doppler technique is preferred. The sample volume should cover the inlet of the ductus venosus.

The examination is done during fetal quiescence since fetal movements, and especially respiratory activity, have a substantial impact on the velocities. The time span of the examination should be sufficient to record the Doppler shift for at least four heart cycles. The examination should be repeated to ensure reproducibility.

The velocities recorded at the smallest angle of insonation are selected for analysis. If good visualization of the flow direction by color Doppler is achieved, then the signals collected at a large angle of interrogation (>30°) will still give acceptable results (38).

To ensure the recording of the maximum velocity in the vessel, a liberal sample volume should be applied. However, this applies to only the last half of pregnancy when the ductus venosus gives a distinct Doppler signal at high velocity levels. In early pregnancy the small di-

mensions of the vasculature and the low-velocity pattern increase the risk of interference and misinterpretation (Fig. 6). Accordingly, during early pregnancy the sample volume should be kept as small as possible.

Sample Site

To achieve uniformity of the technique and good reproducibility, a standardized site of recording is recommended at the inlet portion of the ductus venosus. A comparison between the inlet portion to the midportion and the proximal outlet portion showed that the best agreement was achieved between the inlet and the midportion (Table 1) (38). The midportion of the ductus venosus is an acceptable alternative as a sampling site whereas the outlet portion is poorer, with lower peak velocity and wider confidence limits.

Pitfalls and Limitations

Care should be taken to establish a sound routine of identifying the ductus venosus. The ductus venosus is situated in an area densely covered with vessels and the

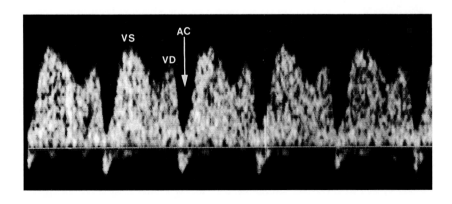

FIG. 6. Pulsed Doppler velocimetry of the ductus venosus in a normal fetus of 13 weeks. The velocities are generally at a lower level than later in pregnancy, but the characteristic profile is still maintained. Note the low velocity during atrial contraction (AC) with even negative components. Passive filling during ventricular diastole (VD). VS, ventricular systole.

TABLE 1. *Velocimetric reproducibility according to site of recording*

Site of sampling[a]	Inlet	Midportion	Outlet
V_{peak} (cm/sec)	76	76	68
SD	14	13	13
Mean difference to inlet		0.1	6.3
SD		10	15
Correlation coeff.		0.7	0.4
Coeff. of variation (%)		13	21
Limits of agreement		(−20; 20)	(−24; 36)
True limits of agreement		(−21; 26)	(−21; 50)

From Kiserud et al. (38).

[a] In 33 sets of observations of the ductus venosus peak velocity (V_{peak}), the recording site at the midportion and the outlet were compared to the standard inlet site by calculating the mean, the SD, the mean difference to the inlet, the SD of the difference, the correlation coefficient, the coefficient of variation, and the limits of agreement.

danger of examining the wrong vein is real. Notably, the inferior vena cava and the left and medial hepatic veins are close to the ductus venosus and have much the same direction (Fig. 4). A normal blood velocity profile in a hepatic vein represents a grossly abnormal finding if it is attributed to the ductus venosus. Such a possibility emphasizes the need for an accurate identification of the ductus venosus. It is prudent to visualize the outlet of the left and medial hepatic veins in the same section as intended for the ductus venosus velocimetry in order to avoid including those veins in the sample volume (Figs. 2–4).

In addition to the risk of examining the wrong vessel, there is a risk of including neighboring vessels in the sample volume. Such interference from neighboring vessels may mask an abnormal velocity profile. This is particularly so in cases of reduced or reversed velocity during atrial contraction. Superimposed signals from the hepatic veins may mimic a reversed blood flow during atrial contraction. And the positive velocity in the umbilical vein may cover a low velocity of the ductus venosus.

In early pregnancy (before week 17) low velocities are normally seen in the ductus venosus, especially during atrial contraction (Fig. 6). Thus, the criteria used in late pregnancy cannot be applied in early second trimester.

Fetal movements, especially respiratory movements (Fig. 7), may cause profound changes in the velocity (38). Adhering to standard conditions when doing the recordings will eliminate this problem.

The diameter of the ductus venosus at the narrow inlet is 1–2 mm. Any variation of the diameter due to a sphincter function will escape assessment due to the limitations in the ultrasound equipment (47). So, by the above-mentioned methods there seems to be no possibility of calculating volume flow or of including a variation of the diameter to evaluate the function of the ductus venosus.

DUCTUS VENOSUS VELOCITY CHARACTERIZATION

Velocity Profile

To avoid the problem of interference of low-velocity signals from other vessels, a standardized reporting system based on the maximum velocity envelope seems to be the best solution. Usually the ductus venosus blood flow is distinguished by a high velocity and a typical velocity profile reflecting the cardiac cycle (Figs. 5 and 6) (37,38). The highest velocity (peak velocity) is recorded during the ventricular systole. A second peak is regularly (86%) seen during the passive filling of the ventricles (38). During the active filling of the ventricles (atrial contraction) the minimum velocity is recorded. In contrast to the velocity in the inferior vena cava and the hepatic veins, this minimum velocity has a positive direction in normal fetuses (37,38,46).

For clinical use a simple documentation consists of the calculated peak velocity, the minimum velocity, and the time-averaged maximum velocity during the heart cycle.

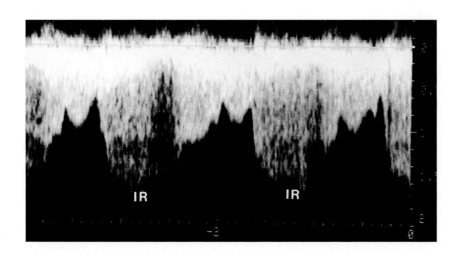

FIG. 7. Pulsed Doppler velocimetry of the ductus venosus in a normal fetus of 35 weeks. Respiratory movements may profoundly alter the velocity. In the present case a peak velocity of 175 cm/sec is recorded during inspiration (IR).

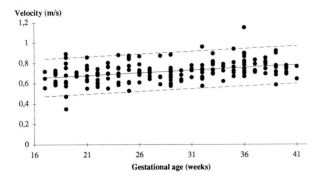

FIG. 8. Ductus venosus peak velocity recorded during the ventricular systole in a longitudinal study of 29 normal pregnancies with 184 observations (*filled circles*). Regression line (——) and 95% CI (- - - -). From Kiserud et al. (38).

The time-averaged maximum velocity seems particularly suitable since it is applicable even in the few cases (3%) that do not have a well-defined peak during the ventricular systole or a minimum during the atrial contraction (38).

The magnitude of the variations during the heart cycle has led to a suggested ratio (S/D) between the peak velocity recorded during the ventricular systole (S) and the peak velocity during the passive filling of the ventricle (D) (37). Such a ratio could reflect hemodynamic properties of the heart and hopefully be of diagnostic value.

Normal Ranges and Reproducibility

Figures 8–10 illustrate normal values of the ductus venosus velocimetry (38). As can be appreciated, the velocities are high and comparable to velocities otherwise seen in arteries. The biological variations, however, are wide as signified by the wide 95% CI. Using the present-

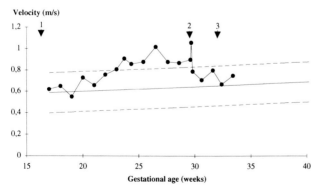

FIG. 9. Ductus venosus time-averaged maximum velocity recorded during the ventricular systole. An example of a longitudinal surveillance of a fetus with anemia due to a hemoglobinopathy (*filled circles*) unsuccessfully treated with a stem cell infusion (1) but improving after regular transfusions (2–3). Regression line (——) and 95% CI (- - - -) for a normal population.

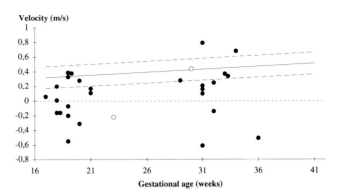

FIG. 10. Ductus venosus minimum velocity recorded during the atrial contraction in 28 fetuses with congenital heart defects (*filled circles*) and two cases of supraventricular tachycardia (*empty circles*). Note the large number of low velocities and in many cases even negative velocities. Regression line (——) and 95% CI (- - - -) for a normal population. From Kiserud et al. (5).

ly described technique of examination, the limits of agreement for the intraobserver variation will roughly be [−13; 13] (Table 2) (38). The *true* limits of agreement include the 95% CI for these limits and indicate the reproducibility of the study. These ranges are applicable after week 17. Before week 17, however, the velocities are lower and separate ranges should be established to evaluate the early fetal hemodynamics (46).

CLINICAL APPLICATION

The ductus venosus is heavily involved in the distribution of oxygenated blood and has accordingly attracted an increasing clinical interest. The nature of this vessel as a direct link between the peripheral umbilical and the central venous system furnishes the opportunity to study an important pressure gradient in the fetus. This pressure gradient across the ductus venosus is reflected in the high velocities that are well suited for Doppler examination. Altered pressures could be associated with a variety of diseases.

TABLE 2. *Intraobserver variation for ductus venosus velocimetry*

Reproducibility[a]	V_{peak}	V_{min}
Correlation coeff.	0.9	0.9
Coeff. of variation (%)	8.7	15.0
Mean of differences (cm/sec)	−0.7	−1.7
SD	6.5	6.9
Limits of agreement	(−13; 12)	(−15; 12)
True limits of agreements	(−16; 14)	(−18; 14)

From Kiserud et al. (38).
[a] Variation for the peak velocity (V_{peak}) during ventricular systole and the minimum velocity (V_{min}) during atrial contraction in 27 pairs of observations.

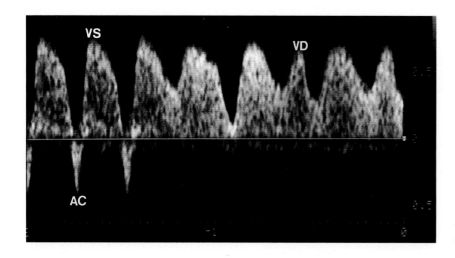

FIG. 11. Pulsed Doppler velocimetry of the ductus venosus in a fetus of 26 weeks with a supraventricular tachycardia. The conversion from tachycardia to sinus rhythm improves the velocity as the reversed flow during atrial contraction (AC) disappears and the peak during ventricular diastole (VD) reappears. VS, ventricular systole.

Raised central venous pressure is expected to occur in congestive heart disease either due to an increased afterload, congenital heart defect, arrhythmia, myocardial disease, or hypoxia. A generally reduced ductus venosus velocity is reported in congestive heart disease (4). Atrioventricular regurgitation influences the atrial pressure and may be the direct cause of the reduced ductus venosus velocity (4,5).

Tachyarrhythmia often alters hemodynamics. In the ductus venosus, a supraventricular tachycardia may cause a reversed ductus venosus blood flow during the atrial contraction (4,5). Once a conversion to sinus rhythm occurs, the hemodynamic improvement can clearly be recorded in the ductus venosus (Fig. 11). In such a case, the conversion increases the time-averaged maximum velocity in the orthogonal direction and may accordingly improve the preferential blood flow through the foramen ovale.

Structural cardiac malformations are associated with altered hemodynamics in the fetus. This is clearly reflected in the ductus venosus velocimetry (5). In 28 cases of antenatally detected congenital heart defects, the ma-

jority managed to maintain an adequate peak velocity. During atrial contraction, however, more than half of the fetuses demonstrated a reduced ductus venosus velocity (Fig. 10). In the cases of malformations involving the atrioventricular valves and great arteries, four out of five had a reduced velocity during atrial contraction, and half of the cases even had a reversed flow (Fig. 12).

Other causes of raised central venous pressure may equally well influence the ductus venosus blood velocity as, for instance, arteriovenous malformations.

Reduced umbilical vein pressure will necessarily lead to a reduced ductus venosus velocity. Such a situation is expected to occur in placental compromise, but may occur during fetal hemorrhage or obstruction of the umbilical vein as well. We know from the fetal lamb studies that during such stress the ductus venosus receives an increasing proportion of the umbilical blood at the expense of the liver circulation (39–43). By increasing the vascular resistance in the liver it seems possible to improve umbilical pressure and maintain a high blood flow through the ductus venosus. Probably the human fetus tries to maintain central oxygenation in the same

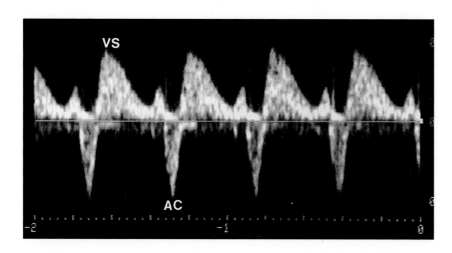

FIG. 12. Pulsed Doppler velocimetry of the ductus venosus in a fetus of 17 weeks with Ebstein's anomaly of the heart. Note the reversed blood flow velocity during the atrial contraction (AC). VS, ventricular systole.

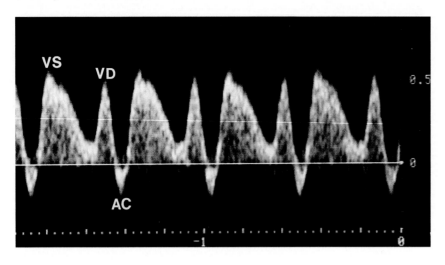

FIG. 13. Pulsed Doppler velocimetry of the ductus venosus in a stuck twin pregnancy of 19 weeks showing reversed flow during atrial contraction (AC) in the hydropic twin. The fetus has a holosystolic mitral regurgitation and polyhydramnion. Passive filling during ventricular diastole (VD). VS, ventricular systole.

way during stress. This is one of the most interesting examples of studies on the ductus venosus opening possibilities of additional diagnostic signs of fetal decompensation.

Raised umbilical vein pressure in fetal lambs has been caused by experimentally induced hypoxia (39–43). A similar mechanism probably operates in the human fetus during hypoxia due to anemia, hemoglobinopathies, or general infections. In such cases a relative hypoxia due either to a reduced capacity to transport oxygen or to an increased oxygen demand in the tissues induces a hyperkinetic circulation. For the ductus venosus this implies a raised umbilical pressure and an increased velocity (Fig. 9).

The liver is a major organ in fetal development. It is connected to the umbilical vein and the ductus venosus by the portal system, and to the inferior vena cava by the hepatic veins. Increased resistance in the liver would reduce flow to the liver and subsequently require increased portal pressure to maintain the perfusion. Portal hypertension is known to cause ascites. In the fetus, portal hypertension means raised umbilical venous pressure, which leads to an increased velocity in the ductus venosus. Thus, ductus venosus velocimetry has diagnostic possibilities in fetal hepatomegaly and in the inflammatory diseases of the liver causing increased portal pressure to the fully developed ascites.

In the twin–twin transfusion syndrome and the stuck twin syndrome, pressure differences in the umbilical circulation may play an important role. Ductus venosus Doppler velocimetry may detect differences in pressures and indicate other underlying causes (Fig. 13).

Repeated examinations for surveillance of a risk pregnancy is another possible way of applying ductus venosus velocimetry (Fig. 9). This method seems to reduce some of the problems of a wide biological variation.

Combining ductus venosus velocimetry with umbilical vein measurements will give a more complete understanding of the umbilical venous distribution. Adding

umbilical venous pressure whenever cordocentesis is done may augment the value of ductus venosus velocimetry, paving the way for an estimation of the central venous pressure in the fetus.

CONCLUSION

The ductus venosus seems to play a central role in the distribution of oxygenated blood during a major period of intrauterine life. This narrow vessel acts by directing a high-velocity jet into the foramen ovale. The high velocity makes it ideal for Doppler evaluation. The position between the umbilical vein and the inferior vena cava makes the ductus venosus an indicator of normal and altered gradient between the peripheral pressure in the umbilical vein and the central venous pressure. Accordingly, in a variety of conditions ductus venosus blood velocity may reflect the hemodynamic alteration, such as in hydrops, anemia, placental complications, liver diseases, twin–twin transfusion syndrome, and cardiac diseases. When natural variation and technical limitations are considered in the evaluation, the method gives an exciting possibility to monitor an essential hemodynamic parameter in the fetus.

ACKNOWLEDGMENT

The text was revised by Nancy Lea Eik-Nes.

REFERENCES

1. Dawes GS. Physiological changes in the circulation after birth. In: Fishman AP, Richards DW, eds. *Circulation of the blood. Men and ideas.* Bethesda: American Physiological Society; 1982:743–816.
2. Barcroft J. *Researches on prenatal life.* Oxford: Blackwell Scientific; 1946.
3. Barclay AE, Franklin KJ, Prichard MM. *The foetal circulation.* Oxford: Blackwell Scientific; 1944.
4. Kiserud T, Eik-Nes SH, Blaas H-G, Hellevik LR. Ultrasonographic velocimetry of the fetal ductus venosus. *Lancet* 1991;338: 1412–1414.

5. Kiserud T, Eik-Nes SH, Hellevik LR, Blaas H-G. Ductus venosus blood velocity changes in fetal cardiac diseases. *J Mat-Fet Invest* 1993;3:15–20.
6. Chacko AW, Reynolds SR. Embryonic development of the sphincter of the ductus venosus. *Anat Rec* 1953;115:151–73.
7. Dickson AD. The development of the ductus venosus in man and the goat. *J Anat* 1957;91:358–368.
8. Lassau JP, Bastian D. Organogenesis of the venous structures of the human liver: A hemodynamic theory. *Anat Clin* 1983;5:97–102.
9. Chinn DH, Filly RA, Callen PW. Ultrasonic evaluation of fetal umbilical and hepatic vascular anatomy. *Radiology* 1982;144:153–157.
10. Champetier J, Yver R, Tomasella T. Functional anatomy of the liver of the human fetus: Applications to ultrasound. *Surg Radiol Anat* 1989;11:53–62.
11. Kiserud T, Eik-Nes SH, Blaas H-G, Hellevik LR. Foramen ovale: A sonographic study of its relation to the inferior vena cava, ductus venosus and hepatic veins. *Ultrasound Obstet Gynecol* 1992;2:356–389.
12. Leonidas JC, Fellows RA. Congenital absence of the ductus venosus: With direct connection between the umbilical vein and the distal inferior vena cava. *AJR* 1976;126:892–895.
13. Barron DH. The changes in the foetal circulation at birth. *Physiol Rev* 1944;24:277–295.
14. Barclay AE, Franklin KJ, Prichard MM. The mechanism of closure of the ductus venosus. *Br J Radiol* 1942;15:66–71.
15. Meyer WW, Lind J. The ductus venosus and the mechanism of its closure. *Arch Dis Child* 1966;41:597–605.
16. Salzer P. Beitrag zur kenntnis des ductus venosus. *Z Anat Entwickl-Gesch* 1970;130:80–90.
17. Pearson AA, Sauter RW. The innervation of the umbilical vein in human embryos and fetuses. *Am J Anat* 1969;125:345–352.
18. Ehinger B, Gennser G, Owman C, Persson H, Sjöberg N-O. Histochemical and pharmacological studies on amine mechanisms in the umbilical cord, umbilical vein and ductus venosus of the human fetus. *Acta Physiol Scand* 1968;72:15–24.
19. Zink J, van Petten RG. The effect of norepinephrine on blood flow through the fetal liver and ductus venosus. *Am J Obstet Gynecol* 1980;137:71–77.
20. Edelstone DI, Merick RE, Caritis SN, Mueller-Heubach E. Umbilical venous blood flow and its distribution before and during autonomic blockade in fetal lambs. *Am J Obstet Gynecol* 1980;138:703–707.
21. Adeagbo AS, Coceani F, Olley PM. The response of the lamb ductus venosus to prostaglandins and inhibitors of prostaglandin and thromboxane synthesis. *Circ Res* 1982;51:580–586.
22. Adeagbo AS, Bishai I, Lees J, Olley PM, Coceani F. Evidence for a role of prostaglandin I_2 and thromboxane A_2 in ductus venosus of the lamb. *Can J Physiol Pharmacol* 1985;63:1101–1105.
23. Adeagbo AS, Breen CA, Cutz E, Lees JG, Olley PM, Coceani F. Lamb ductus venosus: Evidence of a cytochrome P-450 mechanism in its contractile tension. *J Pharmacol Exp Ther* 1990;252:875–879.
24. Coceani F, Adeagbo AS, Cutz E, Olley PM. Autonomic mechanisms in the ductus venosus of the lamb. *Am J Physiol* 1984;247:H17–24.
25. Coceani F, Olley PM. The control of cardiovascular shunts in the fetal and perinatal period. *Can J Pharmacol* 1988;66:1129–1134.
26. Paulick RP, Meyers RL, Rudolph CD, Rudolph AM. Venous and hepatic vascular responses to indomethacin and prostaglandin E_1 in the fetal lamb. *Am J Obstet Gynecol* 1990;163:1357–1363.
27. Paulick RP, Meyers RL, Rudolph CD, Rudolph AM. Umbilical and hepatic venous responses to circulating vasoconstrictive hormones in fetal lamb. *Am J Physiol* 1991;260(*Heart Circ Physiol* 29):H1205–1213.
28. Loberant N, Barak M, Gaitini D, Herkovits M, Ben-Elisha M, Roguin N. Closure of the ductus venosus in neonates: Findings on real-time gray-scale, color-flow Doppler, and duplex Doppler sonography. *AJR* 1992;159:1083–1085.
29. Dawes GS. The umbilical circulation. *Am J Obstet Gynecol* 1962;84:1634–1648.
30. Dawes GS. *Foetal and neonatal physiology.* Chicago: Year Book; 1968.
31. Peltonen T, Hirvonen L. Experimental studies on fetal and neonatal circulation. *Acta Paediat* 1965;44(Suppl.161):1–55.
32. Rudolph AM. Distribution and regulation of blood flow in the fetal and neonatal lamb. *Circ Res* 1985;57:811–821.
33. Lind J. Human fetal and neonatal circulation. *Eur J Cardiol* 1977;5:265–281.
34. Edelstone DI, Rudolph AM, Heymann MA. Liver and ductus venosus blood flows in fetal lamb in utero. *Circ Res* 1977;42:426–433.
35. Edelstone DI, Rudolph AM. Preferential streaming of ductus venosus blood to the brain and heart in fetal lambs. *Am J Physiol* 1979;237(6):H724–729.
36. Edelstone DI. Regulation of blood flow through the ductus venosus. *J Dev Physiol* 1980;2:219–238.
37. Huisman TW, Stewart PA, Wladimiroff JW. Ductus venosus blood flow velocity waveforms in the human fetus: A Doppler study. *Ultrasound Med Biol* 1992;18:33–37.
38. Kiserud T, Eik-Nes SH, Hellevik LR, Blaas H-G. Ductus venosus: A longitudinal Doppler velocimetric study of the human fetus. *J Mat-Fet Invest* 1992;2:5–11.
39. Behrman RE, Lees MH, Peterson EN, de Lannoy CW, Seeds AE. Distribution of the circulation in the normal and asphyxiated fetal primate. *Am J Obstet Gynecol* 1970;108:956–969.
40. Edelstone DI, Rudolph AM, Heymann MA. Effect of hypoxia and decreasing umbilical flow on liver and ductus venosus flows in fetal lambs. *Am J Physiol* 1980;(*Heart Circ Physiol* 7):H656–663.
41. Itskovitz J, LaGamma EF, Rudolph AH. Effect of cord compression on fetal blood flow distribution and O_2 delivery. *Am J Physiol* 1987;252(*Heart Circ Physiol* 21):H100–109.
42. Paulick RP, Meyers RL, Rudolph CD, Rudolph AM. Venous responses to hypoxemia in the fetal lamb. *J Dev Physiol* 1990;14:81–88.
43. Meyers RL, Paulick RP, Rudolph CD, Rudolph AM. Cardiovascular responses to acute, severe haemorrhage in fetal sheep. *J Dev Physiol* 1991;15:189–97.
44. Rudolph CD, Meyers RL, Paulick RP, Rudolph AM. Effects of ductus venosus obstruction on liver and regional blood flow in the fetal lamb. *Pediatr Res* 1991;29:347–352.
45. Brinkman CR, Kirschbaum TH, Assali NS. The role of the umbilical sinus in the regulation of placental vascular resistance. *Gynecol Invest* 1970;1:115–127.
46. Huisman TW, Stewart PA, Wladimiroff JW. Doppler assessment of the normal early fetal circulation. *Ultrasound Obstet Gynecol* 1992;2:300–305.
47. Eik-Nes SH, Marsal K, Brubakk AO, Kristoffersen K, Ulstein M. Ultrasonic measurement of fetal blood flow. *J Biomed Eng* 1982;4:28–36.

Doppler Ultrasound in Obstetrics and Gynecology,
edited by Joshua A. Copel and Kathryn L. Reed.
Raven Press, Ltd., New York © 1995.

CHAPTER 31

The Fetal Pulmonary Circulation

Donald S. Emerson and Mark S. Cartier

The newborn's first gasp of air initiates a series of events that decisively alters the fetal pulmonary vasculature. Arterial resistance falls dramatically, accompanied by a marked increase in pulmonary blood flow and the onset of closure of two vascular shunts that had limited the extent of cardiac output supplying the fetal lungs. Factors controlling vascular resistance and flow within the fetal lungs have been extensively studied to better explain the regulation of normal extrauterine pulmonary circulation. The presence of serious pediatric pulmonary vascular conditions, whether independent of or secondary to cardiac and great vessel disease, provides another powerful incentive to probe the dramatic changes occurring in pulmonary blood flow at birth.

Until recently, physiologic knowledge of the fetal pulmonary circulation has been acquired only through invasive means and primarily in species other than human. The advent of color and pulsed Doppler ultrasound, however, opened a new noninvasive window on the fetal pulmonary vasculature allowing for noninstrumented evaluation of normal and abnormal human fetuses. After a brief review of the anatomy and physiology of the fetal pulmonary vasculature, this chapter will present normal Doppler findings and will conclude with a discussion of the current and future roles of Doppler in the diagnosis of abnormalities affecting the pulmonary circulation.

DEVELOPMENT, STRUCTURE, AND PHYSIOLOGY OF THE FETAL PULMONARY CIRCULATION

The main vascular connections of the pulmonary circulation are established between 32 and 50 days gestation at which time intrapulmonary arteries and veins

D. S. Emerson, and M. S. Cartier: Department of Radiology, University of Tennessee at Memphis, Memphis, TN 38163.

lose their connection to the central circulation and become connected to the developing main pulmonary artery and proximal pulmonary vein. The major (preacinar) intrapulmonary arteries assume their definitive branching pattern by 16 weeks gestation and grow in size later in pregnancy and after birth (1). After 16 weeks, small pulmonary arteries ramify extensively, increasing in number dramatically until term (2) (Fig. 1a,b). Some intraacinar arterial growth occurs during late gestation, but most of it accompanies the massive alveolar growth of early childhood (3). Growth of the pulmonary veins parallels that of the arteries in the fetus with the exception that the venous system of the lungs is more extensive than the arterial system (4).

There is muscle in the walls of the fetal pulmonary arteries to the level of the terminal bronchioles, and only after birth does muscle extend more distally to the level of the alveolar ducts and beyond (1,3). Nevertheless, in those arteries where there is a muscular wall, it is thicker in the fetus than in the child, thereby producing a narrower vascular lumen (1,3). An immediate fall in muscular wall thickness occurs over the first three days of life, probably due to vascular dilatation induced by a number of stimuli, including altered gas tension (3). A slower decrease in wall thickness follows over the first 4 months of life, probably due to decreased muscular growth rate induced by lower arterial pressures (3).

The pulmonary vascular circuit is a high-resistance, high-pressure, low-flow system *in utero*. Only 3.7% of total cardiac output supplies the lungs in early gestation, rising to 7% near term (5). Because the ductus arteriosus is patent *in utero*, pulmonary arterial pressure is believed to be maintained at least equal to systemic arterial pressure (6). Thus, regulation of fetal pulmonary flow, i.e., maintenance of a low-flow vascular circuit, depends on the high resistance of the pulmonary vasculature. Factors responsible for maintaining this high resistance *in utero* and those responsible for the dramatic fall in resistance at birth have been studied extensively and are the

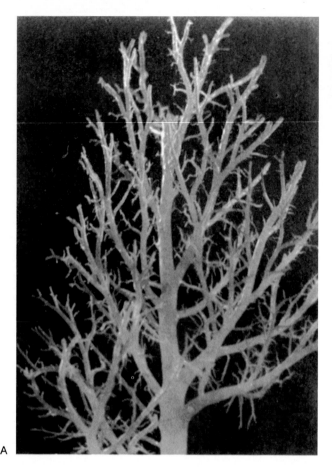

A

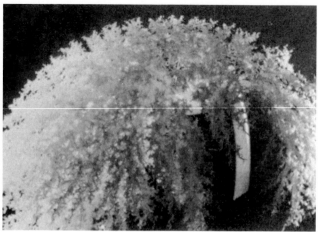

B

FIG. 1. Pulmonary arterial casts from fetal lambs at 0.65 (**A**) and 0.95 (**B**) gestation. Interval change reflects, in particular, growth of small muscular arteries. From Levin DL et al. (2).

subject of a comprehensive review by Long (7). A low total cross-sectional pulmonary vascular area appears to be the major final factor responsible for this high resistance. Cross-sectional area can be regulated by controlling both the absolute number of vessels and the caliber of these vessels. The absolute number of vessels present in the fetus may be genetically predetermined but vascular caliber can be altered in response to changing metabolic and physical conditions (8,9). Furthermore, pulmonary vascular resistance may be increased also by limiting flow to certain subsets of the pulmonary arteries (10), or, conversely, reduced by recruiting additional previously quiescent vessels (8).

The reactivity of fetal intrapulmonary arterial branches to various stimuli, the ability to dilate or narrow and thereby alter vascular resistance, increases with gestational age of the fetus. The presence of increasing pulmonary vasoactivity could be explained by a progressive thickening of the arterial wall of muscular resistance arteries. Actually, however, wall thickness of resistance arteries has been shown not to increase with advancing gestation (1,2). Furthermore, the absolute fall in pulmonary vascular resistance occurring over the course of gestation seems to contradict the concept of increased vascular wall thickness. Levin and coworkers resolved this apparent contradiction by discovering a 40-fold increase

in the number of pulmonary resistance arteries from 0.59 to 0.97 gestation in the fetal lamb (2). Both the total vascular cross-sectional area and the total amount of vascular wall muscular tissue increased significantly (2). The increased cross-sectional area of the pulmonary vascular bed produces a lower total resistance, while the greater number of small vessels with muscular walls provides a more widespread mechanism for controlling resistance. Nevertheless, while absolute pulmonary flow increases over the course of gestation, Morin and Egan determined that when corrected for wet weight of the lungs, pulmonary flow actually fell somewhat and total pulmonary resistance rose (11). In other words, rising pulmonary blood flow does not keep pace with the increase in pulmonary vascularity. Hyperbaric oxygen treatment, however, produces a 10-fold increase in pulmonary flow in mature fetal lambs (11). This suggests that the normal relatively hypoxic status of the fetus induces pulmonary vasoconstriction, which has the effect of limiting the absolute increase in pulmonary blood flow thereby protecting the fetal heart from unnecessary increases in output (11).

Flow studies using radiolabeled microsphere injection, direct pressure measurements, and electromagnetic flow transducers have significantly expanded our understanding of fetal vascular physiology (5,12,13). Never-

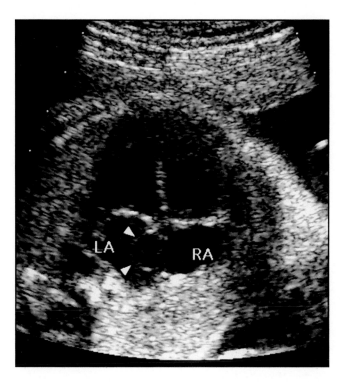

FIG. 2. Two-dimensional sonogram provides indirect evidence of the right-to-left shunt at the foramen ovale, one of two pathways allowing blood to bypass the fetal pulmonary circulation. Four-chamber view of the heart reveals bowing of the septum primum (*arrowheads*) into left atrium (LA) indicating direction of current from right atrium (RA) to LA.

theless, differences in experimental technique have yielded some contradictory findings, and conclusions have been predicated on measurements in instrumented animals. These conclusions may not be entirely applicable to normal noninstrumented human fetuses. For instance, using pulsed Doppler sonography, we have discovered flow patterns in the ductus venosus of normal human fetuses that are significantly different from those found in instrumented lambs (14). It is hoped, therefore, that the use of color and pulsed Doppler as noninvasive tools will supplement our understanding of normal human fetal pulmonary vascular flow. Nevertheless, contribution of multiple factors to the shape of the arterial velocity waveform and inherent errors in calculation of flow in very small vessels will of necessity limit some of the inferences that can be drawn from Doppler studies.

COLOR AND PULSED DOPPLER FLOW OF THE NORMAL PULMONARY CIRCULATION

Two-dimensional real-time ultrasound clearly delineates the proximal and distal limbs of the pulmonary circulation. In fact, much can be learned about the nature of fetal lung flow by simply examining this sonographic anatomy. The septum primum can be seen bowing into the left atrium, an obvious directional indication of the shunting of blood currents from the right side of the heart to the left side of the heart, thereby bypassing the lungs (Fig. 2). The pulmonary artery can be followed until it trifurcates into the right and left pulmonary arteries and the ductus arteriosus. It is obvious from two-dimensional sonography that the ductus arteriosus is the major outflow from the pulmonary artery in the fetus, shunting blood away from the lungs and into the descending aorta (Fig. 3a,b). Two-dimensional sonography can identify the main pulmonary veins joining at the back of the left atrium. Their narrow caliber is an indication of the low volume of flow passing through the lungs (Fig. 4). Nevertheless, while all of these anatomic indicators of pulmonary vascular physiology are useful, the actual vessels within the lung parenchyma and the time-velocity waveforms within these vessels are hidden from two-dimensional ultrasound.

Color Doppler sonography reveals the pulmonary circulation to a much fuller extent than does gray scale sonography. The arterial circulation is demonstrated from the main pulmonary artery to the main right and left pulmonary arteries and through the next several divisions out at least three-fourths of the hemithoracic diameter (Fig. 5a,b). In opposite color coding, pulmonary veins can be traced for a similar distance back to the left atrium (Fig. 5c). Despite the dramatic appearance of these vessels on the color map, color Doppler generally plays a subordinate role to pulsed Doppler in the study of the fetal pulmonary circulation. Color Doppler quickly identifies vessels for pulsed Doppler interrogation and accurately guides Doppler angle adjustment (Fig. 5d).

The pulmonary arterial bed of the fetus possesses a unique pulsed Doppler waveform that we have not found elsewhere in the fetus (Fig. 5d). It is characterized by an extremely rapid initial flow acceleration followed by a very early and rapid deceleration phase producing a unique needle-like systolic peak (15). This is followed by

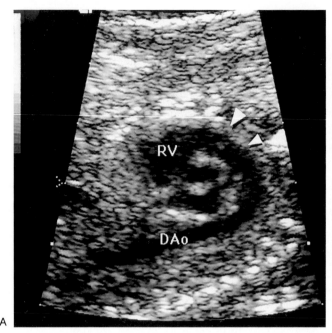

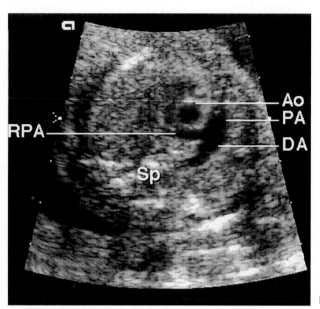

FIG. 3. Sonographic anatomic evidence of the shunting of right ventricular output past the lungs via the ductus arteriosus. **A:** Sagittal view of pulmonary artery–ductus arteriosus arch. The ductus arteriosus continues straight along the main axis of the pulmonary artery (thereby minimizing vascular resistance). This is in agreement with the general observation that the major branching vessel at an arterial juncture continues on most closely with the main axis of the parent vessel (45). The preferential flow through the ductus arteriosus is also suggested by its large caliber, only slightly less than that of the pulmonary artery, and its direct drainage into the descending aorta. RV, right ventricle; DAo, descending aorta. *Large arrowhead,* pulmonary valve; *small arrowhead,* beginning of ductus arteriosus. **B:** Transverse view of the pulmonary artery. The steep angle of the right pulmonary artery (RPA) off the main pulmonary artery (PA) introduces increased resistance to flow. Compare with the axis of the ductus arteriosus (DA). Ao, ascending aorta; Sp, spine.

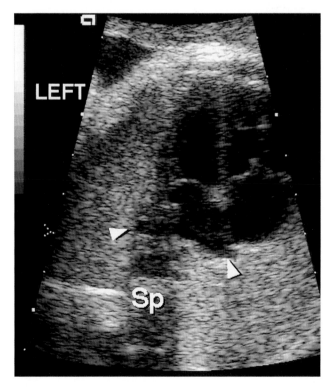

FIG. 4. Transverse view of pulmonary veins (*arrowheads*) draining into the back of the left atrium. Sp, spine.

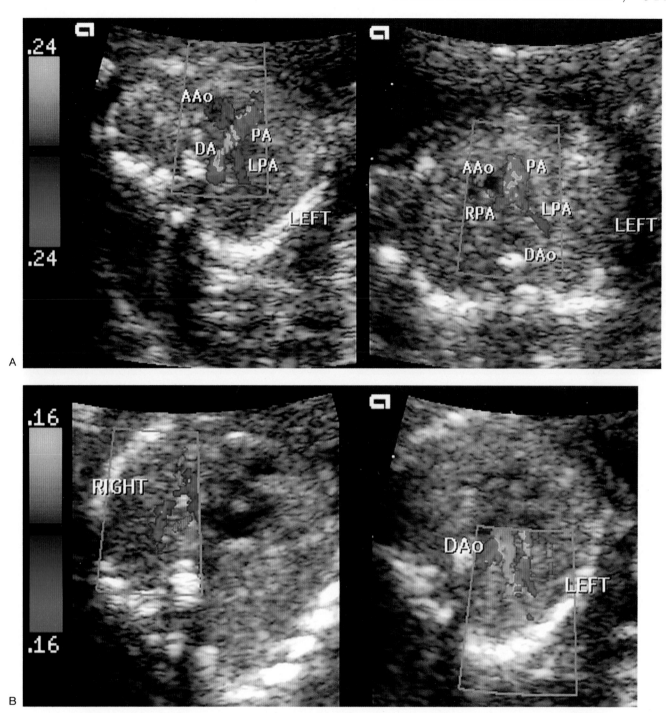

FIG. 5. Color Doppler depiction of the fetal pulmonary circulation. **A: Left:** Transverse view demonstrating continuation of the main pulmonary artery into the ductus arteriosus (DA) and the left pulmonary artery (LPA) in a fetus at 18 weeks gestation. **Right:** Slightly different view of the same fetus demonstrating main pulmonary artery (PA) and its main left (LPA) and right (RPA) branches. AAo, ascending aorta; DAo, descending aorta. **B:** Color maps following pulmonary vasculature deeper into the lungs in the same fetus. Color coding indicates the nature of the vessels, with arterial flow away from and venous flow to the mediastinum.

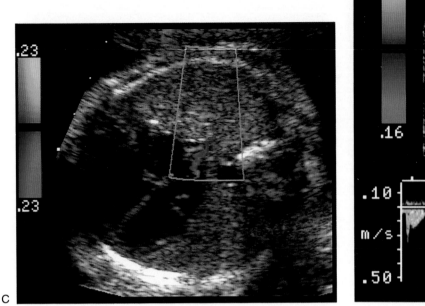

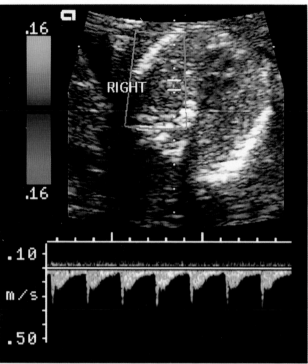

C

D

FIG 5. (*Continued.*) **C:** Color flow map of right pulmonary venous drainage into the left atrium of a fetus at 29 weeks gestation. **D:** Characteristic pulmonary arterial branch time–velocity waveform in a fetus at 18 weeks gestation. Color Doppler greatly facilitates pulsed Doppler interrogation of the fetal pulmonary circulation.

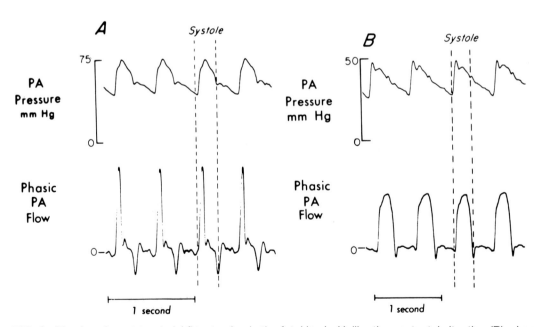

FIG. 6. Phasic pulmonary arterial flow tracing in the fetal lamb. Unlike the postnatal situation (**B**) when forward flow occurs throughout systole and there is minimal reversed flow, forward flow in the fetal pulmonary artery (**A**) is limited to the first third of systole and there is a greater amount of reversed flow in late systole. From Lewis AB et al. (13).

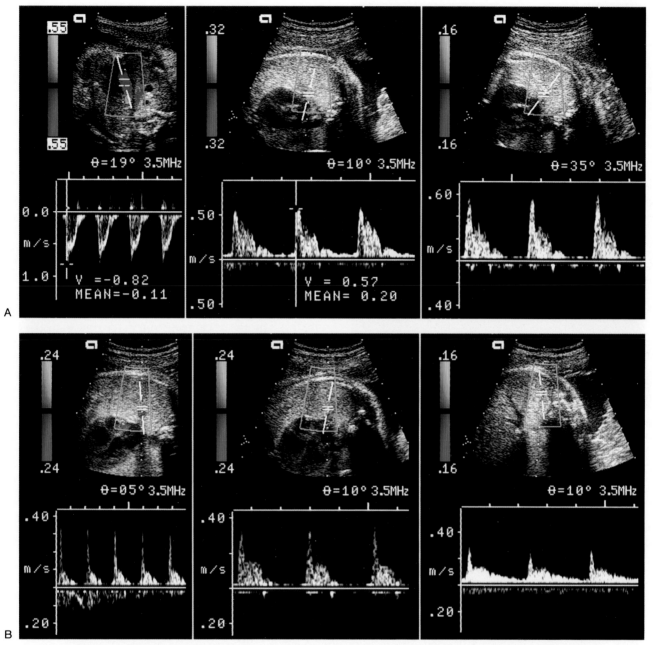

FIG. 7. Series detailing the changes in pulsed Doppler flow characteristics from proximal to distal in the fetal pulmonary circulation. (Fetus at 30 weeks gestation. Markers on pulsed Doppler strip define 200-msec segments.) **A:** From left to right, flow velocity waveforms in the main pulmonary artery, right pulmonary artery, and a proximal branch of the right pulmonary artery. **B:** Left images show arterial waveforms (at different sweep speeds) in pulmonary arterial branches distal to those in 7A. Right image demonstrates a typical waveform in a very distal pulmonary arterial branch.

a short but relatively stable systolic flow segment culminating in a gradual decay in systolic flow and no diastolic flow. A number of systolic flow notches (possibly followed by secondary acceleration spikes) may be found. This fetal pulmonary artery flow velocity waveform is similar to tracings obtained by direct flow measurements in fetal sheep (13) (Fig. 6).

The actual waveform patterns observed vary at partic-

ular sites along the pulmonary arterial tree. The very characteristic needle-like waveform is identified only from the right and left pulmonary arteries and distally. Upstream, in the main pulmonary artery, the waveform is primarily composed of a dominant, relatively broad-based triangular systolic component and a minor low-velocity diastolic component (Fig. 7a). Downstream from the right and left pulmonary arteries, in the main

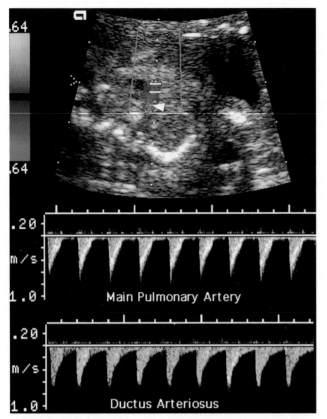

FIG. 8. Comparison of main pulmonary arterial and ductus arteriosus waveforms in an 18-week fetus. (Sites of sampling are seen on the transversely oriented color map above: pulmonary artery waveform from within the pulsed Doppler range gate and the ductus arteriosus waveform at the level of the arrowhead.) The upslope of initial systolic acceleration is straight and comes to a needle-like point in the pulmonary artery. In contrast, the systolic velocity peak is delayed and more rounded in the ductus arteriosus. Notice also the presence of greater diastolic flow in the ductus. Although not demonstrated in this case, peak velocities are typically greater in the ductus arteriosus than in the pulmonary artery.

hilar branches, there is a longer and steeper deceleration slope of the initial systolic flow spike (Fig. 7a). Branch arteries, found further downstream in the lungs, manifest similar waveforms although with a progressive fall in peak systolic velocity and a reduction in the time course of the entire systolic component as pulsed Doppler interrogation proceeds more distally (Fig. 7a,b). In contrast, the ductus arteriosus manifests no needle-like systolic spike but rather a full triangular-shaped systolic peak (with the highest velocity of the pulmonary arterial tree) and continuous forward flow during diastole (Fig. 8). Figure 9 presents a schematic comparison of the different arterial waveforms found in the pulmonary circulation. The pulmonary venous flow pattern is characterized largely by forward flow modulated by pressure changes in the left atrium (Fig. 10).

The physical basis for the shape of the fetal pulmonary arterial flow–velocity waveform remains a matter of speculation. Arterial flow velocity characteristics derive from multiple factors, including vascular pressure, resistance, capacitance, impedance, and distensibility, and ventricular contractility (dependent on ventricular preload and afterload). Studies directly relating pulsed Doppler flow–velocity waveforms with actual pressure and flow measurements in fetal lungs in baseline and altered conditions are needed before one can draw absolute physiologic conclusions from these waveforms.

Nevertheless, it is tempting to infer from pulsed Doppler data in children and adults with pulmonary hypertension that high resistance in the pulmonary circuit and elevated pulmonary arterial pressure are responsible for normal fetal pulmonary artery waveform characteristics. The degree to which the normal adult pulmonary artery waveform evolves in pulmonary hypertension into a waveform similar to that of the normal fetus is directly related to the pulmonary arterial pressure (16,17). Thus, there is a proportional reduction in the time to peak systolic velocity (acceleration time) and in systolic ejection period with rising pulmonary arterial pressures (16,17). Machado and coworkers applied this concept to the fetal circulation and studied normal human fetuses with pulsed Doppler between 16 and 30 weeks gestation (18). They demonstrated a consistently shorter acceleration time in the main pulmonary artery (32.1 msec) com-

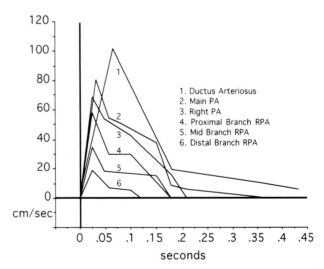

FIG. 9. Schematized comparative diagram of central to peripheral pulmonary arterial waveforms based on measurements obtained in a 22-week fetus. Peak velocity, percentage of cycle with forward systolic flow, and extent of measurable diastolic flow diminish as pulsed Doppler beam interrogation proceeds further into the lung periphery. Notice also the unique characteristics of the ductus arteriosus compared with the main pulmonary artery: longer initial systolic acceleration time, later peak velocity, slower decay in forward flow, and presence of major diastolic flow component.

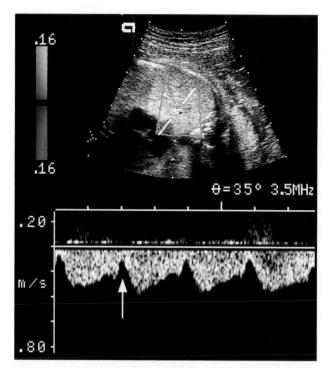

FIG. 10. Pulmonary venous waveform demonstrated in a 30-week fetus. Flow modulations are produced by changes in left atrial pressures over the course of the cardiac cycle. *Arrow* defines the beginning of one such cycle, with the largest trough in forward flow occurring during atrial contraction. Moving to the right, forward flow picks up during atrial relaxation and reaches peak velocity during early atrial diastole. Forward flow then begins to fall as atrial capacitance diminishes. Forward flow stabilizes and increases as the mitral valve opens. The cycle then begins again with another deep trough at atrial systole.

pared with that in the proximal ascending aorta (43.7 msec) and interpreted this to indicate higher mean pressures in the fetal pulmonary artery than in the aorta (18).

The fall in pulmonary artery pressure occurring at birth (19) provides an additional window into the relationship between pulmonary arterial pressure and acceleration time. Wilson and coworkers performed serial Doppler studies of the pulmonary artery from the last 24 hr of fetal life through 3–4 days of postnatal life and found progressively rising acceleration times (20). The increase in acceleration time from fetal life to less than 6 hr after birth was not statistically significant (46 ± 14 msec to 51 ± 13 msec) although the increase became significant at 6–24 hr of life (69 ± 14 msec) (20). They attributed this change to the dramatic fall in pulmonary arterial pressure occurring secondary to falling pulmonary vascular resistance in the transition from fetal to early neonatal life (20). Pulmonary artery peak systolic velocities remained constant during this time frame (20). Shiraishi and Yanagisawa found that the pulmonary arterial waveform became less triangular and more dome-

like with lengthening acceleration and systolic ejection times in the first several days of life, and arrived at similar conclusions as Wilson et al. (21). The aortic flow-velocity waveform showed no significant change during this same time period (21).

Further evidence for the relationship between pulmonary arterial pressure (and resistance) and the flow-velocity waveform comes from animal studies in which the fetus is challenged with changes to its normal environment. The fetal lamb pulmonary artery phasic flow curve changes dramatically following intravenous administration of acetylcholine, which causes pulmonary arterial resistance and pressure to drop (13). Instead of forward flow occurring only in the initial very brief systolic spike as it does in the normal fetal pulmonary artery, the flow curve becomes significantly widened and forward flow continues throughout systole (13) (Fig. 11).

There are problems with inferring too much about the fetal pulmonary vascular circuit from pulmonary arterial Doppler waveforms. Groenenberg and coworkers identified technical limitations in analysis of Doppler flow–velocity waveforms in the fetal cardiac outflow tracts (22). Measurements of acceleration time in the pulmonary artery and aorta had coefficients of variation between tests within patients of 10% and 11%, respectively, indicating only moderate reproducibility (22). Other authors have pointed out that varying the location of the pulsed Doppler sampling site within the adult pulmonary artery alters the flow–velocity waveform, significantly altering the measured acceleration time and systolic ejection time (23,24). Even without consideration of technical limitations, there are differences of opinion regarding analysis of the fetal pulmonary artery waveform. Silverman suggested that fetal and adult car-

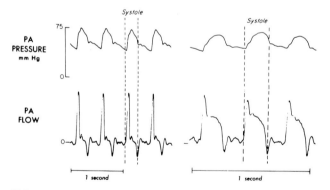

FIG. 11. Fetal lamb pulmonary arterial pressure and phasic flow curves. **Left:** Baseline conditions. Forward flow occurs only briefly at the very beginning of systole under normal conditions. **Right:** After intravenous acetylcholine injection. The pulmonary arterial tracing of forward flow is widened to encompass the entire systolic period when resistance falls. It is possible that the duration of forward systolic flow may prove to be a useful Doppler ultrasound indicator of human pulmonary arterial resistance. From Lewis et al. (13).

diovascular physiology are sufficiently different that one should reject imposition on the fetus of conclusions regarding the adult acceleration–time–pulmonary arterial pressure relationship (25). He suggested that the shorter acceleration time of the fetal pulmonary artery flow–velocity waveform described by Machado does not indicate higher pressure in the pulmonary artery because animal studies have demonstrated equal pressures in both the fetal aorta and pulmonary artery (25). He claimed, in addition, that main pulmonary artery pulsed Doppler measurements must reflect a combination of the lower resistance of the placenta and the higher resistance of the lower body as well as the higher pulmonary vascular resistance since the ductus arteriosus is widely patent *in utero* (25). This concept is bolstered by a pulsed Doppler study by Groenenberg and coworkers of pulmonary arterial and aortic peak systolic velocities in normal and growth-retarded fetuses (26). Pulmonary arterial peak systolic velocity fell significantly in 95% of fetuses with growth retardation whereas aortic velocity fell in only 57% of these fetuses (26). This difference was attributed to the fact that although both ventricles had an elevated afterload caused by elevated placental resistance, the increased afterload of the left ventricle was decreased somewhat by reduced cerebral vascular resistance in some of the fetuses (26). Thus, the pulmonary artery flow–velocity waveform is markedly affected by changes in placental resistance, possibly even more so than by changes in pulmonary vascular resistance. A pulsed Doppler study of human fetal right and left ventricular function by St. John Sutton and coworkers additionally strengthened the belief that pressures are equal in both great arteries of the human fetus (27). They found that despite a right ventricular stroke volume 24% greater than the left, both ventricles develop similar force during myocardial shortening. They indicated that their observation of similar right and left ventricular force *in utero* agreed well with equality of pressures in the pulmonary artery and aorta determined in the fetal lamb (27).

Experimental evidence indicates that in the fetal lamb pulmonary arterial pressure is equal to or just very slightly greater than aortic pressure (28). The conflict over equivalence of human fetal pulmonary and aortic pressures, however, hinges not only on the relevance of animal data but possibly also on the degree of ductus arteriosus patency. A "widely patent" ductus, as stated by Silverman (25), implies that pulmonary and aortic pressures are equal (29). However, ductus arteriosus velocities are normally rather high, certainly higher than in the pulmonary artery (30). Huhta suggested that this velocity difference indicates the presence of at least mild obstruction to pulmonary outflow into the descending aorta (30). This could then argue for higher pulmonary arterial pressures than in the aorta. Application of the

Bernoulli equation ($\Delta P = 4[V_{da}^2 - V_{pa}^2]$) to a number of our cases from the third trimester, however, yielded a maximum peak instantaneous systolic pressure gradient of only 5–7 mm Hg between the pulmonary artery and aorta. This gradient is so small compared with normal peak systolic pressures in the fetal pulmonary artery (approximately 70–75 mm Hg [13]) that it seems unlikely to represent the basis for the shorter acceleration time found by Machado et al. (18) and St. John Sutton et al. (27) in the fetal pulmonary artery.

Although falling pressures may be responsible for (or at least associated with) changes in the pulmonary arterial waveform at birth, it seems unlikely that pulmonary arterial pressure alone can be used to explain the uniqueness of the fetal pulmonary artery waveform (such as the shorter acceleration time) since pulmonary arterial and aortic pressures appear to be nearly equivalent *in utero*. Furthermore, since intrapulmonary flow represents only up to 8–10% of total fetal cardiac output or 10–15% of right ventricular output (28), it seems unlikely that pulmonary vascular resistance will exert a greater influence on main pulmonary arterial flow than do placental and lower body resistance. It may be useful to consider again the change in the flow–velocity waveform occurring as pulsed Doppler sampling proceeds from the main pulmonary artery into the right and left main pulmonary arteries. The initial unique spike-like systolic peak becomes first recognizable in the main right and main left branches. In concert with this obvious waveform change, the acceleration time further shortens as one proceeds from the main to the main left and right pulmonary arteries. Since arterial pressure is likely to be the same in the main pulmonary artery and its major branches, arterial pressure, once again, is not likely to be responsible for the unique waveform of the fetal pulmonary artery. Consideration should be given to several interrelated factors, such as pulmonary vascular resistance as well as capacitance and distensibility of the pulmonary bed. Furthermore, the potential for these factors to cause earlier systolic deceleration may be amplified by more rapid return of reflection waves from the lung periphery due to increased vascular resistance and rigidity of the fetal pulmonary circuit. That there must be some proximal extension of these effects back into the main pulmonary artery is strongly suggested by the shorter acceleration time of the main pulmonary artery compared with the ductus arteriosus and aorta.

Flow studies in fetal lambs have documented a fall in absolute pulmonary resistance over the course of gestation (11,31). We have used the pulsatility index (PI) as a measure of downstream arterial resistance in the right and left main pulmonary arteries of human fetuses and found a mean PI value of 2.97, consistent with the high degree of vascular resistance in the fetal pulmonary cir-

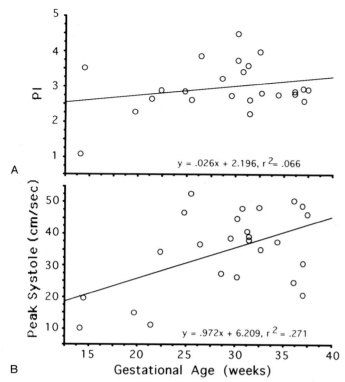

$$y = .026x + 2.196, r^2 = .066$$

$$y = .972x + 6.209, r^2 = .271$$

FIG. 12. A: Pulsed Doppler measurements in the main right or main left pulmonary arteries in 25 normal human fetuses between 15 weeks and term. Pulsatility index (PI) measurements show a slight but not significant increase over gestation ($p < 0.5$). **B:** Peak systolic velocity increases with gestation ($p < .01$). The slight rise in PI probably occurs because of the combination of absent diastolic flow and rising peak systolic velocity.

culation (15). The small and insignificant rise in PI over the course of gestation was probably secondary to the progressive rise in peak systolic velocity in the pulmonary arteries (Fig. 12). Failure to identify a fall in resistance in the pulmonary arteries via the PI calculation may be due more to insensitivity of the PI to small changes in resistance in this high-resistance circuit than to the constancy of resistance in the pulmonary circulation of the developing human fetus. It is possible that other Doppler data may identify the expected gestational age-related change in resistance in the human fetal pulmonary circulation. Although the physiologic basis for the difference in acceleration times between the pulmonary artery and ascending aorta in the fetus is not clear, it may be due to higher resistance in the pulmonary vascular bed and in the lower body. The initial report of acceleration time in the fetal pulmonary artery demonstrated no change from 16 to 30 weeks gestation (18), but a subsequent communication indicated that the acceleration time in both vessels became equal later in pregnancy (32). This change was interpreted to be secondary to the progressive fall in placental resistance (32). It is

worth speculating as to whether it may reflect also, in part, falling pulmonary vascular resistance.

COLOR DOPPLER SONOGRAPHY OF FETAL PULMONARY CIRCULATION: CLINICAL UTILITY

Current analysis of pulmonary vascular flow characteristics for clinical purposes is based on recognition of gross changes in the color map and the spectral waveform. While detection of subtle homeostatic changes may have to await the application of more sensitive quantitative analysis of the pulmonary arterial time–velocity waveform, qualitative information from color and pulsed Doppler sonography already provides diagnostic information in the workup of certain fetal abnormalities. We have found five general situations in which color Doppler sonography offers new information (33):

1. *Abnormal heart and abnormal pulmonary vascular flow.* Pulmonary arterial and venous waveforms may be discovered that do not correlate with the recognized lesions of an abnormal fetal heart. These abnormal waveforms thus can indicate the presence of an additional unrecognized cardiac lesion. We have seen two cases with hypoplastic left ventricle in which an additional lesion, a constricted foramen ovale, was suspected only after color and pulsed Doppler sonography revealed a markedly dampened pulmonary venous waveform (Fig. 13).

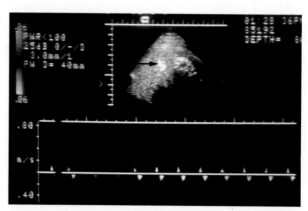

FIG. 13. Pulmonary venous waveform in a fetus at 34 weeks with prenatal diagnosis of hypoplastic left ventricle, mitral atresia, and double-outlet right ventricle. This unusual, extremely dampened to-and-fro venous blood flow pattern indicates extremely high downstream resistance to flow. (It is not seen in usual cases of hypoplastic left heart because of a reversal of the normal flow pattern across the foramen ovale in this condition.) The etiology for the abnormal venous flow pattern in this case was revealed postnatally with identification of a constricted foramen ovale. Pulmonary arterial peak systolic velocity was also reduced in this case, possibly due to venous hypertension.

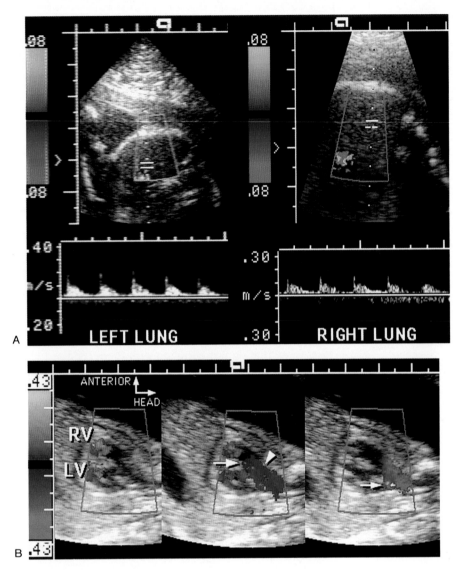

FIG. 14. Fetus at 21 weeks with a large VSD and a single large overriding outflow artery on two-dimensional sonography. The differential diagnosis based on the available sonographic findings included pulmonary atresia, tetralogy of Fallot, and truncus arteriosus. **A:** Normal peripheral pulmonary arterial waveforms were found in both lungs, indicating that a central pulmonary arterial supply was present and should be identifiable. **B:** Using color Doppler sonography, the main pulmonary artery was found to originate from the posterior aspect of the single ascending outflow vessel, thereby narrowing the diagnosis to truncus arteriosus. **Left:** Diastole—inflow into each ventricle is coded red on this short-axis outflow view. **Middle:** Early systole—biventricular outflow is coded blue as it traverses an overiding ventricular septal defect (*arrow*) and enters the single truncal vessel (*arrowhead*). **Right:** End-systole—main pulmonary artery (*arrow*) is seen arising from the back wall of the truncus. LV, left ventricle; RV, right ventricle. From Emerson and Cartier (47).

2. *Nonvisualized pulmonary artery and normal pulmonary arterial flow.* Detection of normal pulmonary arterial waveforms in the lung periphery of a fetus with an absent main pulmonary artery on two-dimensional imaging strongly suggests the existence of (anatomically displaced) central pulmonary arteries. This information encourages the sonographer to search for the aberrant central pulmonary artery[ies] arising from either the ductus arteriosus (through retrograde flow) or the truncus arteriosus (Fig. 14). The status of the pulmonary arteries is a significant factor in determining prognosis.

3. *Color flow mapping of anomalous pulmonary venous return.* The color flow map can be used to trace the course of the abnormally draining common pulmonary vein and to determine whether there is infradiaphragmatic, intracardiac, or supracardiac drainage (34) (Fig. 15a–c). Identification of subdiaphragmatic drainage signifies nearly complete likelihood of pulmonary venous

obstruction whereas the presence of intracardiac drainage indicates only a 20% chance of obstruction.

4. *Intrathoracic mass and altered pulmonary arterial or venous flow.* Pulmonary arterial and venous flow are dampened in compressed lung due to an intrathoracic mass such as a cystic adenomatoid malformation of the lung or a diaphragmatic hernia. Doppler manifestations of this include poor visualization of the pulmonary vasculature on the color map and very low velocities on recordable vascular waveforms (Fig. 16). The reduction in flow is proportional to the degree of lung compression: there is greater dampening of pulmonary flow in association with a large diaphragmatic hernia than with a small cystic adenomatoid malformation. Additionally, flow may be altered even in normal uncompressed lung segments when a centrally located thoracic or lung mass obstructs venous flow from that portion of the lung returning to the heart (Fig. 17a,b).

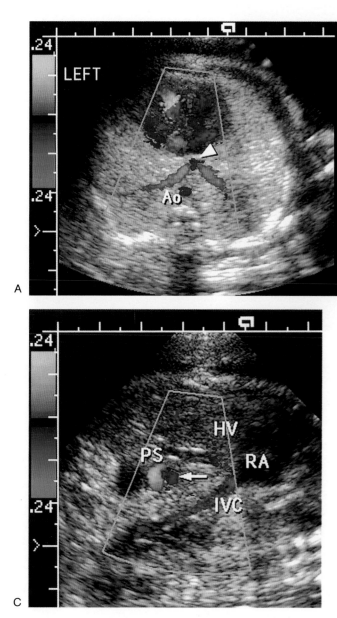

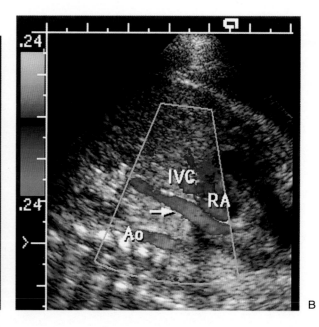

FIG. 15. Infradiaphragmatic total anomalous pulmonary venous return in a fetus at 30 weeks. **A:** Transverse color Doppler flow map demonstrating right and left pulmonary veins (*in red*) draining into a common pulmonary vein (*arrowhead*) that is coded blue, similar to the aorta, indicating caudally directed flow. **B:** Longitudinal color Doppler flow map reveals similar color coding of abdominal aorta (Ao) and common pulmonary vein (*arrow*), indicating flow from the chest into the abdomen. **C:** Longitudinal color Doppler sonogram identifies the ultimate drainage of the blue-coded common pulmonary vein (*arrow*) into the red-coded portal sinus (PS) in the liver. IVC, inferior vena cava; RA, right atrium. From Emerson et al. (34).

5. *Rebounding pulmonary arterial flow after reduction of an intrathoracic mass.* The pulmonary vasculature reappears on the color flow map immediately after pulmonary compression is relieved, possibly with even greater intensity than in the normal lung. This rebound in pulmonary flow is marked also by a dramatic increase in both arterial and venous velocity on the pulsed Doppler spectrum (Fig. 18a–c). These findings probably directly reflect a significant fall in resistance to blood flow as lung compression is relieved.

Color and pulsed Doppler sonography of pulmonary blood flow are potentially useful in the evaluation of other abnormal conditions of the fetus:

1. *Providing a more specific sonographic diagnosis of bronchopulmonary sequestration.* Since color Doppler sonography is well equipped to identify flow in otherwise unapparent small vessels, it may be used to detect the small aortic branch supplying a lung mass, which can help confirm the diagnosis of bronchopulmonary sequestration.

2. *Predicting severity of pulmonary underdevelopment due to intrathoracic masses and to oligohydramnios.* The sonographic prediction of pulmonary hypoplasia based on chest circumference has had variable success (35,36). Theoretically it may be possible to use prenatal Doppler to predict the degree of pulmonary hypoplasia since underdevelopment of the pulmonary vascular bed

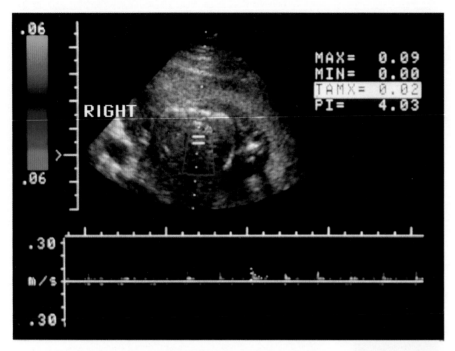

FIG. 16. Diminished peripheral pulmonary arterial flow in a fetus at 18 weeks due to lung compression by a right-sided diaphragmatic hernia. Pulmonary flow is more compromised on the side of the hernia (shown here) than in the contralateral lung, possibly indicating a gradient of the pulmonary compression (46). We have noted less dampening of the pulmonary waveform in conjunction with smaller intrathoracic masses.

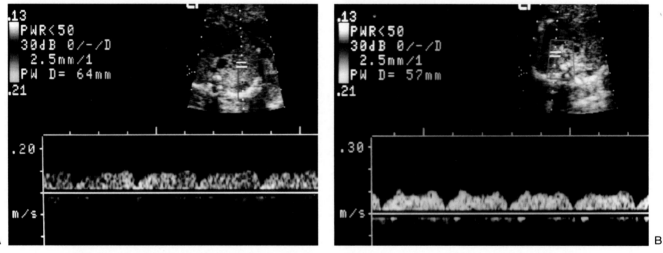

A   B

FIG. 17. Changes in venous flow due to small cystic adenomatoid malformation of the right posterior lung base without global lung compression in a 22-week fetus. **A:** Abnormally diminished modulation of pulmonary venous flow is seen in venous drainage from the right lung base. The waveform is less pulsatile and less reflective of intracardiac pressure changes. Real-time color Doppler sonography revealed that the pulmonary vein draining this lung segment was deviated ventrally by the lung mass as the vein headed toward the left atrium. These Doppler findings suggest mild segmental obstruction to pulmonary venous return. **B:** Normal venous waveforms were identified from all other regions of the lungs. This image demonstrates normal venous flow from the contralateral lung segment.

accompanies pulmonary hypoplasia (37). And failure of the pulmonary vascular bed to properly ramify and grow may prevent, or possibly even reverse, the normal absolute fall in pulmonary vascular resistance occurring over gestation. Nevertheless, while color and pulsed Doppler have successfully detected the diminution in fetal pulmonary vascular flow secondary to intrathoracic masses, this effect probably occurs secondarily to increased resis-

tance caused directly by lung compression rather than by pulmonary vascular underdevelopment. Currently we do not know which aspects of the Doppler flow data will prove most clinically sensitive and predictive. If any approach ultimately proves useful, it will probably be dependent on more quantitative analysis of intrapulmonary Doppler flow data than is currently available.

3. *Identifying changes in fetal pulmonary arterial flow*

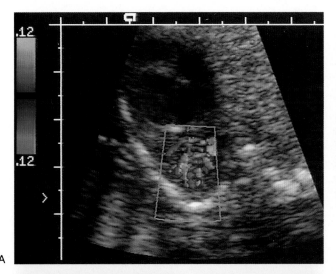

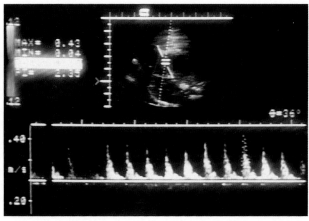

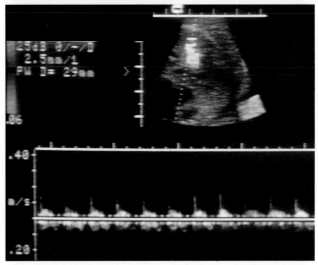

FIG. 18. Color and pulsed Doppler sonography of pulmonary vascularity immediately following percutaneous drainage of a large cystic adenomatoid malformation of the lung. **A:** Color flow map depicts markedly increased vascularity in the ipsilateral lung just above the cystic mass. This is considerably greater flow than is typically revealed in normal fetuses. From Emerson and Cartier (47). **B:** Pulsed Doppler sonography identifies increased peak systolic velocity and a longer period of forward flow immediately after drainage compared with the predrainage waveform as seen in **C.**

predicting development of persistent pulmonary hypertension or persistent pulmonary circulation in the newborn. Etiologies for development of persistent pulmonary hypertension range from meconium aspiration and fetal hypoxia to indomethacin-induced ductus arteriosus narrowing to an assortment of cardiac disorders (38). Owing to the range of vascular structural abnormalities associated with persistent pulmonary circulation in the newborn, there may be a variety of altered pulmonary flow patterns to be discovered with pulsed Doppler in the fetus. Constriction of the ductus arteriosus *in utero* can cause persistent pulmonary circulation in the newborn. Doppler has detected ductal constriction *in utero* through identification of elevated ductus arteriosus systolic and diastolic velocities (30), but Doppler findings in the lung flow have not been described. Invasive studies involving fetal lambs have shown that as the ductus arteriosus becomes constricted, pulmonary vascular resistance falls, pulmonary arterial pressure rises, and flow increases (39,40). It may be possible to demonstrate

some of these intrapulmonary effects with color and pulsed Doppler.

4. *Predicting the status of the pulmonary circulation in pulmonary atresia.* Evidence of diminished fetal pulmonary arterial pressure in pulmonary atresia (41) may be identifiable by pulsed Doppler study. The peak velocity of right-to-left ductus arteriosus shunting in newborns and pediatric patients with patent ductus arteriosus yields reasonable estimates of pulmonary artery pressures (42,43). Thus, it may be possible to estimate the systemic-to-pulmonary pressure difference in the fetus with pulmonary atresia by Doppler assessment of retrograde ductal flow. Detection of a greater pressure gradient could indicate a narrow ductus but could also indicate a larger vascular capacity in the fetal pulmonary bed. Increased pulmonary bed vascular capacity might predict a more developed peripheral pulmonary circulation (despite central pulmonary atresia) capable of handling the increase in flow after surgery in the newborn period.

5. *Predicting pulmonary maturity.* Since fetal lungs have been shown to become considerably more reactive to certain stimuli closer to term (44), it is possible that a safe challenge test could precipitate sufficient change in pulmonary arterial flow to cause an altered pulmonary waveform. If this change in pulmonary flow could be measured, one might correlate the degree of change with pulmonary maturity and thereby develop a relatively noninvasive test for lung maturity.

CONCLUSION

Color and pulsed Doppler ultrasound offer the possibility of new insights into the pulmonary vascular physiology of normal noninstrumented human fetuses. Doppler sonography is already providing valuable qualitative information in the workup of fetal abnormalities affecting the lungs and the pulmonary vasculature. It is anticipated that the development of more quantitative methods of analysis of the spectral time–velocity waveform will increase the diagnostic effectiveness of Doppler in the pulmonary circulation.

REFERENCES

1. Hislop A, Reid L. Intrapulmonary arterial development during fetal life: Branching pattern and structure. *J Anat* 1972;113:35–48.
2. Levin D, Rudolph A, Heymann M, Phibbs R. Morphological development of the pulmonary vascular bed in fetal lambs. *Circulation* 1976;53:144–151.
3. Hislop A, Reid L. Pulmonary arterial development during childhood: Branching pattern and structure. *Thorax* 1973;28:129–135.
4. Hislop A, Reid L. Fetal and childhood development of the intrapulmonary veins in man: Branching pattern and structure. *Thorax* 1973;28:313–319.
5. Rudolph AM, Heymann MA. Circulatory changes during growth in the fetal lamb. *Circ Res* 1970;26:289–299.
6. Heymann MA, Rudolph AM. Control of the ductus arteriosus. *Physiol Rev* 1975;55:62–78.
7. Long W. Developmental pulmonary circulatory physiology. In: Long W, ed. *Fetal and neonatal cardiology.* Philadelphia: WB Saunders; 1990.
8. Haworth S, Hislop A. Adaptation of the pulmonary circulation to extrauterine life in the pig and its relevance to the human heart. *Cardiovasc Res* 1981;15:108–119.
9. Heymann MA. Regulation of the pulmonary circulation in the perinatal period and in children. *Intensive Care Med* 1989;15:9–12.
10. Lipsett J, Hunt K, Carati C, Gannon B. Changes in the spatial distribution of pulmonary blood flow during the fetal/neonatal transition: An in vivo study in the rabbit. *Pediatr Pulmonol* 1989;6:213–222.
11. Morin FC III, Egan EA. Pulmonary hemodynamics in fetal lambs during development at normal and increased oxygen tension. *J Appl Physiol* 1992;73:213–218.
12. Rudolph AM, Heymann MA. The circulation of the fetus in utero. Methods for studying distribution of blood flow, cardiac output and organ blood flow. *Circ Res* 1967;21:163–184.
13. Lewis AB, Heymann MA, Rudolph AM. Gestational changes in pulmonary vascular responses in fetal lambs in utero. *Circ Res* 1976;39:536–541.
14. Emerson D, Cartier M, Brown D, Felker R, Smith W. Shunting of umbilical vein blood via the ductus venosus: Fetal Doppler study. *Radiology* 1989;173(P):249.
15. Emerson D, Cartier M, DeVore G, Altieri L, Felker R, Smith W. Distal pulmonary artery branches in the fetus: New observations with color flow and pulsed Doppler. *J Ultrasound Med* 1991;10: S19.
16. Okamato M, Miyatake K, Kinoshita N, Sakakibara H, Nimura Y. Analysis of blood flow in pulmonary hypertension with the pulsed Doppler flowmeter combined with cross sectional echocardiography. *Br Heart J* 1984;51:407–415.
17. Kitabatake A, Inoue M, Asao M, Masuyama T, Tanouchi J, Morita T. Noninvasive evaluation of pulmonary hypertension by a pulsed Doppler technique. *Circulation* 1983;68:302–309.
18. Machado MV, Chita SC, Allan LD. Acceleration time in the aorta and pulmonary artery measured by Doppler echocardiography in the midtrimester normal human fetus. *Br Heart J* 1987;58:15–18.
19. Emmanouilides G, Moss A, Duffie E, Adams F. Pulmonary arterial pressure changes in human newborn infants from birth to 3 days of age. *J Pediatr* 1964;65:327–333.
20. Wilson N, Reed K, Allen H, Marx G, Goldberg S. Doppler echocardiographic observations of pulmonary and transvalvular velocity changes after birth and during the early neonatal period. *Am Heart J* 1987;113:750–758.
21. Shiraishi H, Yanagisawa M. Pulsed Doppler echocardiographic evaluation of neonatal circulatory changes. *Br Heart J* 1987;57: 161–167.
22. Groenenberg IA, Hop WC, Wladimiroff JW. Doppler flow velocity waveforms in the fetal cardiac outflow tract: Reproducibility of waveform recording and analysis. *Ultrasound Med Biol* 1991;17: 583–587.
23. Panadis I, Ross J, Mitz G. Effect of sampling site on assessment of pulmonary artery blood flow by Doppler echocardiography. *Am J Cardiol* 1986;58:1145–1147.
24. Shaffer E, Snider R, Serwer G, Peters J, Reynolds P. Effect of sampling site on Doppler derived right ventricular systolic time intervals. *Am J Cardiol* 1990;65:950–952.
25. Silverman NH. Acceleration time in the aorta and pulmonary artery measured by Doppler echocardiography in the midtrimester normal human fetus. *Br Heart J* 1988;59:639–640.
26. Groenenberg IA, Stijnen T, Wladimiroff JW. Blood flow velocity waveforms in the fetal cardiac outflow tract as a measure of fetal well-being in intrauterine growth retardation. *Pediatr Res* 1990;27:379–382.
27. St. John Sutton M, Gill T, Plappert T, Saltzman DH, Doubilet P. Assessment of right and left ventricular function in terms of force development with gestational age in the normal human fetus. *Br Heart J* 1991;66:285–289.
28. Rudolph AM. Fetal and neonatal pulmonary circulation. *Am Rev Resp Dis* (Comroe Symposium) 1977;115:11–18.
29. Rudolph AM. The changes in the circulation after birth. Their importance in congenital heart disease. *Circulation* 1970;41:343–359.
30. Huhta JC, Moise KJ, Fisher DJ, Sharif DS, Wasserstrum N, Martin C. Detection and quantitation of constriction of the fetal ductus arteriosus by Doppler echocardiography. *Circulation* 1987;75: 406–412.
31. Rudolph AM. Fetal and neonatal pulmonary circulation. *Annu Rev Physiol* 1979;41:383–395.
32. Allan L, Machado V. Acceleration time in the aorta and pulmonary artery measured by Doppler echocardiography in the midtrimester normal human fetus. *Br Heart J* 1988;59:639–640.
33. Cartier M, Emerson D, Felker R, et al. Color flow Doppler for evaluation of abnormal fetal pulmonary blood flow. *J Ultrasound Med* 1993;12:S54.
34. Emerson D, Becker J, Felker R, et al. Pulmonary venous connection, total anomalous. *Fetus* 1993;3:7474-1–7474-6.
35. Blott M, Greenough A, Nicolaides KH, Campbell S. The ultrasonographic assessment of the fetal thorax and fetal breathing movements in the prediction of pulmonary hypoplasia. *Early Hum Dev* 1990;21:143–51.
36. Ohlsson A, Fong K, Rose T, et al. Prenatal ultrasonic prediction of autopsy-proven pulmonary hypoplasia. *Am J Perinatol* 1992;9: 334–337.
37. Kitigawa M, Hislop A, Boyden E, Reid L. Lung hypoplasia in congenital diaphragmatic hernia: A quantitative study of airway, artery, and alveolar development. *Br J Surg* 1971;58:341–346.

38. Long W. Persistent pulmonary hypertension of the newborn syndrome (PPHNS). In: Long W, ed. *Fetal and neonatal cardiology.* Philadelphia: WB Saunders; 1990:627–655.

39. Morin FC III, Egan EA. The effect of closing the ductus arteriosus on the pulmonary circulation of the fetal sheep. *J Dev Physiol* 1989;11:283–287.

40. Abman SH, Accurso FJ. Acute effects of partial compression of ductus arteriosus on fetal pulmonary circulation. *Am J Physiol* 1989;257:H626–634.

41. Haworth S, Reid L. Quantitative structural study of the pulmonary circulation in the newborn with pulmonary atresia. *Thorax* 1977;32:129–133.

42. Hiraishi S, Horiguchi Y, Misawa H, et al. Noninvasive Doppler echocardiographic evaluation of shunt flow dynamics of the ductus arteriosus. *Circulation* 1987;75:1146–1153.

43. Musewe NN, Poppe D, Smallhorn JF, et al. Doppler echocardiographic measurement of pulmonary artery pressure from ductal Doppler velocities in the newborn. *J Am Coll Cardiol* 1990;15:446–456.

44. Morin FC III, Egan EA, Ferguson W, Lundgren CE. Development of pulmonary vascular response to oxygen. *Am J Physiol (Heart and Circulatory Physiol)* 1988;23:H542–H546.

45. Von Hayek H. *The human lung.* New York: Hafner; 1960;234–263.

46. Nakamura Y, Yamamoto I, Fukuda S, Hashimoto T. Pulmonary acinar development in diaphragmatic hernia. *Arch Pathol Lab Med* 1991;115:372–376.

47. Emerson DS, Cartier MS. Fetal abnormalities and malformations. In: Fleischer AC, Emerson DS, eds. Color Doppler sonographer in obstetrics and gynecology. New York: Churchill Livingstone; 1993.

Doppler Ultrasound in Obstetrics and Gynecology,
edited by Joshua A. Copel and Kathryn L. Reed.
Raven Press, Ltd., New York © 1995.

CHAPTER 32

The Fetal Ductus Arteriosus

James C. Huhta

The fetal ductus arteriosus is a muscular tube connecting the descending aorta immediately distal to the left subclavian artery with the main pulmonary artery at the origin of the left pulmonary artery. The fetal ductus arteriosus is in a pivotal position in the fetal circulation and its patency results in equal pressures in the right and left ventricles in the fetus after aortopulmonary and ventricular septation are completed during the fourth to eighth menstrual weeks of gestation. This equivalency of pressure also results in parallel circulations with linking of the preloads and afterloads of both ventricles.

The histology of the ductus is unique in the developing circulation because it has no intimal layer and behaves differently than other great vessels such as the aortic wall. Later in gestation, there is the development of focal cushions of tissue that are related to the development of ductal maturity and are seen by 32 weeks gestation in pathologic studies. During constriction and natural closure after birth, there is simultaneous shortening and thickening of the ductus with narrowing of its lumen at the midportion toward the pulmonary end. The aortic end of the ductus may remain open long after ductal closure creating the so-called ductal diverticulum. In the preterm infant, the ductus may close temporarily and reopen to create hemodynamic difficulties.

The ductus arteriosus is known to close, in part, due to withdrawal of the prostaglandin stimulation that is present during fetal life. Some authors have suggested that the ductus is under a constant state of physiologic dilation, which is withdrawn naturally after a normal birth. There is also evidence that the sensitivity of the ductus to withdrawal of prostaglandin stimulation either naturally or pharmacologically by inhibition of prostaglandins, such as with indomethacin, increases with gestational age. These *in vitro* observations combined with several anecdotal observations in neonates exposed to aspirin or indomethacin have led to the clinical practice of avoiding the use of prostaglandin inhibitors in pregnancy after 32 weeks gestation. While that is the case, one now sees increasing use of this class of drugs as a tocolytic agent. There are compelling reasons to believe that the only class of drugs at the present time that are effective in inhibiting preterm labor is the prostaglandin inhibitors and that their use may be a vital part of the prevention of prematurity (1).

NATURAL HISTORY OF CLOSURE AFTER BIRTH

Finally, the knowledge of the natural closure of the ductus arteriosus after birth has enhanced the understanding of the timing and morphology of this process (2). The use of pulsed, color, and continuous wave Doppler in this setting has improved the detection of ductal patency, which may persist as long as 72 hr postnatally. In addition, assessment of the gradient from the right ventricle to the right atrium and between the aorta and the pulmonary artery while the ductus is open using continuous wave Doppler and the modified Bernoulli assumption has allowed the noninvasive measurement of changes in right-sided pressures during normal ductal constriction in both the neonate and the fetus (3). Most authors agree that the major factor controlling the pressure in the subpulmonary ventricle in the neonate is the status of the ductus arteriosus. Stated another way, the larger the size of the ductus arteriosus, the higher the pressure that is transmitted to the pulmonary artery from the aorta and the higher the subpulmonary ventricular pressure.

J. C. Huhta: Departments of Pediatrics and Obstetrics and Gynecology, University of Pennsylvania, and Department of Perinatal Cardiology, Pennsylvania Hospital, Philadelphia, PA 19107.

PRETERM DUCTAL CONSTRICTION

Data from the preterm neonate also confirms that indomethacin use can cause a major constriction, if not closure, of the ductus in most neonates (4). Its use has been advocated and promoted even more strongly since the use of artificial surfactants has given clinicians the ability to improve the pulmonary mechanics in even extremely premature infants less than 1000 g in birthweight. Constriction of the ductus, though associated with inhibition of systemic prostaglandins, may also be linked to prostaglandins intrinsic to the ductus.

BASICS OF DOPPLER INTERROGATION

The normal fetal ductus arteriosus carries a significant portion of the fetal right ventricular stroke volume, thereby supplying the lower body and the placenta. The velocity of blood through this site is the result of a complex interaction between several factors including the right ventricular stroke volume, ductal wall compliance, and the pulmonary artery and placental resistances. It is known from fetal lamb studies that there is a small (3–5 mm Hg) gradient across the ductus during ventricular systole with the pulmonary artery higher than the aorta (5). The fetal ductal velocity reflects this by being directed toward the aorta in systole and diastole (6). The latter suggests that the stored energy in the main and branch pulmonary arteries is released during ventricular diastole causing pulmonary-to-aortic flow at this time. This also confirms the concept that the pulmonary vascular resistance is higher than the systemic resistance *in utero*.

The human fetal ductus is interrogated by imaging the ductal flow using color Doppler and placing the pulsed or continuous wave Doppler position tangential to the ductal arch in the area of increased velocity (Fig. 1).

HEMODYNAMICS OF DUCTAL CONSTRICTION

During artificial constriction of the ductus using a ligature in fetal lamb experiments, there is an elevation of

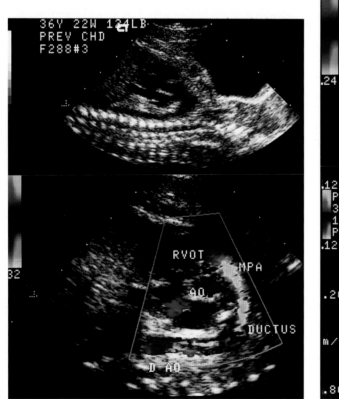

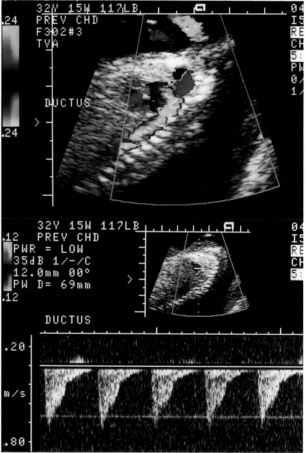

FIG. 1. A: Normal ductal arch at 22 weeks gestation (**upper**). Color Doppler shows aliasing in right ventricular outflow tract (RVOT), main pulmonary artery (MPA), and the ductus DAo = descending aorta. **B:** Normal ductal arch with color Doppler at 15 weeks gestation (**upper**). The peak systolic and diastolic velocities are in the same direction (**lower**).

systolic and diastolic velocities to numbers that reflect the peak instantaneous pressure gradients that can be developed by the immature myocardium. In our experience, the fetal right ventricular pressure can be elevated to 90 mm Hg consistently, but seldom higher, and the ductal instantaneous gradient averages maximally 65–70 mm Hg. Consistent with this, the maximal peak systolic velocity by continuous wave Doppler under these conditions is 4–4.5 m/sec (7). There is an excellent correlation between the predicted gradients instantaneously and those measured in such experiments (6). By applying the modified Bernoulli equation one may calculate the pressure gradient in mm Hg by squaring the maximal velocity measured by Doppler and multiplying by 4. Calculations of the mean velocity may be accomplished by integrating the transformed velocities (pressure gradients at each instant) and averaging. It is known that anything that increases the cardiac output of the fetal right ventricle will increase the systolic velocity but not usually the diastolic velocity. Therefore, with several caveats, one may extrapolate from a blood velocity in the circulation measured noninvasively with Doppler to a decrease in cross-sectional area of the ductus. In an attempt to use the continuity equation to calculate the ratio of mean velocities before and in the ductus, the ratio of the ductal area to that of the main pulmonary artery was estimated to be approximately 70% in normal fetuses. Constriction can be estimated to be present when both the systolic and the diastolic velocities are increased above normal and when the mean velocity is also elevated. This can be simplified by utilizing the pulsatility index of Gosling (8) to describe the waveform utilizing the formula:

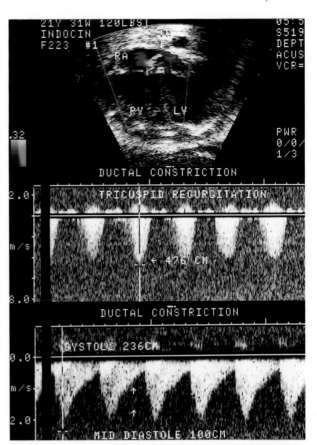

FIG. 3. Ductal constriction in a 31-week fetus with tricuspid valve regurgitation on color Doppler (**upper**). Tricuspid valve regurgitation (peak velocity 4.8 m/sec) is measured with continuous wave Doppler (**middle**). Ductal constriction with high systolic and diastolic velocities is shown in the lower panel.

$$PI = \frac{\text{maximal velocity} - \text{end-diastolic velocity}}{\text{mean velocity}}$$

The pulsatility index (PI) provides a measure of ductal hemodynamics that does not vary during gestation in normal fetuses (mean $\pm$ 2 SD: 2.46 $\pm$ 0.52). Fetal ductal constriction appears as an increase in systolic and diastolic velocity above the normal ranges for age. Diagnosis is simplified using the pulsatility index (Fig. 2) (10). Values less than 1.9 are consistent with constriction of the ductus and values less than 1.0 suggest severe constriction and are usually associated with significant tricuspid valve regurgitation (Fig. 3). In this way, changes in the velocity can be correlated with changes in the cross-sectional area of the ductus arteriosus. So far, we know that in narrowing of the ductus, and one systolic and diastolic gradient across it, the mean velocity will be increased and the pulsatility index will decrease.

DUCTAL OCCLUSION

To assess fetal right ventricular and hemodynamic responses to acute occlusion of the ductus arteriosus, five

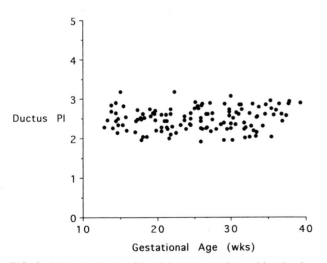

FIG. 2. Normal charts of fetal ductus arteriosus blood velocity pulsatility index vs. gestational age (GA) in weeks. The region of increased pulsatility (PI > 3) suggests increased fetal cardiac output. Fetal ductal constriction manifests as decreased pulsatility (PI < 2). Note the constant normal range between 2 and 3 over the second and third trimesters of gestation.

fetal lambs were instrumented to measure pulmonary pressure, right and left ventricular outputs, and right ventricular dimensions with simultaneous echocardiographic monitoring (7). Ductal occlusion resulted in a rise in pulmonary arterial pressure, a decrease in right ventricular output by 68%, an increase in left ventricular output by 18%, and a fall in combined ventricular output of 34%. The right ventricular systolic dimension increased while the shortening fraction decreased from 0.41 to 0.14. Tricuspid regurgitation started within two heartbeats after ductal occlusion and resolved immediately when the occlusion was released. Acute fetal ductal occlusion imposes a marked increase in the right ventricular afterload resulting in reversible tricuspid regurgitation. This animal model demonstrated that tricuspid regurgitation occurred immediately following an increase in right ventricular afterload. Main pulmonary artery flow decreased as pulmonary artery pressure rose. This was consistent with an inverse relationship between the afterload and stroke volume of the ventricle. At the same time there was a significant increase in left ventricular output, probably due to right-to-left shunting across the foramen ovale, and perhaps increased pulmonary arteriolar flow. In fetal rats, ductal closure has been shown to cause right ventricular hypertrophy (9).

HUMAN DATA

Normal values for the human fetal ductus are now available from the first trimester onward (6). These data show several consistent characteristics of blood flow at this site during development: (a) the systolic velocities increase progressively from less than 50 cm/sec to greater than 130–160 cm/sec near term, (b) the diastolic velocity is always toward the aorta and increases from near zero early in gestation to 30–40 cm/sec, (c) the mean velocity increases with gestational age, and (d) the pulsatility index remains constant throughout gestation, between 1.9 and 3.0 (10) (Fig. 2). Therefore, one may refer to ductal constriction as a ductal pulsatility index less than 1.9 with an elevated mean ductal velocity and signs of decreased right ventricular ejection.

There are several technical details that will ensure success in obtaining similar data:

1. The ductal arch should be visualized in sagittal scans and the entire arch interrogated using either pulsed Doppler with a sample volume 5–10 mm in length or continuous wave Doppler. This is because the ductal velocity is the highest velocity normally found in the fetal circulation and can be differentiated from the aortic arch. The only exception to this, namely, occlusion of the ductus, will be discussed separately.
2. Color Doppler may be useful to identify the site of maximal velocity and is especially helpful in recognizing the presence of continuous diastolic turbu-

lence in the ductus and upper descending aorta during constriction (Fig. 3).
3. Decreased right ventricular shortening and tricuspid valve regurgitation often accompany ductal constriction or occlusion, and may aid in diagnosis when the arch is difficult to visualize (Fig. 3) (see below).

When the pulsatility index of the ductus is less than 1.0 and the mean velocity is increased, the increase in the right ventricular work is significant enough to consistently cause tricuspid valve regurgitation. For this reason, we have referred to this type of constriction as severe. The pulmonary artery Doppler waveform during constriction shows evidence of increased forward flow in diastole due to the increase in diastolic pulmonary artery pressure.

HUMAN DATA ON FETAL DUCTAL CONSTRICTION WITH INDOMETHACIN

Exposure to nonsteroidal antiinflammatory agents, with the prototype being indomethacin, can lead to constriction of the ductus and alterations in human cardiovascular physiology. The majority of experience in fetal changes secondary to drugs has been obtained with indomethacin when it has been administered to the pregnant mother to treat preterm labor or, less commonly, uterine fibroids or polyhydramnios. Typically, fetuses with structurally normal hearts presenting with preterm labor refractory to other agents with a gestational age 23–32 weeks are treated with indomethacin in doses ranging from 25 to 50 mg every 6–12 hr (11–13). After 24 hr on indomethacin, increased ductal velocities consistent with constriction are found in 25–30% of fetuses and the others show no significant changes. Naturally, treatment with any nonsteroidal antiinflammatory agent can cause a decrease in urine flow and amniotic fluid due to fetal renal effects and this must also be monitored. Blood velocity evidence of constriction resolves within 24–48 hr after discontinuation of indomethacin. Thus far, follow-up of newborn infants having short-term constriction before birth has failed to show any deleterious effects.

It now appears that indomethacin-induced inhibition of prostaglandins is reversible, and the effects of a short period of ductal constriction are well tolerated by the fetus. To investigate why this was the case, we measured the right and left ventricular outputs of fetuses during and after resolution of ductal constriction. Another group exposed to indomethacin without signs of ductal constriction were used as controls. Using pulsed Doppler at the aortic and pulmonary valves and comparing the product of the time–velocity integral and the heart rate at each, a measure of change in cardiac output was obtained. Ductal constriction in the fetus caused a significant change in the distribution of the cardiac output between the ventricles. In six fetuses with constriction, the left ventricular output increased significantly (average 21%) relative to baseline ($p < 0.0005$). The ratio of aortic to pulmonary valve flow (time–velocity integral/heart rate product) increased ($p < 0.033$) whereas the group exposed to indomethacin without constriction had no significant change in flow distribution. We may conclude that the fetal circulation tolerates short-term constriction well since there is probably little impact on total combined ventricular output, because the foramen ovale allows flow to be redistributed to the left ventricle. We may then add that an additional sign of ductal constriction in the fetus is an increase in aortic valve and a decrease in pulmonary valve flow indices. This redistribution of flow is similar to that measured in the fetal lamb and also in morphologic experiments in fetal rats.

TRICUSPID VALVE REGURGITATION

It has been observed that constriction of the ductus arteriosus could be associated with regurgitation of the tricuspid valve. Although this finding is common after birth in the low-pressure right ventricle, it is extremely rare in fetal Doppler examinations of normal babies *in utero* where the right ventricular geometry is optimized for systemic pressure. This sign has also been associated with a poor prognosis in fetuses with congenital heart disease (14) and may be a sign of myocardial dysfunction in some fetuses. In order to investigate this manifestation of ductal constriction we set out to perform several studies that would help clarify the clinical significance of tricuspid valve regurgitation. First, to determine the incidence of tricuspid regurgitation in fetuses who had ductal constriction from maternal indomethacin therapy and whether the severity of this tricuspid regurgitation correlated with degree of ductal constriction, 147 echocardiographic studies were reviewed in 44 fetuses, gestational age 20–36 weeks, during and after indomethacin therapy (15). One-half of these fetuses manifested ductal constriction during therapy. This was consistent with our previous series where 35–50% of fetuses manifested constriction depending on the gestational age. Five (11%) had severe (defined as ductal Doppler PI $\leq$ 1) and 18 (41%) had mild (1 < PI $\leq$ 1.9) constriction. Tricuspid valve Doppler showed significant regurgitation (holosystolic and velocity > 2 m/sec) in 14 fetuses (32%) and trace in 5 (11%). There was significant tricuspid regurgitation in all 8 studies (100%) with severe ductal constriction, in 13 of 44 (30%) with mild ductal constriction, and in 3 of 95 (3%) without ductal constriction (Fig. 4). Tricuspid regurgitation continued 1–4 days after the disappearance of ductal constriction in 10 fetuses. We concluded that: (a) as many as 83% of fetuses with ductal constriction by these criteria manifested tricuspid regurgitation, (b) the severity of tricuspid regurgitation correlated with the degree of ductal constriction (and

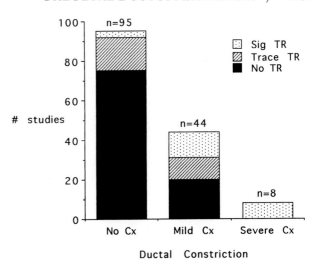

FIG. 4. Doppler-detected tricuspid valve regurgitation (TR) in patients during indomethacin therapy with no ductal constriction (No Cx), mild constriction (Mild Cx), or severe constriction (Severe Cx). By definition, all those with severe constriction had significant TR.

presumably with the degree of elevation of right ventricular pressure), (c) in some cases, tricuspid regurgitation with normal ductal Doppler indicated previous ductal constriction, and (d) tricuspid regurgitation was a reversible effect of ductal constriction.

The upstroke of tricuspid valve regurgitation gives information about the myocardial function because it is possible in some cases to calculate the ventricular pressure change first derivative, or the so-called dP/dt, from this jet. Calculations of this type in human fetuses showed normal values of dP/dt even when the right ventricular shortening was markedly decreased (15%) (15). Therefore, we may conclude that the right ventricle maintains its contractility in spite of an increased workload leading to increased wall thickness, decreased shortening, and tricuspid regurgitation.

The finding of tricuspid valve regurgitation on color Doppler sometimes shows a long and easily detectable jet extending into the back of the right atrium. To assess color Doppler and its accuracy in assessment of tricuspid regurgitation, we correlated the severity by pulsed Doppler (as described above), by jet length compared to right atrial length, and jet area compared to right atrial area (16). We found that jet length overestimated the severity of regurgitation, jet area underestimated it, and pulsed Doppler had the best correlation with constriction severity. We concluded that the severity of this side effect is difficult to assess and may not be clinically significant in terms of volume overload. However, signs of right atrial enlargement with ductal constriction and tricuspid regurgitation would be a concern and lead us to alter therapy.

DUCTAL OCCLUSION

Recently, it was observed that occlusion of the ductus arteriosus in the human fetus can be associated with indomethacin therapy. In our practice ductal *closure* of unknown duration was observed in four fetuses, all exposed to some form of nonsteroidal antiinflammatory agent:

A. Singleton 31 weeks gestation; mother on indomethacin 50 mg q6h; ductus reopened off indomethacin and delivered normally at term.
B. Singleton 32 weeks gestation; indomethacin 50 mg q12h; documented closure for 48 hr resolved in 36 hr.
C. Monoamniotic twins 32 weeks gestation; mother on indomethacin; one twin had ductal constriction and the other had closure with hydrops and a restrictive foramen ovale; hydropic twin died intrapartum.
D. Singleton 35 weeks gestation; mother taking an ibuprofen analog chronically; delivered electively after partial reopening of the ductus over 2 days off medicine.

Neither A, B, nor D had pulmonary hypertension on postnatal examination. Fetal echocardiographic signs that were associated with ductal closure included the following: (a) right atrial enlargement with tricuspid valve regurgitation (velocity > 4 m/sec), (b) decreased right ventricular shortening, (c) increased main and branch pulmonary artery sizes, and (d) increased left ventricular shortening and aortic arch velocity. We noted that ductal closure could have been missed because the aortic arch velocity on Doppler resembled a normal blood velocity tracing in the ductus arteriosus. Careful examination by color Doppler showed no flow in the ductus.

We may conclude from these few patients that if the foramen ovale is adequate, human fetal ductal closure is compatible with normal physiology due to redistribution of cardiac output to the left heart. Hydrops fetalis with right heart failure may occur with an inadequate foramen ovale. Removal of the medication causing prostaglandin inhibition resulted in ductal reopening and is the optimal treatment if the gestation is premature. The single fetus delivered with ductal constriction did well and we have observed this previously in one other 35-week-gestation newborn. In one case of ductal closure from indomethacin, withdrawal resulted in reopening, but constriction persisted for 7 days. We believe that this is further evidence that the ductus matures with increasing gestational age and that with closure it begins to effect sealing. We have observed a single fetus near term with ductal constriction without any obvious cause who tolerated delivery and had mild pulmonary hypertension for 3–4 days postnatally.

OTHER AGENTS

Mild increases in ductal velocity have been observed with low-dose aspirin therapy during pregnancy but ductal constriction has not (17). We are aware of changes that may occur in the ductal velocities during treatment with steroids (18).

CONCLUSIONS

Many questions remain concerning indomethacin therapy for preterm labor and its fetal side effects. It is clear, however, that short-term constriction of the ductus is well tolerated and reversible. Like decreased amniotic fluid, it is a common side effect of treatment, but with surveillance it can be factored into treatment and allow indomethacin to be used in many problem pregnancies. How long can ductal constriction be allowed to continue without inducing any significant clinical result? It is known that animals exposed to ductal ligation develop pulmonary vascular changes as soon as one week (19). When there is ultrasound evidence of ductal constriction we notify the obstetricians and coordinate a plan of monitoring that leads to a decision regarding the prostaglandin inhibitor within 5 days.

DEFINITIONS

Degree of ductal constriction:

No constriction = ductal PI is within the range of normal control group (1.9–3.0)
Mild constriction = 1 < ductal PI < 1.9
Severe constriction = ductal PI ≤ 1.0

Degree of tricuspid regurgitation (Fig. 1):

Significant = presence of holosystolic flow across tricuspid valve, its maximal velocity exceeding 2 m/sec
Trivial = other tricuspid regurgitation not fulfilling the above criteria (i.e., not holosystolic, incomplete waveform, or low-amplitude signal)

REFERENCES

1. Higby K, Xenakis Elly M-J, Pauerstein CJ. Do tocolytic agents stop preterm labor? A critical and comprehensive review of efficacy and safety. *Am J Obstet Gynecol* 1993;4:1247–1258.
2. Huhta JC, Cohen M, Gutgesell HP. Patency of the ductus arteriosus in normal neonates: Two-dimensional echocardiography versus Doppler assessment. *J Am Coll Cardiol* 1984;4:561–564.
3. Huhta JC, Cohen A, Wood DC. Premature constriction of the ductus arteriosus. *J Am Soc Echo* 1990;3:30–34.
4. Ramsay JM, Murphy DJ, Vick GW, Courtney JT, Garcia-Prats

JA, Huhta JC. Response of the patent ductus arteriosus to indomethacin treatment. *AJDC* 1987;141:294–297.

5. Rudolph A. Fetal and neonatal pulmonary circulation. *Annu Rev Physiol* 1979;41:383–395.

6. Huhta JC, Moise KJ, Fisher DJ, Sharif DS, Wasserstrum N, Martin C. Detection and quantitation of constriction of the fetal ductus arteriosus by Doppler echocardiography. *Circulation* 1987;75:406–412.

7. Tulzer G, Gudmundsson S, Rotondo KM, Wood DC, Yoon GY, Huhta JC. Acute fetal ductal occlusion in lambs. *Am J Obstet Gynecol* 1991;165:775–778.

8. Gosling RG, Dunbar G, King DH, et al. The quantitative analysis of occlusive peripheral arterial disease by a non-intrusive ultrasonic technique. *Angiology* 1971;22:52–55.

9. Momma K, Takao A. Right ventricular concentric hypertrophy and left ventricular dilatation by ductal constriction in fetal rats. *Circ Res* 1989;64:1137–1146.

10. Tulzer G, Gudmundsson S, Sharkey AM, Wood DC, Cohen AW, Huhta JC. Doppler echocardiography of fetal ductus arteriosus constriction versus increased right ventricular output. *J Am Coll Cardiol* 1991;18:532–536.

11. Niebyl JR, Blake DA, White RD, et al. The inhibition of premature labor with indomethacin. *Am J Obstet Gynecol* 1980;136:1014–1019.

12. Dudley DKL, Hardie MJ. Fetal and neonatal effects of indomethacin used as a tocolytic agent. *Am J Obstet Gynecol* 1985;151:181–184.

13. Niebyl JR. Prostaglandin synthetase inhibitors. *Semin Perinatol* 1981;5:274–287.

14. Silverman NH, Kleinman CS, Rudolph AM, et al. Fetal atrioventricular valve insufficiency associated with nonimmune hydrops: A two-dimensional echocardiographic and pulsed Doppler ultrasound study. *Circulation* 1985;72:825–832.

15. Tulzer G, Gudmundsson S, Rotondo KM, Wood DC, Cohen AW, Huhta JC. Doppler in the evaluation and prognosis of fetuses with tricuspid regurgitation. *J Mat–Fet Invest* 1991;1:15–18.

16. Khowsathit P, Tian Z-Y, Wood DC, Tulzer G, Cohen AW, Huhta JC. Color doppler versus pulsed doppler in fetal tricuspid regurgitation. Abstract presented at the Fourth International Congress of Perinatal Doppler Society, Malino, Sweden, August 1991.

17. Forouzan I, Cohen AW, Lindenbaum C, Samuels P. Umbilical artery and ductal blood flow velocities in patients treated with aspirin and prednisone for presence of anticardiolipin antibody. *J Ultrasound Med* 1993;12:135–138.

18. Wasserstrum N, Huhta JC, Mari G, Sharif DS, Willis R, Neal NK. Betamethasone and the human fetal ductus arteriosus. *Obstet Gynecol* 1989;74:897–900.

19. Wild LM, Nickerson PA, Morin FC III. Ligating the ductus arteriosus before birth remodels the pulmonary vasculature of the lamb. *Pediatr Res* 1989;25:251–257.

Subject Index

Note: Page numbers followed by f refer to illustrations; page numbers followed by t refer to tables.